Orthopedic

Adam E. M. Eltorai • Craig P. Eberson
Alan H. Daniels
Editors

Orthopedic Surgery Clerkship

A Quick Reference Guide for Senior Medical Students

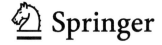 Springer

Editors
Adam E. M. Eltorai
Warren Alpert Medical School
Brown University
Providence, RI
USA

Alan H. Daniels
Department of Orthopaedic Surgery
Division of Spine Surgery
Rhode Island Hospital
Providence, RI
USA

Craig P. Eberson
Department of Orthopedic Surgery
Division of Pediatric Surgery
Warren Alpert Medical School
  of Brown University
Providence, RI
USA

ISBN 978-3-319-52565-5   ISBN 978-3-319-52567-9   (eBook)
DOI 10.1007/978-3-319-52567-9

Library of Congress Control Number: 2017943119

Printed on acid-free paper

This Springer imprint is published by Springer Nature
The registered company is Springer International Publishing AG
The registered company address is: Gewerbestrasse 11, 6330 Cham, Switzerland

Preface

This quick-reference review is the first book written specifically for third- and fourth-year medical students completing orthopedic surgery rotations. Organized by body part, *Orthopedic Surgery Clerkship* focuses on diagnosis and management of the most common pathologic entities. Each chapter covers history, typical presentation, relevant anatomy, physical examination, imaging, options for nonoperative and operative management, and expected outcomes.

Orthopedic Surgery Clerkship is the ideal on-the-spot reference for those seeking fast facts on diagnosis and management. Its bullet-pointed outline format makes this book a perfect addition to a white coat pocket, allowing busy students to find the information they need rapidly. Its content breadth covers the most commonly encountered orthopedic problems in practice.

Students can read the text from cover to cover to gain a general foundation of orthopedic knowledge and then reread specific chapters for more focused subspecialty review. This book will serve as tool to propel students to the next level and help them start their journey as orthopedists on the right foot.

Providence, USA   Adam E. M. Eltorai
Craig P. Eberson
Alan H. Daniels

Acknowledgments

This collaborative project would not have been possible without the thoughtful comments, insights, and advice of the many orthopedic residents and members of faculty, whom we gratefully acknowledge for their support in the development of *Orthopedic Surgery Clerkship*. Our special thanks to Kristopher Spring, Prakash Jagannathan, and the contributing authors.

Contents

Contributors

Robert Ablove, MD Department of Orthopaedics, Jacobs School of Medicine and Biomedical Sciences, Buffalo, NY, USA

Eildar Abyar Orthopedics, University of South Florida Morsani Center, Tampa, FL, USA

Amiethab A. Aiyer Department of Orthopaedic Surgery, University of Miami, Miami, FL, USA

John Alexander, MD Department of Orthopaedics, Hand and Upper Extremity Center, The Ohio State University Wexner Medical Center, Columbus, OH, USA

Tonya W. An Orthopedics, Cedars-Sinai Medical Center, Los Angeles, CA, USA

Christopher Arena Department of Orthopaedics and Rehabilitation, Penn State Milton S. Hershey Medical Center, Hershey, PA, USA

David Arsanious University of Vermont College of Medicine, Burlington, VT, USA

Hisham M. Awan, MD Hand and Upper Extremity Center, The Ohio State University Wexner Medical Center, Columbus, OH, USA

Navkirat Bajwa Department of Orthopaedic Surgery, University of South Alabama, Mobile, AL, USA

Karl Balch, MD Orthopaedic Surgery, The Ohio State University Wexner Medical Center, Columbus, OH, USA

Domenico Barbuti Imaging Department, Bambino Gesù Children's Hospital, Rome, Italy

Giulia Battafarano Bone Physiopathology Group, Multifactorial Disease and Complex Phenotype Research Area, Rome, Italy

Patrick F. Bergin, MD Department of Orthopedic Surgery, University of Mississippi Medical Center, Jackson, MS, USA

Geoffrey Bernas, MD Department of Orthopaedics, Jacobs School of Medicine and Biomedical Sciences, Buffalo, NY, USA

Matthew Binkley, MD Department of Orthopedic Surgery, Erie County Medical Centre, Buffalo, NY, USA

Charles Bishop, MD Department of Orthopaedics, Marshall University School of Medicine, Huntington, WU, USA

Leslie J. Bisson Jacobs School of Medicine and Biomedical Sciences, University at Buffalo, Amherst, NY, USA

Richard Boe Department of Orthopaedics, Marshall University Medical Center, Huntingston, WV, USA

Chad S. Boomershine, MD, PhD Rheumatology and Immunology, Vanderbilt University, Nashville, TN, USA

Allen Borne, MD Department of Orthopaedic Surgery, University of Arkansas for Medical Sciences, Little Rock, AR, USA

Phillip A. Bostian, MD Department of Orthopedics, West Virginia University, Health Science Center South, Morgantown, WV, USA

Erik Bowman, MD Department of Orthopaedic Surgery and Rehabilitation, University of Nebraska Medical Center, Omaha, NE, USA

Keely Boyle, MD Department of Orthopaedics Surgery, SUNY University at Buffalo, Buffalo, NY, USA

Matthew J. Brown, MD Department of Orthopaedics, Jacobs School of Medicine and Biomedical Sciences, Buffalo, NY, USA

Timothy P. Bryan, MD Department of Orthopaedics, State University of New York at Buffalo, Buffalo, NY, USA

Grant S. Buchanan, MD Department of Orthopaedic Surgery, Joan C. Edwards School of Medicine, Marshall University, Huntington, WV, USA

Andrew Campbell, MD Hand Upper Extremty Center, The Ohio State University Wexner Medical Center, Columbus, OH, USA

Brian Carpenter Department of Orthopaedic Surgery, John Peter Smith Hospital, Fort Worth, TX, USA

Department of Orthopaedic Surgery, UNT Health Science Center, Fort Worth, TX, USA

David Cealrey, MD Augusta University, Augusta, GA, USA

Michael J. Chambers, MD Marshall University Orthopaedics, King's Daughters Medical Center, Ashland, KY, USA

Nileshkumar M. Chaudhari, MD Division of Orthopaedic Surgery, Department of Surgery, University of Alabama – Birmingham, Birmingham, AL, USA

Anne Marie Chicorelli, DO, MPH Orthopaedics and Sports Medicine, The Ohio State University Wexner Medical Center, Wooster, OH, USA

Nicolette Clark Department Orthopaedics and Sports Medicine, University of South Florida, Tampa, FL, USA

Corey T. Clyde, MD Department of Orthopaedic Surgery, University at Buffalo, Buffalo, NY, USA

Jenna Cooley, DO Division of Rheumatology, Cooper University Hospital, Camden, NJ, USA

Aristides I. Cruz Jr, MD Warren Alpert Medical School at Brown University, Rhode Island Hospital/Hasbro Children's Hospital, Providence, RI, USA

Scott D. Daffner, MD Department of Orthopaedics, West Virginia University, Morgantown, WV, USA

D. Daniel Rotenberg Desert Orthopaedic Center, Las Vegas, NV, USA

Alan H. Daniels, MD Department of Orthopaedic Surgery, Division of Spine Surgery, Rhode Island Hospital, Providence, RI, USA

Department of Orthopedic Surgery, Warren Alpert Medical School, Brown University, Providence, RI, USA

James B. Day, MD, PhD Director of Orthopaedic Trauma, Department of Orthopaedics, Joan C. Edwards School of Medicine, Marshall University, Huntington, WU, USA

Andrea Del Fattore Bone Physiopathology Group, Multifactorial Disease and Complex Phenotype Research Area, Imaging Department, Bambino Gesù Children's Hospital, Rome, Italy

J. Mason DePasse, MD Department of Orthopedic Surgery, Division of Pediatric Surgery, Warren Alpert Medical School of Brown University, Providence, RI, USA

Alex C. DiBartola Department of Orthopaedics, The Ohio State University Wexner Medical Center, Columbus, OH, USA

Kyle Duncan Department of Orthopaedic Surgery, John Peter Smith Hospital, Fort Worth, TX, USA

Thomas Duquin, MD Department of Orthopaedics, State University of New York at Buffalo, Buffalo, NY, USA

Craig P. Eberson, MD Department of Orthopedic Surgery, Division of Spine Surgery, Warren Alpert Medical School of Brown University, Providence, RI, USA

Hossein Elgafy, MD, FRCSEd, FRCSC Department of Orthopedic Surgery, University of Toledo Medical Center, Toledo, OH, USA

Jordan Ernst Orthopedics, John Peter Smith, Fort Worth, TX, USA

Paul Esposito Department of Orthopaedic Surgery, University of Nebraska Medical Center, Children's Hospital and Medical Center, Omaha, NE, USA

Reed Estes, MD Department of Surgery, Division of Orthopedic Surgery, University of Alabama at Birmingham, Birmingham, AL, USA

Joshua S. Everhart Department of Orthopaedics, The Ohio State University Wexner Medical Center, Columbus, OH, USA

Michael R. Ferrick, MD Department of Orthopaedic Surgery, SUNY Buffalo, Women and Children's Hospital of Buffalo, Amherst, NY, USA

Brooks W. Ficke, MD Division of Orthopedic Surgery, University of Alabama at Birmingham, Birmingham, AL, USA

Marc Fineberg, MD University of SUNY Buffalo, Buffalo, NY, USA

Department of Orthopaedics, University at Buffalo, Buffalo, NY, USA

David C. Flanigan Department of Orthopaedics, The Ohio State University Wexner Medical Center, Columbus, OH, USA

Joseph Fox, MD Department of Orthopaedic Surgery, Jacobs School of Medicine, University at Buffalo, Buffalo, NY, USA

John France Department of Orthopaedic Surgery, West Virginia University, Stewart Hall, Morgantown, WV, USA

Dominic J. Gargiulo, DO Pediatric Orthopedics, Children's Hospital New Orleans, New Orleans, LA, USA

Orthopedic Department, Louisiana State University School of Medicine, New Orleans, LA, USA

Lauren E. Geaney, MD Department of Orthopaedic Surgery, UCONN Health, Farmington, CT, USA

Daniel J. Gehling Department of Orthopaedic Surgery, University of Toledo – Health Science Campus, Toledo, OH, USA

Thomas Gill, MD Department of Orthopedic Surgery, Marshall University/ Cabell Huntington Hospital, Huntington, WV, USA

Jonathan Gillig, MD Department of Orthopaedic Surgery, University of South Alabama, Mobile, AL, USA

Andrew H. Glassman, MD, MS Orthopaedic Surgery, The Ohio State University Wexner Medical Center, Columbus, OH, USA

Akshay Goel, MD Department of Orthopaedics, Three Rivers Medical Center, Louisa, KY, USA

Kanu Goyal, MD Ohio State University Wexner Medical Center, Columbus, OH, USA

Bobby Kwanghoon Han, MD Division of Rheumatology, Cooper University Hospital, Camden, NJ, USA

Andrew E. Hanselman, MD Department of Orthopedics, Health Sciences South, Morgantown, WV, USA

Jared L. Harwood, MD Department of Orthopaedics, The Ohio State University wexner Medical Center, Columbus, OH, USA

Michael Heffernan, MD Orthopedic Department, Children's Hospital Of New Orleans, Louisiana State University, New Orleans, LA, USA

Henry C. Hilario, DPM Department of Orthopedics, John Peter Smith Hospital, Fort Worth, TX, USA

Ilia Iliev Department of Orthopaedic Surgery, Joan C. Edwards School of Medicine, Marshall University, Huntington, WV, USA

Carlos Isales Regenerative Medicine, Orthopaedic Surgery, Medical College of Georgia, Augusta, GA, USA

Rajiv J. Iyengar, BS Warren Alpert Medical School, Brown University, Providence, RI, USA

Aprajita Jagpal, MBBS Division of Clinical Immunology and Rheumatology, School of Medicine, University of Alabama at Birmingham, Birmingham, AL, USA

Margaret Jain Hand and Upper Extremity Surgery, University of Toledo School of Medicine, Toledo, OH, USA

David Johannesmeyer, MD Department of Surgery, Division of Orthopedic Surgery, University of Alabama at Birmingham, Birmingham, AL, USA

Anna Johnson Department of Orthopedic Surgery, University of South Alabama Medical Center, Mobile, AL, USA

Brock Johnson, MD Department of Orthopedic Surgery, Marshall University/Cabell Huntington Hospital, Huntington, WV, USA

Michael D. Johnson, MD Department of Orthopaedics, University of Alabama – Birmingham, Birmingham, AL, USA

Grant L. Jones Department of Orthopaedics, The Ohio State University Wexner Medical Center, Columbus, OH, USA

Paul J. Juliano, MD Department of Orthopaedics and Rehabilitation, Penn State Health Milton S. Hershey Medical Center, Hershey, PA, USA

Jonathan M. Karnes, MD Department of Orthopedics, West Virginia University, Morgantown, WV, USA

Daniel C. Kim, MD Department of Orthopaedic Surgery, University of South Alabama Hospitals, Mobile, AL, USA

Jeffrey Kim, MD Department of Orthopaedic Surgery, Cabell Huntington Hospital/Marshall University School of Medicine, Huntington, WV, USA

Joseph J. King, MD Orthopaedics and Rehabiliation, UF Health Shands Hospital, Gainesville, FL, USA

Alexander J. Kish, MD Department of Orthopaedic Surgery, University of Maryland Medical Center, Baltimore, MD, USA

Alan R. Koester, MD Department of Orthopaedic Surgery, Joan C. Edwards School of Medicine, Marshall University, Huntington, WV, USA

Sean Kraekel, MD Department of Orthopedic Surgery, The George Washington University, Washington, DC, USA

Kafai Lai Orthopaedics, The University of Toledo Medical Center, Toledo, OH, USA

Darin Larson, MD Department of Orthopaedic Surgery and Rehabilitation, University of Nebraska Medical Center, Omaha, NE, USA

Tracye J. Lawyer, MD, PhD Department of Orthopedic Surgery, University of Mississippi Medical Center, Jackson, MS, USA

Benjamin Leger-St. Jean, MD Department of Orthopaedics, The Ohio State University Wexner Medical Center, Columbus, OH, USA

Nathaniel Lempert, MD Department of Orthopedic Surgery, University of Toledo Medical Center, Toledo, OH, USA

S. Louis Bridges Jr, MD, PhD Division of Clinical Immunology and Rheumatology, School of Medicine, University of Alabama at Birmingham, Birmingham, AL, USA

John P. Lubicky, MD Department of Orthopaedics, West Virginia University, Morgantown, WV, USA

Jonathan Ludwig, MD Orthopedic Surgery, University of Alabama at Birmingham Hospital, Birmingham, AL, USA

Dana Lycans, MD Department of Orthopaedic Surgery, Marshall University/Cabell Huntington Hospital, Huntington, WV, USA

Adam Martin, MD Hand and Upper Extremity Center, The Ohio State University Wexner Medical Center, Columbus, OH, USA
Warren Alpert Medical School, Brown University, Providence, RI, USA

John M. Marzo, MD Department of Orthopaedics, Jacobs School of Medicine and Biomedical Sciences, Buffalo, NY, USA

J. Mason DePasse, MD Department of Orthopaedic Surgery, Warren Alpert Medical School of Brown University, Rhode Island Hospital, Providence, RI, USA

John R. Matthews, MD Department of Orthopaedic Surgery, SUNY University of Buffalo, Buffalo, NY, USA

Robert C. Matthias, MD University of Florida, Gainesville, FL, USA

Joel Mayerson, MD Department of Orthopaedics, The Ohio State University wexner Medical Center, Columbus, OH, USA

James L. McFadden, MD Orthopaedic Surgery, University of Alabama at Birmingham, Birmingham, AL, USA

Ryan J. McNeilan Department of Orthopaedics, The Ohio State University Wexner Medical Center, Columbus, OH, USA

Nicole Meschbach Warren Alpert Medical School, Brown University, Providence, RI, USA

Joseph Meyerson, MD Hand and Upper Extremity Center, The Ohio State University Wexner Medical Center, Columbus, OH, USA

Amit Momaya, MD Department of Surgery, Division of Orthopedic Surgery, University of Alabama at Birmingham, Birmingham, AL, USA

Steven R. Niedermeier, MD Hand and Upper Extremity Center, The Ohio State University, Wexner Medical Center, Columbus, OH, USA

Thomas E. Niemeier University of Alabama at Birmingham, Birmingham, AL, USA

Mark Oliver, MD Orthopaedic, University of Toledo Medical Center, Toledo, OH, USA

Dana Olszewski, MD, MPH Childrens Orthopaedics of Atlanta, Atlanta, GA, USA

Howard Y. Park, MD Department of Orthopedic Surgery, UCLA Medical Center, Santa Monica, CA, USA

Viral Patel, MD Orthopedic Department, Gillette Children's Hospital, University of Minnesota, St. Paul, MN, USA

Albert Pearsall, MD Department of Orthopedic Surgery, University of South Alabama Hospitals, Mobile, AL, USA

Jeffery Pearson Orthopedic Surgery, UAB, Birmingham, AL, USA

Noah Porter, MD Department of Orthopaedic Surgery and Rehabilitation, University of Nebraska Medical Center, Omaha, NE, USA

Brien Rabenhorst University of Arkansas for Medical Sciences, Little Rock, Arkansas, USA

Viorel Raducan, MD Department of Orthopaedic Surgery, Marshall University/Cabell Huntington Hospital, Huntington, WV, USA

Satheesh K. Ramineni Orthopaedic Surgery, University of Toledo Medical Center, Toledo, OH, USA

Erin F. Ransom, MD Division of Orthopaedic Surgery, Department of Surgery, University of Alabama – Birmingham, Birmingham, AL, USA

Raj Rao, MD Department of Orthopedic Surgery, The George Washington University, Washington, DC, USA

James Reagan, MD Department of Orthopaedic Surgery, CabellHuntington Hospital/Marshall University School ofMedicine, Huntington, WV, USA

Brady W. Rhodes, DPM Department of Orthopedics, John Peter Smith Hospital, Fort Worth, TX, USA

Yoseph A. Rosenbaum, MD Hand and Upper Extremity Center, The Ohio State University Wexner Medical Center, Columbus, OH, USA

Michela Rossi Bone Physiopathology Group, Multifactorial Disease and Complex Phenotype Research Area, Rome, Italy

Shane D. Rothermel Department of Orthopaedics and Rehabilitation, Penn State Health Milton S. Hershey Medical Center, Hershey, PA, USA

Robert D. Santrock, MD Department of Orthopedics, Health Sciences South, Morgantown, WV, USA

Sylwia Sasinowska, MD Division of Rheumatology, Cooper University Hospital, Camden, NJ, USA

Anthony A. Scaduto, MD Department of Orthopaedic Surgery, Orthopaedic Institute for Children/UCLA, Los Angeles, CA, USA

Susan A. Scherl, MD The University of Nebraska, Department of Orthopaedic Surgery, Omaha, NE, USA

Edward Schleyer, MD Department of Orthopaedics, University at Buffalo, Buffalo, NY, USA

Francisco A. Schwartz-Fernandes Department Orthopaedics and Sports Medicine, University of South Florida, Tampa, FL, USA

Ryan Scully, MD Department of Orthopaedic Surgery, George Washington University Medical Center, Washington, DC, USA

Megan N. Severson, MD Division of Orthopedic Surgery, Department of Surgery, University of Alabama – Birmingham Hospital, Birmingham, AL, USA

Jyoti Sharma, MD Orthopaedic Surgery, Penn State Hershey Medical Center, Hershey, PA, USA

Kevin Shepet, MD Department of Orthopaedics, West Virginia University, Health Science Center – South, Morgantown, WV, USA

Evan Sheppard, MD Department of Surgery, Division of Orthopedic Surgery, University of Alabama at Birmingham, Birmingham, AL, USA

Franklin D. Shuler, MD, PhD Department of Orthopaedic Surgery, Joan C. Edwards School of Medicine, Marshall University, Huntington, WV, USA

Justin Siebler, MD Department of Orthopaedic Surgery and Rehabilitation, University of Nebraska Medical Center, Omaha, NE, USA

Martin Skie, MD Orthopedic Surgery, University of Toledo Medical Center, Toledo, OH, USA

Amy Speeckaert, MD Hand and Upper Extremity Center, The Ohio State University Wexner Medical Center, Columbus, OH, USA

John M. Stephenson, MD Department of Orthopaedic Surgery, University of Arkansas for Medical Sciences, Little Rock, AR, USA

Christopher Sugalski, MD Department of Orthopaedic Surgery, The Ohio State University Wexner Medical Center, Columbus, OH, USA

Anne C. Sullivan, MD Department of Orthopaedic Surgery, The Ohio State University Wexner Medical Center, Columbus, OH, USA

Steven M. Theiss Orthopedic Surgery, UAB, Birmingham, AL, USA

John Tidwell Department of Orthopaedics, UCSF Fresno, Fresno, CA, USA

LeeAnne Torres, MD Department of Orthopaedic Surgery, Marshall University/Cabell Huntington Hospital, Huntington, WV, USA

Christopher Treager Regenerative Medicine, Orthopaedic Surgery, Medical College of Georgia, Augusta, GA, USA

Joshua Troyer Department of Orthopaedics, The Ohio State University Wexner Medical Center, Columbus, OH, USA

Christopher E. Urband, MD Department of Orthopaedics, Jacobs School of Medicine and Biomedical Sciences, Buffalo, NY, USA

John W. Uribe Department of Orthopedic Surgery, Herbert Wertheim College of Medicine at Florida International University, Coral Gables, FL, USA

Matthew A. Varacallo, MD Department of Orthopaedic Surgery, Hahnemann University Hospital, Philadelphia, PA, USA

Surahbhi S. Vinod, BS Division of Clinical Immunology and Rheumatology, School of Medicine, University of Alabama at Birmingham, Birmingham, AL, USA

James Vogler University of South Florida, Tampa, FL, USA

Ettore Vulcano Department of Orthopedics, Mount Sinai Health System, New York, NY, USA

M. Wade Shrader, MD Department of Orthopedic Surgery, Children's of Mississippi, University of MS Medical Center, Jackson, MS, USA

Maegen Wallace, MD Department of Orthopaedic Surgery, University of Nebraska Medical Center/Omaha Children's Hospital, Omaha, NE, USA

Colleen Watkins, MD Department of Orthopedics, West Virginia University, Health Science Center South, Morgantown, WV, USA

Eric Wherley Herbert Wertheim College of Medicine at Florida International University, Miami, FL, USA

Stephen White, MD Department of Orthopaedic Surgery, University of South Alabama, Mobile, AL, USA

Erik White Hand and Upper Extremity Surgery, University of Toledo School of Medicine, Toledo, OH, USA

Brad Wills, MD Surgery – Orthopaedics, University of Alabama at Birmingham, Birmingham, AL, USA

William M. Wind Jacobs School of Medicine and Biomedical Sciences, University at Buffalo, Amherst, NY, USA

Megan R. Wolf, MD Department of Orthopaedic Surgery, UCONN Health, Farmington, CT, USA

Theresa Wyrick, MD Department of Orthopaedic Surgery, University of Arkansas for Medical Sciences, Little Rock, AR, USA

Gautam P. Yagnik Department of Orthopedics, West Kendall Baptist Hospital, Miami, FL, USA

Part I

The Basics

General Orthopedic Terminology

Anne C. Sullivan and Christopher Sugalski

Introduction

- Orthopedic surgery encompasses the breadth of surgical and medical management of musculoskeletal injuries and disorders.
- Orthopedic surgeons work closely with a variety of ancillary support staff:
  - Physical and occupational therapists and athletic trainers
  - Physician assistants
  - Nurses and orthopedic/cast techs
- Orthopedics, not unlike other medical specialties, has its own language, with a substantial vocabulary. This makes it particularly important to come to your orthopedic rotation or clerkship prepared.
- There are many definitive and authoritative texts and online sites with which to familiarize oneself with the terminology as well as with the study of orthopedics. For brevity and efficiency, we present the basics here.

A.C. Sullivan, MD (✉) • C. Sugalski, MD
Department of Orthopaedic Surgery,
The Ohio State University Wexner Medical Center,
Columbus, OH, USA
e-mail: suileabhainac@gmail.com;
sullivan.63@osu.edu

Subspecialties

Adult Reconstruction (Joint Replacement/Arthroplasty)

- Expertise in joint replacement, traditionally for management of hip and knee arthritis, includes partial and total hip and knee arthroplasty, as well as revision total hip and knee arthroplasty.
- The need for hip and knee arthroplasty in the United States is projected to increase 174 % and 673 % between 2005 and 2030 [1].
- Replacement of other joints (elbow, ankle, shoulder) often falls to specialists in areas of regional expertise or may be included in arthroplasty practice.

Trauma

- Expertise in care of complex articular fractures, pelvic fractures, and polytrauma, including sequelae of trauma such as nonunion/malunion and infections.
- Most orthopedic surgeons, regardless of specialty, utilize a base of trauma knowledge to care for fractures they encounter while on call.
- Treatments include casting, splinting, open/closed reduction, internal fixation, external fixation, intramedullary nailing, and fracture plating. Trauma surgeons may do variable amounts of arthroplasty and reconstruction.

© Springer International Publishing AG 2017
A.E.M. Eltorai et al. (eds.), *Orthopedic Surgery Clerkship*, DOI 10.1007/978-3-319-52567-9_1

Shoulder and Elbow

- Comprehensive surgical treatment of acute and chronic shoulder and elbow conditions.
- Manage rotator cuff tears, shoulder and elbow instability, arthritis, and fractures.
- Utilize both open and arthroscopic surgical techniques.
- May also include shoulder and elbow arthroplasty and complex reconstructive techniques.

Hand

- A subspecialty shared with both plastic and general surgeons who have completed an additional year of fellowship training in hand surgery
- Concerned with the intricate and vital function of the hand and wrist, including chronic and traumatic conditions
- Surgically manage fractures, instability, arthritis, and nerve compression and have the microsurgical skills to perform digit replantation and various other procedures

Spine

- Surgically treat acute and chronic neck and back pathology and trauma.
- Often work closely with nonsurgical spine physicians to manage and treat chronic neck and back pain.
- Surgeries include deformity correction for scoliosis, lumbar decompression and fusion, cervical decompression and fusion, and lumbar microdiscectomy.
- Share a scope of practice which overlaps spinal neurosurgeons.

Foot and Ankle

- Experts in foot and ankle biomechanics and gait.
- Manage complex fractures of the distal tibia, talus, and calcaneus, along with other foot and ankle trauma.
- Manage degenerative conditions and deformities of the foot and ankle, frequently performing ankle, hindfoot, and midfoot fusions or arthroplasty, tendon transfers, and nerve decompression.
- Share a scope of practice that partially overlaps with podiatry.

Sports Medicine

- Assess and manage injuries and conditions of musculoskeletal pathology encountered in athletes and the active population.
- For arthroscopy specialists, procedures are designed to be minimally invasive to allow the quickest possible return to sport or activity.
- Depending on the population served, sports medicine specialists may also use minimally invasive or cartilage preservation techniques to allow older persons to remain active by addressing early degenerative conditions with less surgical trauma.
- Often focus on the knee and shoulder, tendons, ligaments, and cartilage. Other joint foci are per surgeon preference.
- Nonoperative sports medicine specialists may be family practice physicians, pediatricians, or physical medicine and rehabilitation specialists who have done an additional fellowship (usually 1 year).

Oncology

- Diagnose and surgically treat musculoskeletal tumors, both benign and malignant.
- Perform a wide variety of procedures ranging from minor open biopsies to hemipelvectomies.
- Frequently perform large tumor resections coupled with limb salvage procedures such as bulk allograft or prosthetic replacement of major joints.

Pediatrics

- The general orthopedist for the pediatric population.
- Sports injuries, forearm fractures, scoliosis, neuromuscular disorders, and developmental problems such as hip disorders and club foot are among the common conditions seen by pediatric orthopedists.
- Often, pediatric orthopedists will develop a subspecialty niche within general pediatric orthopedics (sports, spine, etc.).

General Anatomy and Motion

Anatomy

- Anterior: front.
- Volar: front, especially referring to the front of the forearm or hand when in anatomic position. This is a convenient reference plane which is fixed relative to the hand, despite rotation of the forearm.
- Posterior: back.
- Dorsal: back, sometimes referring to the thoracic region of the spine but commonly used in hand surgery, referring to the back of the forearm or hand, opposite side of the limb to volar, above. Also, top of the foot.
- Plantar: bottom of the foot (analogous to volar in the hand).
- Medial: toward midline.
- Lateral: away from midline.
- Superior: up.
- Inferior: down.
- Proximal: closer to the center of the body.
- Distal: farther from the center of the body.
- Supra: above.
- Infra: below.
- Intra: within.
- Inter: between.
- Extra: outside of.
- Meta: adjacent or near.
- Retro: reverse or behind.
- Antero: front or forward.
- Mid: middle.

Postural/Positional or Deformity Descriptions

- Varus: curvature or bowing of a long bone or joint with apex relatively lateral
- Valgus: curvature or bowing of a long bone with apex relatively medial
- Procurvatum: curvature or bowing of a long bone or joint with apex anterior
- Recurvatum: curvature or bowing of a long bone or joint with apex posterior
- Kyphosis: curvature of the spine with apex posterior
- Lordosis: curvature of the spine with apex anterior
- Cavus: high-arched foot
- Equinus: plantar flexed foot or ankle (like a horse that walks on its toes)

Motion Descriptors

- Elevation: upward movement
- Depression: downward movement
- Anterograde: moving or directed from proximal to distal
- Retrograde: moving or directed from distal to proximal
- Extension: bending movement that increases angle of joint (or fracture site) or moves toward the 180 degree or maximally open position
- Flexion: bending movement that decreases angle of joint (or fracture site) from the maximally open or 180 degree position
- Internal rotation: rotating toward midline
- External rotation: rotating away from midline
- Pronation: turning palm of the hand or arch of the foot down
- Supination: turning palm up or raising the arch of the foot
- Adduction: movement toward midline of the body or limb
- Abduction: movement away from midline of the body or limb
- Eccentric: muscle lengthening against resistive force

- Concentric: muscle shortening against resistive force
- Isometric: muscle contraction without a change in length

Bone Growth and Anatomy

- Epiphysis: end of bone closest to joint.
- Metaphysis: the portion of a long bone between the physis or physeal scar and the diaphysis, seen as the "flared" portion of the bone, largely cancellous in structure.
- Diaphysis: the shaft of a long bone.
- Trochanter: a large protruding knob of bone, specifically at the proximal extent of the shaft of the femur.
- Tuberosity: a medium-sized normal knob or protrusion of bone, often serves as a tendon attachment.
- Tubercle: a smaller knob of bone, often a tendon attachment.
- Malleolus: a moderate sized knob of bone, specifically on the medial and lateral sides of the ankle.
- Sesamoid: a relatively small bone which is largely contained within a tendon and serves to enhance tendon function. The patella is the largest sesamoid bone and the sesamoid bones of the hand are variably present.
- Facet: a relatively small and flat cartilage-covered surface of a bone, one of the gliding surfaces of the joint in focus.
- Foramen: a normal hole in a bone, through which a traversing structure, such as a nerve or blood vessel, passes.
- Canal: a longer tunnel or hole through a bone.
- Medulla: central portion of a structure, often relatively soft and protected by some surrounding resilient structure.

Bone Types

- Woven: immature, disorganized bone deposition
- Lamellar: mature, organized bone deposition, having layered histologic appearance

- Cortical: strong, compact, outer layer, usually lamellar
  - Layers (lamellae) of bone surrounding multiple central canaliculi (channels) which allow communication between osteocytes.
  - Haversian unit is the (histologic) canaliculus surrounded by a set of lamellae of cortical bone.
- Cancellous: porous, spongy inner core of bone consisting of interconnected trabeculae

Bone Cells

- Ostcoblasts: form bone and regulate bone metabolism
- Osteocytes: mature bone cells surrounded by osteoid matrix
- Osteoclasts: macrophage-like cells responsible for bone resorption and turnover

Bone Growth and Healing

- Intramembranous ossification
  - Bone forms without cartilage intermediary.
- Endochondral ossification
  - Initial cartilage model is replaced by woven bone and then remodeled to lamellar bone.
  - Replicated in fracture healing.
- Physis: Growth plate. Site of bone growth
  - Organized into zones
    ∘ Reserve
    ∘ Proliferative
    ∘ Hypertrophic
    ∘ Bone deposition
  - Physeal Scar: a variable anatomic landmark which marks the position of the physis in mature bone after it is fused and no longer growing
  - Generally located transversely at the point of maximum width of each end of the bone
- Fracture healing
  - Primary healing
    ∘ Rigid fixation/absolute stability without fracture gap

- ∘ Facilitated by lag screw fixation or compression plates
- ∘ Intramembranous, direct bone healing without callous via Haversian remodeling
- Secondary fracture healing
  - Less rigid fixation/relative stability.
  - Seen after application of a cast, intramedullary nail, external fixator, or bridge plating.
  - Stages as below with cartilage model:
    - ∘ Blood clot and hematoma
    - ∘ Callus (cartilage)
    - ∘ Woven, immature bone
    - ∘ Remodeling to lamellar, compact, and mature bone
  - Optimal fracture healing produces bone that is identical to the original tissue in histology and biomechanics.
  - Bone healing is true healing, not scar formation.

Cartilage

Hyaline Cartilage

- Covers smooth articular surfaces.
- Proteoglycans retain water and provide resistance against compression.
- Type II collagen.
- Chondrocytes.

Fibrocartilage

- Menisci, labrum, annulus fibrosus, and pubic symphysis
- Proteoglycans and water
- Type I collagen
- Chondrocytes

Pharmacology

Anticoagulation

- Venous thromboembolism (VTE) = blood clot
  - Deep venous thrombosis (DVT)
  - Pulmonary embolism (PE)

- Orthopedic patients are at an increased risk for VTE in the perioperative period
  - ∘ Virchow's triad: stasis, endothelial injury, and hypercoagulability
- Often prescribed medications to decrease their risk of VTE
  - Risk of VTE has been weighed against the risk of bleeding while taking these medications.
- Sequential compression devices (SCDs) decrease stasis by actively promoting venous return from the distal limb and may decrease the need for pharmacologic VTE prophylaxis.
- Heparin
  - Activates antithrombin III which inactivates thrombin, factor Xa
  - 5000 units SQ TID to prevent VTE
- Enoxaparin (Lovenox, low-molecular-weight heparin, LMWH)
  - Same mechanism of action of heparin, more predictable anticoagulant effects
  - 30 mg SQ BID or 40 mg qday
  - Generally the preferred method of anticoagulation for patients at significant VTE risk
- Warfarin
  - Inhibits vitamin K-dependent factors II, VII, IX, X, protein C, and protein S.
  - International normalized ratio (INR) must be monitored.
  - Used when long-term anticoagulation is required.
- Aspirin (ASA)
  - Irreversibly binds to cyclooxygenase (COX), decreasing prostaglandin and thromboxane synthesis and platelet aggregation
    - ∘ Fondaparinux (Arixtra)
    - ∘ Related to LMWH, injected
  - Activates antithrombin III to inhibit factor Xa
- Newer oral anticoagulants:
  - Do not require coagulation monitoring
  - Limited orthopedic indications currently in US, some bleeding concerns
  - Rivaroxaban (Xarelto); apixaban (Eliquis) Direct factor Xa inhibitors
  - Dabigatran (Pradaxa) Direct thrombin inhibitor

Antibiotics

- Ancef/cefazolin, first-generation cephalosporin
  - Typical pre-/postoperative antibiotic utilized during orthopedic surgical procedures and in open fractures
  - Blocks cell wall synthesis, modest activity against gram-negative organisms
- Clindamycin
  - Utilized in cases of penicillin or cephalosporin allergy
  - Interferes with function of 50S ribosomal subunit and subsequent protein synthesis
- Vancomycin
  - Indicated when methicillin-resistant *Staph aureus* (MRSA) is suspected
- Aminoglycosides
  - Gentamycin, tobramycin
  - Added in more severe open fractures, grade III, for synergistic effects and gram-negative coverage
- Penicillins
  - Added in farm injuries or if there is concern for anaerobic organisms such as clostridium

NSAIDs (nonsteroidal anti-inflammatory drugs)

- Ibuprofen, naproxen, meloxicam, and others Inhibit COX1/2 decreasing inflammation and platelet aggregation
- Celebrex Inhibit COX2 selectively Spares gastrointestinal side effects (bleeding) and decreases platelet effect

Bisphosphonates

- Inhibit osteoclast bone resorption
- Nitrogen containing bisphosphonates
  - Inhibit farnesyl pyrophosphate synthase
  - Disrupt function of ruffled border and osteoclast ability to resorb bone
- Primarily utilized in treatment of osteoporosis
- Also indicated in other conditions such as metastasis to bone and Paget's disease

Orthopedic Implants

Screws

- Cortical screws
  - Utilized for hard cortical bone
  - Less thread required for equal pullout strength
- Cancellous screws
  - Increased thread depth theoretically increases pullout strength in weaker, less dense cancellous bone; wider spaced threads so thread number is compromised.
- Lag screws
  - Threads only engage the far cortex/aspect of the fracture. This allows the near side to slide and compress across the fracture site.
  - Can be by:
    ○ Design: base of screw does not have threads.
    ○ Technique: fully threaded screw, but near cortex is overdrilled to the outer diameter of the screw, to prevent thread engagement in the near cortex and pull the far cortex in to compress the fracture line.
- Locking screws
  - Head of the screw locks into the plate.
  - Provides an "internal fixator," fixed angle device.
  - Utilized for osteoporotic bone, comminuted fractures, and other situations with compromised bone quality.
- Cannulated screws
  - Central core of screw is hollow.
  - Screw is placed over a wire, allowing for fine-tuning of trajectory.
  - Not as strong as similar-sized solid core screws.

Intramedullary Nails

- Placed within long bone for treatment of fracture or, less commonly, prevention of impending pathologic fracture due to weakened bone
- Commonly utilized for the femur and tibia
- Also available for the humerus, radius, ulna, clavicle, and fibula

External Fixator

- Pins are placed into bone and left protruding external to skin:
  - Can cause irritation or be portal for infection
  - Connected to an external frame providing stability across a fracture or unstable joint
- Often utilized as a temporizing measure in polytrauma or when the soft tissue is not amenable to internal fixation, as in the case of massive soft tissue injury or open wounds
- Can be utilized as definitive fixation until fracture healing or for definitive correction of limb deformity

Percutaneous Pins

- Threaded or smooth pins, placed through skin and across fractures or joints to provide either temporary or permanent fixation
- Can be left protruding outside the skin for ease of later removal
- Can cause irritation, or be portal for infection, especially if placed through abundant, mobile soft tissue

Arthroplasty

- Joint replacement or resurfacing aims to preserve motion and reduce pain at a joint that has been damaged by trauma or degenerative disease.
- Commonly performed for the knee, hip, shoulder, ankle, and elbow utilizing metal, polyethylene, and/or ceramic implants.
- Hemiarthroplasty refers to the replacement of the ball of the hip or shoulder with preservation of the native socket.
- Unicompartmental arthroplasty is a partial (knee) replacement, which resurfaces the femur and the tibia on only the medial or lateral side of joint. Reserved for cases when degenerative changes are isolated to one compartment.
- Total joint arthroplasty refers to replacement of both sides of the articular surface.
- Resurfacing arthroplasty is less common and replaces surface of joint with minimal intramedullary fixation.

- Metal, polyethylene, silicone, and soft tissue interposition arthroplasty are often utilized for the hand and wrist.
- Disc replacement is performed for degenerative disc disease in the cervical and lumbar spine.

Miscellaneous

- Autograft: tissue transferred from self to repair damage tissue such as tendon, ligament, or bone.
- Allograft: cadaver tissue.
- Arthrocentesis: aspiration of a joint.
- Arthrodesis: joint fusion.
- Arthroscopy: minimally invasive surgery where cameras are utilized to visualize and perform intra-articular surgery.
- Bursa: synovial tissue sac that reduces friction between two surfaces.
- Crepitus: grating, grinding, and popping caused by friction from the bone, cartilage, or other soft tissues.
- Curettage: scrape out.
- Dislocation: disruption of normal relationship of bones meeting in a joint, usually requiring significant trauma and soft tissue disruption, often maintained in abnormal position by geometry of the joint and spasm of surrounding muscles. Interposed tissue may prevent reduction.
- Effusion: increase in joint swelling or fluid.
- Fascia: fibrous tissue separating the subcutaneous layer from the deep muscular layer. Also separates muscular compartments.
- Fluoroscopy: live X-ray imaging.
- Fracture: broken bone. May or may not be visible on X-ray.
- Iatrogenic fracture: unintentional fracture caused by event in the course of treatment.
- Lavage: irrigation and washing.
- Malunion: improperly healed fracture.
- Nonunion: failure of fracture healing.
- Occult fracture: not readily visible on X-ray.
- Open fracture: fracture which communicates with a break in skin that allows physical continuity between fracture and the outside environment, presumed contaminated with bacteria.

- Osteotomy: cutting of bone.
- Paresthesia: altered sensation.
- Pathologic fracture: fracture caused by weakened bone.
- Reduce: restore normal alignment and position of a structure, such as a bone or joint that has been disrupted by injury.
- Sprain: ligament injury.
- Strain: muscle injury.
- Stress fracture: repetitive use injury causing microfractures to bone with resultant pain. May lead to a true displaced fracture if weakened bone is overloaded.
- Subluxation: incomplete joint dislocation.

References

1. Kurtz S, Ong K, Lau E, Mowat F, Halpern M. Projections of primary and revision hip and knee arthroplasty in the United States from 2005 to 2030. J Bone Joint Surg Am. 2007;89(4):780–5.
2. Terry Canale S, Beaty JH. Campbell's operative orthopedics. 12th ed. St. Louis: Mosby; 2012.
3. Tornetta P III, Court-Brown C, et al. Rockwood, Green, and Wilkins' 'Fractures in adults' and 'fractures in children'. 8th ed. Philadelphia, PA: LWW; 2014.
4. Flynn JM. OKU 10 : orthopedic knowledge update. Rosemont, IL: American Academy of Orthopedic Surgeons; 2011.
5. Hoppenfeld S, de Boer P, Buckley R. Surgical exposures in orthopedics: the anatomic approach. 4th ed. Philadelphia, PA: LWW; 2009.

Radiology: The Basics

Anne Sullivan, Christopher Sugalski, and D. Daniel Rotenberg

Types (Modalities) of Musculoskeletal Imaging

- Plain X-ray = radiograph = roentgenogram = plain film, in common use "X-ray" or "film"
  - Standard, two-dimensional image, generated when X-rays travel through a substance (tissue) and are variably absorbed, reflected, or transmitted by the tissue to a receiving plate of unexposed photographic film, or digitally recorded by a fluorescent receiving grid.
  - Views: AP (or PA), lateral, and oblique; views correspond to the projection of (the shadow of) the structure, relative to anatomic position, against the receiving device; special named or anatomic views may provide specialized anatomic information to help understand the pathology more specifically for surgical planning.
- Ultrasound = sonogram = sonographic image
  - Image generated by the relative transmission versus reflection of high-frequency sound energy as it travels through tissues, related to tissue density; the reflected waves are received by a transducer and electronically interpreted to produce an image.
  - Musculoskeletal ultrasound is improving in quality and finding new applications, for example, in assessing integrity of tendons and other structures, as well as providing guidance for percutaneous procedures.
- Nuclear medicine scan = radioisotope-labeled scan, may also be named isotope, e.g., indium-111 or technicium-99
  - Image created by measurement of radioisotope labeling:
    - A substance or cell used by the body is radiolabeled and injected into the circulation, allowing the isotope to pass through the circulation and be metabolized, concentrating in areas which accumulate more of the radiolabeled substance.
    - The whole body or region of interest is then imaged by a radiation receiver (essentially a Geiger counter), and areas of isotope concentration are recorded, formatted to produce an image, and

A. Sullivan, MD (✉) • C. Sugalski, MD
Department of Orthopaedic Surgery,
The Ohio State University Wexner Medical Center,
Columbus, OH, USA
e-mail: suileabhainac@gmail.com;
anne.sullivan@osu.edu

D. Daniel Rotenberg
Desert Orthopaedic Center,
Las Vegas, NV, USA

© Springer International Publishing AG 2017
A.E.M. Eltorai et al. (eds.), *Orthopedic Surgery Clerkship*, DOI 10.1007/978-3-319-52567-9_2

interpreted in the context of the clinical situation.

  ◦ Reliability and resolution are variable, often used for screening or confirmation of diagnosis, in conjunction with other modalities.

• Computed (axial) tomography images = CT scan = CAT scan

  – Three-dimensional imaging technology involving X-rays transmitted from a source revolving around the body or structure and striking a revolving receiver that is 180 degrees opposed.
  – This data is then reformatted to generate complementary series of high-resolution thin slice/section images of the structure or region of interest for diagnosis and treatment decision-making.
  – Views: axial, coronal, sagittal, and special anatomic reconstruction.
  – Three-dimensional CT reconstructions may be very detailed and may be used to pattern physical models for surgical planning.

• Magnetic resonance imaging = MRI

  – High-resolution three-dimensional imaging generated by the signal generated by the excitation and relaxation of protons of water molecules in response to perturbations of their alignment in a high-strength magnetic field (pulse sequences). The signal generated by the protons in the changing field is characteristic to the tissue and its water content and is used to generate a high-resolution gray-scale image of the structure being imaged. MRI scanners come in different magnet field strengths measured in teslas or T, usually between 0.5 T and 3.0 T. They also come in varying sizes, including open and wide bore. Higher-tesla magnets typically result in higher-resolution images.
  – MR images are well suited to visualize soft tissues and soft tissue pathologic processes, as well as subtle changes in bone marrow.
  – Planes of reconstruction: axial, coronal, sagittal, special anatomic (e.g., longitudinal or radial with respect to an axis), or

three-dimensional reconstruction, similar to CT scanning.

  – Different pulse sequences of excitation-relaxation cycles produce different characteristic signal patterns which are contrasted and compared to identify pathologic processes:

    ◦ T1 sequences can be identified by fatty tissues showing bright or white signal and water showing dark signal representation, particularly useful for visualizing fine anatomic detail.
    ◦ T2 sequences are identified by water showing bright signal and fat showing dark signal, useful for demonstrating edema and related pathologic processes.
    ◦ "Fat suppression" and other advanced pulse sequences enhance visualization of various tissue characteristics.

Types/Patterns of Fractures

• Fracture – break in the bone.
• Closed fracture – fracture in which the skin is intact.
• Open fracture – fracture in which the zone of injury communicates with a break or laceration of the skin or mucosa (anus, vagina), exposing the broken bone to air and potential bacterial contamination.

  – Gustilo classification:
  – Grade 1 – relatively low-energy injury; the skin wound is 1 cm or less, often an inside-out injury resulting from piercing of the skin by a spike of bone.
  – Grade 2 – moderate injury fracture with wound <10 cm and no neurovascular compromise, minimal accompanying deep soft tissue damage, and the ability to close the defect with local tissues.
  – Grade 3 – more severe open fracture with major soft tissue damage, characterized by wound >10 cm in length or similar soft tissue compromise:

    ◦ 3a no neurovascular injury, local soft tissue coverage possible without flap
    ◦ 3b flap coverage required
    ◦ 3c (neuro)vascular injury requiring immediate repair/reconstruction

- Stress fracture = fatigue fracture = fracture that is the result of repetitive stress (fatigue) over time, which exceeds the bone's ability to heal and therefore results in cycle of partial healing and repeated cumulative injury and weakened bone.
  - Often not visible on plain film or may be visible as incomplete fracture or sclerotic incomplete healing response.
  - The "dreaded black line" is a radiographic appearance of a radiolucent line surrounded by sclerotic callus, representing a stress fracture which may complete in the near future.
  - May eventually become complete fracture.
- Torus/buckle fracture – incomplete fracture with a buckling of the cortex, no obvious fracture "line" through the cortex, usually in pediatric/immature bone which is relatively flexible.
- Greenstick fracture – incomplete, angulated fracture. Break in outer cortex (tension side), with the inner cortex intact or showing plastic deformation, usually in pediatric/immature, or sometimes pathologic bone which is relatively flexible.
- Compression fracture is structural failure of bone under compressive load, often resulting in decreased volume of bone, common in osteoporotic or compromised bone, especially in areas that are mostly cancellous (vertebral body).
- Burst fracture (vertebrae) is fracture occurring under compressive load, in which the bone is resilient enough to partially resist the load and ultimately fail in a propulsive manner, resulting in the fracture fragment propulsion approximately 90 degrees to the direction of the load.
- Stable fracture is fracture configuration that remains anatomically aligned and resists displacement under normal physiologic load in a normal loading direction and may often be treated nonoperatively with external bracing or support.
- Pathologic fracture – any fracture occurring under normal physiologic load, indicative of abnormality of bone strength, or other compromise. Common causes include destructive lesion of bone such as metastasis or infection, metabolic bone disease such as osteoporosis, or genetic abnormality.

- Common eponyms
  - *Bennett* fracture is an unstable fracture of the base of the first metacarpal.
  - *Colles* fracture – a distal radius fracture with apex pointing volar.
  - *Charcot* fracture or joint (neuropathic arthropathy) is a destructive process due to neuropathy; lack of protective sensation impairs the ability of the structure to resist harmful loading and heal micro- or macro-injuries, leading to catastrophic failure.
  - *Galeazzi* fracture is a forearm fracture consisting of radial fracture and dislocation of the distal radial ulnar joint (DRUJ).
  - *Lisfranc* joint is the tarso-metatarsal joint, named for the Napoleonic era surgeon who described (eponymously named) fracture dislocation injuries to this area.
  - *Maisonneuve* fracture (complex) is a pronation-external rotation injury to the ankle syndesmosis, which disrupts the entire length of the interosseous (tibiofibular) membrane and produces an oblique or spiral fracture of the proximal fibula, usually requiring operative stabilization at the ankle mortise. The fibular fracture heals secondarily.
  - *Monteggia* fracture is a forearm and elbow injury involving an ulno-humeral dislocation, and usually radial forearm injury requires imaging of the elbow and wrist to look for associated injury.
  - *Jones* fracture is an acute or chronic or completed stress fracture of the proximal end of the fifth metatarsal, at the watershed area of blood supply in the meta-diaphyseal region of the bone.

Steps to Reading Musculoskeletal Imaging from an Orthopedic Perspective

- Name the imaging modality, and view(s) or plane represented, if cross-sectional imaging.
- Name the skeletal region, joint, bone, or region of bone (e.g., proximal or distal portion of long bone), which is represented in the image, and laterality if appropriate.

- Describe the skeletal maturity: if able to be determined:
  - "This is an AP view plain film of the right shoulder of a skeletally mature individual."
  - "These are AP and frog-leg lateral views of the pelvis of a skeletally immature individual."
- (Optional) describe any technique details if appropriate: image quality, completeness, and sequence type (T1- or T2-type sequences):
  - "These are T1-weighted axial images of the right knee."
  - "This is a swimmer's view lateral c-spine film which appears underpenetrated and the C7–T1 junction is not visible."
- Begin to list pathologic findings:
  - Special appearance or characteristics of bone or bone quality, even if unable to completely characterize them:
    - Osteopenia – decreased density, darker on plain film
    - Sclerosis – increased density, whiter on plain film
    - Calcifications – represented by white appearance which may be irregular or correspond to a known structure
    - Callus – bone deposition at fracture site
    - Other obvious deformities or abnormalities
  - Beware of general appearance/expectations of appropriate penetration for analog films or appropriate contrast window in digital films.
  - Tip: If the bone looks clearly abnormal, note it; start by stating that the bone looks abnormal; if more details are possible (e.g., osteopenia, subtle bone destruction due to other pathologic processes), think about it, as you may be asked.
  - Special characteristics of soft tissue:
    - Foreign bodies such as gravel or glass.
    - Disruption of or air in tissues, which can indicate either open wound or gas production by an organism.
    - Calcification or ossification may be subtle difference.
    - Edema (extra-articular swelling).
    - Effusion – intra-articular swelling.
  - Soft tissue envelope may be notable for its dimensions.
  - Presence of implants/hardware or foreign bodies:
    - A radiopaque implant or replacement prosthesis is best described as "hardware" initially; further description may be given, e.g., a plate, prosthesis, or screw, if needed. Describing hardware incorrectly may be an unnecessary source of embarrassment!
    - Tip: Avoid overstating – it is safest to "under call" it and state that, for example, "a hip prosthesis is present," unless you are sure whether a hip arthroplasty is a "total hip" with a femoral stem with a small femoral head and a hemispheric metallic or polyethylene acetabular component or a "hemiarthroplasty" if there is a large spherical prosthetic head which fills the native acetabulum.
    - Tip: Beware of objects external to the body which may appear on X-rays such as coins in a pocket, body piercings, zippers or buckles, jewelry, EKG leads or monitors, external bracing or bandaging, and foreign bodies, e.g., gravel in a wound.
  - Traumatic or focal findings:
    - Fractures – see below for how to describe.
    - Subluxations and dislocations.
    - Malunions, deformities, and malalignments.
    - More subtle deformities and lesions of bone, joint, or soft tissue.
    - Other soft tissue defects or lesions.
- How to describe a fracture:
  - State brief demographics of patient: gender and age.
  - One or two noteworthy facts if known, e.g., mechanism of injury, significant history, or comorbidities.
- Name the bone that is fractured and if it is open or closed.
- Name the approximate direction and configuration of the fracture line(s):

- Name the region of the bone where the fracture is located:
  - Is the fracture articular (the fracture line enters a joint) or non-articular?
  - Is it a physeal fracture (does the fracture line communicate with a physis)?
- Note the characteristics of fracture pattern:
  - Displacement, bone loss, angulation, and shortening if present.
  - State the direction of the APEX if angulated, on both AP and lateral view.
  - Note the fracture pattern: transverse, long or short oblique, spiral, or comminuted.
  - Note if segmental – more than two major fragments along length of bone.
- "These are AP and lateral view X-rays of the distal radius and ulna (or wrist) of a skeletally immature individual. There is a complete, transverse, non-articular fracture of the distal radius with apex volar angulation. The fracture line involves the distal radial physis."
- Bonus: If it is a physeal fracture, which type is it per the Salter-Harris classification?
  - I. Nondisplaced disruption of the physis itself.
  - II. The fracture line involved the physis, where there is displacement, and the fracture line exits through the metaphysis, so that a small portion of the metaphysis, known as the "Thurstan-Holland fragment," remains attached to the physeal fragment.
  - III. The fracture is articular, and the fracture line is actually through the epiphysis, but not the metaphysis.
  - IV. The fracture line travels through the metaphysis, crosses the physis, and continues through the epiphysis to exit into the joint.
  - V. The fracture line is not visible and the physis is impacted.

Example

How to Describe a Fracture

Used with permission from D. Daniel Rotenberg, M.D.

A _ _ Y.O. [male/female] with a [open/closed] fracture of [which bone].

The fracture is an [intra-articular/extra-articular].

[spiral/oblique/transverse/greenstick/buckle/segmental/comminuted]

fracture of the [proximal third/middle third/distal third/__cm from the joint].

On the AP view, the fracture is angulated ___ degrees apex [medial/lateral].

On the lateral view, there is ___ degrees of angulation apex [anterior/posterior].

On the AP view, the fracture is displaced ___ percent [medially/laterally]

[with __ cm of shortening].

On the lateral view, the fracture is displaced ___ percent [anterior/posterior]

[with __ cm of shortening].

Angulation: the angle described by drawing a line through the center of fracture fragments, i.e., 30° apex anterior (pictured below).

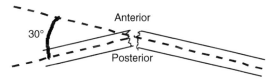

Displacement: described in terms of percent of bone width, where the distal fragment is shifted with respect to the proximal fragment, i.e., the distal fragment is 50% displaced medially.

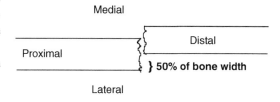

Suggested Readings

1. Terry Canale S, Beaty JH, Campbell WC. Campbell's operative orthopedics. 12th ed. St. Louis/London: Mosby; 2012.

2. Tornetta III P, Court-Brown C, et al. Rockwood, Green, and Wilkins' 'Fractures in adults' and 'fractures in children'. 8th ed. Philadelphia: LWW; 2014.
3. Flynn JM. OKU 10 : orthopedic knowledge update. Rosemont: American Academy of Orthopedic Surgeons; 2011.
4. Daniel Rotenberg D. "How to describe a fracture" teaching unit. Columbus, OH: Personal communication; 1994.
5. Herring W. Learning radiology: recognizing the basics. 3rd ed. Philadelphia, USA: Saunders (Elsevier); 2016. http://www.learningradiology.com.
6. Yochum TR, Rowe LJ, editors. Essentials of skeletal radiology, vol. 2. 3rd ed. Philadelphia: Wolters Kluwer Health ; 2012. ISBN-13: 978-0781739467.
7. Chew FS. Skeletal radiology: the bare bones; hardcover. Baltimore: Williams & Wilkins; 1997. ISBN-13: 978-0683016802.

Fractures

3

Tracye J. Lawyer and Patrick F. Bergin

Bone Composition [4]

- Bone consists of cells and a blend of mineral and matrix that coexist in a very exact relationship. The matrix phase consists of collagen and glycosaminoglycans.
- Calcium hydroxyapatite is the basic mineral crystal in bone. The bulk of calcium in the skeletal reservoir is bound in the crystals of hydroxyapatite. The organic component of the bone matrix, primarily type 1 collagen, contributes to bone strength.
- Osteoblasts are bone-forming cells that secrete the matrix components. As ossification occurs, the osteoblasts become trapped in the matrix they produce and are then referred to as osteocytes.
- Osteocytes represent terminally differentiated osteoblasts and function within syncytial networks to support bone structure and metabolism.
- Osteoclasts are the only cells that are known to be capable of resorbing bone. Their primary function is the degradation and removal of mineralized bone. They are derived from mononuclear precursor cells of the monocyte-macrophage lineage.

T.J. Lawyer, MD, PhD • P.F. Bergin, MD (✉)
Department of Orthopedic Surgery, University of Mississippi Medical Center, Jackson, MS, USA
e-mail: pbergin@umc.edu

Anatomy [3]

- Microscopically, bone is described as either mature or immature.
- Mature bone has an ordered lamellar arrangement of haversian systems or osteons and canalicular communications.
- Immature bone has much more random appearance of collagen in a matrix with irregularly spaced cells. Immature bone is seen in the adult skeleton only under pathologic conditions like fracture callus or osteogenic sarcoma.
- Macroscopically, the lamellar bone is configured either as dense cortical bone or as spicules called trabeculae.
- Cortical bone is dense and solid and surrounds the marrow space, whereas trabecular bone is composed of a honeycomb-like network of trabecular plates and rods interspersed within the bone marrow compartment.
- Cortical bone has an outer periosteal surface and inner endosteal surface. Periosteal surface activity is important for appositional growth and fracture repair.
- Both cortical and trabecular bone are composed of haversian systems. Cortical and trabecular bone are normally formed in a lamellar pattern, in which collagen fibrils are laid down in alternating orientations.
- The normal lamellar pattern is absent in woven bone.

- The periosteum is a fibrous connective tissue sheath that surrounds the outer cortical surface of bone, except at joints where bone is lined by articular cartilage.
- The periosteum is tightly attached to the outer cortical surface of the bone by thick collagenous fibers called Sharpey's fibers.
- The endosteum is a membranous structure covering the inner surface of cortical bone, trabecular bone, and Volkmann's canal present in the bone. The endosteum contains blood vessels, osteoblasts, and osteoclasts.

Vascularity [1]

- The vascularity of bone is very important when it comes to fracture repair.
- In an intact adult long bone, there are three major sources of blood.
- The nutrient artery enters the cortical diaphysis and divides proximally and distally within the endosteal canal.
- Smaller metaphyseal arteries enter the bone near its ends. These arteries supply the metaphyseal region and form an anastomotic system with the endosteal blood supply coming from the nutrient artery.
- The bone is also perfused by small vessels from the periosteum that are adherent to the outer surface of the bone.
- The endosteal circulation perfuses approximately the inner two-thirds of the cortex. Most of the metaphyseal bone is also perfused by the endosteal circulation rising from the metaphyseal arteries.
- The outer one-third of the cortex is perfused by the periosteal vasculature.

Bone Healing [2]

- The primary goal of fracture healing is to reestablish the integrity of the injured bone, restoring function of the affected limb.

- Fracture healing is classically categorized into two types: direct bone healing and secondary bone healing.
- Direct bone healing refers to direct cortical healing of two fractured ends of a bone. There is no transitional cartilaginous stage. This process primarily occurs between rigidly opposed cortical fracture ends.
- Secondary bone healing involves healing processes within the bone marrow, periosteum, and the soft tissues surrounding the bone. A transitional cartilaginous or fibrocartilaginous stage precedes bone formation. This type of healing dominates when the fracture is held less rigidly, like seen when a fracture is treated with a cast.
- Direct bone healing occurs primarily after the fractured ends of cortical bone are directly reduced and rigidly opposed under compression. Rigid compression fixation of the opposed cortical ends creates a mechanical environment with minimal interfragmentary motion.
- Direct appositional bone healing must occur across the gaps before contact healing can proceed. However, on a microscopic scale, perfect apposition of the fractured cortices is not achieved. Cortical ends are connected with a series of contact points and gaps.
- Gap healing is primarily characterized by direct bone formation between the ends of the bone, thus enclosing the gap. Smaller gaps fill with mature lamellar bone. Larger gaps fill more slowly primarily with primitive woven bone.
- These gaps that have filled with primitive woven bone during the initial phase of gap healing require remodeling to achieve prefracture strength, which is achieved by contact healing.
- Contact healing occurs in a series of events controlled by basic multicellular units. They facilitate bone resorption and then direct formation in the tunnels spanning the fracture. These multicellular components form a cutting cone with osteoclast leading the path.

- The cutting cones burrow through the fracture cortices and across the fracture plane, creating a void. Osteoblasts then follow along the edges of the cutting cone and begin bone formation.
- Fractures treated by closed methods, intramedullary fixation, external fixation, or less than rigid plate unite by secondary bone healing.
- The fracture causes localized bleeding with formation of a hematoma. This initiates a set of inflammatory events.
- Secondary bone healing employs a combination of direct intramembranous bone formation and endochondral ossification, similar to bone formation processes seen in skeletal growth.
- In both mechanisms, mesenchymal cells migrate to the wound site in response to locally increased levels of growth factors and cytokines, where they differentiate into chondrocytes or osteoblasts. The mechanical environment influences this cell fate decision.
- Secondary bone healing initially produces primary woven bone. Following the initial repair, remodeling transforms the primitive woven bone into a more efficient secondary structure which restores the bony architecture to its normal state.

Inflammatory Phase [4]

- Fracture healing is a natural process that can reconstitute injured tissue and recover its original function and form.
- It is a very complex process that involved the coordinated participation of migration, differentiation, and proliferation of inflammatory cells, angioblasts, fibroblasts, chondroblasts, and osteoblasts which synthesize and release bioactive substance of extracellular matrix components.
- The inflammatory phase occurs shortly after a bone is fractured.

- The fracture includes injury not only to the osseous structures but also to the marrow elements, periosteum, and soft tissue surrounding the bone.
- These structures are all well vascularized in comparison with bone, and disruption of their vascular supplies leads to the accumulation of hematoma.
- Local cell death accompanies the damage to the vascular elements. The hematoma and necrotic tissue elicit an immune response that attracts cellular elements through chemotaxis.
- The process of chemotaxis gives rise to primitive mesenchymal elements that then begin to accumulate in the area of the fracture.
- The inflammatory response has two beneficial effects, hydraulic splinting of the limb and voluntary immobilization from pain and swelling, and mesenchymal cells proliferate and differentiate into osteoblasts.

Reparative Phase [4]

- The reparative phase of fracture healing is marked by changes in the microenvironment of the fracture itself.
- Changes in oxygen tension and acidity of the microenvironment lead to differentiation of the primitive mesenchymal cells into more differentiated cellular elements.
- These pluripotential mesenchymal cells differentiate into a variety of cell types. Granulation tissue develops, bringing with it new blood supply into the area of the fracture.
- Islands of cartilage formation are evident which eventually undergoes endochondral ossification as the fracture unites.
- Damage to the periosteum activates the cambium layer of the periosteum, and some new bone formation occurs.
- Altogether these changes are referred to as callus formation. Once callus is observed to be bridging the fracture site, the bone fragments are usually stable.

- As the callus matures, it is remodeled to its normal configuration. In this process, the newly formed bone in the area of the fracture undergoes osteoclastic resorption and osteoblastic deposition of mature lamellar bone (Fig. 3.1).

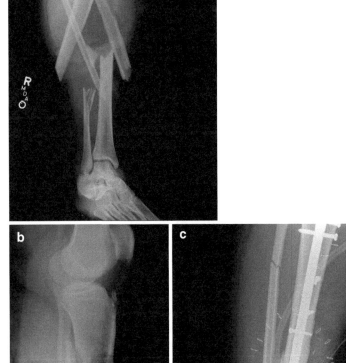

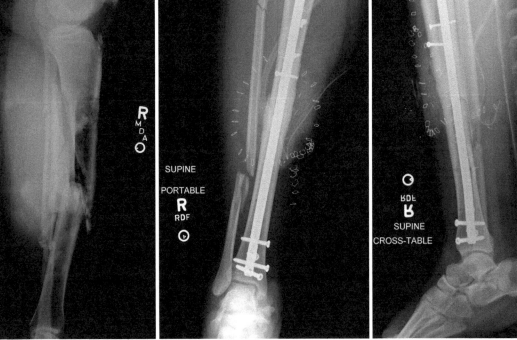

Fig. 3.1 (**a, b**) Show orthogonal views of a comminuted and displaced open tibial shaft fracture. (**c, d**) Reveal the same injury after reconstruction with interfragmentary screws and a tibial nail

References

1. Copenhaver WM, Kelly DE, Wood RL. The connective tissues: cartilage and bone. In: Bailey's textbook of histology. Philadelphia: Williams and Wilkins; 1978.
2. Dee R. Bone healing. In: Principles of orthopedic practice. New York: McGraw-Hill; 1988.
3. Recker RR. Embryology, anatomy, and microstructure of bone. In: Disorders of bone and mineral metabolism. New York: Raven; 1992.
4. Wicscl SW, Delahay JN, Conell MC. Essentials of orthopedic surgery: Philadelphia, Pennsylvania: WB Saunders Co.; 1993.

Dislocations

4

Tracye J. Lawyer and Patrick F. Bergin

Definition

- A dislocation is a complete disruption of a joint so that the articular surfaces are no longer in appropriate contact.

Etiology

- Most often, the cause of the dislocation is a traumatic event, and the result is a loss of structural stability of the joint. Traumatic dislocation usually causes pain, deformity of the involved extremity, and limited joint motion.

Management

- Appropriate treatment of a dislocation involved careful neurovascular evaluation, radiographic studies, and prompt reduction of the involved joint.

T.J. Lawyer, MD, PhD • P.F. Bergin, MD (✉)
Department of Orthopedic Surgery, University of Mississippi Medical Center, Jackson, MS, USA
e-mail: pbergin@umc.edu

Complications [1]

- Complications and long-term sequelae of traumatic dislocation include neurovascular injuries, avascular necrosis, heterotopic bone formation, posttraumatic arthritis, musculotendinous injuries, joint instability, and joint stiffness.

Neurovascular Injuries [2]

- Vascular injury can occur in the involved extremity because the joint is forcibly displaced from its anatomic location.
- For example, in the shoulder, the humeral head dislocates anteriorly most often, and the axillary artery becomes taut and is displaced forward. Since the artery is relatively fixed at the lateral margin of the pectoralis minor muscle, this forward displacement causes the pectoralis minor muscle to act as a fulcrum over which the artery is deformed and ruptured.
- Patients with axillary artery injuries resulting from shoulder dislocations experience pain, an expanding hematoma, pulse deficit, peripheral cyanosis, pallor, and neurological dysfunction.

- Treatment requires emergent vascular repair.
- The most common dislocation resulting in vascular injury is dislocation of the knee [3].
- Anatomically, the popliteal artery is tethered proximally to the femur in the adductor hiatus and distally to the fibula by the fibrous bands of the soleus fascia [3].
- Posterior dislocations (posterior displacement of the tibia) can result in complete transection of the artery because the vessel impacts the posterior rim of the tibia plateau [3].
- Anterior dislocations (anterior displacement of the tibia) typically cause a contusion of the vessel with intimal injury [3].
- The axillary nerve is the neural structure most commonly injured in association with shoulder dislocations.
- The axillary nerve lies directly across the anterior surface of the subscapularis muscle. As the humeral head displaces the subscapularis muscle and tendon move forward and anterior in glenohumeral dislocations, traction and direct pressure are produced on the axillary nerve and result in injury to neural structures.
- Popliteal artery injuries are a surgical emergency requiring immediate repair.
- Circulation to the extremity needs to be restored within 6–8 hours if the risk of amputation is to be minimized.
- Treatment involves a thorough physical and radiographic examination followed by a prompt reduction.
- In addition to vascular injuries, neural structures can be contused, stretched, or even lacerated in the event of the joint being dislocated.
- The sciatic nerve, specifically the peroneal component, is injured in 10–20% of patients who sustain a posterior dislocation of the hip.
- As the hip dislocates posteriorly, it directly entraps or contuses the nerve which results in a peroneal nerve palsy.
- These nerve injuries must be recognized early because nerve tissue does not tolerate pressure well and permanent ischemic changes occur quickly.
- Most axillary nerve injuries are traction neurapraxias and will recover completely.

Avascular Necrosis (Hip) [4]

- Avascular necrosis of the femoral head is a well-recognized complication after posterior dislocation of the hip.
- Both the degree of initial trauma and the time during which the hip remains dislocated have been found to directly correlate with the likelihood of avascular necrosis.
- Reduction within 6 hours of injury substantially decreases the incidence of avascular necrosis. Therefore, prompt reduction is mandated in all cases of hip dislocations.
- Careful monitoring and follow-up must be maintained after reduction if possible avascular changes are to be detected.
- If avascular necrosis is not diagnosed early, femoral head collapse and traumatic arthritis will result.
- Reduction of any dislocated joint helps to reduce pain, improves circulation within the surrounding soft tissues, removes pressure on the chondral surfaces, and allows for better radiographic imaging.
- Avascular necrosis is a devastating complication that results in death of the osteocytes in the femoral head, subsequent chondral collapse, and secondary degenerative osteoarthritis of the hip joint.
- Death of these osteocytes is thought to occur because of ischemia from damage to the blood supply to the femoral head.
- Early reduction may reverse ischemic changes that occur in the femoral head at a cellular level.

Heterotopic Ossification (Elbow and Hip Most Common) [1]

- Heterotopic ossification of the surrounding soft tissue can occur as a result of traumatic joint dislocation.
- This condition is most frequently noted after elbow dislocations.
- The most common sites of periarticular calcification are the anterior elbow region and the collateral ligaments.

- Ectopic bone formation is associated with delayed surgical intervention, closed head injury, and aggressive passive elbow manipulation after dislocation.
- If heterotopic bone formation is limiting joint motion, resection of the involved bone should be delayed until the ossification appears mature on plain radiographs.
- Radiographic maturation is characterized by well-defined cortical margins with linear trabeculations.
- Ectopic bone formation has also been reported after hip dislocations.
- The ectopic bone formation can be a result from the initial muscle damage, the formation of hematoma, and the influx of inflammatory mediators.
- The severity of the traumatic dislocation seems to be the best predictor of the occur-rence of bone formation in the surrounding tissue.
- Treatment is based on symptoms, and the recommended excision time of the extraosseous tissue correlates with the maturity of the ectopic bone.

Articular Cartilage [1]

- The traumatic process of a joint dislocation can permanently and irreversibly injure the articular cartilage lining of the involved joint.
- This injury to the cartilage can lead to the development of osteoarthritis.
- The severity of the initial trauma and the structural damage to the articular surface are the primary factors in determining the later development of posttraumatic arthritis (Fig. 4.1).

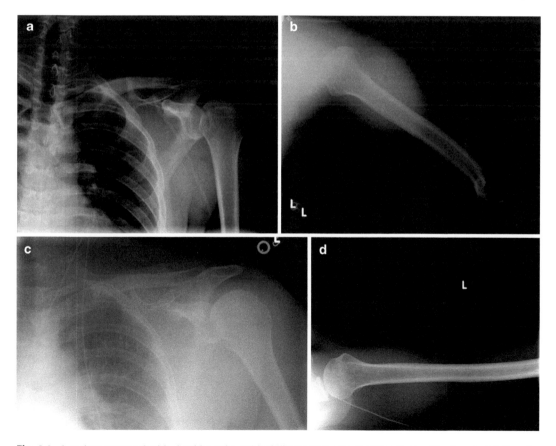

Fig. 4.1 A patient presented with shoulder pain and inability to move the shoulder in any direction. (**a, b**) Reveal a perched posterior shoulder dislocation. (**c, d**) Are similar images after a closed reduction was performed

References

1. Cohn SM. Complications in surgery and trauma. Boca Raton: Taylor and Francis Group; 2013.
2. Cornwall R, Radomisli TE. Nerve injury in traumatic dislocation of the hip. Clin Orthop Relat Res. 2000;377:84–91.
3. Hegyes MS, Richardson MW, Miller MD. Knee dislocation: complications of nonoperative and operative management. Clin Sports Med. 2000;9:519–43.
4. Rodriguez-Merchan EC, Goddard NJ. Traumatic dislocation of the hip. Clin Orthop Relat Res. 2000;377:2–3.

Orthopedic Emergencies

5

Ilia Iliev, Grant Buchanan, and Franklin Shuler

Compartment Syndrome

- Overview
  - Increased pressure in a closed fascial space impairing perfusion
  - Causes irreversible nerve and muscle damage
- Anatomy
  - Most common in the leg
- Etiology
  - Intracompartmental
    ◦ Fractures (most common)
    ◦ Soft tissue injury
    ◦ Arterial injury
    ◦ Revascularization
  - Extracompartmental
    ◦ Circumferential burns
    ◦ Tight/constrictive cast
- Presentation
  - The five Ps of compartment syndrome.
    ◦ Pain with passive stretch (most sensitive finding)
    ◦ Paresthesia
    ◦ Poikilothermia (different temperatures of affected versus unaffected limb)
    ◦ Pallor
    ◦ Paralysis (late finding)
  - Pulselessness is a late finding usually associated with irreversible damage.
- Diagnosis
  - In the absence of unequivocal clinical findings, diagnosis is made using compartment pressure measurements.
    ◦ Pressures taken from each compartment.
    ◦ Measurements taken closer to the fracture site associated with the highest manometry readings.
    ◦ Pressure >30 mmHg or within 30 mmHg of diastolic pressure is diagnostic and warrants emergent fasciotomy [1].
- Treatment
  - Loosen constrictive casts or dressing.
  - Ice and elevate.
  - Definitive treatment is emergent fasciotomy of affected compartments.
  - Fascial released in a late missed compartment syndrome is controversial and may increase risk of infection [2].

Unstable Pelvic Fracture

- Etiology
  - High-energy blunt trauma, usually associated with multiple long bone fractures and spine and chest injury.

I. Iliev • G. Buchanan, MD (✉)
F. Shuler, MD, PhD
Department of Orthopaedic Surgery, Joan C. Edwards School of Medicine, Marshall University, Huntington, WV, USA
e-mail: buchanang@marshall.edu

© Springer International Publishing AG 2017
A.E.M. Eltorai et al. (eds.), *Orthopedic Surgery Clerkship*, DOI 10.1007/978-3-319-52567-9_5

- These injuries are associated with significant morbidity and mortality of up to 25% for closed fractures and 50% for open fractures.
- Anatomy
  - Pelvic ligaments
    ∘ Anterior and posterior sacroiliac ligaments
      - Most important for pelvic stability
    ∘ Sacrospinous ligaments
    ∘ Sacrotuberous ligaments
    ∘ Symphyseal ligaments
- Signs and symptoms
  - Pelvic instability on palpation
  - Local swelling, hematoma, ecchymosis, and scrotal hematoma
  - Gross hematuria
  - Chest injury, low BP, and higher ISS
- Imaging
  - AP, inlet, and outlet views.
  - CT will better show extent of injury.
- Classification
  - Tile classification [3]
    ∘ Type A
      - Stable
    ∘ Type B
      - Rotationally unstable and vertically stable
    ∘ Type C
      - Rotationally and vertically unstable
  - Young-Burgess classification [4]
    ∘ AP compression
    ∘ Lateral compression
    ∘ Vertical shear
- Treatment
  - Airway, breathing, and circulation
  - Emergent or in field placement of pelvic binder
  - External and/or internal fixation
- Complications
  - Life-threatening internal hemorrhage
  - Neurologic injury
  - DVT/PE
  - Fat emboli
  - Urogenital injury

Necrotizing Fasciitis

- Overview
  - Life-threatening infection of deeper skin and subcutaneous tissues
  - Spreads along fascial planes
  - Mortality rate >30%
- Risk factors
  - Immunocompromised due to AIDS, cancer, and diabetes
  - IV drug use
- Classification [5]
  - Type 1
    ∘ Polymicrobial
      - Most common type
      - At least one anaerobe
      - +/− facultative anaerobes
  - Type 2
    ∘ Monomicrobial
      - Seen in healthy patients
      - Group A *Strep* most common
  - Type 3
    ∘ Marine *Vibrio* (gram-negative rods)
    ∘ Due to marine exposure
- Signs and symptoms
  - Early
    ∘ Pain at site
    ∘ Generally normal appearance of skin
  - Late
    ∘ Progressively intense pain
    ∘ Fever and tachycardia
    ∘ Skin discoloration and edema
    ∘ Crepitus from subcutaneous emphysema
- Diagnosis
  - Emergent presentation to the operating room.
  - Biopsy can provide early diagnosis usually completed intraoperatively with emergent frozen biopsy of tissue sample.
  - Laboratory Risk Indicator for Necrotizing Fasciitis (LRINEC) score [6].
    ∘ White blood cell (WBC) count.
      - <15 per mm^3 = 0 points
      - 15–25 per mm^3 = 1 point

- – >25 per mm^3 = 2 points
  - ○ Hemoglobin (Hb).
    - – <11 g/dL = 2 points
    - – 11–13.5 g/dL = 1 point
    - – >13.5 g/dL = 0 points
  - ○ Sodium (Na$^+$).
    - – >135 mEq/L = 0 points
    - – <135 mEq/L = 2 points
  - ○ Glucose (Glu).
    - – <180 mg/dL = 0 points
    - – >180 mg/dL = 1 point
  - ○ Creatinine (Cr).
    - – <1.6 mg/dL = 0 points
    - – >1.6 mg/dL = 2 points
  - ○ C-reactive protein (CRP).
    - – <150 mg/L = 0 points
    - – >150 mg/L = 4 points
  - ○ WBC + Hb + Na$^+$ + Glu + Cr + CRP = LRINEC score.
  - ○ Score ≥ 6 should be treated for necrotizing fasciitis (PPV = 92%).
- Treatment
  - – Early broad-spectrum IV antibiotics
  - – Urgent and aggressive surgical debridement
  - – Generally require multiple trips to the operating room for reexploration and repeat debridement

Septic Arthritis

- Overview
  - – More common in large joints
  - – Most common in knee
  - – Risk factors: rheumatoid arthritis, osteoarthritis, prosthetic joint, intravenous drug abuse, alcoholism, and diabetes [7]
- Etiology
  - – Common organisms: *Staphylococcus* and *Streptococcus* > gram negatives (*Neisseria gonorrhoeae, Escherichia coli*)
- Presentation

- – Acutely painful, warm, erythematous, and swollen joint with limited range of motion and refusal to bear weight
- Diagnosis
  - – Synovial fluid aspiration [8]
    - ○ Appearance (opaque, purulent).
    - ○ Gram stain.
    - ○ WBC count >50,000–100,000 cells/mm^3 in native joint.
    - ○ Positive culture is definitive.
  - – Labs
    - ○ Elevated WBC count with left shift
    - ○ Elevated erythrocyte sedimentation ratio (ESR) and CRP
  - – Prosthetic joint infection [9]
    - ○ Diagnosed by having one major criterion:
      - – Two positive synovial cultures with same organism
      - – Sinus tract communicating with joint
    - ○ Or having three minor criteria:
      - – Elevated CRP (>10 mg/L) and ESR (>30 mm/hr)
      - – Elevated synovial WBC count (>3000 cells/mm^3)
      - – Positive synovial leukocyte esterase test
      - – Elevated polymorphonuclear neutrophil percentage (PMN% > 80)
      - – Positive tissue histology
      - – Single positive culture
- Treatment
  - – Intravenous antibiotics
  - – Irrigation and debridement
  - – Prosthetic joint infection
    - ○ Two-stage revision – most common and effective method
      - – Stage I – irrigation and debridement, removal of components, placement of antibiotic cement spacer, and intravenous antibiotics until all clinical signs of infection have cleared
      - – Stage II – removal of antibiotic cement spacer and placement of revision components

Cauda Equina Syndrome

- Definition
  - Compression of terminal lumbosacral (L1-S5) nerve roots
- Anatomy
  - Conus medullaris terminates around T12-L1
  - Cauda equina formed by L1-S5 nerve roots
- Causes
  - Lumbar disc herniation – most common
  - Mass (tumor, epidural abscess, hematoma, fracture fragment)
  - Spinal stenosis
- Presentation
  - Red flag symptoms [10]
    ∘ Severe lower back pain
    ∘ Sciatica
    ∘ Saddle anesthesia
    ∘ Bowel, bladder, and sexual dysfunction
- Imaging
  - MRI
- Treatment
  - Urgent surgical decompression
    ∘ Significantly better neurological outcome if treated within 48 h of symptom onset [11]

Open Fracture

- Overview
  - Fracture with exposed bone
  - Typically caused by high-energy trauma
- Gustilo-Anderson classification [12]
  - Type I – wound <1 cm, simple fracture pattern, minimal contamination, and soft tissue injury
  - Type II – wound 1–10 cm, moderate fracture comminution, soft tissue injury, and contamination
  - Type III – wound >10 cm, severely comminuted or segmental fracture, extensive soft tissue damage, and contamination
    ∘ A. Adequate soft tissue for local coverage
    ∘ B. Requiring rotational or free flap for soft tissue coverage
    ∘ C. Vascular injury requiring repair

- Treatment
  - Prompt irrigation and debridement and fracture stabilization.
  - Administer intravenous antibiotics and provide tetanus prophylaxis [13].
    ∘ Gram-positive coverage is evidence-based management – typically a first-generation cephalosporin.
    ∘ Benefit of gram-negative or anaerobe coverage is controversial and is beneficial for larger wounds.

Hip Dislocation

- Overview
  - Often caused by high-energy trauma.
  - Associated musculoskeletal and solid organ injuries are common.
    ∘ Sciatic nerve injury in 10% [14]
- Classification
  - Posterior dislocation
    ∘ 90% of hip dislocations.
    ∘ Caused by axial force on femur with hip in flexion and adduction (knee hitting dashboard).
    ∘ Patients present shortened, flexed, adducted, and internally rotated hip.
  - Anterior dislocation
    ∘ 10% of hip dislocations.
    ∘ Caused by posterior force on knee with hip in abduction.
    ∘ Patients present shortened, abducted, and externally rotated hip.
- Diagnosis
  - X-ray
    ∘ AP pelvis
      - Shenton's line – parabolic line drawn along inferior border of obturator foramen and inferior femoral neck
        • Shows discontinuity when there is a dislocation
    ∘ Cross-table lateral
  - CT
    ∘ Improved visualization of associated fractures and intra-articular fragments [15]

- ○ Typically performed following closed reduction
- Treatment
  - Nonoperative
    - ○ Urgent reduction within 6 h to prevent avascular necrosis of the femoral head [16]
  - Operative
    - ○ Open reduction recommended for irreducible dislocation or incarcerated fragment
    - ○ Fixation of associated fractures

Knee Dislocation

- Overview
  - Caused by high- or low-energy trauma (motor vehicle, athletics)
  - High incidence of vascular injury (popliteal artery injury in 32%) [17]
  - High incidence of nerve injury (peroneal > tibial) [18]
  - High incidence of ligamentous injury (ACL, PCL, MCL, LCL, PLC)
- Classification
  - Classified by position of the tibia relative to the femur, low vs. high velocity, and acute vs. chronic
  - Order of commonality: anterior > posterior > lateral > medial > rotatory [19]
- Diagnosis
  - Thorough neurovascular examination is critical.
    - ○ Doppler ultrasound and ankle brachial index.
    - ○ Routine arteriogram is controversial – absolutely indicated with clinical evidence of vascular injury [20].
  - Examine compartments, joint congruity, and ligamentous status.
  - Radiographs – AP, lateral, and oblique view of the knee.
    - ○ Rule out associated fractures with AP and lateral views of the hip, femur, tibia, and ankle.

- MRI – assess for ligamentous, cartilaginous, and bony injuries.
- Treatment
  - If the limb is ischemic, an emergent reduction should be performed, and vascular status should be reassessed. If pulses do not return, emergent surgical exploration by a vascular surgeon is required.
  - If limb is not ischemic, careful reduction under sedation should be performed. Repeat neurovascular examination and apply long leg splint.
  - Ligamentous injuries should be repaired 2–3 weeks following injury.

References

1. McQueen MM, Court-Brown CM. Compartment monitoring in tibial fractures. The pressure threshold for decompression. J Bone Joint Surg Br. 1996;78(1):99–104.
2. Reis ND, Michaelson M. Crush injury to the lower limbs. Treatment of the local injury. J Bone Joint Surg Am. 1986;68(3):414–8.
3. Tile M. Acute pelvic fractures: I. causation and classification. J Am Acad Orthop Surg. 1996;4(3):143–51.
4. Burgess AR, Eastridge BJ, Young JW, Ellison TS, Ellison Jr PS, Poka A, et al. Pelvic ring disruptions: effective classification system and treatment protocols. J Trauma. 1990;30(7):848–56.
5. Lancerotto L, Tocco I, Salmaso R, Vindigni V, Bassetto F. Necrotizing fasciitis: classification, diagnosis, and management. J Trauma Acute Care Surg. 2012;72(3):560–6.
6. Wong CH, Khin LW, Heng KS, Tan KC, Low CO. The LRINEC (Laboratory Risk Indicator for Necrotizing Fasciitis) score: a tool for distinguishing necrotizing fasciitis from other soft tissue infections. Crit Care Med. 2004;32(7):1535–41.
7. Mathews CJ, Kingsley G, Field M, Jones A, Weston VC, Phillips M, et al. Management of septic arthritis: a systematic review. Ann Rheum Dis. 2007;66(4):440–5.
8. Visser S, Tupper J. Septic until proven otherwise: approach to and treatment of the septic joint in adult patients. Can Fam Physician. 2009;55(4): 374–5.
9. Parvizi J, Gehrke T, Chen AF. Proceedings of the international consensus on periprosthetic joint infection. Bone Joint J. 2013;95-b(11):1450–2.

10. Gardner A, Gardner E, Morley T. Cauda equina syndrome: a review of the current clinical and medico-legal position. Eur Spine J. 2011;20(5):690–7.

11. Ahn UM, Ahn NU, Buchowski JM, Garrett ES, Sieber AN, Kostuik JP. Cauda equina syndrome secondary to lumbar disc herniation: a meta-analysis of surgical outcomes. Spine. 2000;25(12):1515–22.

12. Gustilo RB, Anderson JT. Prevention of infection in the treatment of one thousand and twenty-five open fractures of long bones: retrospective and prospective analyses. J Bone Joint Surg Am. 1976;58(4):453–8.

13. Hauser CJ, Adams Jr CA, Eachempati SR. Surgical Infection Society guideline: prophylactic antibiotic use in open fractures: an evidence-based guideline. Surg Infect (Larchmt). 2006;7(4):379–405.

14. Cornwall R, Radomisli TE. Nerve injury in traumatic dislocation of the hip. Clin Orthop Relat Res. 2000;377:84–91.

15. Brooks RA, Ribbans WJ. Diagnosis and imaging studies of traumatic hip dislocations in the adult. Clin Orthop Relat Res. 2000;377:15–23.

16. Clegg TE, Roberts CS, Greene JW, Prather BA. Hip dislocations--epidemiology, treatment, and outcomes. Injury. 2010;41(4):329–34.

17. Green NE, Allen BL. Vascular injuries associated with dislocation of the knee. J Bone Joint Surg Am. 1977;59(2):236–9.

18. Goitz RJ, Tomaino MM. Management of peroneal nerve injuries associated with knee dislocations. Am J Orthop. 2003;32(1):14–6.

19. Brautigan B, Johnson DL. The epidemiology of knee dislocations. Clin Sports Med. 2000;19(3):387–97.

20. Klineberg EO, Crites BM, Flinn WR, Archibald JD, Moorman CT. The role of arteriography in assessing popliteal artery injury in knee dislocations. J Trauma. 2004;56(4):786–90.

Principles of Trauma

6

Thomas Gill and Brock Johnson

Overview: Trauma

- Fourth leading cause of death
- 2:1 male-to-female ratio
- Mechanism
  - Motor vehicle accident: 38%
  - Falls: 30%
  - Blunt trauma: 86%
  - Penetrating trauma: 11%
- Cause of death
  - 40–50% neurologic injury
  - 30–35% hemorrhage
- Mortality
  - 50% within minutes
    - Neurologic injury
    - Hemorrhage
  - 30% within days
    - Neurologic injury
  - 20% after weeks
    - Infection
    - Multi-organ failure

Management of the Trauma Patient

- ABCs: airway, breathing, and circulation
- Imaging

T. Gill, MD (✉) • B. Johnson, MD
Department of Orthopaedics, Marshall University,
Huntington, WV, USA
e-mail: gillth@marshall.edu

- Focused assessment with sonography for trauma (FAST)
  - Radiographs
    - AP chest
    - AP pelvis
    - Lateral C-spine
  - Computed tomography
- Resuscitation
  - Crystalloid.
  - PRBC, FFP, and platelets in 1:1:1 ratio.
  - Failure to respond to crystalloid and blood requires further intervention (exploratory laparotomy, embolization, thoracotomy).
- Hypovolemic shock stages
  - I
    - Volume loss: < 15% (750 mL)
    - HR and BP normal
  - II
    - Volume loss: 15–30% (750–1500 mL)
    - Tachycardiac
    - BP normal
  - III
    - Volume loss: 30–40% (1500–2000 mL)
    - Tachycardiac
    - Hypotensive
    - Lactic acid >2.5
    - Lethargic
  - IV
    - Volume loss: > 40% (>2000 mL)
    - Life-threatening
    - Tachycardiac
    - Hypotensive
    - Comatose

© Springer International Publishing AG 2017

A.E.M. Eltorai et al. (eds.), *Orthopedic Surgery Clerkship*, DOI 10.1007/978-3-319-52567-9_6

- Markers of adequate resuscitation
  - Urine output: 0.5–1 mL/kg/h
  - Lactic acid:
    ∘ Normal <2.5 mmol/L
    ∘ Most sensitive
  - Base excess: −2 to +2

- Polytrauma
- Head injury
- Hemodynamic instability
- Hypothermia
- Coagulopathy
- Pulmonary contusions

Damage Control Orthopedics

- Delay definitive fixation to prevent additional injury to patient (fractures should be stabilized with external fixator, splint, or traction).
- Acute inflammatory window.
  - Days 2–4
  - Systemic inflammatory response
  - Increased inflammatory markers
  - Increased risk or acute respiratory distress syndrome (ARDS)
- Stages.
  - Temporary fixation (external fixation, traction, splint)
  - Resuscitation
  - Definitive fixation
- Patient selection.

Indicators for Early Total Care

- Hemodynamic stability
- Lactic acid <2 mmol/L
- Urine output >1 mL/kg/h
- No coagulopathy

Open Fractures

- Gustilo-Anderson classification
  - I: wound <1 cm
  - II: 1–10 cm (Fig. 6.1)
  - III: > 10 cm
    ∘ III A: adequate soft tissue envelope
    ∘ III B: need for flap coverage
    ∘ III C: vascular injury requiring repair

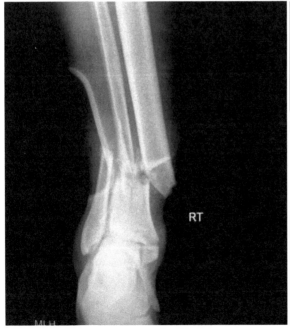
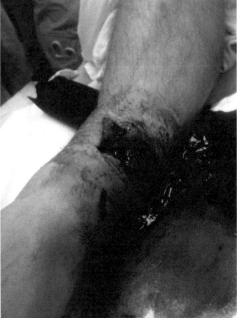

Fig. 6.1 Gustilo-Anderson type II open distal tibia fracture

- Automatic type III injuries
  - Segmental fracture
  - High-velocity gunshot wound
  - Severely contaminated wound
  - Extensive periosteal stripping
- Treatment
  - Antibiotics
    - Type I and II: first-generation cephalosporin (cefazolin).
    - Type III: first-generation cephalosporin and aminoglycoside (cefazolin + gentamycin).
    - Add penicillin for barnyard injury (anaerobic coverage).
    - Add fluoroquinolone for water injury.
  - Tetanus booster
  - Surgical debridement
  - External versus internal fixation

Gunshot Wounds (GSW)

- Low velocity.
  - Muzzle velocity < 2000 ft./s
  - Local wound care, tetanus, and oral antibiotics for nonoperative fractures
  - ORIF for unstable fractures
- High velocity.
  - Muzzle velocity > 2000 ft./s
  - Close-range shotgun
  - Extensive zone of injury
  - External fixation
  - Aggressive debridement

- Definitive fixation when soft tissues allow
- Remove intra-articular bullet due to potential for lead toxicity.
- GSW to spine.
  - IV antibiotics for 7–14 days if bullet perforated viscous
  - Decompression and bullet removal for neurologic injury with retained bullet in spinal canal

Suggested Readings

1. Rockwood CA, Green DP, Bucholz RW. Rockwood and Green fractures in adults, vol. 1. 7th ed. New York: J. B. Lippincott; 1991.
2. Boyer MI. Comprehensive orthopedic review 2, vol. 1. Rosemont: Amer Academy of Orthopedic; 2014.
3. Browner BD. Skeletal trauma, basic science, management, and reconstruction. 4th ed. Philadelphia: Elsevier Health Sciences; 2009.
4. Gustilo RB, Anderson JT. JSBS classics. Prevention of infection in the treatment of one thousand and twenty-five open fractures of long bones. Retrospective and prospective analyses. J Bone Joint Surg Am. 2002;84-A(4):682.
5. Bartlett CS, Helfet DL, Hausman MR, Strauss E. Ballistics and gunshot wounds: effects on musculoskeletal tissues. J Am Acad Orthop Surg. 2000;8(1):21–36.
6. Gustilo RB, Mendoza RM, Williams DN. Problems in the management of type III (severe) open fractures: a new classification of type III open fractures. J Trauma. 1984;24(8):742–6.
7. Kim PH, Leopold SS. In brief: Gustilo-Anderson classification. [corrected]. Clin Orthop Relat Res. 2012;470(11):3270–4.

Part II

The Upper Extremity

Physical Exam of the Shoulder

7

Navkirat Bajwa and Albert Pearsall

Four Aspects

- Inspection: atrophy, hypertrophy, scar, erythema, skin abnormalities, and swelling.
- Palpation: palpate all around the shoulder including the sternoclavicular joint, acromioclavicular joint, glenohumeral joint, acromion, coracoid, clavicle, and scapula/scapular spine.
- ROM: both active and passive ROM should be documented (Table 7.1).
- Neurovascular exam:
  - Sensations: axillary n. (C5–C6), lateral cutaneous nerve of the forearm (C5–C7), medial brachial/antebrachial cutaneous n. (C8–T1), median n. (C5–T1), radial n. (C5–T1), and ulnar n. (C7–T1)
  - Motor: deltoid, biceps, triceps, EPL, FDS, FDP, and intrinsics

- Reflexes: biceps (C5), triceps (C7), and brachioradialis (C6)
- Vascular: brachial artery, radial artery, and ulnar artery
- Tests for shoulder function (Table 7.2)
  - Evaluation of rotator cuff
    - Supraspinatus
    - Infraspinatus
    - Teres minor
    - Subscapularis
    - Superior labrum anterior posterior (SLAP) lesions
  - Biceps
  - Impingement
  - AC pathology
  - Instability

Table 7.1 ROM of the shoulder

Motion	Normal range (°)
Flexion	0–180
Extension	0–60
Abduction	0–180
Internal rotation	0–70
External rotation	0–90

N. Bajwa (✉) • A. Pearsall
Department of Orthopaedic Surgery, University of South Alabama, Mobile, AL, USA
e-mail: drbajwans@gmail.com

© Springer International Publishing AG 2017
A.E.M. Eltorai et al. (eds.), *Orthopedic Surgery Clerkship*, DOI 10.1007/978-3-319-52567-9_7

Table 7.2 Tests for shoulder function

Muscle Tests	Technique
Supraspinatus	
Jobe test	Abduct the arm to 90°, forward flex to 30° (bringing it into the scapular plane), and internally rotate (the thumb pointing to floor). Then press down on the arm. Weakness or pain while maintaining position is a positive test
Drop sign	Abduct the arm to 90° and forward flex to 30°. Then slowly lower the arm. The test is positive when weakness or pain causes the arm to drop to its side
Supraspinatus strength	Assessed using Jobe test
Infraspinatus	
External rotation lag sign	Flex the elbow to 90, 0° abduction, and rotate the shoulder to maximal external rotation. Inability to hold the arm in that externally rotated position/drifting into internal rotation is a positive test
Infraspinatus strength	External rotation strength tested while the arm is in neutral abduction/adduction
Teres minor	
Hornblower's sign	Abduct the shoulder to 90°, ER 90°. Inability to hold this position/drifting into IR is a positive test
Teres minor strength	External rotation strength tested with the arm held in 90° of abduction
Subscapularis	
Internal rotation lag sign	*Most sensitive and specific test* Flex the elbow to 90°, extend the shoulder to 20°, and elevate 20° (place the hand over lumbar spine). Passively lift the dorsum of the hand away from the lumbar spine. Support the elbow. Inability to maintain position without touching the spine is a positive test
Lift off test	Same position as the previous test. Inability to lift the hand away from the back (internal rotation) indicates subscapularis pathology
Belly press test	Press the abdomen with the palm of the hand; maintain the shoulder in internal rotation with the elbow in front of the trunk. Inability to maintain the elbow in front of the trunk is a positive test
Subscapularis strength	Flex the elbow to 90° and test ability to internally rotate against resistance
SLAP lesion	
Active compression test ("O'Brien's test")	Flex the arm to 90° and adduct 10–15°, with the elbow fully extended. Then pronate the forearm (so the thumb is pointing down) and apply downward force to the wrist while the patient resists. Then do the same with the forearm fully supinated. Pain in pronation but not in supination is a positive test
Crank test	Abduct the arm to 160° and forward flex to 30°. Apply internal/external rotation with simultaneous axial rotation stress. Click or pain indicates a positive test
Biceps	
Speed test	Extend the elbow, and supinate the forearm. Flex the shoulder against resistance while maintaining this position. Pain in the proximal biceps region is a positive test
Yergason sign	Flex the elbow to 90°, and pronate the forearm. Attempt to supination against resistance. Pain in the bicipital groove is a positive test
Popeye	Swelling in the area of the biceps muscle belly unaffected by flexion/supination of the elbow. Consistent with long head of biceps proximal tendon rupture

Table 7.2 (continued)

Muscle Tests	Technique
Impingement tests	
Neer impingement sign and test	Place the patient's hand on unaffected shoulder. Gradually flex the shoulder with one hand, while the other hand prevents motion of the scapula. The greater tuberosity impinges against the acromion (between 70–110°). Pain signifies positive sign Marked reduction in pain from above impingement maneuver following subacromial lidocaine injection is a positive test
Hawkins Test	Flex the shoulder to 90°, flex the elbow to 90°, and forcibly internally rotate the shoulder driving the greater tuberosity under the CA ligament Pain means positive test
Jobe Test	Abduct the arm to 90°, forward flex to 30°, and internally rotate (the thumb pointing to floor). Press down on the arm while patient attempts to maintain position. Weakness or pain is a positive test
AC pathology	
Cross body abduction	Flex the arm to 90°, and adduct the arm 10–15° (bring the arm across the midline). Pain at the AC joint is a positive test
O' Brien's test (active compression test)	As described above
Anterior instability	
Anterior load and shift	Abduct the shoulder to 40–60°, and flex to 90° in a supine position. Axially load with anterior/posterior translation is applied through the humerus shaft. Increased anterior translation compared to the contralateral side is a positive test
Apprehension and relocation	Abduct the shoulder to 90° and full ER in a supine position. Sense of instability is a positive apprehension test Apply a posterior force on the humeral head in the same position Reduction of sense of instability is a positive relocation test
Anterior release	Same position as the apprehension/relocation test. Remove the posterior force on the shoulder. Humerus subluxates anteriorly causing sense of instability
Posterior instability	
Posterior load and shift	
Jerk test	Flex the shoulder to 90° and IR to 90°. Axial load to the humerus is applied and maintained while adducting the shoulder. Pain or clunk is a positive test
Multidirectional instability	
Sulcus sign	Place the arm by the side while standing. Inferior pull through the elbow is applied. A sulcus/step-off between the acromion and humeral head is a positive test

Rotator Cuff Pathology

Daniel C. Kim and Albert Pearsall

Anatomy

- Rotator cuff (RTC) consists of four muscles originating on the scapula that insert on the tubercles of the proximal humerus.

that includes the capsule, superior glenohumeral ligament, and coracohumeral ligament.
- Blood supply from five arteries [2, 3]:
  - Anterior humeral circumflex a. Anterior cuff

Muscle	Origin	Insertion	Function	Innervation
Supraspinatus	Supraspinous fossa	Superior/middle facet of greater tubercle (GT)	Abduct humerus	Suprascapular nerve (C5)
Infraspinatus	Infraspinous fossa	Posterior facet GT	Externally rotate humerus	Suprascapular nerve (C5)
Teres minor	Lateral border of scapula	Inferior facet GT	Externally rotate humerus	Axillary nerve (C5)
Subscapularis	Subscapular fossa	Lesser tubercle	Internally rotate humerus	Upper and lower subscapular nerve (C5–6)

- The rotator cuff muscles form a common tendon that covers the superior, anterior, and posterior aspects of the humeral head [1].
- Insertion of tendon on tubercles referred to as "footprint."
- "Rotator interval" = Region between tendinous junction of supraspinatus and subscapularis

- Posterior humeral circumflex a. Posterior cuff
- Suprascapular a. Superior and posterior cuff
- Thoracoacromial a. Supraspinatus
- Subscapular a.

D.C. Kim, MD
Department of Orthopaedic Surgery, University of South Alabama Hospitals, Mobile, AL, USA

A. Pearsall, MD (✉)
Orthopaedic Surgery, University of South Alabama, Department of Orthopaedics, Mobile, AL, USA
e-mail: apearsal@health.southalabama.edu

Function

- RTC muscles provide stability to the glenohumeral joint by compressing the humeral head in the shallow glenoid fossa, resisting translation of the head during movement.

- Cuff muscles activate individually to counterbalance each other and keep the humerus centered in the glenoid (i.e., subscapularis and infraspinatus). Also, interior RTC balances the superior moment generated by the deltoid.
- In abduction, the subscapularis provides static stability to anterior translation, while the infraspinatus and teres minor limit posterior translation [4].

Epidemiology

- Rotator cuff disease is the most common shoulder disorder treated by orthopedic surgeons, with over 17 million people in the USA alone at risk for disabilities caused by the disease.
- Studies show surgically demonstrable full-thickness RTC tears present in about 20% of elderly patients; MRI studies show up to 40% prevalence [5].
- RTC show correlation with increasing age
  - 30% cuff tears in patients >40 years old and up to 80% prevalence in patients >60 years old [6]
- Asymptomatic tears are very common
  - Over 10% of full-thickness tears in population above 50yo are asymptomatic.
  - Limited healing potential in RTC leads to increase in tear size and progression of partial-thickness tears to full thickness [7].

Etiology

- Rotator cuff pathology is a continuum of disease typically beginning with subacromial or subcoracoid impingement (75%)
  - Internal impingement in overhead throwing athletes causes partial-thickness RTC tears [8]
  - Chronic degenerative tears in older patients involving SIT (supraspinatus, infraspinatus, teres minor)
    ° Natural history is progression of tear in size and symptoms [7].
  - Genetic component; strong relationship between RTC tears and family history established [9]

- Can also be due to shoulder instability (15%)
  - Acute SIT tears in patients >40 yo with a shoulder dislocation
- Trauma (10%)
  - Acute subscapularis tears seen in younger patients (hyperabduction/external rotation injury) [10].
  - Greater tuberosity fx is a RTC tear equivalent.

Pathology

- Impingement syndromes cause calcification and tendon degeneration near the RTC insertion (calcific tendonitis):
  - Most often associated with the supraspinatus due to its location between the superior humeral head and acromion
  - Tears most common on articular side, not bursal side [11]
- Disease progression leads to chronic degenerative tears or acute avulsion injuries of the RTC.
- Can lead to rotator cuff arthropathy:
  - Shoulder arthritis in setting of RTC dysfunction
  - Combination of chronic massive RTC tear, glenohumeral cartilage destruction, subchondral osteoporosis, and humeral head collapse

Presentation

- Insidious onset of pain anterior/anterolateral shoulder pain, especially with overhead activities
- Limited active range of motion (especially elevation in scapular plane) and passive range of motion usually preserved
- Night pain = poor indicator for successful nonoperative treatment
- Instability of shoulder
  - Massive RCT can present with pseudoparalysis of shoulder (active forward flexion less than 90°, limited active abduction, passive ROM intact)

Exam

- Impingement tests
  - Neer impingement sign
  - Hawkins modification
  - Impingement test
  - Jobe's test
- Subscapularis (weakness to IR at 0° abduction)
  - Internal rotation lag sign
  - Lift-off test
  - Belly press
- Supraspinatus (weakness to elevation in scapular plane)
  - Jobe's test
  - Drop sign
- Infraspinatus (weakness to ER at 0° abduction)
  - External rotation lag sign
- Teres minor (weakness to ER at 90° abduction)
  - Hornblowers sign

Workup

- Radiographs
  - AP
  - Shoulder outlet view
- MRI
  - Gold standard.
  - Evaluate muscle quality, degree/shape/size of tear, and retraction.
  - Often see humeral head cysts in chronic RCT tear.
- Ultrasound
  - Inexpensive, allows for dynamic testing
  - Similar sensitivity/specificity to MRI but highly user dependent [12]

Classification

- RTC tear size
  - Small: 0–1 cm
  - Medium: 1–3 cm
  - Large: 3–5 cm
  - Massive: >5 cm, involving multiple tendons

- Tear shape
  - Crescent: Mobile, can be repaired to bone with minimal tension
  - U shape: Similar to cresent but with deeper medial extension of tear
  - L shape: Similar to U shape but with one leaf that is more mobile than the other

Treatment

- Nonoperative – 1st line for most tears. Partial tears have good outcomes with therapy, ranging from 45% to 82% satisfactory results in studies. 1^0 tx for all asymptomatic tears.
  - Physical therapy – immobilization > passive movement > RTC and scapular stabilization strengthening
  - NSAIDS
  - Subacromial corticosteroid injections
- Surgical management
  - Arthroscopic repair
    - Single row suture anchor repair preferred in smaller tears
    - Double row repairs for larger tears with poor quality tissue.
      - No clinical advantage but may improve structural integrity [13]
  - Open repair
    - Less preferred due to deltoid detachment, larger incision, and higher complication rate
  - Tendon transfers
    - Pectoralis major – Reserved for massive RTC tears in young patients with anterior rotator cuff insufficiency
    - Latissimus dorsi – Patients with massive RTC, posterior rotator cuff insufficiency, and intact subscapularis
  - Reverse shoulder arthroplasty
    - RTC arthropathy with intact deltoid
    - Massive RCT with shoulder ROM <90o abd/fflex
    - Patient age >70 years

Postoperative Course

- Initial immobilization in sling for 6 weeks
  - Early passive motion with strengthening at 1.5–3 months post-op.
  - Full return to activity at 4–5 months.
  - Large and massive tears have longer course of recovery.

Complications

- Axillary (posterior portal) and musculocutaneous (anterior) nerve injury
- Excessive swelling of tissues due to fluid extravasation from arthroscope fluid
- Postoperative stiffness (more common in open technique)
- Infection (rare in arthroscopic procedure)

References

1. Clark JM, Harryman 2nd DT. Tendons, ligaments, and capsule of the rotator cuff. Gross and microscopic anatomy. J Bone Joint Surg Am. 1992;74(5):713–25.
2. Terabayashi N, Watanabe T, Matsumoto K, et al. Increased blood flow in the anterior humeral circumflex artery correlates with night pain in patients with rotator cuff tear. J Orthop Sci. 2014;19(5):744–9.
3. Chansky HA, Iannotti JP. The vascularity of the rotator cuff. Clin Sports Med. 1991;10(4):807–22.
4. Lee SB, Kim KJ, O'Driscoll SW, Morrey BF, An KN. Dynamic glenohumeral stability provided by the rotator cuff muscles in the mid-range and end-range of motion. A study in cadavera. J Bone Joint Surg Am. 2000;82(6):849–57.
5. Maman E, Harris C, White L, Tomlinson G, Shashank M, Boynton E. Outcome of nonoperative treatment of symptomatic rotator cuff tears monitored by magnetic resonance imaging. J Bone Joint Surg Am. 2009;91(8):1898–906.
6. Safran O, Schroeder J, Bloom R, Weil Y, Milgrom C. Natural history of nonoperatively treated symptomatic rotator cuff tears in patients 60 years old or younger. Am J Sports Med. 2011;39(4):710–4.
7. Keener JD, Galatz LM, Teefey SA, et al. A prospective evaluation of survivorship of asymptomatic degenerative rotator cuff tears. J Bone Joint Surg Am. 2015;97(2):89–98.
8. Lazarides ALA-GE, Choi JH, Stuart JJ, Lo IK, Garrigues GE, Taylor DC. Rotator cuff tears in young patients: a different disease than rotator cuff tears in elderly patients. J Shoulder Elbow Surg. 2015;24(11):1834–43.
9. Tashjian RZFJ, Albright FS, Teerlink CC, Cannon-Albright LA. Evidence for an inherited predisposition contributing to the risk for rotator cuff disease. J Bone Joint Surg Am. 2009;91(5):1136–42.
10. Dilisio MFNC, Noble JS, Bell RH. Traumatic supraspinatus tears in patients younger than 25 years. Orthopedics. 2015;38(7):613–34.
11. Modi CS, Smith CD, Drew SJ. Partial-thickness articular surface rotator cuff tears in patients over the age of 35: etiology and intra-articular associations. Int J Shoulder Surg. 2012;6(1):15–8.
12. Teefey SA, Hasan SA, Middleton WD, Patel M, Wright RW, Yamaguchi K. Ultrasonography of the rotator cuff. A comparison of ultrasonographic and arthroscopic findings in one hundred consecutive cases. J Bone Joint Surg Am. 2000;82(4):498–504.
13. Dines JS, Bedi A, ElAttrache NS, Dines DM. Single-row versus double-row rotator cuff repair: techniques and outcomes. J Am Acad Orthop Surg. 2010;18(2):83–93.

Adhesive Capsulitis

9

Christopher E. Urband and John M. Marzo

Epidemiology

- Females >> males
- 40–60-year-olds affected more than others

Etiology (See Table 9.1 for Risk Factors)

Table 9.1 Risk factors

A. Primary
1. Diabetes mellitus
2. Autoimmune disorder/hypothyroidism
3. Prolonged disuse or immobilization, including from neurologic disease
4. Cardiovascular disease
B. Secondary
1. Trauma
2. Postsurgical (including after thoracic or upper extremity surgery)
C. History of contralateral adhesive capsulitis is a strong risk factor

Pathology

- Inflammation of the synovium and fibrosis of the capsule

C.E. Urband, MD • J.M. Marzo, MD (✉)
Department of Orthopaedics, Jacobs School of
Medicine and Biomedical Sciences, Buffalo, NY, USA
e-mail: chris.urband@gmail.com; jmmarzo@buffalo.edu

- Cytokines, including TGF-β, PDGF, IL-1β, and TNF-α, are increased.
- Contracture of the glenohumeral capsule
  - Coracohumeral ligament contracted and rotator interval thickened
  - Results in decreased volume of the GH joint

Diagnosis

- History and physical examination
  - Pain with ROM, which has occurred gradually
  - Decreased passive ROM (and therefore active ROM as well)
    - External rotation <50 % of contralateral
    - Forward flexion <100°
  - Normal strength/neurovascular exam
- Imaging
  - XR (Fig. 9.1)
    - Overall normal
    - Disuse osteopenia seen in some cases
    - Used to rule out differential diagnoses
  - MRI/MRA (Fig. 9.2)
    - Not critical for diagnosis
    - Capsule thickened, especially rotator interval, coracohumeral ligament, and axillary recess
    - Loss of axillary recess (from capsule contracture)

© Springer International Publishing AG 2017
A.E.M. Eltorai et al. (eds.), *Orthopedic Surgery Clerkship*, DOI 10.1007/978-3-319-52567-9_9

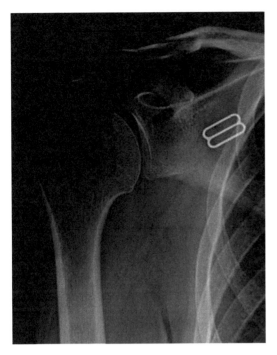

Fig. 9.1 Normal AP radiograph

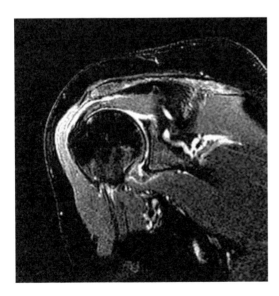

Fig. 9.2 Coronal MRI, fat suppressed showing thickened capsule

Natural History/Clinical Stages (Table 9.2): 3 to 4 Months Each

Arthroscopic/Descriptive Stages

- Fibrinous synovitis (patchy)
- Capsule contracted, with synovitis and adhesions
- Capsular contraction increased, but synovitis improving
- Severe contraction (no further synovitis)

Treatment

- Nonsurgical (12–16-week trial)
    - Physical Therapy (PT)
        ○ Home exercise programs work as well as formal therapy
        ○ Avoid intense stretching in early phases
    - NSAIDs
        ○ Symptomatic pain relief, but not proven to be effective

Table 9.2 Natural history/clinical stages

	Inflammation	Contraction
Inflammatory	Severe Diffuse pain – with any motion and at night Gradual onset	Minimal
Frozen	Decreased Pain only at extremes of motion	Increased Noted as capsular stiffness, decreased ROM ADLs are severely affected
Thawing	Inflammation continues to decrease	Contraction decreases ROM returns gradually Function improves

- Oral steroids
  - Short-term use only for pain relief and ROM improvement
- Corticosteroid injections
  - Better than oral steroids at relieving pain and improving motion
- Hydrodilatation
  - Injection of large amounts of saline into the joint to stretch the capsule
- Surgical (if failure of 12–16-week nonoperative trial)
  - Manipulation under anesthesia (MUA)
    - Proven to be a safe option
    - Risk of humeral fracture is increased in secondary adhesive capsulitis (after trauma, surgery) or after severe cases of primary disease
  - Arthroscopic or open debridement and fibrinolysis
    - Components
      - Rotator interval tissue
      - Anterior capsule
      - Inferior capsule: Accomplished through manipulation or directly
      - Posterior capsule: If IR limited also. Less reliable results
  - Open release
    - Rarely performed.
    - Useful in postoperative cases and for hardware removal at time of release.
    - Subscapularis tendon must be taken down for complete assessment of capsule.

Outcomes

- Nonoperative:
  - PT, MUA, hydrodilatation, and corticosteroid injections are similar in the long term.
    - GH injections: better than subacromial in short term. Long term, both are similar to placebo.
  - Benefits of MUA have been shown to last up to at least 1.5 years.
- Operative:
  - Younger patients tend to do better with surgical options.
  - Arthroscopic or open fibrinolysis provides relief of pain and stiffness.

Suggested Readings

1. Baumfeld J, Hart J, Miller M. Sports medicine. In: Miller M, editor. Review of orthopedics. 5th ed. Philadelphia: Elsevier; 2008. p. 282.
2. Neviaser A, Hannafin J. Adhesive capsulitis: a review of current treatment. Am J Sports Med. 2010;38(11):2346–56.
3. Keener J. Adhesive capsulitis. In: Boyer M, editor. AAOS comprehensive orthopedic review, vol. 2. Rosemont: AAOS; 2014. p. 943–6.
4. Lynch T, Edwards S. Adhesive capsulitis: current concepts in diagnosis and treatment. Curr Orthop Pract. 2013;24(4):365–9.
5. Favejee M, Huisstede B, Koes B. Frozen shoulder: the effectiveness of conservative and surgical interventions – systematic review. Br J Sports Med. 2011;45:49–56.

Calcific Tendonitis

10

Christopher E. Urband, William M. Wind, and Leslie J. Bisson

Definition

Shoulder disorder noted for:

- Severe pain, usually worse in the a.m.
- Sometimes with loss of motion (ROM)
  - Secondary to pain
- Calcific lesion located within the tendon

Epidemiology

- Women > men (slightly)
- Ages 40–60 more common

Etiology

- Unknown etiology
- Metabolic and endocrine disorders have been implicated:
  - Thyroid

The original version of this chapter was revised. An erratum to this chapter can be found at https://doi.org/10.1007/978-3-319-52567-9_159

C.E. Urband, MD
Department of Orthopaedics, Jacobs School of Medicine and Biomedical Sciences, Buffalo, NY, USA

W.M. Wind, MD • L.J. Bisson (✉)
Jacobs School of Medicine and Biomedical Sciences, University at Buffalo, 4949 Harlem Road, Amherst, NY 14226, USA
e-mail: ljbisson@buffalo.edu

- Diabetes
- Genetic predisposition

Pathology

- Degenerative calcification
  - Long-term impingement, aging, and decreased vascularity changes to microstructure of tendon fibers.
  - Degeneration of fibers results in necrosis and calcification.
  - Supraspinatus most commonly affected.
- Reactive calcification
- Calcification occurs within the tendon itself typically 1.5–2.0 cm from tendon insertion

Diagnosis

- History and physical exam
  - Severe pain
- Spontaneous onset
- Usually worse in the morning and/or at night
- May also have stiffness and decreased ROM
  - Usually secondary to pain
- Radiographs (Fig. 10.1)
  - Calcification seen in area of the tendon, most often in supraspinatus
  - Two radiographic types:
    - Type 1 – fluffy appearance with poorly defined periphery
    - Type 2 – discrete homogeneous deposits

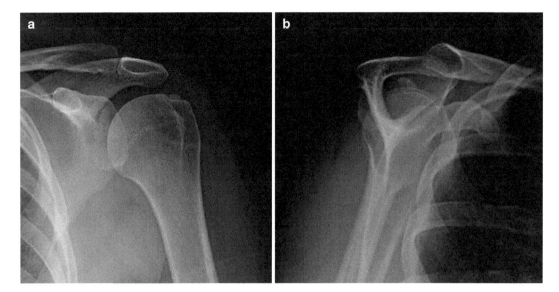

Fig. 10.1 Shoulder radiographs. (**a**) AP; (**b**) scapular Y, axillary lateral

- Osteolysis of greater tuberosity seen in a variant form of the condition
- MRI
  - If rotator cuff tear suspected
  - T1 – calcifications manifest as decreased signal
  - T2 – increased intratendinous signal with edema
  - May help localize for barbotage procedure if performed intraoperatively during rotator cuff repair

Stages: Reactive Calcification

- Precalcific
  - No symptoms yet
  - Fibrocartilaginous metaplasia of tendon tissue
- Calcific
  - Formative phase
    ∘ Appearance of chondrocytes within tendon tissue
    ∘ Well-delineated, dense homogeneous calcification
    ∘ Calcium excreted from cells into chalky form

  - Resting phase
    ∘ Fibrocartilaginous tissue borders calcium deposit indicating calcium deposition has stopped
    ∘ Painless
  - Resorptive phase
    ∘ Spontaneous resorption of calcium.
    ∘ Vascular invasion at periphery with calcium granuloma.
    ∘ Most painful. Calcification appears like toothpaste.
- Postcalcific
  - Calcification disappears with appearance of vascular channel remodeling calcium granulation tissue with maturing fibroblasts.
  - Rotator cuff tendon replaces the void.
  - Painless.

Treatment

- Nonoperative
  - Physical therapy
    ∘ Prevent loss of motion
    ∘ Strengthen cuff
    ∘ Therapy modalities:

- Heat
- Cryotherapy
- ROM
- Pendulum
  - NSAIDs
  - Corticosteroid subacromial injections (SAI)
  - Needling (barbotage)
    - Performed with U/S guidance
    - Can be combined with subacromial injection
- Operative
  - Indicated for failure of conservative management especially during the formation phase
  - Arthroscopic or open debridement with extraction of the deposit:
    - Palpate rotator cuff for calcium deposits.
    - Rotator cuff should be assessed at the time of surgery for competency after removal of large deposits.
    - Postoperative pain may continue for weeks.

Outcomes

- In a 2013 study comparing barbotage + SAI vs. isolated SAI, the barbotage group had decreased calcification size (11.6 mm vs 5.1 mm decrease), more cases of total resorption (13 vs 6), improved constant score at 1 year (86 vs 74), lower rates of secondary barbotage, and similar DASH and WORC scores.
- Outcomes worse in the osteolysis variant.

References

1. Baumfeld J, Hart J, Miller M. Sports medicine. In: Miller M, editor. Review of orthopedics. 5th ed. Philadelphia: Elsevier; 2008. p. 282.
2. Carli ADE, Pulcinelli F, Rose G, Pitino D, Ferretti A. Calcific tendinitis of the shoulder. Joints. 2014;3(2):130–6.
3. de Witte P, Selten J, Navas A, Nagels J, Visser C, Nelissen R, Reijnierse M. Calcific tendinitis of the rotator cuff: a randomized controlled trial of ultrasound-guided needling and lavage versus subacromial corticosteroids. Am J Sports Med. 2013;41(7):1665–73.
4. Uthoff H, Loehr J. Calcific tendinopathy of the rotator cuff: Pathogenesis, diagnosis, and management. J Am Acad Orthop Surg. 1997;5:183–91.
5. Kachewar S, Kulkarni D. Calcific tendinitis of the rotator cuff: a review. J Clin Diagn Res. 2013;7(7): 1482–5.

Proximal Humerus Fractures

11

Anna Johnson and Albert Pearsall

Abbreviations

AN   Anatomical neck
CRPP   Closed reduction percutaneous pinning
GT   Greater tuberosity
IMN   Intramedullary nail
LT Lesser tuberosity
ORIF   Open reduction internal fixation
SN   Surgical neck

Epidemiology

- Proximal humerus fractures are relatively rare and represent 4–5% of all fractures [1]:
  - The majority of proximal humerus fracture are not significantly displaced, and do not require surgery.
  - Can be associated with shoulder dislocation and rotator cuff tears.
- Patient population: Trauma, young individuals with high-velocity mechanism of injury, such as MVC

A. Johnson, MD
Department of Orthopedic Surgery, University of South Alabama Medical Center, Mobile, AL, USA

A. Pearsall, MD (✉)
Department of Orthopedic Surgery, University of South Alabama, Mobile, AL, USA
e-mail: apearsal@health.southalabama.edu

- Associated injuries: soft tissue destruction, injuries to thorax such as rib fractures and pnuemothorax, and distracting injuries to other extremities
- Individuals >50 years of age with fall as mechanism of injury, osteoporotic bone
  - 4:1 Female to male ratio [11]

Anatomy

- The humeral head is retroverted 30–45° [6, 14].
- Deforming forces to the 4 osseous segments of the proximal head occur. Understanding the osseous segments and deforming forces is key to fracture classification and treatment.
  - *4 proximal humerus osseous segments:*
    - *Humeral head.*
    - *Lesser tuberosity (LT):* attachment site of the subscapularis tendon; will displace medially.
    - *Greater tuberosity (GT):* attachment site of supraspinatus, infraspinatus, and teres minor; will displace superiorly and posteriorly.
    - *Humeral shaft:* attachment site of deltoid, proximal segment will displace medially; attachment site for pectoralis major; shaft will displace medially [4, 6, 9, 11].
  - Other osteology:
    - *Anatomic neck (AN):* area below humeral articular surface, above tuberosities

- ○ *Surgical neck (SN):* begins at metaphyseal flare below tuberosities [6, 14]
- – Neurovascular supply:
  - ○ Vascular: rich vascular supply makes osteonecrosis secondary to fracture a rare complication
    - – Anterior humeral circumflex artery: includes anterolateral ascending branch and terminal arcuate artery
      - • *Pearl:* fractures of anatomic neck, "danger area" due to blood supply
    - – Posterior humeral circumflex artery: runs in quadrangular space
      - • May play a greater role in perfusion to humeral head than previously believed [1, 9, 14]
  - • Neuro: Axillary nerve, more susceptible to injury with anterior dislocations
    - – Course off posterior cord, anterior inferior to glenoid humeral joint, lies posterior to axillary artery, anterior to subscapularis muscle, then courses through quadrangular space with posterior humeral artery
      - • Motor: deltoid and teres minor
      - • Sensory: superficial lateral cutaneous nerve of arm [6, 9, 14]

Presentation and Evaluation

- • Presentation: Patient may present with arm held close, swelling, tenderness, ecchymosis, and decreased range of motion
- • Evaluation: a neurovascular exam is crucial, especially with respect to the axillary nerve:
  - – Axillary nerve: motor may be unable to obtain secondary to pain, but sensation over lateral proximal arm and deltoid can be tested, Hornblower's test.
  - – Distal upper extremity neurovascular exam should also be obtained and documented.
- • Radiographs: 3 views
  - – AP shoulder
  - – Axillary
    - ○ Velpeau and West point are alternative views if axillary unobtainable secondary to pain.

- – Scapular Y
- – CT scan: indicated for preoperative planning, fractures with significant intra-articular involvement, and fracture patterns where location of displaced tuberosity or humeral head is unclear on plain films [6, 4, 9, 11, 16]

Classification and Treatment

- • Several different classification schemes have been created, but the Neer classification is the most commonly and consistently used system.
- • *Neer classification*: based on humeral osseous segments, parts, and displacement (see Table 11.1)
  - – *Part*: fragment with >1 cm displacement or 45° of angulation
    - ○ One-part fractures are almost exclusively treated nonoperatively, whereas two-part and greater fractures generally have operative indications.
  - – Valgus impacted: not in original Neer classification, four-part fracture, humeral articular surface impacted on shaft in valgus position [4, 6, 9, 11, 14, 16].
- • Fracture-dislocations: occur, anterior most common, attempt closed reduction although may not be possible
- • Nonoperative treatment
  - – Closed reduction and sling immobilization 2–3 weeks (see section V.), surgeon preference for initiation of range or motion exercises.
  - – Patient's age, pre-injury shoulder function, bone quality, compliance, activity level, dominance, occupation, and associated injuries should all be taken into account [4, 6].
- • Operative treatment
  - – CRPP (closed reduction percutaneous pinning)
  - – ORIF plate fixation most common
    - ○ locking screws options, possible fixation of rotator cuff with sutures through plate
    - ○ IMN less commonly used

Table 11.1 Neer classification of proximal humerus fractures

Part	Description and segment(s)	Treatment
One (85%) [11] No displaced fragments, proximal humerus appears to be in "one part," can have several fracture lines present	Any proximal osseous segment	Nonoperative
Two	Surgical neck *Most common* [4, 9]	Operative, CRRP vs. ORIF based on fracture reducibility and bone quality
	Greater tuberosity *Anterior dislocation often associated*	Nonoperative and operative- operative treatment indicated for >5 cm displacement [4, 6, 7, 9]
	Lesser tuberosity *Rule out posterior dislocation*	Nonoperative and operative- closed reduction unless fragment prevents internal rotation, may need ORIF or excision of fragment
	Anatomic neck *Rare, higher incidence of osteonecrosis* [4, 9]	Operative, ORIF vs. hemiarthroplasty based on patient age and bone quality
Three Unstable, obtaining and maintaining reduction difficult	SN + GT Often associated with longitudinal rotator cuff tear	Operative, CRPP vs. ORIF
3–14% osteonecrosis	SN + LT Often has associated with longitudinal rotator cuff tear [1, 11]	Operative, CRPP vs. ORIF
Four-part 45% osteonecrosis [9]	Valgus impacted Less osteonecrosis, 11% [4], blood supply from posterior humeral circumflex artery maintained	Operative, ORIF, minimally displaced due to rotator cuff
	Articular surface and head splitting	Operative, ORIF vs. hemiarthoplasty based on patient age and bone quality, humeral head split

- Deltopectoral approach (shoulder anterior)
  - Positioning: supine with bump under medial scapula
  - Internervous plane: deltoid muscle and pectoralis major (axially nerve, medial and lateral pectoral nerve, respectively)
  - *Dangers:*
    1. Axillary nerve
    2. Musculocutaneous nerve
    3. Anterior circumflex artery
    4. Cephalic vein
- Deltoid splitting approach (shoulder lateral)
  - Positioning: supine with bump under ipsilateral scapula or "beach chair" with arm at edge of table
  - Internervous plane: no true plane, deltoid spilt
  - *Dangers:*
    1. Axillary nerve [1, 4, 6, 9, 11]
- *Pearl:* Axillary nerve runs 5–7 cm distal to tip of acromion [2].

- Arthroplasty: Hemiarthroplasty vs. reverse shoulder arthroplasty
  - Indicated for older patients with poor bone quality, complex fractures involving articular surface, and humeral head split [1, 6, 16]

- Nonunion
  - *Pearl:* Humeral height, the top of prosthesis head should sit 5.6 cm cephalad to tip of pectoralis major tendon insertion [12, 15].

Posttreatment Rehabilitation

- Frequent x-rays assure no increase in displacement, proper bone healing, and hardware placement.
- Sling or sling with abduction pillow.
- Begin motion early, advance in phases, surgeon preference:
  - Pendulum swings
  - Passive range of motion exercises, especially wrist and elbow
  - Active range of motion at 4–6 weeks
  - Resistance work at 6–12 weeks
  - Full function normally within 1 year [4, 6, 9, 11, 16]

Complications

- Axillary nerve injury
  - Initial injury: 5–30% complex fractures, especially with anterior fracture-dislocation [11]
  - Iatrogenic causes, lateral pin placement in CRPP [9]
- Vascular injury
- Osteonecrosis
- Nonunion
  - Treat with revision ORIF with allograft versus autograft bonegrafting, arthroplasty in older patients [1, 3, 5, 16]. Treatment based on patient level of pain, function, overall health.
- Malunion
  - Varus deformity in younger patient, treated with revision ORIF and osteotomy [13].
  - Greater tuberosity malunion treated with hemiarthroplasty [8].
- Infection
  - Rare due to rich vascular supply
  - *Pearl:* Propionibacterium infections may occur more with hemiarthroplasty [16].

- Adhesive capsulitis
- Myositis ossificans
- Stiffness and decreased range of motion
  - Secondary to prolonged immobilization
- Intra-articular screw penetration
  - Most common complication with locking plate use [10]

References

1. Bohsali K, Wirth M, Lippett S. Hemiarthoplasty for proximal humerus fractures. In: Wiesel SW, et al., editors. Operative techniques in orthopedic surgery. 2nd ed. Philadelphia: Wolters Kleuwer; 2015. p. 3757–66.
2. Cetik O, Uslu M, Acar HI, Comert A, Tekdemir I, Cift H. Is there a safe area for the axillary nerve in the deltoid muscle? A cadaveric study. J Bone Joint Surg Am. 2006 Nov;88(11):2395–9.
3. Cheung EV, Sperling JW. Management of proximal humeral nonunions and malunions. Orthop Clin North Am. 2008 Oct;39(4):475–82.
4. Dillon M, Torres S, Gilotra M, Glaser D. Open reduction and internal fixation of proximal humerus fractures. In: Wiesel SW, et al., editors. Operative techniques in orthopedic surgery. 2nd ed. Philadelphia: Wolters Kleuwer; 2015. p. 3731–9.
5. Dines D, Warren R, Altchek D, Moeckel B. Posttraumatic changes of the proximal humerus: Malunion, nonunion, and osteonecrosis. Treatment with modular hemiarthroplasty or total shoulder arthroplasty. J Shoulder Elbow Surg. 1993;2(1):11–21.
6. Egol K, Koval K, Zuckerman J. Handbook of Fractures, vol. 4. Philadelphia: Wolters Kleuwer; 2010. p. 193–202.
7. Flatow E, Cuomo F, Maday M, Miller S, McIlveen S, Bigliani L. Open reduction and internal fixation of two-part displaced fractures of the greater tuberosity of the proximal part of the humerus. J Bone Joint Surg Am. 1991 Sep;73(8):1213–8.
8. Frankle M, Mighell M. Techniques and principles of tuberosity fixation for proximal humeral fractures treated with hemiarthoplasty. J Shoulder Elbow Surg. 2004;13:239–47.
9. Galatz L. Percutaneous pining for proximal humerus fractures. In: Wiesel SW, et al., editors. Operative techniques in orthopedic surgery. 2nd ed. Philadelphia: Wolters Kleuwer; 2015. p. 3722–9.
10. Konrad G, Bayer J, Hepp P, Voigt C, Oestern H, Kääb M, Luo C, Plecko M, Wendt K, Köstler W, Südkamp N. Open reduction and internal fixation of proximal humeral fractures with use of the locking proximal humerus plate. Surgical technique. J Bone Joint Surg Am. 2010;92(Suppl 1 Pt 1):85–95.

11. Morrey N, Boileau P, Cole J, d'Ollonne T. Intramedullary fixation of proximal humerus fractures. In: Wiesel SW, et al., editors. Operative techniques in orthopedic surgery. 2nd ed. Philadelphia: Wolters Kleuwer; 2015. p. 3741–56.

12. Murachovsky J, Ikemoto RY, Nascimento LG, Fujiki EN, Milani C, Warner JJ. Pectoralis major tendon reference (PMT): a new method for accurate restoration of humeral length with hemiarthroplasty for fracture. J Shoulder Elbow Surg. 2006;15(6):675–8.

13. Siegel J, Dines D. Techniques in managing proximal humerus malunions. J Shoulder Elbow Surg. 2003;12:69–78.

14. Thompson J. Netter's concise orthopedic anatomy. 2nd ed. Philadelphia: Saunders Elsevier; 2010. p. 75–107.

15. Torrens C, Corrales M, Melendo E, Solano A, Rodríguez-Baeza A, Cáceres E. The pectoralis major tendon as a reference for restoring humeral length and retroversion with hemiarthroplasty for fracture. J Shoulder Elbow Surg. 2008;17(6):947–50.

16. Warner J, Costouros J, Gerber C. Fracture of the Proximal Humerus. In: Bucholz R, Heckman J, Court-Brown C, editors. Rockwood & Green's fractures in adults. 6th ed. New York: Lippincott Williams & Wilkins; 2006. p. 1117–209.

Clavicle Fractures

12

Daniel C. Kim and Albert Pearsall

Epidemiology

- The clavicle is the most commonly broken bone in the human body, accounting for up to 5–10% of all fractures seen in hospital emergency admissions [1].
- Incidence of clavicle fractures ranges worldwide from 24 fractures per 100,000 population per year to 71 per 100,000 and has been increasing over recent years [2, 3].
- Clavicle fractures are most common in younger patients, often associated with direct trauma to the clavicle, as in contact sports and motor vehicle accidents.
  - Males are affected more than females.
  - Prevalence declines progressively with age, although traumatic falls in elderly patients cause a bimodal peak in age distribution [4].

Associated Injuries

- Ipsilateral scapular fractures
- Scapulothoracic dissociation
- Rib fracture

D.C. Kim, MD • A. Pearsall, MD (✉)
Department of Orthopaedic Surgery, University of South Alabama Hospitals, Mobile, AL, USA
e-mail: apearsal@health.southalabama.edu

- Pneumothorax
- Neurovascular injury (brachial plexus, subclavian a.)
- Pediatric patients may have physeal injury (medial physis may not close till age 27 in some adults) [5]

Anatomy

- The clavicle is a long, dual curved bone that forms the only direct link between the axial and upper appendicular skeletons.
- It is the first bone in the body to be ossified (begins at 5–6-week gestation) and the last bone to complete ossification (the medial epiphysis completes ossification as late as 27 years of age) [6].
- Highly variable structure in terms of length, although many studies have shown the length to be around 140–150 mm [7]. Mean cortical thickness only around 2 mm at the midpoint [8].
- Two main articulations:
  - Medial: Sternoclavicular joint with the manubrium sternum
  - Lateral: Acromioclavicular joint with the acromion of the scapula
- Important muscles/ligaments that surround or attach to the clavicle:
  - Deltoid, trapezius, subclavius, pectoralis major, and sternocleidomastoid muscles
  - Coracoclavicular ligaments (vertical stability of AC joint)

© Springer International Publishing AG 2017   61
A.E.M. Eltorai et al. (eds.), *Orthopedic Surgery Clerkship*, DOI 10.1007/978-3-319-52567-9_12

- ∘ Trapezoid (3 cm from lateral end) and conoid (4.5 cm)
  - Acromioclavicular ligament (horizontal stability of AC joint)
- Deforming forces in fractures:
  - Medial fragments: Sternocleidomastoid pulls cranially and posteriorly.
  - Lateral fragments: Pulled inferiorly and rotated anteriorly by the weight of the shoulder.
  - Pull of trapezius, pectoralis, and latissimus on the shoulder also medially shortens the fractured clavicle.

Classification

- Allman classification [9]
  - Group 1 – middle third (80% of all clavicle fractures)
  - Group 2 – lateral third (15%)
  - Group 3 – medial third (5%)

Presentation and Exam

- Careful examination for asymmetry, ecchymosis, deformity, skin integrity, skin tenting, and swelling.
- Lacerations or skin tenting should alert the examiner to the possibility of an open or impending open fracture.
- Palpate for assessed for crepitus, instability, and location of tenderness.
- Complete neurovascular exam should be completed distal to the injured clavicle, including:
  - Palpation of distal radial and ulnar pulses; sensory examination of the radial, median, ulnar, and axillary nerve distributions; and a motor exam of the affected extremity.
- Evaluate for associated injuries including:
  - Scapular fractures, rib fractures, acromioclavicular or sternoclavicular injury or dislocation, pneumothorax, brachial plexus injury, and flail limb

Imaging

- Radiographs
  - AP view bilateral shoulders, 20 downward tilt (to determine amount of shortening) [10]
  - 45 cephalic tilt to assess superior/inferior displacement
- CT
  - May further elucidate nonunion, comminution, articular involvement, or physeal injury

Treatment

- Nonoperative
  - Sling vs figure of eight brace
    - ∘ No difference in healing times or alignment between the two, but figure of eight has higher rates of discomfort
  - Begin ROM at 2–4 weeks, strengthening at 10 weeks
  - Complications:
    - ∘ Nonunion
      - 15% of midshaft fractures [11, 12], up to 28% of lateral third [13]
    - ∘ Poor cosmesis
    - ∘ Decreased shoulder strength
- Operative
  - Indications
    - ∘ Group 3 with >2 cm shortening or 100% displacement
    - ∘ Unstable Group 2 fractures (Type IIA, IIB, V)
    - ∘ Group 3 fractures with posterior displacement
    - ∘ Open fracture
    - ∘ Skin tenting
    - ∘ Neurovascular involvement (brachial plexus, subclavian artery or vein)
    - ∘ Floating shoulder (clavicle and scapular neck fracture)
    - ∘ Symptomatic nonunion

– Open Reduction Internal fixation
  ○ Results in improved shoulder function, faster union, less pain, better cosmetic, and overall shoulder satisfaction [14]
  ○ Slightly higher complications (usually hardware related)
  ○ Compression plating
    – 3.5 mm recon plate, locking plate, or precontoured anatomic plates
    – Superior plating: Higher biomechanical stability but more symptomatic hardware/prominence [15]
    – Anteroinferior placement: Safer screw trajectory and decreased plate prominence [16]
  ○ Intramedullary screw/pin fixation
    – Dangerous complication: pin migration into thorax [17].
    – Studies show it may have faster time to union with less complication rates than plating [18].
    – Performed more in Europe.
    – Smaller skin incision.
    – Often must remove hardware.

References

1. Postacchini F, Gumina S, De Santis P, Albo F. Epidemiology of clavicle fractures. J Shoulder Elbow Surg. 2002;11(5):452–6.
2. Robinson CM. Fractures of the clavicle in the adult. Epidemiology and classification. J Bone Joint Surg Br. 1998;80(3):476–84.
3. Nordqvist A, Petersson C. The incidence of fractures of the clavicle. Clin Orthop Relat Res. 1994;300:127–32.
4. Khan LA, Bradnock TJ, Scott C, Robinson CM. Fractures of the clavicle. J Bone Joint Surg Am. 2009;91(2):447–60.
5. Schulz RMM, Mutze S, Schmidty S, Reisinger W, Schmeling A. Studies on the time frame for ossification of the medial epiphysis of the clavicle as revealed by ct scans. Int J Leg Med. 2005;119(3):142–5.
6. Garzon-Alvarado DA, Gutierrez ML, Calixto LF. A computational model of clavicle bone formation: a mechano-biochemical hypothesis. Bone. 2014;61:132–7.
7. Mathieu PA, Marcheix PS, Hummel V, Valleix D, Mabit C. Anatomical study of the clavicle: endomedullary morphology. Surg Radiol Anat. 2014;36(1):11–5.
8. Andermahr J, Jubel A, Elsner A, et al. Anatomy of the clavicle and the intramedullary nailing of midclavicular fractures. Clin Anat. 2007;20(1):48–56.
9. Allman Jr FL. Fractures and ligamentous injuries of the clavicle and its articulation. J Bone Joint Surg Am. 1967;49(4):774–84.
10. Axelrod DSO, Axelrod T, Whyne C, Lubovsky O. Fractures of the clavicle: Which x-ray projection provides the greatest accuracy in determining displacement of the fragments? J Orthop Trauma. 2013;3:1–3.
11. Hill JM, McGuire MH, Crosby LA. Closed treatment of displaced middle-third fractures of the clavicle gives poor results. J Bone Joint Surg Br. 1997;79(4):537–9.
12. McKee RC, Whelan DB, Schemitsch EH, McKee MD. Operative versus nonoperative care of displaced midshaft clavicular fractures: a meta-analysis of randomized clinical trials. J Bone Joint Surg Am. 2012;94(8):675–84.
13. van der Meijden OA, Gaskill TR, Millett PJ. Treatment of clavicle fractures: current concepts review. J Shoulder Elbow Surg. 2012;21(3):423–9.
14. Robinson CM, Goudie EB, Murray IR, et al. Open reduction and plate fixation versus nonoperative treatment for displaced midshaft clavicular fractures: a multicenter, randomized, controlled trial. J Bone Joint Surg Am. 2013;95(17):1576–84.
15. Partal G, Meyers KN, Sama N, et al. Superior versus anteroinferior plating of the clavicle revisited: a mechanical study. J Orthop Trauma. 2010;24(7):420–5.
16. Formaini N, Taylor BC, Backes J, Bramwell TJ. Superior versus anteroinferior plating of clavicle fractures. Orthopedics. 2013;36(7):e898–904.
17. Grassi FATM, D'Angelo F. Management of midclavicular fractures: comparison between nonoperative treatment and open intramedullary fixation in 80 patients. J Trauma. 2001;50(6):1096–100.
18. Houwert RM, Wijdicks FJ, Steins Bisschop C, Verleisdonk EJ, Kruyt M. Plate fixation versus intramedullary fixation for displaced mid-shaft clavicle fractures: a systematic review. Int Orthop. 2012;36(3):579–85.

Acromioclavicular Joint Separation

13

Stephen White and Albert Pearsall

Anatomy

- Diarthrodial synovial joint
- Contains round intra-articular meniscus composed of fibrocartilage
- Surrounding ligaments stabilize joint
  - Acromioclavicular (AC) ligaments
    ◦ Provide anterior/posterior stability to AC joint.
    ◦ Include superior, inferior, anterior, and posterior components.
    ◦ Superior ligament is strongest; posterior is second strongest [1].
  - Coracoclavicular (CC) ligaments
    ◦ Provide vertical stability to distal clavicle
    ◦ Include trapezoid and conoid
      - Trapezoid inserts 3 cm from distal clavicle.
      - Conoid inserts 4.5 cm from distal clavicle.

Mechanism

- Direct blow to the shoulder, e.g., falls directly onto shoulder.

S. White, MD • A. Pearsall, MD (✉)
Department of Orthopaedic Surgery, University of
South Alabama, Mobile, AL, USA
e-mail: apearsal@health.southalabama.edu

Presentation/Exam

- AC joint swelling and tenderness
- Possible visual and palpable step-off at AC joint depending on severity
- Pain with overhead movement or arm adduction
- Check for stability
  - If patient tolerates, anterior/posterior movement of distal clavicle checks AC ligaments
  - Downward pressure of distal clavicle tests vertical stability which can indicate CC ligament injury

Imaging

- Bilateral AC joint AP radiograph [2]
  - Useful for comparison to check for anatomic variants
- Zanca view [3]
  - Most accurate for AC joint pathology.
  - Tilt x-ray beam 10–15° toward cephalic direction.
  - Use only 50% of standard penetration strength.

Classification

- Rockwood classification [4] (Fig. 13.1)

© Springer International Publishing AG 2017
A.E.M. Eltorai et al. (eds.), *Orthopedic Surgery Clerkship*, DOI 10.1007/978-3-319-52567-9_13

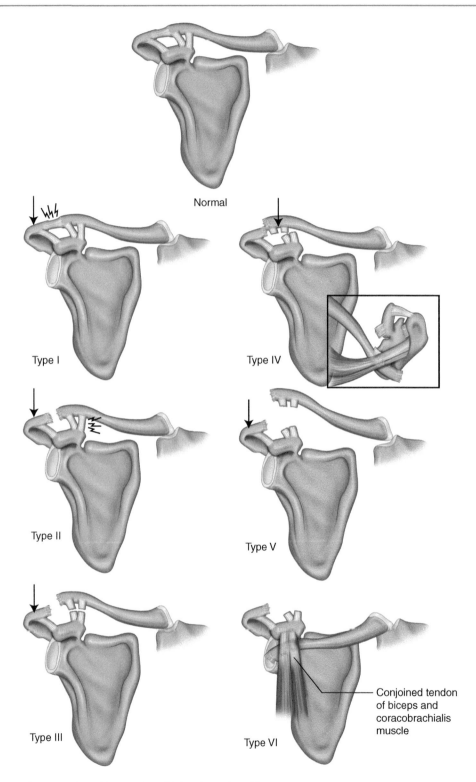

Fig. 13.1 Rockwood classification for AC joint dislocation [7]

- Type I
  - AC ligament sprained, CC ligaments intact.
  - Radiograph is normal.
- Type II
  - AC ligament torn, CC ligaments sprained.
  - Radiograph shows <25% vertical displacement compared to contralateral side.
  - Measured by coracoclavicular distance (CCD)
    - CCD: undersurface of clavicle to superior cortex of coracoid process
- Type III
  - AC and CC ligament torn.
  - Radiographs show 25–100% vertical displacement.
- Type IV
  - AC and CC ligaments torn.
  - Radiographs show distal clavicle posteriorly displaced.
    - Usually seen on axillary lateral x-ray
- Type V
  - AC and CC ligaments torn.
  - Radiograph shows >100% vertical displacement.
  - Associated deltotrapezial fascia rupture.
- Type VI
  - AC and CC ligaments torn.
  - Inferior displacement of distal clavicle.
  - Often distal clavicle is underneath acromion or coracoid.

Treatment

- Nonoperative
  - Indications
    - Types I, II [5], and most cases of Type III
  - Technique
    - Usually consists of sling for comfort for 2–3 weeks during acute phase of pain
    - Early range of motion

  - Should regain motion by 6 weeks
  - Most able to return to full activity by 3 months
- Operative
  - Indications
    - Types IV, V, and VI [6]
      - Some Type III injuries, e.g., high-performance athlete or laborer
  - Technique
    - Open reduction internal fixation
      - CC screw fixation
      - Hook plate
      - CC suture fixation
    - Ligament reconstruction
      - CC ligament reconstruction (modified Weaver-Dunn)
        - Distal clavicle excision
        - Transfer coracoacromial ligament to distal clavicle
          - Recreates CC ligament
      - Free tendon reconstruction of CC ligament
        - Sling created around coracoid and then free ends passed through tunnels drilled in clavicle
        - Recreates native strength of CC ligaments

Postoperative Protocol

- Shoulder immobilizer 6–8 weeks.
- Gentle ROM started at 2–6 weeks.
- Passive/active ROM begins at 6 weeks.
- Strength training at 12 weeks.

Complications

- Loss of reduction
- Excessive distal clavicle excision
- Osteolysis due to nonbiologic fixation material
- Coracoid fracture
- Infection

References

1. Debski RE, Parsons 4th IM, Woo SL, Fu FH. Effect of capsular injury on acromioclavicular joint mechanics. J Bone Joint Surg Am. 2001;83-A(9):1344–51. PMID:11568197
2. Bradley JP, Elkousy H. Decision making: operative versus nonoperative treatment of acromioclavicular joint injuries. Clin Sports Med. 2003;22:277–90.
3. Mazzocca AD, Arciero RA, Bicos J. Evaluation and treatment of acromioclavicular joint injuries. Am J Sports Med. 2007;35:316–29. PMID:17251175
4. Rockwood CA, Williams GR, Youg DC. Disorders of the acromioclavicular joint. In: Rockwood CA, Masten II FA, editors. The shoulder. Philadelphia: Saunders; 1998. p. 483–553.
5. Mouhsine E, Garofalo R, Crevoisier X, Farron A. Grade I and II acromioclavicular dislocations: results of conservative treatment. J Shoulder Elbow Surg. 2003;12(6):599–602.
6. Bradley JP, Elkousy H. Decision making: operative versus nonoperative treatment of acromioclavicular joint injuries. Clin Sports Med. 2003 Apr;22(2): 277–90.
7. Rockwood Jr CA, Young DC. Disorders of the acromioclavicular joint. In: Rockwood Jr CA, Matsen III FA, editors. The shoulder. 2nd ed. Philadelphia: WB Saunders; 1998. p. 495.

Glenohumeral Pathology

14

Matthew J. Brown and Geoffrey Bernas

Osteoarthritis (OA)

Epidemiology

- Primary: no known cause, may have genetic predisposition, and 5–10% of patients with full-thickness rotator cuff tears
- Secondary: post-traumatic, postsurgical, and instability

Pathoanatomy

- Primary OA: posterior glenoid wear with posterior humeral head subluxation in 45% of shoulders
- Inferior joint space narrowing and periarticular osteophytes

History

- Pain with activity, pain at night, decreased range of motion (ROM), and progressive loss of function

Physical Exam

- May see atrophy of entire shoulder girdle, crepitus, painful ROM, and limited ROM. Strength may be preserved.

Imaging

- X-ray (Fig. 14.1) /CT: joint space narrowing, subchondral sclerosis, osteophytes, posterior glenoid erosion, and humeral head subluxation

Classification: Walch Primary OA Glenoid Morphology

- Type A: Concentric wear with no subluxation (59%)
- Type B: A biconcave glenoid with posterior humeral subluxation and posterior glenoid wear (32%)
- Type C: Glenoid retroversion >25° with posterior humeral head subluxation (9%)

Inflammatory Arthritis

Epidemiology

- Rheumatoid arthritis most prevalent, with history >5 years. 91% have shoulder symptoms.

M.J. Brown, MD (✉) • G. Bernas, MD
Department of Orthopaedics, Jacobs School of
Medicine and Biomedical Sciences, Buffalo, NY, USA
e-mail: mjb9rc@mail.missouri.edu;
gabernas@buffalo.edu

© Springer International Publishing AG 2017
A.E.M. Eltorai et al. (eds.), *Orthopedic Surgery Clerkship*, DOI 10.1007/978-3-319-52567-9_14

Fig. 14.1 X-ray: glenohumeral joint osteoarthritis (Image courtesy of Dr. Thomas Duquin)

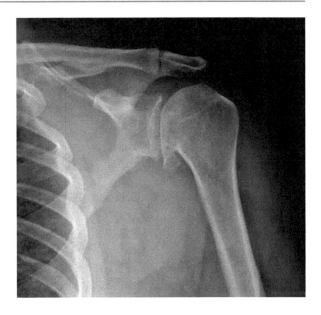

Pathoanatomy

- Cytokine release leads to erosive pannus formation, cartilage damage, and bony resorption.
- Seventy-five percent of patients can have rotator cuff tear pathology; 25–30% of surgical patients have full-thickness tears at surgery.

Physical Exam

- Early: warmth around joint and limited ROM
- Later: crepitus, weakness, and peri-scapular atrophy if there is rotator cuff involvement

Labs

- ESR, CRP, CBC, uric acid level, rheumatoid factor, serum complement, HLA-B27, and ANA.
- Aspirate: analyze for crystals, cell count, gram stain, and culture.

Imaging

- X-ray/CT:
  - Early: osteopenia, marginal erosions, and cyst formation
  - Later: concentric joint space narrowing and medial glenoid wear
- If there is large rotator cuff tear, superior migration humeral head with "acetabularization" of acromion can be seen.

Classification: Neer

- Dry: joint space narrowing, erosions with marginal osteophytes, and subchondral cysts
- Wet: marginal erosions with pointed contour of proximal humerus
- Resorptive: rapid bone and cartilage loss with medialization, possibly to the level of the coracoid

Osteonecrosis

Epidemiology

- Post-traumatic: four-part fracture dislocations with almost 100% rate, displaced four-part fractures 45%, and three-part 10–15%
- Atraumatic: systemic corticosteroid use as the most common cause (5–25%)
  - Also associated with alcohol abuse, sickle cell, systemic lupus erythematosus,

syringomyelia, Charcot arthropathy, and caisson disease

Pathoanatomy

- Main blood supply to humeral head from ascending branch of anterior circumflex humeral artery.
- Insufficient blood flow results in bony death and resorption with subchondral collapse.

History

- Early, pain and weakness; late, crepitus with loss of motion. Insidious symptom onset with history of risk factors

Physical Exam

- Early: unremarkable other than pain with ROM. Late: crepitus, weakness, and limited ROM

Imaging

- X-ray/CT/MRI: most common site of osteo-necrotic lesions is the superior-middle portion of humeral head. MRI preferred.

- If osteonecrosis of humeral head is confirmed, obtain X-ray of hips.

Classification: Cruess

- Stage 1: no changes on X-ray, only on MRI.
- Stage 2: wedge-shaped sclerotic area on X-ray, spherical head.
- Stage 3: "crescent sign" subchondral fracture on X-ray.
- Stage 4: "flattening" with collapse of joint surface collapse.
- Stage 5: arthritic change involves humeral head and glenoid.

Treatment

- Nonsurgical: NSAIDs, physical therapy, and intra-articular corticosteroids
- Surgical:
  - Osteoarthritis/inflammatory arthritis/osteo-necrosis (Fig. 14.1)
    ○ Total shoulder arthroplasty (TSA) (Fig. 14.2)
    ○ Hemiarthroplasty
  - Irreparable rotator cuff tear/rotator cuff arthropathy (Fig. 14.3)
    ○ Reverse total shoulder arthroplasty (rTSA) (Fig. 14.4)

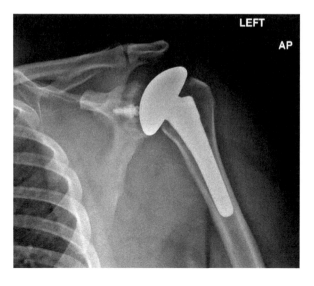

Fig. 14.2 X-ray: total shoulder arthroplasty for glenohumeral osteoarthritis (Image courtesy of Dr. Thomas Duquin)

Fig. 14.3 X-ray: rotator cuff arthropathy (Image courtesy of Dr. Thomas Duquin)

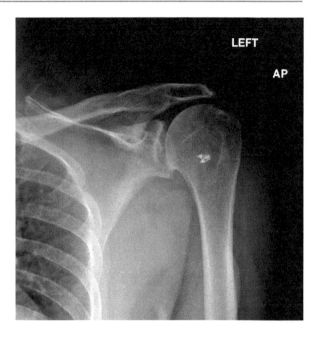

Fig. 14.4 X-ray: reverse total shoulder arthroplasty for rotator cuff arthropathy (Image courtesy of Dr. Thomas Duquin)

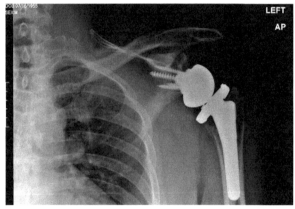

References

1. Boyer et al. AAOS Comprehensive orthopedic review 2. Chapter 81. Arthritis and arthroplasty of the shoulder. AAOS. p. 949–57.
2. Harreld KL, et al. Osteonecrosis of the humeral head. J Am Acad Orthop Surg. 2009;17:345–55.
3. Izquierdo R, et al. Treatment of glenohumeral osteoarthritis. J Am Acad Orthop Surg. 2010;18:375–82.
4. Miller, et al. Review of orthopedics. 6th ed. Adult reconstruction: section 20: shoulder arthroplasty. Elsevier. p. 417–21.
5. van der Zwaal P. The natural history of the rheumatoid shoulder: a prospective long-term follow-up study. Bone Joint J. 2014;96-B:1520–4.

Arthroplasty of the Shoulder

15

Matthew Binkley and Robert Ablove

Work-Up

- History
- Physical examination
- Plain XR to evaluate for signs of osteoarthritis (cysts, joint space narrowing, osteophytes, subchondral sclerosis) and fractures
- CT scan to evaluate for glenoid bone stock and version
- MRI is helpful to evaluate the integrity of the rotator cuff tendons and musculature

Types

- Hemiarthroplasty
- Total shoulder arthroplasty (TSA)
- Reverse total shoulder arthroplasty (RTSA)

M. Binkley, MD (✉)
Department of Orthopedic Surgery, Erie County Medical Centre, Buffalo, NY, USA
e-mail: w104mtb@gmail.com

R. Ablove, MD
Department of Orthopaedics, Jacobs School of Medicine and Biomedical Sciences, Buffalo, NY, USA

Hemiarthroplasty

- Prosthetic components
  - Humeral articular surface replaced with prosthetic implant
- Indications
  - Complex proximal humerus fractures (3 or 4 part fractures) with reconstructable rotator cuff
  - Osteoarthritis
    - Young, active patient (risk of accelerated glenoid component failure)
  - Avascular necrosis with little or no glenoid disease
    - May occur secondary to proximal humeral head fracture, corticosteroid use, radiation, alcohol abuse, endocrine disorders, sickle cell disease, and caisson disease [1]
  - Cuff tear arthropathy
    - Used with rotator cuff deficiency in young patients with functional elevation
- Contraindications
  - Infection
  - Coracoacromial ligament incompetence (risk of anterosuperior escape)
  - Neuropathic joint

A.E.M. Eltorai et al. (eds.), *Orthopedic Surgery Clerkship*, DOI 10.1007/978-3-319-52567-9_15

- Complications and treatment
  - Progressive glenoid arthrosis, treated with conversion to total shoulder arthroplasty
  - Tuberosity malunion/nonunion (when used for fracture), treated with revision open reduction internal fixation versus reverse total shoulder arthroplasty
  - Overstuffing the joint, which can lead to stiffness or accelerated arthrosis
  - Anterosuperior escape, which occurs secondary to rotator cuff and coracoacromial ligament insufficiency and treated with conversion to a reverse total shoulder arthroplasty

Total Shoulder Arthroplasty (TSA)
(Fig. 15.1)

- Prosthetic components
  - Replacement of the humeral articular surface
  - Glenoid articular surface replaced with complete or composite polyethylene glenoid component
- Indications
  - Glenohumeral arthritis with an intact rotator cuff and adequate glenoid bone stock and version
  - Primarily performed for glenohumeral osteoarthritis
  - Inflammatory arthritis
  - Osteonecrosis with glenoid involvement
  - Post-traumatic degenerative joint disease
- Contraindications
  - Rotator cuff arthropathy
  - Irreparable rotator cuff
  - Insufficient glenoid bone stock
  - Active infection
  - Brachial plexus palsy
- Complications
  - Glenoid loosening (most common cause of failure).
  - Humeral stem loosening.
  - Subscapularis failure.

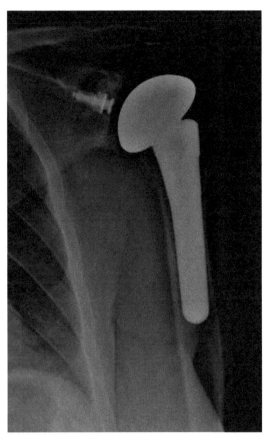

Fig. 15.1 Total shoulder arthroplasty with polyethylene glenoid component

  - Rotator cuff failure.
  - Neurologic injury. Axillary nerve palsy is most common.

Reverse Total Shoulder Arthroplasty (RTSA) (Fig. 15.2)

- Prosthetic components
  - Humeral articular surface replaced with a concave polyethylene socket.
  - Glenoid replaced with metal ball (glenosphere).
  - Center of rotation is moved and stabilized to enable deltoid to elevate shoulder.

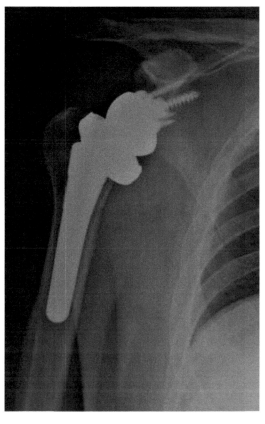

Fig. 15.2 Reverse shoulder arthroplasty

- Indications
  - Rotator cuff arthropathy
  - Pseudoparalysis
  - 4 Part proximal humerus fracture in elderly individual
  - Failed total shoulder/hemiarthroplasty secondary to rotator cuff failure, tuberosity nonunion, or superior escape
- Contraindications
  - Deltoid deficiency
  - Infection
  - Inadequate glenoid bone stock
- Complications
  - Dislocation
  - Infection
  - Neuropraxia and hematoma
  - Acromial stress fracture
  - Notching/glenoid failure

Reference

1. Neer C, Watson K, Stanton F. Recent experience in total shoulder replacement. J Bone Joint Surg Am. 1982;64:319–37.

Glenoid Superior Labrum Anterior to Posterior (SLAP) Lesions

16

Matthew Binkley and Marc Fineberg

Anatomy and Function

- The superior labrum is the attachment site for the long head of the biceps with the labrum anchored medial to the superior glenoid rim.
- Glenoid labrum is made of fibrous or fibrocartilaginous tissue.
- Vascular supply for the labrum is from the suprascapular artery, the circumflex scapular branch of the subscapular artery, and the posterior humeral circumflex artery [1]. Blood supply derives from capsule and periosteal vessels. No bloody supply received from bone.
- Three normal variants of the anterosuperior labrum have been identified and include a sublabral foramen, a cord-like middle glenohumeral ligament, and an absent anterosuperior labrum with a cord-like middle glenohumeral ligament (Buford complex). Erroneously fixing these normal variants can result in loss of external rotation.
- The superior labrum/biceps complex acts to improve joint stability and torsional rigidity of the abducted and externally rotated shoulder [2].

M. Binkley, MD (✉)
Department of Orthopedic Surgery, Erie County
Medical Centre, Buffalo, NY, USA
e-mail: w104mtb@gmail.com

M. Fineberg, MD
University of SUNY Buffalo, Buffalo, NY, USA

Pathology

- Mechanisms of injury include forced traction to the arm, direct compressive loads, and repetitive overhead throwing activities.
- May be associated with internal impingement, articular-sided partial rotator cuff tears, or glenohumeral instability.
- Throwers may develop increased external rotation and decreased internal rotation in the throwing position from anterior capsular laxity and posterior capsular contracture. These adaptive changes increase the shear forces on the superior labrum/biceps anchor and result in the peel back injury to the labrum.

Snyder's Original Classification [3]

- Type I lesions include superior labral fraying and degeneration with an intact biceps anchor. Generally asymptomatic in middle-aged individuals.
- Type II lesions exhibit a detached superior labrum/biceps anchor. Increased mobility and soft tissue failure between the superior labrum/biceps anchor and superior glenoid rim. Most common clinically significant lesions.
- Type III lesions have a bucket-handle tear of the central portion of the superior labrum with an intact biceps anchor. Mechanical symptoms due to labral displacement may be present.

A.E.M. Eltorai et al. (eds.), *Orthopedic Surgery Clerkship*, DOI 10.1007/978-3-319-52567-9_16

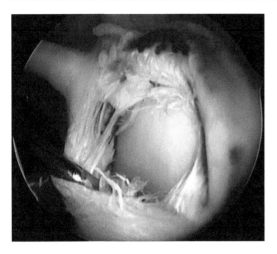

Fig. 16.1 Bucket-handle tear of the labrum with tear extending into the biceps anchor

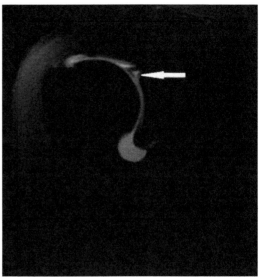

Fig. 16.2 Coronal MR image of SLAP tear

- Type IV lesions include a bucket-handle tear of the superior labrum with a split into the biceps. The biceps may remain partially anchored (Fig. 16.1).

Clinical Presentation

- Frequently coexisting pathology in the shoulder.
- Onset may be traumatic or insidious.
- Pain is commonly deep although often non-specific in location and pattern.
- Symptoms typically worse with overhead motions, lifting, or pushing activities.
- Pain often present with abduction, external rotation of the shoulder. Internal rotation deficits should be noted as this may predispose the patient to internal impingement and SLAP tears [4].
- Inspection of the patient's posterior rotator cuff musculature for atrophy and testing for external rotation weakness are important to identify underlying suprascapular nerve compression from a paralabral cyst.
- Range of motion and strength may be normal.
- Biceps-specific tests (Speed, Yergason) may recreate symptoms, and testing should be done for glenohumeral instability.
  - Dynamic shear testing, O'Brien's test, and apprehension test all may be helpful in determining the diagnosis.

Imaging

- X-rays are typically normal.
- MRI arthrogram is the preferred imaging technique, but accuracy is variable (Fig. 16.2).
  - Paralabral cysts may be present and are strongly associated with adjacent labral tears.
- Arthroscopy is the definitive method for diagnosis.

Management

- Nonsurgical management includes rotator cuff and periscapular strengthening and posterior capsular stretching. Intra-articular injections may play a role in the diagnosis and treatment of SLAP tears.
- Surgical management is considered after failure of nonsurgical management. Earlier intervention may be warranted in patients with evidence of suprascapular nerve compression secondary to spinoglenoid notch cysts. Nerve conduction and electromyographic studies may be helpful in evaluating nerve damage and following recovery after cyst decompression.

- Surgical treatment is performed arthroscopically with treatment depending on the type of lesion present:
  - Type I lesions are debrided.
  - Type II lesions are often reattached, but degenerative tears may not require repair. Proximal biceps tenotomy or tenodesis may be considered when significant degenerative changes extend into the proximal biceps tendon.
  - Type III lesions are usually treated with resection of the bucket-handle component.
  - Type IV lesions are most commonly treated with resection of the bucket-handle component with proximal biceps tenotomy or tenodesis. Whether to reattach the residual superior labrum remains questionable. Anatomic repair of acute type III or IV lesions may also be considered.
- Labral fixation with suture anchors is the most common method of repair with proper portal placement essential to facilitating the repair.
- Paralabral cyst formation should be addressed at time of surgery with cyst decompression and labral repair with expected cyst resolution [5].

- Associated shoulder pathology including rotator cuff tears and subacromial impingement can be addressed at time of surgery.
- Physical therapy with graduated range of motion and progressive strengthening in the months following surgery.

References

1. Anders J, Carson W, McLead W. Glenoid labrum tears related to the long head of the biceps. Am J Sports Med. 1985;13:337–41.
2. Rodosky M, Harner C, Fu F. The role of the long head of the biceps muscle and superior glenoid labrum in anterior stability of the shoulder. Am J Sports Med. 1994;22:121–30.
3. Mileski R, Snyder S. Superior labral lesions in the shoulder: pathoanatomy and surgical management. J Am Acad Orthop Surg. 1998;6:121–31.
4. Burkart S, Morgan C, Kibler W. The disabled throwing shoulder: spectrum of pathology Part I: pathoanatomy and biomechanics. Arthroscopy. 2003;19:404–20.
5. Youm T, Matthews P, El Attrache NS. Treatment of patients with spinoglenoid cysts associated with superior labral tears without cyst aspiration, debridement, or excision. Arthroscopy. 2006;22:548–52.

Biceps Brachii Tendon Injuries: Biceps Tendon Rupture

17

Edward Schleyer and Marc Fineberg

Proximal Biceps Tendon Injuries

Anatomy

- Short head originates from the coracoid process, long head originates from the supraglenoid tubercle and superior labrum.
- Intra-articular portion of the long head is extrasynovial, enveloped in a synovial sheath and curves approximately 30° as it enters the intertubercular groove.
- Branches of the musculocutaneous nerve provide innervation. The ascending branch of the anterior circumflex humeral artery provides main blood supply.

Proximal Biceps Rupture

- Often associated with rotator cuff disorders
- Most often treated with benign neglect
- May have residual cosmetic defect, loss of forearm supination and elbow flexion strength

Proximal Biceps Instability

- Long head tendon may be injured as it runs in the intertubercular groove by trauma, repetitive loads, and abrasive wear. The tendon may develop an inflammatory response with fraying and partial tearing.
- Structures responsible for restraint of the tendon may fail, causing subluxation or dislocation out of the groove.
- Instability is most frequently medial involving compromise of the medial biceps pulley which is a confluence of the supraspinatus, subscapularis, superior glenohumeral ligament, and rotator interval tissues.
- Complete medial dislocation involves tearing of the subscapularis tendon.

Presentation

- Onset may be traumatic or insidious.
- Popeye deformity with distal retraction of muscle belly confirms a proximal rupture.
- Elbow flexion weakness often not present with intact short head. May have pain elicited with throwing, lifting, or extending arm with daily activities.
- May have tenderness over intertubercular groove, positive Speed's and Yergason's tests.
- May have signs of rotator cuff involvement including empty can and lift off tests along with impingement signs such as Neer and Hawkins signs.

E. Schleyer, MD (✉) • M. Fineberg, MD
Department of Orthopaedics,
University at Buffalo, Buffalo, NY, USA
e-mail: Edward.schleyer@gmail.com

© Springer International Publishing AG 2017
A.E.M. Eltorai et al. (eds.), *Orthopedic Surgery Clerkship*, DOI 10.1007/978-3-319-52567-9_17

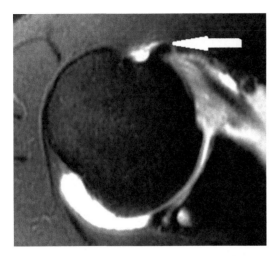

Fig. 17.1 Axial MRI arthrogram image showing medial subluxation of the proximal biceps tendon (*white arrow*) out of the intertubercular groove

Imaging

- X-ray is usually normal but may show subtle changes associated with any related rotator cuff disorders and impingement.
- MRI may show edema surrounding or within an inflamed tendon along with any tendon splitting, partial tearing, rupture, or static instability (Fig. 17.1).
- Ultrasound is gaining popularity and adds a dynamic assessment and needle guidance for injections but remains highly dependent on operator experience.

Management

- Nonoperative management
  - A course of rest, ice, NSAIDs, and activity modification is the initial treatment for most proximal biceps tendon injuries.
  - Intra-articular and bicipital groove intra-sheath steroid injections may be beneficial.
  - Formal rehabilitation may be indicated for strengthening and coordination of surrounding supportive structures.
- Operative management

  - For acute proximal biceps ruptures, a subpectoral tenodesis may be considered in young, active patients to restore length and strength and prevent the "Popeye" deformity.
  - Proximal biceps tenodesis
    ○ In addition to the repair of any associated subscapularis pathology, proximal biceps tenodesis is appropriate in the young, active individual with instability or partial tearing of the tendon.
    ○ Proximal biceps tendon is released at superior labrum and reattached to proximal humerus.
    ○ Tenodesis may be performed open or arthroscopically, with soft tissue fixation or osseous fixation, and either above (intra-articular), within ("in the groove"), or below (subpectoral) the bicipital groove.
    ○ Fixation techniques vary and include suture anchors, interference screws, flip buttons, and bone tunnels.
    ○ Advantages of tenodesis compared to tenotomy or benign neglect of acute ruptures include minimal loss of elbow flexion and supination strength, decreased risk of postoperative cramping, and improved cosmesis.
    ○ Disadvantages include a more complex operation, a period of postoperative immobilization, and lengthier rehabilitation.
  - Proximal biceps tenotomy
    ○ It is recommended in older, sedentary individuals.
    ○ Release the tendon just distal to its insertion on the glenoid and superior labrum.
    ○ Advantages include technically easier to perform and reliably improves pain from proximal tendon pathology, there is no need for postoperative immobilization, and rehabilitation is minimal.

  ° Disadvantages include increased risk of "Popeye" deformity, possible forearm supination and elbow flexion weakness, cramping, fatigue, and soreness.

Distal Biceps Injuries

Anatomy

- Distal biceps tendon inserts onto the bicipital tuberosity on the proximal portion of the radius.
- The distal portion of the short-head contribution inserts more distally and acts to flex the elbow, whereas the distal portion of the long-head contribution inserts further from the central axis of the forearm and provides a strong supination force.
- The lacertus fibrosus (bicipital aponeurosis) helps to stabilize the tendon as it originates at the myotendinous junction and blends with the fascia of the forearm.
- There is an approximate 2 cm hypovascular zone in the distal tendon between the proximal supply off the brachial artery and distal supply off the posterior interosseous recurrent artery.
- The lateral antebrachial cutaneous nerve runs superficially between the biceps and the brachialis.

Presentation

- Injuries most commonly occur in the dominant elbow of men in their 40s.
- Patients usually report feeling a painful pop with eccentric loading of biceps muscle.
- May report weakness with elbow flexion but more markedly with forearm supination.
- Typically present with positive hook test, biceps squeeze test, and varying levels of proximal retraction (Popeye deformity).

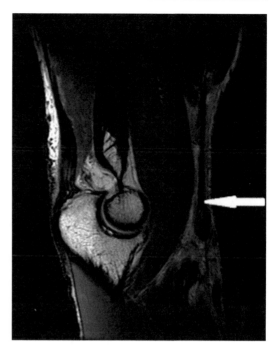

Fig. 17.2 Sagittal MR image showing complete tear of the distal biceps tendon (*white arrow*) with several cm of proximal migration

Imaging

- XR is usually normal but may show small bony avulsion and helps rule out associated injuries.
- MRI indicated if clinical diagnosis is unclear, concern for rare myotendinous junction tear, evaluation of chronic tear, suspected partial tear (Fig. 17.2).
  - FABS (flexion abducted supinated) position is helpful to delineate the tendon on MR (90° elbow flexion, 180° shoulder abduction, forearm supination).

Management

- Nonoperative management generally limited to sedentary patients who do not require elbow flexion or supination strength or those medically unfit for surgery.
- Operative intervention superior to nonoperative intervention in restoring supination strength,

flexion strength, upper extremity endurance, cosmesis, and functional outcome scores.

- Single-incision repair
  - Limited antecubital fossa incision using the interval between brachioradialis and pronator teres
  - Increased risk of lateral antebrachial cutaneous nerve injury and resultant paresthesia which are often temporary. Usually due to aggressive retraction
- Dual-incision repair
  - A second incision over the posterior lateral aspect of the elbow is used to identify the radial tuberosity and reattach the distal biceps.
  - Increased risk of heterotopic ossification and radioulnar synostosis.
- Several methods of fixation include sutures through drill holes, flip button, suture anchor, and interference screw techniques with some surgeons combining techniques for secondary fixation.
  - Flip button fixation has increased pullout strength.
  - Radial placement of interference screw pushes tendon into a more ulnar and anatomic position.

- Partial distal biceps tendon tears that fail nonoperative management with period of rest, NSAIDs, and physical therapy may be indicated for conversion into a complete tear with reinsertion into the radial tuberosity
- Postoperative protocols vary with physical therapy aimed at graduated return of range of motion and progressive strengthening.

References

1. Busconi BB, DeAngelis N, Guerrero PE. The proximal biceps tendon: tricks and pearls. Sports Med Arthrosc. 2008;16(3):187–94.
2. Friedman DJ, Dunn JC, Higgins LD, Warner JJ. Proximal biceps tendon: injuries and management. Sports Med Arthrosc. 2008;16(3):162–9.
3. Miyamoto RG, Elser F, Millett PJ. Distal biceps tendon injuries. J Bone Joint Surg Am. 2010;92(11): 2128–38.
4. Quach T, Jazayeri R, Sherman OH, Rosen JE. Distal biceps tendon injuries—current treatment options. Bull NYU Hosp Jt Dis. 2010;68(2):103–11.
5. Sutton KM, Dodds SD, Ahmad CS, Sethi PM. Surgical treatment of distal biceps rupture. J Am Acad Orthop Surg. 2010;18(3):139–48.

Humeral Shaft Fractures

18

Alan R. Koester

Anatomy

Multiple muscle attachments include:

- Pectoralis major, deltoid, coracobrachialis, latissimus dorsi, brachialis, triceps, and brachioradialis.
- The radial nerve runs in spiral groove posteriorly and courses laterally approximately 14 cm to lateral epicondyle.
- Median nerve is anterior-medial; ulnar nerve travels medially.

Fracture Classification

Describe by location: proximal, middle, or distal third

Characteristics

- Short oblique is more difficult to reduce.
- Long oblique heals faster due to increased surface area.
- Fractures with gaps may have muscle interposed (higher chance of nonunion).

Exam

AP and lateral x-rays may need a shoot though lateral to prevent rotation through fracture:

- CT or MRI generally not needed.
- Need a good neuro assessment (especially radial nerve).
- Check pulses.

AO Classification	1	2	3
A: Simple	Spiral A1	Oblique A2	Transverse A3
B: Wedge – butterfly fragment	Spiral B1	Bending wedge B2	Fragmented B3
C: Complex – multiple fragments	Spiral C1	Segmental C2	Irregular C3

A.R. Koester, MD
Department of Orthopaedic Surgery, Joan C. Edwards
School of Medicine, Marshall University,
Huntington, WV, USA
e-mail: koestera@marshall.edu

© Springer International Publishing AG 2017
A.E.M. Eltorai et al. (eds.), *Orthopedic Surgery Clerkship*, DOI 10.1007/978-3-319-52567-9_18

Treatment

- Nonoperative: most can be treated non-op:
  - Long arm splint
  - Coaptation splint
  - Hanging arm cast (may increase chance of nonunion)
  - Functional bracing (94.5% healing rate) varus angulation rarely exceeded $10°$
- Acceptable non-op alignment: $20°$ anterior, $30°$ varus, $15°$ malrotation, and 3 cm shortening
- Operative indications:
  - Absolute: open fractures, vascular injuries, floating elbow, and intra-articular extension
  - Relative: failure of closed treatment (compliance, body habitus), segmental fractures, bilateral fractures, brachial plexus injury, nerve injury after reduction, delayed union, nonunion, malunion, infection, pathologic fracture, neuromuscular disease, and skin compromise
- Operative techniques:
  - Plate fixation: usually 4.5 LCDCP plate, 96% healing rate, lowest complications, and best outcomes
  - IM Nail: equivalent healing rates, shoulder pain, and possible nerve injury with locking screws
  - External fixator: usually reserved for open fractures, burns, bone loss, or infected nonunions

Special Fractures

- Holstein–Lewis: spiral fracture at distal 1/3 of humerus (22% incidence of neuropraxia of radial nerve).

- Compression plating with bone graft is superior to IM nail with graft or plating without graft.

Radial Nerve Palsy

- 8–15% with closed fractures, and 85% improve with observation over 3–4 months.
- Explore if nerve goes out *after* reduction.
- Explore if no improvement with conservative treatment after 3–6 months (EMG fibrillation = bad prognosis).

Suggested Readings

1. Sarmiento A, Zagorski JB, Zych GA, Latta LL, Capps CA. Functional bracing for the treatment of fractures of the humeral diaphysis. J Bone Joint Surg Am. 2000;82:478–86.
2. Vander Griend R, Tomasin J, Ward EF. Open reduction and internal fixation of humeral shaft fractures. Results using AO plating techniques. J Bone Joint Surg Am. 1986;68(3):430–3.
3. Matuszewski PE, Kim TW, Gay AN, Mehta S. Acute operative management of humeral shaft fractures: analysis of the national trauma data bank. Orthopedics. 2015;38(6):e485–9. doi:10.3928/01477447-20150603-56.
4. Ekholm R, Adami J, Tidermark J, Hansson K, Törnkvist H, Ponzer S. Fractures of the shaft of the humerus. An epidemiological study of 401 fractures. J Bone Joint Surg Br. 2006;88(11):1469–73.
5. Weatherford B. Humeral shaft fractures. 2016. Orthobullets, 21. Retrieved from http://www.orthobullets.com/trauma/1016/humeral-shaft-fractures.
6. Wheeless textbook of orthopedics. Humeral shaft fractures. 2015. Retrieved from http://www.wheelesonline.com/ortho/humeral_shaft_fractures.
7. Schaller T. Miller review course 2015. Upper extremity fractures.
8. Denard Jr A, Richards JE, Obremskey WT, Tucker MC, Herzog GA. Outome of nonoperative vs operative treatment of humeral shaft freactue: a retrospective study of 213 patients. Orthopedics. 2010;33(8).

Tennis and Golfer's Elbow: Epicondylitis

19

John Matthews and Keely Boyle

Overview

- Epicondylitis is seen in laborers (carpenters, plumbers), athletes (pitchers, javelin throwers, golfers, bowlers, weight lifters, and racket sports), as well as individuals that play recreational sports [1].
- Frequently affects the dominant extremity.
- Lateral epicondylitis was originally described by Major in 1883 as lateral elbow pain in tennis players [2].
- Peak incidence of lateral epicondylitis is between 1% and 3%.
- In a 2015 study published by the Mayo Clinic, the prevalence of lateral epicondylitis was noted to have decreased over the past 15 years; however, the recurrence rate remained constant at 8.5% within 2 years [3].
- Medial epicondylitis occurs less frequently and may be associated with ulnar neuropathies or ulnar collateral ligament (UCL) injuries, which must be ruled out at time of diagnosis.

Anatomy and Pathophysiology

- Epicondilitis commonly occurs during repetitive elbow/wrist activity including pronation/supination with the elbow in near extension [4]. In throwing athletes, repeated valgus force on the elbow is absorbed by the flexor-pronator mass and ulnar collateral ligament [11].
- In lateral epicondylitis, the pathology arises at the origin of the ECRB but may extend to other tendons within the common extensor origin in up to 50% of cases [5, 6]. Common extensor tendons include extensor carpi radialis brevis (ECRB), extensor carpi radialis longus (ECRL), extensor digitorum communis (EDC), and extensor carpi ulnaris (ECU). Of note, the anconeus shares the same attachment site at ECRB.
- The medial epicondyle provides the origin for pronator teres and wrist/finger flexors: pronator teres (PT), flexor carpi radialis (FCR), palmaris longus (PL), flexor carpi ulnaris (FCU), and flexor digitorum superficialis (FDS).
- In medial epicondylitis, the PT and FCR are affected most [1, 7].
- Innervation of pronator-flexor mass: median nerve, except FCU which is ulnar nerve.

J. Matthews, MD • K. Boyle, MD (✉)
Department of Orthopaedics, SUNY University at Buffalo, Buffalo, NY, USA
e-mail: keelyboyle@gmail.com

© Springer International Publishing AG 2017
A.E.M. Eltorai et al. (eds.), *Orthopedic Surgery Clerkship*, DOI 10.1007/978-3-319-52567-9_19

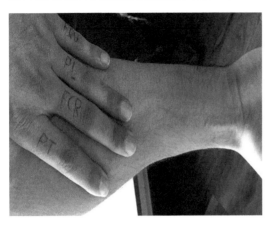

(Memorization technique: "pass, fail, pass, fail" referring to order **PT/FCR/PL/FCU**)

Pathology

- The definitive pathology of epicondylitis has been debated for years, however, current literature describes micro-trauma at the origin of the tendons secondary to repetitive wrist flexion/extension which predisposes to tears. This micro-trauma results in prostaglandin release resulting in local tenderness/swelling and may result in ulnar nerve irritation.
- Epicondylitis is a misnomer as histologic evaluation of the pathologic tissues reveals angio-fibroblastic hyperplasia, vascular proliferation and focal hyaline degeneration of the tendon without inflammatory cells [4, 8].
- It has also been postulated that the relative hypo-vascular regions of the lateral elbow may play a role in the pathogenesis of lateral epicondylitis [2, 7].

Presentation and Physical Exam Findings

Presentation [1, 7, 12]

- Most patients report pain over the affected epicondyle or just distally and may complain of subjective weakness in wrist flexion/extension.

- In lateral epicondylitis, pain worsens with gripping activities or wrist extension.
- In medial epicondylitis, elbow/wrist flexion results in worsening of symptoms. Patients may also complain of ulnar nerve symptoms.

Evaluation

History: As with every patient encounter, begin with obtaining relevant information:

- OPQRS ADA – onset of sx, position (location) of pain, quality (dull/ache/sharp), radiation of pain, severity, aggravating/alleviating factors, duration of sx, associated complaints
- Extremity involved
- New activities/hobbies
- Repetitive use of elbow/motions/gripping
- Important to ask about ulnar nerve symptoms: paresthesia in ulnar digits and grip strength

Physical Exam

- Begin every physical exam with simple inspection:
  - Obvious injury? Ecchymosis/erythema? Swelling?
- With medial epicondylitis, patient will be tender slightly anterior and distal to the medial epicondyle, over origins of PT and FCR.
- With lateral epicondylitis, patients will be tender over the lateral epicondyle or just distally:
  - Reminder: micro-trauma at insertion site leads to PG release pain.
  - Irritated tendons are painful with use especially when motion is resisted. With medial epicondylitis, resisted wrist flexion/forearm pronation exacerbates sx verse resisted wrist extension/supination in lateral epicondylitis.
- Always perform neuro (sensory/motor) and vascular exam of the involved extremity.
- Do not forget to examine the ulnar collateral ligament (compare with contralateral extremity).

Work-Up

- Differential:
  - MCL/LCL injury
  - Cubital tunnel syndrome
  - Occult fx
  - Cervical radiculopathy
  - Triceps tendinitis
  - Shingles
- Plain radiographs (AP/lateral of the elbow):
  - Need to rule out osseous defect. Usually unremarkable in epicondylitis
- MRI: rarely obtained since diagnosed clinically:
  - Demonstrates increased signal intensity at insertion sites of pronator teres/FCR in medial epicondylitis vs ECRB in lateral
  - May demonstrate ligamentous injury
- Consider EMG/NCS for ulnar nerve dysfunction

Treatment

*Medial epicondylitis is usually more difficult to treat than lateral.

Nonoperative (First Line) [7, 9, 12]

- As with most overuse injuries, common techniques to resolve symptoms included:
  - Rest/ice – allowing time for tissue irritation/micro-trauma to resolve.
  - Activity modification – prevent reoccurring micro-trauma to involved tendons.
  - Bracing – provide additional support/stability.
  - NSAIDs – decreases pain and PG production.
  - Corticosteroid injections – decreases pain/inflammation locally:
    ◦ Repeat injections should be avoided as steriods may increase risk of tendon rupture/tear.
  - Physical therapy – flexor-pronator stretching/strengthening.
  - Alternative options – botulinum toxin, blood (ABI or autologous blood injection), and blood products such as platelet-rich

plasma (PRP) are newer injection alternatives currently being offered to patients. There is no evidence to date showing that these treatments have better efficacy than the other nonoperative treatments described.

Operative Treatment

- Indications:
  - Repeated failure of conservative management in reliable/compliant patients with severe symptoms affecting ADL's for >6 months

Lateral Epicondylitis

- Debridement and release of the ECRB tendon with or without tendon repair [4]:
  - Open and arthroscopic techniques described.
  - 85–90% improvement in pain with most surgical techniques [4].
- Complications:
  - Iatrogenic LUCL injury leading to instability
  - Neurovascular injury
  - Persistent or recurrent pain

Medial Epicondylitis

- Debridement pathologic tissue and epicondyle decortication with reattachment of flexor muscle masses [7, 10, 12]:
  - If symptoms of cubital tunnel syndrome present, perform decompression or transposition of ulnar nerve concomitantly.
- Complications:
  - Similarities to most surgeries: infection/bleeding
  - Neuropathy:
    ◦ Injury to medial antebrachial cutaneous nerve
    ◦ Injury to ulnar nerve

Post-op

- Immobilization for short period of time.
- ROM exercises (to prevent elbow stiffness but avoid wrist flexion/extension in the immediate post-op period as causes strain at repair site).

- Strength training begins at 6 weeks post-op.
- Return to sports at 3–4 months:
  - Outcome: less successful than with lateral epicondylitis but good to excellent in >80% patients

References

1. Boyer MI. Comprehensive orthopedic review. American Academy of Orthopedic Surgeons. 2014;2: 988–90, 1027–8. ISBN: 978–0–89203-845-9.
2. Whaley AL, Baker CL. Lateral epicondylitis. Clin Sports Med. 2004;23(4):677–91. x
3. Sanders Jr TL, et al. The epidemiology and health care burden of tennis elbow: a population-based study. Am J Sports Mcd. 2015;43(5):1066–71.
4. Morrey BF. The elbow and it's disorders. 3rd ed. Philadelphia: W.B. Saunders Company. 2000; p. 543–48. 103, 105.
5. Gabel GT, Morrey BF. Tennis elbow. Instr Course Lect. 1998;47:165–72.
6. Greenbaum B, et al. Extensor carpi radialis brevis. An anatomical analysis of its origin. J Bone Joint Surg Br. 1999;81(5):926–9.
7. Jobe FW, Ciccotti MG. Lateral and medial epicondylitis of the elbow. J Am Acad Orthop Surg. 1994;2(1):1–8.
8. Bunata RE, Brown DS, Capelo R. Anatomic factors related to the cause of tennis elbow. J Bone Joint Surg Am. 2007;89(9):1955–63.
9. Calfee RP, et al. Management of lateral epicondylitis: current concepts. J Am Acad Orthop Surg. 2008; 16(1):19–29.
10. Gabel GT, Morrey BF. Operative treatment of medical epicondylitis: influence of concomitant ulnar neuropathy at the elbow. J Bone Joint Surg Am. 1995;77(7):1065–9.
11. Park MC, Ahmad CS. Dynamic contributions of the flexor-pronator mass to elbow valgus stability. J Bone Joint Surg Am. 2004;86-A(10):2269–74.
12. Amin NH, Kumar NS, Schickendantz MS. Medial epicondylitis: evaluation and management. J Am Acad Orthop Surg. 2015;23(6):348–55. Review. PubMed PMID: 26001427

Olecranon Bursitis

20

Joseph Fox and Thomas Duquin

Olecranon Bursitis: "Student's Elbow," "Baker's Elbow," and "Swellbow"

- Olecranon bursa is a small fluid-filled sac between the olecranon and skin.
- Normally not palpable.
- Bursitis = excess fluid within the bursa.

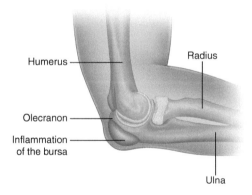

Reproduced and modified from The Body Almanac. (c) American Academy of Orthopaedic Surgeons, 2003

J. Fox, MD
Department of Orthopaedic Surgery, Jacobs School of Medicine, University at Buffalo, Buffalo, NY, USA

T. Duquin, MD (✉)
Department of Orthopaedics, State University of New York at Buffalo, Buffalo, NY, USA
e-mail: trduquin@buffalo.edu

Epidemiology/Demographics [1, 2]

- True incidence unknown
- Minimum annual incidence of 10/100,000
- 0.01–0.1% of overall hospital admissions
- More common in males 30–60

Etiology

- Post-traumatic, inflammatory (RA, CREST syndrome), or crystal-induced.
- Direct trauma to the olecranon most common.
- Prolonged pressure on a hard surface can cause gradual swelling of the bursa and is especially common in students or jobs involving crawling or leaning such as plumbers and HVAC technicians.
- Infection via a break in the skin, commonly from trauma or insect bites.
- *S. aureus* is the most common organism [2–4].
- Systemic conditions, such as gout and rheumatoid arthritis as well as long-term hemodialysis, have higher rates of olecranon bursitis.
- Bone spurs at olecranon may predispose to developing olecranon bursitis.

Signs/Symptoms

- Patients usually notice swelling first, followed by pain as the bursa stretches.

© Springer International Publishing AG 2017
A.E.M. Eltorai et al. (eds.), *Orthopedic Surgery Clerkship*, DOI 10.1007/978-3-319-52567-9_20

- The inflamed bursa is boggy and tender to palpation and, if large enough, may limit elbow flexion.
- Overlying erythema and warmth will develop if the bursa becomes infected but can be difficult to distinguish from aseptic bursitis.

Treatment

- No clear consensus on optimal treatment regimen for aseptic bursitis.
- Aseptic olecranon bursitis
  - Nonoperative "benign neglect."
  - Avoid direct pressure, NSAIDs, and padded compressive dressings.
  - Needle aspiration +/− corticosteroid injection (CSI) if not resolved.
  - Majority will resolve with time, but some may become chronic.
- Septic olecranon bursitis
  - Aspiration of bursal fluid for cell count, culture, crystals, and Gram stain.
  - Open or arthroscopic irrigation, debridement, and bursectomy if not resolved on IV antibiotics.
  - Bursa will regrow.

Complications

- Skin atrophy from corticosteroid injection
- Persistent drainage:
  - Aspirate obliquely to avoid creating direct sinus tract.
- Chronic bursitis

References

1. Baumbach SF, Lobo CM, Badyine I, Mutschler W, Kanz K-G. Prepatellar and olecranon bursitis: literature review and development of a treatment algorithm. Arch Orthop Trauma Surg. 2014;134(3):359–70.
2. Abzug JM, Chen NC, Jacoby SM. Septic olecranon bursitis. J Hand Surg. 2012;37(6):1252–3.
3. Garcia-Porrua C, Gonzalez-Gay MA, Ibanez D, Garcia-Pais MJ. The clinical spectrum of severe septic bursitis in northwestern Spain: a 10 year study. J Rheumatol. 1999;26(3):663–7.
4. Laupland KB, Davies HD. Olecranon septic bursitis managed in an ambulatory setting. The calgary home parenteral therapy program study group. Clin Invest Med. 2001;24(4):171–8.

Distal Humeral Fractures

21

Joseph Fox and Thomas Duquin

Anatomy

- Distal humerus can be conceptualized as a triangle, composed of medial and lateral columns connected by articular surface of capitellum and trochlea.
- Condyle = articular, epicondyle = non-articular:
  - Medial epicondyle: ulnar collateral ligament attachment
  - Lateral epicondyle: extensor-supinator mass attachment
- Articular surface is in 5–7° of internal rotation, projects anteriorly 30–40° and has a valgus "carrying angle" of 5–8° [1].

Epidemiology/Demographics

- Bimodal incidence – young (high energy) and old (low energy):
  - Peak in 12–19-year-old males and 80+-year-old females

- Rare fracture overall (<7% of all fractures, 30% of all elbow fractures) [2]

Signs/Symptoms/Exam

- Swelling and ecchymosis at the elbow.
- Detailed neurovascular exam critical as the fracture fragments may injure the brachial artery, median nerve, ulnar nerve and radial nerve.
- Range of motion may reveal instability and crepitus but should not be tested with a known fracture.
- AP, lateral and oblique as well as traction view x-rays delineate fracture fragments, CT scan useful in preoperative planning.

Intercondylar Fractures

- Most common [1]

Classification

- Riseborough and Radin: [3]
  - I: Nondisplaced
  - II: Displaced, but no rotation between condyles
  - III: Displaced, rotation between condyles
  - IV: Severe articular comminution

J. Fox, MD • T. Duquin, MD (✉)
Department of Orthopaedics, State University
of New York at Buffalo, Buffalo, NY, USA
e-mail: joseph.fox100@gmail.com; trduquin@buffalo.edu

© Springer International Publishing AG 2017
A.E.M. Eltorai et al. (eds.), *Orthopedic Surgery Clerkship*, DOI 10.1007/978-3-319-52567-9_21

- AO/OTA Classifications:
  - A: Extra-articular
  - B: Partial articular
  - C: Complete articular

Treatment [1, 2]

- Nonoperative:
  - "Bag of bones" treatment reserved only for low-demand patients unfit for surgery
- Open reduction internal fixation:
  - Approaches:
    ° Triceps sparing (paratricipital or Alonso-Llames):
      - Bryan-Morrey modification: triceps reflection subperiosteally with anconeus radially
    ° Triceps splitting (Campbell):
      - Radial nerve limits exposure to distal 15 cm of humerus.
    ° Transolecranon:
      - Chevron osteotomy with apex distal
      - Pre-drill and pre-tap
  - Reduction of articular surface paramount:
    ° Provisional fixation with K-wires or minifragment screws
  - Fixation – locked plating:
    ° 90–90 plating, medial and posterior
    ° Parallel plating (180 Plating), medial and lateral:
      - Biomechanically superior
- Total elbow replacement:
  - Indicated for comminuted fractures in elderly, osteoporotic, low-demand patients or patients with inflammatory arthritis (i.e. RA)
  - Postoperative lifting restriction: <5 lbs for life

Capitellum Fractures

Classification

- Type 1: complete fracture, does not extend to trochlea (Hahn-Steinthal fragment)

- Type 2: osteochondral fragment (Kocher-Lorenz fragment)
- Type 3: severely comminuted (Morrey)
- Type 4: extension into trochlea (McKee)

Treatment

- Nonoperative:
  - Non-displaced fractures
- Operative:
  - Approach (in isolated capitellum fractures):
    ° Lateral extensile via posterior or lateral incision.
    ° Elevation of wrist extensor and capsule proximally. Distal interval is the Kocher (ECU/anconeus) interval.
- Fixation:
  - Headless screws in anterior to posterior direction or posterior to anterior screws

Complications

- Stiffness: key to motion preservation is early motion postoperatively.
- Nonunion: rates vary from 2 to 10% and may require revision fixation, bone grafting, contracture release and ulnar nerve adhesiolysis.
- Ulnar nerve palsy: up to 15% in transcondylar fractures after ORIF.
- Failure of fixation.
- Infection: low rate, but suspect if persistent drainage or nonunion.
- Heterotopic ossification:
  - Risk factors include head injury, delayed ORIF, use of bone graft, extended immobilization and method of fixation.
  - Excision of HO should be considered in the first 6–9 months following injury to avoid joint degeneration.
  - After excision, HO prophylaxis with indomethacin or low-dose radiation in conjunction with continuous passive motion (CPM).
  - Routine prophylaxis not recommended.

References

1. Miller AN. Intra-articular distal humerus fractures. Orthop Clin N Am. 2013;44(1):35–45.

2. Mighell MA. Distal humerus fractures: open reduction internal fixation. Hand Clin. 2015;31(4):591.

3. Riseborough EJ, Radin EL. Intercondylar T fractures of the humerus in the adult. J Bone Joint Surg Am. 1969;51(1):130–41.

Olecranon Fracture

22

Timothy P. Bryan and Thomas Duquin

Overview

- Incidence of isolated olecranon fractures in adults is 1.15 per 10,00 person-years [1]
- Triceps tendon avulsion off the olecranon may present with similar complaints

Anatomy

- Coronoid process and the olecranon form the greater sigmoid notch
- Greater sigmoid notch articulates with the trochlea of the distal humerus
- Triceps tendon inserts on the olecranon

Classification

Colton Classification [2]

- Type I – nondisplaced fracture:
  - Stable fracture with less than 2 mm of displacement with elbow flexed to 90° or extension against gravity
  - Preservation of elbow extension against gravity
- Type II – displaced fracture, subdivided into avulsion, oblique, transverse, comminuted, or fracture dislocation

The Mayo Classification [3]

- Type I – undisplaced fracture, subdivided into noncomminuted or comminuted
- Type II – displaced, stable fracture (Fig. 22.1), subdivided into noncomminuted or comminuted
- Type III – unstable fracture dislocations (Fig. 22.2), subdivided into noncomminuted or comminuted

T.P. Bryan, MD (✉) • T. Duquin, MD
Department of Orthopaedics, State University of
New York at Buffalo, Buffalo, NY, USA
e-mail: tpbryan1@gmail.com

© Springer International Publishing AG 2017
A.E.M. Eltorai et al. (eds.), *Orthopedic Surgery Clerkship*, DOI 10.1007/978-3-319-52567-9_22

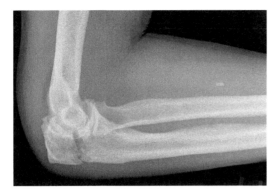

Fig. 22.1 Mayo type II displaced-stable fracture of the olecranon

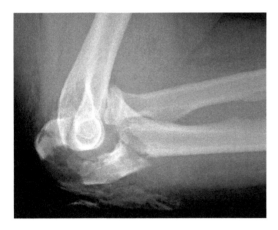

Fig. 22.2 Mayo type III fracture dislocation of the olecranon

Evaluation

History

- Often low-energy trauma such as a fall, direct blow, or forced hyperextension [3]
- Commonly presents with pain and swelling over the posterior aspect of the elbow

Physical Examination

- Inspection often reveals ecchymosis, oedema, or open wounds over the posterior aspect of the elbow
- Palpation of the olecranon is often possible because of the subcutaneous nature of the ulna and may elicit pain or crepitus

- Absence of elbow extension may be present
- Neurovascular examination with particular attention evaluating ulnar nerve

Imaging

- Typically orthogonal plain radiographs are sufficient for diagnosis and determining treatment.
- Lateral radiograph will clearly demonstrate displacement, comminution, and dislocation.
- Radiocapitellar view can be helpful to evaluate for radial head fractures.
- Rarely is a CT scan indicated in the management of isolated olecranon fractures.

Treatment

Nonoperative

- Reserved for nondisplaced fractures with intact extensor mechanisms
- Some select elderly patients with displaced olecranon fractures may be treated nonoperatively with acceptable functional outcome [4]
- Immobilization long arm cast or splint at 90° of flexion and neutral rotation for 3–4 weeks
- Gentle active motion may be begun with gradual increase in activities while avoiding active resisted elbow extension or weight bearing for 6–8 weeks

Operative

- Fracture fragment excision and advancement of the triceps tendon
  - Indicated in comminuted fractures in older patients with limited functional demands and avulsion type extra-articular fractures
  - Resection should be limited to less than 30–50% of the olecranon [3]
- Open reduction and internal fixation with tension band (Fig. 22.3)

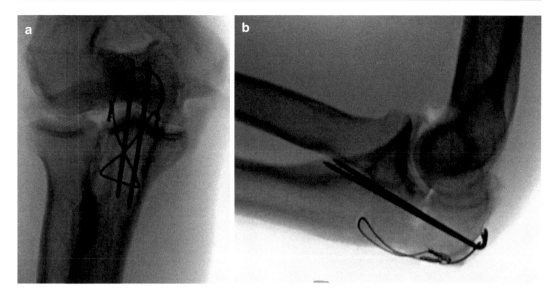

Fig. 22.3 Open reduction and internal fixation of olecranon with tension band construct (**a**) AP and (**b**) lateral

- Indicated for transverse fractures proximal to the coronoid without comminution [3]
- Comminution is a contraindication to a tension band construct
- Approach subcutaneous proximal ulna through a posterior midline incision
- Two 1.6 mm or 2 mm K-wires and 18-guage wire
- Penetration of the anterior cortex of the ulna associated with stronger fixation but over-penetration associated with injury to the anterior interosseous nerve [5]
• Open reduction and internal fixation with dorsal plate and screw fixation (Fig. 22.4)
- Indicated for comminuted fractures or fracture-dislocations of the olecranon
- Precontoured plates are available

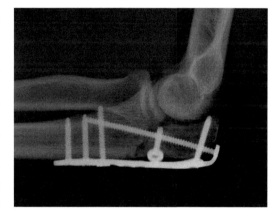

Fig. 22.4 Open reduction and internal fixation of olecranon with dorsal plate and screw construct

Complications

• Hardware prominence
• Elbow stiffness
• Nonunion
• Post-traumatic arthrosis
• Ulnar neuropathy
• Heterotopic ossification

References

1. Karlsson MK, et al. Fractures of the olecranon: a 15-to 25-year followup of 73 patients. Clin Orthop Relat Res. 2002;403:205–12.
2. Colton CL. Fractures of the olecranon in adults: classification and management. Injury. 1974;5:121–9.
3. Adams JE, Steinmann SP. Fractures of the olecranon. In: Morrey BF, editor. The elbow and its disorders. 4th ed. Philadelphia: Saunders Elsevier; 2009. p. 389–400.
4. Duckworth AD, et al. Nonoperative management of displaced fractures in low-demand elderly patients. J Bone Joint Surg Am. 2014;96:67–72.
5. Parker JR, et al. Anterior interosseus nerve injury following tension band wiring of the olecranon. Injury. 2005;36:1252–3.

Radial Head Fracture

23

Timothy P. Bryan and Thomas Duquin

Overview

- Occur in approximately 20% of elbow trauma [1]
- Associated elbow injuries [1]
  - Terrible triad – elbow dislocation, radial head fracture, and coronoid fracture
  - Carpal fractures
  - Essex-Lopresti – distal radioulnar joint and interosseous membrane disruption
  - Monteggia fracture-dislocation
  - Capitellar fracture
  - Associated ligamentous injury about the elbow

Anatomy

- Inherent stability of the elbow conferred with bony articulation.
- Radial head serves as an important valgus stabilizer of the elbow.
- Radial head has two articulations, the radio-capitellar joint and proximal radioulnar joint.

- Medial collateral ligamentous complex and the lateral collateral ligamentous complex are important stabilizers to the elbow.
- Musculotendinous structures, fascia, and capsule also contribute to stability.

Classification

- Mason classification [2] – has been subsequently modified by many authors
  - Type I – nondisplaced fracture
  - Type II – displaced partial articular fracture of radial head (Fig. 23.1)
  - Type III – comminuted and displaced fracture of the radial head (Fig. 23.2)

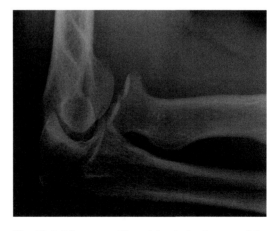

Fig. 23.1 Mason type II partial articular fracture of the radial head

T.P. Bryan, MD (✉) • T. Duquin, MD
Department of Orthopaedics,
State University of New York at Buffalo,
Buffalo, NY, USA
e-mail: tpbryan1@gmail.com

© Springer International Publishing AG 2017
A.E.M. Eltorai et al. (eds.), *Orthopedic Surgery Clerkship*, DOI 10.1007/978-3-319-52567-9_23

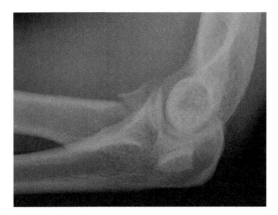

Fig. 23.2 Mason type III comminuted and displaced fracture of the radial head

Evaluation

History

- Vast majority of radial head fractures result from a fall onto an outstretched hand [1].

Physical Examination

- Inspection for ecchymosis, edema, or open wounds over the lateral aspect of the elbow
- Palpation over the radial head may elicit pain
- Limitation of elbow range of motion secondary to pain or mechanical block may be present
- Neurovascular examination
- Radiocapitellar joint aspiration of hematoma and injection of local anesthetic can be helpful to determine if there is a mechanical block to range of motion [1].

Imaging

- Typically orthogonal plain radiographs are sufficient for diagnosis and determining treatment.
- On the lateral radiograph, elevation of the anterior or posterior fat pad from intra-articular hemarthrosis may be the only indication of a nondisplaced radial head fracture [1].

- Radiocapitellar view can be helpful to evaluate for radial head fractures.
- CT scan can be useful to evaluate associated injuries.

Treatment

Nonoperative

- Indicated in isolated nondisplaced to minimally displaced isolated radial head fractures with no mechanical block to range of motion
- Fractures involving less than one third of the articular surface may be treated with early mobilization [1].
- Fractures involving more than one third of the articular surface should be treated with a splint or sling for 2 weeks followed by progressive functional activity [1].

Operative

- Resection of the radial head
  - Indicated in isolated comminuted radial head fractures [2]
  - Remains somewhat controversial and unresolved [3]
  - Contraindicated in complex injury patterns associated with elbow instability
  - Show to alter kinematics and increase laxity in elbows with intact ligamentous structures [4]
- Open reduction and internal fixation (Fig. 23.3)
  - Indicated for minimally comminuted fractures with three or fewer articular fragments [5]
    Approaches
    ° Kocher approach [2]
      - Interval between the anconeus and the extensor carpi ulnaris
      - Provides greater protection of the posterior interosseous nerve than Kaplan approach
      - Lateral collateral ligament complex is at risk
    ° Kaplan approach [2]
      - Interval between the extensor carpi radialis brevis and extensor digitorum communis

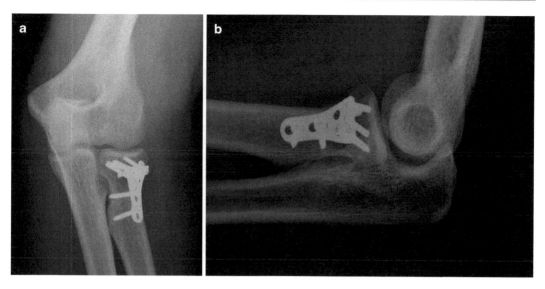

Fig. 23.3   Open reduction and internal fixation of the radial head (**a**) AP and (**b**) lateral

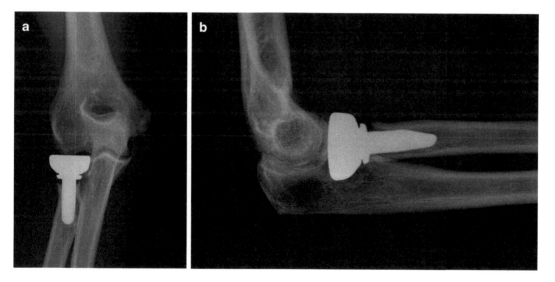

Fig. 23.4   Radial head arthroplasty (**a**) and (**b**) lateral

- Posterior interosseous nerve is at risk
○ Common extensor tendon splitting approach [2]
  - Incise the extensor digitorum communis
  - The radial collateral and annular ligaments are divided longitudinally at the midportion of the radial head
○ Internal Fixation
  - Small screws used for internal fixation should be countersunk to avoid impinging at the proximal radioulnar joint.

- Small plates are available for comminuted head or neck fractures.
- The safe area for placement of implants on the nonarticular surface of the radial head can be defined as the area of the proximal radius corresponding to the region between Lister's tubercle and the radial styloid of the distal radius [6].
- Radial head arthroplasty (Fig. 23.4)
○ Indicated in comminuted, irreparable fractures of the radial head [2]

- ° Cemented or press fit stems are available
- ° Caution should be used to prevent over-stuffing the radiocapitellar joint [7]

Complications

- Elbow stiffness
- Heterotopic ossification
- Posterior interosseous nerve – iatrogenic injury during exposure, may be minimized by maintain the forearm in pronated position [8]
- Avascular necrosis
- Nonunion

References

1. McKee MD, Jupiter JB. Trauma to the adult elbow and fractures of the distal humerus part I trauma to the adult elbow. In: Browner BD, et al., editors. Skeletal trauma. 4th ed. Philadelphia: Saunders Elsevier; 2009. p. 1503–41.
2. Ring D. Elbow fractures and dislocations. In: Bucholz RW, Heckman JD, et al., editors. Rockwood and green's fractures in adults. 7th ed. Philadelphia: Lippincott Williams & Wilkins; 2010. p. 905–44.
3. Van Riet RP, et al. Radial head fracture. In: Morrey BF, editor. The elbow and its disorders. 4th ed. Philadelphia: Saunders Elsevier; 2009. p. 359–88.
4. Beingessner DM, et al. The effect of radial head excision and arthroplasty on elbow kinematics and stability. J Bone Joint Surg Am. 2004;86:1730–9.
5. Ring D, et al. Open reduction and internal fixation of fractures of the radial head. J Bone Joint Surg Am. 2002;84:1811–5.
6. Caputo AE, et al. The nonarticulating portion of the radial head: anatomic and clinical correlations for internal fixation. J Hand Surg [Am]. 1998;23:1082–90.
7. Doornberg JN, et al. Reference points for radial head prosthesis size. J Hand Surg Am. 2006;31:53–7.
8. Diliberti T, et al. Anatomical considerations regarding the posterior interosseous nerve during posterolateral approaches to the proximal part of the radius. J Bone Joint Surg Am. 2000;82:809–13.

Coronoid Fractures

24

Corey T. Clyde

Introduction

Overview

- Pathognomonic for episode of traumatic elbow instability
- Commonly associated with other injuries including radial head fracture, olecranon fracture, and injury to LCL or MCL
  - i.e., terrible triad injury: coronoid fracture, radial head fracture, and elbow dislocation [10]

Epidemiology

- Identified in 2–15% of elbow injuries [2]

Anatomy

- Coronoid process of proximal ulna articulates with coronoid fossa of distal humerus
- Anterior buttress and primary osseous stabilizer that resists posterior elbow subluxation or dislocation [4, 8]

C.T. Clyde, MD
Department of Orthopaedic Surgery, University at Buffalo, Buffalo, NY, USA
e-mail: corey.t.clyde@gmail.com

- Coronoid tip is an intra-articular structure [1]
- Insertion point for medial ulnar collateral ligament, anterior joint capsule, and brachialis [1]

Mechanism

- Tip fracture: shearing force injury, not avulsion injury since nothing inserts on coronoid tip

Pathoanatomy

- Fractured when distal humerus is driven against coronoid typically during episode of posterior subluxation with varus stress
- Anteromedial facet fractures considered a distinct type of coronoid fracture caused by a varus posteromedial rotational force [3]

Presentation

History [7]

- Patient often reports history of dislocation
- Injury occurs with outstretched arm and rotational forces
- Diffuse elbow pain with possible radiation to the forearm and wrist
- Arm held in flexed position

© Springer International Publishing AG 2017
A.E.M. Eltorai et al. (eds.), *Orthopedic Surgery Clerkship*, DOI 10.1007/978-3-319-52567-9_24

Physical Exam [6]

- Visual inspection for open injuries, abrasions, and effusion
- Perform thorough upper extremity motor, sensory, and vascular exam
- Test range of motion: flexion, extension, supination, and pronation
- Test elbow for stability: varus and valgus stress and posterolateral rotatory drawer/pivot shift

Imaging

X-Ray

- Standard AP and lateral radiographs
- Visualize coronoid look for other concomitant osseous injuries

CT

- May be useful for high-grade coronoid fractures and severe comminution
- May assist with surgical planning in some instances

Classification

Reagan and Morrey Classification: Based on Fragment Size [9]

- Type I: Tip fracture
- Type II: Involves less than 50% of coronoid
- Type III: Involves greater than 50% coronoid

Alternate Classification System: O'Driscoll Classification

- Subdivides fractures according to location on coronoid
  - Tip, anteromedial facet, and base

Current Concepts in Treatment

- Operative decision-making based on joint stability and associated injuries including other fractures and ligamentous pathology

Nonoperative Treatment

- Brief period of immobilization (<7–10 days) for pain control with elbow maintained in 90° of flexion with neutral rotation [11]
- Duration of immobilization depends on degree of instability
- Following immobilization start range of motion exercises, but avoid weight bearing or active use for 6 weeks or until elbow clinically stable on examination [11]

Operative Treatment

- Most common treatment course due to high prevalence of chronic instability with untreated coronoid fractures
- Type I and type II coronoid fractures may be repaired with suture fixation [5]
- Large type II and type III coronoid fractures may benefit from retrograde cannulated screws or small buttress plate fixation [5]
- External fixation may be used for grossly unstable injuries or for delay until other definitive fixations
- Medial, lateral, and posterior approaches possible to gain access to coronoid [5]

Potential Complications

- Reoperation rates are high due to [6]:
  - Elbow stiffness
  - Recurrent elbow instability
  - Posttraumatic arthritis
  - Heterotopic ossification

References

1. Ahlove RH, Moy OJ, Howard C, Peimer CA, S'Doia S. Ulnar coronoid process anatomy: possible implications for elbow instability. Clin Orthop Relat Res. 2006;449:259–61.
2. Boyer MI. American academy of orthopedic surgeons: comprehensive orthopedic review 2. 2014;1: 317–28.
3. Doornberg JN, Ring DC. Fracture of the anteromedial facet of the coronoid process. J Bone Joint Surg Am. 2006;88(10):2216–24.
4. Jeon IH, et al. The contribution of the coronoid and radial head to the stability of the elbow. J Bone Joint Surg Br. 2012;94(1):86–92.
5. McKee MD, Pugh DM, Wild LM, Schemitsch EH, King GJ. Standard surgical protocol to treat elbow dislocation with radial head and coronoid fractures: Surgical technique. J Bone Joint Surg Am. 2001;83(8):1201–11.
6. Miller MD, Thompson SR, Hart JA. Review of orthopedics. 6th ed. Philadelphia: Elsevier Saunders; 2012. p. 576–81.
7. Morrey BF. The elbow and its disorders. 3rd ed. Philadelphia: W.B. Saunders Company; 2000.
8. Morrey BF, An KN. Stability of the elbow: osseous constraints. J Shoulder Elbow Surg. 2005;14(1 Suppl S):174S–8S.
9. Regan W, Morrey B. Fractures of the coronoid process of the ulna. J Bone Joint Surg Am. 1989;71:1348–54.
10. Ring D, Jupiter JB, Zilberfarb J. Posterior dislocation of the elbow with fractures of the radial head and coronoid. J Bone Joint Surg Am. 2002;84-A:547–51.
11. Ross G, et al. Treatment of simple elbow dislocation using an immediate motion protocol. Am J Sports Med. 1999;27(3):308–11.

Elbow Dislocation

25

John R. Matthews and Keely Boyle

Overview

- The incidence of elbow dislocations is 5.21 per 100,000 person-years [1].
- Posterolateral dislocations are the most common type.
- Adolescent males involved in sports (football) are at highest risk followed by females involved in gymnastics and skating.

Anatomy and Pathophysiology

- The greater sigmoid notch (formed by the coronoid process and olecranon) articulates with the trochlea of the distal humerus.
- Normal elbow range of motion (ROM): 0–150° of flexion, 85° supination, and 80° pronation.
- Functional ROM: 100° arc (30–130° flexion) and 50° of supination/pronation.

Stabilizers of the Elbow

- The elbow is one of the most stable joints in the body with three articulations (ulnohumeral, radiocapitellar, and radioulnar).

Osseous Stabilizers

- The ulnohumeral joint is the primary stabilizer to the elbow. The humeral trochlea and olecranon sigmoid notch function as a buttress acting as the main stabilizer during varus/valgus stress and rotational movements [2–4].
- The coronoid process of the ulna provides anterior support along with resistance to varus stress.

Soft Tissue Stabilizers

- The medial collateral ligament (MCL), especially the anterior bundle, is also a primary stabilizer of the elbow joint and provides over 50% of valgus stability [5, 6].
- The lateral collateral ligament (LCL) complex provides stability to varus and posterolateral rotatory stress.
  - The primary component of the LCL is the lateral ulnar collateral ligament (LUCL) [7].
- The annular ligament encompasses and secures the radial head to allow for rotational movements of the forearm.
- Dynamic stabilizers of the elbow joint include the muscles that cross the joint: anconeus, brachialis, forearm flexors/extensors, and triceps.

J.R. Matthews, MD • K. Boyle, MD (✉)
Department of Orthopaedic Surgery, SUNY University of Buffalo, Buffalo, NY, USA
e-mail: keelyboyle@gmail.com

© Springer International Publishing AG 2017
A.E.M. Eltorai et al. (eds.), *Orthopedic Surgery Clerkship*, DOI 10.1007/978-3-319-52567-9_25

Mechanism of Injury

- Fall onto an outstretched arm with resultant axial loading, supination, or external rotation of the forearm providing a posterolaterally directed force.
- Failure of capsuloligamentous structures occurs in a complete or near-complete circular manner from lateral to medial [8] as seen in image A. The sequence of failure has recently been challenged with debate of the MCL failing first.
- It is imperative to determine the extent of soft tissue injury and identify associated fractures for proper treatment.
- O'Driscoll described post-traumatic elbow instability according to five criteria: (1) bony articulations involved, (2) direction of displacement, (3) degree of the displacement, (4) timing of injury, and (5) the presence of absence of associated fractures [6].

Evaluation

Presentation

- Pain in affected elbow, usually held in slight flexion. It is important to obtain a complete history regarding mechanism of injury and rule out associated injuries.

Physical Exam

- Inspection: swelling, ecchymosis, abrasions, lacerations, and exposed soft tissue or bone.
- Passive range of motion: assess for mechanical block; it may be limited due to joint effusion/swelling and pain.
- Neurovascular exam: evaluation of motor/sensory functions of the median, radial, and ulnar nerves. Although rare, it is necessary to evaluate for potential compartment syndrome of the forearm.
- Evaluate the joint above and below the level of injury to rule out associated injury.

Imaging

- XR: AP, lateral, radial head, and/or oblique views of the elbow.
- Assess the congruency of the ulnohumeral and radiocapitellar joints.
- Center of the radial head should align with the center of the capitellum on all views.
- Assess for fractures of the coronoid, ulna, radial head, and distal humerus.
- Dislocations associated with one or more intra-articular fractures are at higher risk for recurrent dislocation or chronic instability [13].
- Obtain post-reduction images of the bone/joint proximal and distal to the injury.
- Handbook for fractures [13] (Fig. 25.1).

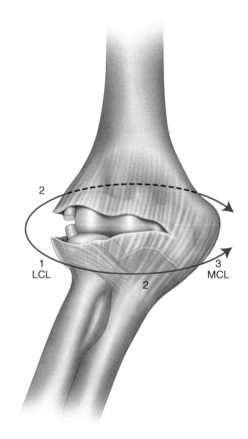

Fig. 25.1 The capsuloligamentous structures of the elbow are injured in a lateral to medial progression during dislocation of the elbow. The elbow can dislocate with the anterior band of the MCL remaining intact (From Bucholz et al. [14])

CT Indications

- Assess fractures or nonconcentric joint reduction evidenced on plain radiographs.
- Preoperative planning.
- 3-D reconstructions may be helpful in further evaluating the injury and developing an appropriate treatment plan.

Classification

Anatomic Description

- Based on the location of the olecranon relative to the humerus [9] as demonstrated in image B.
- As mentioned previously, posterolateral dislocations are the most common encountered variant.

Simple vs Complex

- Simple dislocations = no fractures, purely ligamentous injury
- Complex dislocation = dislocation associated with a fracture
- Terrible triad: elbow dislocation, radial head fracture, and coronoid fracture [8] – very unstable

Treatment

- Initially: reduction under conscious sedation
  - Maneuver: in-line traction of the arm, supination to clear the coronoid from underneath the trochlea, and then flexion of the elbow with direct pressure on the tip of the olecranon [10].
  - Following reduction, assess elbow stability by passive ROM (flexion, extension, pronation, and supination). The treatment algorithm will depend upon degree of instability.
  - Always perform post-reduction neurovascular exam and obtain radiographs.

Handbook for fractures [13] (Fig. 25.2)

Nonoperative Indications

- Stable post-reduction: sling and early range of motion exercises.
- Unstable with extension <30°: splint the elbow at 90° and reevaluate stability in 7–10 days.
- Unstable elbows at <90° or persistent instability may require surgery.
- The elbow joint is relatively sensitive to immobilization, and to avoid stiffness, it is important to initiate progressive range of motion exercises early [11].

Operative Indications

- Open reduction internal fixation (ORIF) of the coronoid/distal humerus and ORIF or replacement of the radial head
  - ORIF is often indicated in complex dislocations secondary to persistent instability or joint incongruity due to interposition of soft tissue or fragmented bone.

Ligamentous Repair or Construction
- LUCL repair or reconstruction and MCL repair or reconstruction if elbow is still unstable

Hinged External Fixator
- External fixation can be used for chronic dislocations or if ORIF and repair of the ligamentous structures fail to maintain a concentric and stable reduction [10].

Potential Complications [12, 13]

- Persistent or recurrent instability
- Neurovascular injury – ulnar/median/radial nerve and brachial artery
- Stiffness – correlated with immobilization for longer than 2–3 weeks
- Loss of motion, particularily loss of terminal extension

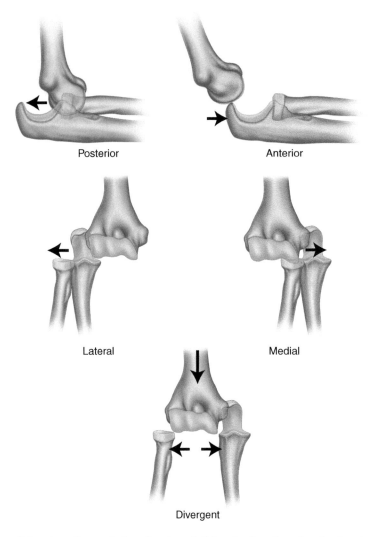

Posterior   Anterior

Lateral   Medial

Divergent

Fig. 25.2 Elbow dislocations. Image depicts direction of dislocation based on the ulna location in relation to the humerus (From Browner et al. [15] with permission)

- Heterotopic ossification
- Post-traumatic arthritis
- Volkmann contracture secondary to ischemia from immobilization >90° flexion

References

1. Stoneback JW, et al. Incidence of elbow dislocations in the United States population. J Bone Joint Surg Am. 2012;94(3):240–5.

2. Englert C, et al. Elbow dislocations: a review ranging from soft tissue injuries to complex elbow fracture dislocations. Adv Orthop. 2013;2013:951397.
3. Morrey BF, An KN. Stability of the elbow: osseous constraints. J Shoulder Elbow Surg. 2005;14(1 Suppl S):174S–8S.
4. Jeon IH, et al. The contribution of the coronoid and radial head to the stability of the elbow. J Bone Joint Surg Br. 2012;94(1):86–92.
5. O'Driscoll SW, et al. Elbow subluxation and dislocation. A spectrum of instability. Clin Orthop Relat Res. 1992;280:186–97.
6. O'Driscoll SW, et al. The unstable elbow. Instr Course Lect. 2001;50:89–102.

7. Miller MD, Thompson SR, Hart JA. Review of orthopedics. 6th ed. Philadelphia: Elsevier; 2012.

8. Mathew PK, Athwal GS, King GJ. Terrible triad injury of the elbow: current concepts. J Am Acad Orthop Surg. 2009;17(3):137–51.

9. Cohen MS, Hastings 2nd H. Acute elbow dislocation: evaluation and management. J Am Acad Orthop Surg. 1998;6(1):15–23.

10. Leiberman JR. AAOS Comprehensive Orthopedic Review in American Academy of Orthopedics Surgeons 2009. p. 865–869.

11. Ross G, et al. Treatment of simple elbow dislocation using an immediate motion protocol. Am J Sports Med. 1999;27(3):308–11.

12. O'Driscoll SW, Bell DF, Morrey BF. Posterolateral rotatory instability of the elbow. J Bone Joint Surg Am. 1991;73(3):440–6.

13. Egol K, et al. Hand book of fractures. 5th ed. Philadelphia: Wolters Kluwer Health; 2015. p. 225–38.

14. Bucholz RW, Heckman JD, Court-Brown C, et al., editors. Rockwood and green's fractures in adults. 6th ed. Philadelphia: Lippincott Williams & Wilkins; 2006.

15. Browner BD, Jupiter JB, Levine AM, editors. Skeletal trauma. Philadelphia: WB Saunders; 1992. p. 1142.

Degenerative Joint Disease of the Elbow

26

Matthew Binkley and Thomas R. Duquin

Degenerative joint disease of the elbow can be subclassified into osteoarthritis, post-traumatic arthritis, inflammatory arthritis, neuropathic arthritis, and septic arthritis. Stiffness, loss of motion, and pain are common symptoms regardless of etiology. Radiographs are often diagnostic with CT scan occasionally helpful.

Osteoarthritis (Refer to Chaps. 2, 3, 4, 5, 6, 7, 8, 9, 10, 11, 12, 13, 14, 15, 16, 17, 18, 19, 20, and 21)

- Osteoarthritis of the elbow is an infrequent but disabling disease process.
- The dominant arm of male laborers in their 50s.
- Nonsurgical: nonsteroidal anti-inflammatories, steroid injections, gentle range of motion activities, and activity modification.
- Surgical: arthroscopic or open ulnohumeral arthroplasty, total elbow arthroplasty, interposition arthroplasty, and arthrodesis are used sparingly as salvage procedures.

M. Binkley, MD (✉)
Department of Orthopedic Surgery, Erie County Medical Center, Buffalo, NY, USA
e-mail: w104mtb@gmail.com

T.R. Duquin, MD
University at Buffalo, Flint Entrance, Amherst, NY 14260, USA

Post-traumatic Arthritis (Refer to Chaps. 2, 3, 4, 5, 6, 7, 8, 9, 10, 11, 12, 13, 14, 15, 16, 17, 18, 19, 20, 21, and 22)

- Post-traumatic arthritis of the elbow is a rare and often debilitating disorder.
- History: fracture/dislocation event, treatment, infections or wound healing complications, and nerve symptoms.
- Nonsurgical treatment: nonsteroidal anti-inflammatories, steroid injections, gentle range of motion activities, and activity modification.
- Surgical treatments: arthroscopy, ulnohumeral arthroplasty with debridement, interposition arthroplasty, total elbow arthroplasty, and arthrodesis.
- Total elbow arthroplasty in patients less than 60 years of age is associated with high complication, failure, and reoperation rates.

Inflammatory Arthritis (Rheumatoid Arthritis)

Etiology

- Prevalence 0.5–2% with 20–50% of rheumatoid patients experiencing elbow involvement [1, 2]
- Rheumatoid more prevalent in females

© Springer International Publishing AG 2017
A.E.M. Eltorai et al. (eds.), *Orthopedic Surgery Clerkship*, DOI 10.1007/978-3-319-52567-9_26

Pathology

- Synovitis is a hallmark of inflammatory arthritis and results in joint effusions and pain.
- Secondary changes including flexion contractures and ligamentous disruption can occur with resulting instability and bony destruction.
- End stages marked by substantial bone loss, loss of joint space, progressive elbow instability, and pain.

Evaluation

- Examination of the ipsilateral hand, wrist, and shoulder important
- Important to delineate the patient's level of pain, motion, stability, and functional capacity [3]

Treatment

- Nonsurgical: intra-articular injections, physical therapy, and hinged elbow braces to help limit painful motions.
- Surgical treatment: synovectomy with or without radial head resection and total elbow arthroplasty.
- Total elbow arthroplasty has been shown to provide durable pain relief and preserve motion but with a high complication rate.

Neuropathic Arthritis

Etiology

- Rare condition which is poorly understood.
- Conditions linked to neurotrophic arthropathy include syringomyelia, diabetes mellitus, tabes dorsalis, and Charcot-Marie-Tooth disease [8].

Pathology

- True pathology is debated.

- Associated with loss of nociception and proprioception resulting in repeated trauma that goes unnoticed by the patient causing joint destruction.

Evaluation

- Identification of underlying cause of the neuropathic joint (syringomyelia, diabetes, and tabes dorsalis common).
- Examine other body parts for evidence of abnormalities.
- Complete neurovascular examination in regard to sensation with investigation into whether autonomic dysfunction symptoms (orthostatic hypotension, loss of sweating, urinary incontinence, and impotence) are present.
- Blood, urine, and genetic tests and nerve conduction studies can be helpful in some instances.

Treatment

- Protection of the joint and treatment of the underlying disorder are the mainstays of treatment.
- Pain is rare, whereas stability and functionality are the primary considerations.
- Nonsurgical treatment: bracing or splint to retain function.
- Surgical treatment: total elbow arthroplasty and arthrodesis (avoided in most cases due to high complication rate).

Septic Arthritis

Etiology

- Rare but does occur more commonly in IV drug abusers, rheumatoid patients, and HIV patients

Pathology

- *S. aureus* inciting organism is two-thirds of patients [5].

Evaluation

- The elbow generally held in 80° of flexion (maximum capsule volume) [4].
- History: fevers, erythema, swelling, pain, loss of motion, open wounds, and immunocompromised patients at higher risk.
- Laboratory: leukocytosis, elevated sedimentation rate, and C-reactive proteins.
- Aspiration of joint hallmark of diagnosis.
- Radiographs may show an anterior or posterior fat pad, while MRI may show a joint effusion.

Treatment

- Joint debridement and irrigation which can be performed through arthroscopic or open approaches.
- Intravenous antibiotics starting with empiric coverage and adjusting based on culture and sensitivity results.
- Delay in diagnosis and treatment is the most important factor regarding prognosis

with loss of function being the most common sequel of septic arthritis of the elbow [6, 7].

References

1. Inglis A, Figgie M. Septic and non-traumatic conditions of the elbow: rheumatoid arthritis. In: Morrey BF, editor. The elbow and its disorders. 2nd ed. Philadelphia: WB Saunders; 1993. p. 751–66.
2. Silman A, Hochberg M. Epidemiology of the rheumatic diseases. Oxford: Oxford University Press; 1993.
3. Morrey B, Adams R. Semiconstrained arthroplasty for the treatment of rheumatoid arthritis of the elbow. J Bone Joint Surg Am. 1992;74:479–90.
4. O'Driscoll S, Morrey B, An K. Intraarticular pressure and capacity of the elbow. Arthroscopy. 1990;6:100.
5. Kelly P, Martin W, Coventry M. Bacterial (suppurative) arthritis in the adult. J Bone Joint Surg. 1970;52A:1595.
6. Goldenberg D, Cohen A. Acute infectious arthritis. Am J Med. 1976;60:369.
7. Argen R, Wilson C, Wood P. Suppurative arthritis. Arch Intern Med. 1966;117:661.
8. Storey G, Stein J, Poppel M. Rapid osseous changes in syringomyelia. Radiology. 1957;69:415.

Osteoarthritis of the Elbow

27

Matt Binkley and Thomas R. Duquin

Incidence and Etiology

- Occurs in men more commonly at a 4:1 ratio to women [1]
- Average age at presentation 50 years of age with range reported from 20 to 65 years of age [3]
- Association with overuse and manual labor
- The dominant arm in 80–90% with bilateral involvement in 25–60% [2]
- May be related to single or multiple trauma or osteochondritis dissecans [4]

Clinical Presentation

- Stiffness is common with average arc of motion from 30° to 120° with forearm rotation that is minimally restricted [2].
- Pain with terminal extension in most patients with pain at terminal flexion in 50%.
- Pain throughout range of motion arc is less common but can be present.

M. Binkley, MD (✉)
Orthopedic Surgery, Erie County Medical Center,
Buffalo, NY, USA
e-mail: w104mtb@gmail.com

T.R. Duquin, MD
University at Buffalo,
Flint Entrance, Amherst, NY 14260, USA

- Radiocapitellar joint arthritis may result in pain with supination and pronation.
- Ulnar nerve pathology is present in 10% of patients [3].

Work-Up

- Elbow radiographs (AP, lateral, radial head):
  - Osteophyte formation present anteriorly on the coronoid and in the coronoid fossa and posteriorly on olecranon process and in the olecranon fossa [5].
  - Radiocapitellar joint involvement is present in 85% with osteophyte formation of the radial head and flattening of the capitellum [6].
  - Loose bodies are common (Fig. 27.1).
- Computerized tomography may be helpful in earlier stages to show subtle osteophytes and loose bodies and is important for preoperative planning.

Non-operative Treatment

- Symptomatic treatment is appropriate early.
- Anti-inflammatory medications and aceta minophen.
- Intra-articular steroid injection.
- Gentle range of motion exercises should be performed to maintain mobility.

© Springer International Publishing AG 2017
A.E.M. Eltorai et al. (eds.), *Orthopedic Surgery Clerkship*, DOI 10.1007/978-3-319-52567-9_27

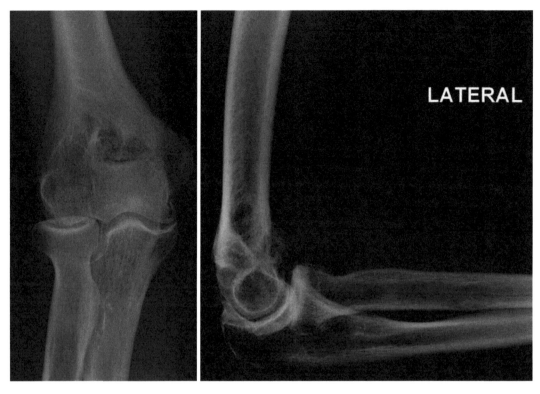

Fig. 27.1 Osteoarthritis of the elbow with osteophyte formation and joint space narrowing present

- Hyaluronic acid has not been shown to be of benefit [7].
- Avoidance of aggravating activities and counseling of the disease course are recommended.

Operative Treatment

Arthroscopic Ulnohumeral Arthroplasty

- Loose body and osteophyte removal with capsular release or resection (simple removal may relieve symptoms and can improve motion up to 15°) [8]
- Indicated for early stages of arthritis with loss of motion or pain with terminal flexion or extension
- Performed as outpatient with rapid return of motion and minimal morbidity

- Potential risks to neurovascular structures due to proximity to operative field
- Generally high patient satisfaction with improved pain and function postoperatively

Open Ulnohumeral Arthroplasty (Outerbridge-Kashiwagi Procedure)

- Indicated for loss of motion and pain at extremes of motion but not mid-arc pain
- Relieves impingement pain and allows improved range of motion
- Performed through a triceps-splitting approach with removal of osteophytes from the posterior elbow with a core osteotomy of the humerus in the olecranon fossa to access to the anterior portion of the joint
- Capsular release performed to improve motion

Total Elbow Arthroplasty (TEA)

- Indicated in patients with advanced arthritis with pain throughout the arc of motion who have failed other treatment modalities.
- Typically reserved for patients over 65 years of age with low functional demands.
- Approximately 3000 total elbow arthroplasties done yearly.
- Prosthetic designs include unconstrained or semi-constrained implants with main complication being instability in the unconstrained and loosening in the constrained implants.
- Lifelong lifting restriction of 5–10 lbs following TEA.
- Most patients achieve functional range of motion and are satisfied with results.
- Complication rate is 27–43% (including infection, ulnar neuropathy, instability, aseptic loosening, triceps insufficiency).

Interposition Arthroplasty

- Indicated in young, high-demand patients with damage to articular surface as alternative to total elbow arthroplasty.
- Contraindications include gross instability/deformity, active infection, and loss of elbow flexor power [3].
- Allograft Achilles tendon used to resurface the distal humerus. No postoperative weight-bearing restrictions after initial post-op phase.
- Technically demanding procedure with variable results in the literature.
- Inadequate bone stock and pain at rest are associated with suboptimal results.

Arthrodesis

- Salvage procedure in face of infection or unreconstructable limb
- May be useful for the young laborer but is controversial
- Incompatible with satisfactory function due to range of motion required by the elbow for hand function
- Nonunion and wound healing problems being common [9]

References

1. Doherty M, Wall I, Dieppe PA. Influence of primary generalized osteoarthritis on development of secondary osteoarthritis. Lancet. 1983;2:8.
2. Doherty M, Preston B. Primary osteoarthritis of the elbow. Ann Rheum Dis. 1989;48:743.
3. Minami M, Kato S, Kashiwagi D. Outerbridge-Kashiwagi's method for arthroplasty of osteoarthritis of the elbow: 44 elbows followed for 8-16 years. J Orthop Sci. 1996;1:11.
4. Kelly WN, Harris ED, Ruddy S, Sledge CP. Textbook of rheumatology. 3rd ed. Philadelphia: W.B. Saunders Co.; 1989.
5. Minami NM, Ishii S. Roentgenological studies of osteoarthritis of the elbow joint. Jpn Orthop Assoc. 1977;51:1223.
6. Delal S, Bull M, Stanley D. Radiographic changes at the elbow in primary osteoarthritis: a comparison with normal aging of the elbow joint. J Shoulder Elbow Surg. 2007;16:358.
7. Van Brakel RW, Eygendaal D. Intra-articular injection of hyaluronic acid is not effective for the treatment of post-traumatic osteoarthritis of the elbow. Arthroscopy. 2006;22:1199.
8. Ozbaydar M, Tonbul M, Altan E, Yalaman O. Arthroscopic treatment of symptomatic loose bodies in osteoarthritis elbows. Acta Orthop Traumatol Turc. 2006;40:371.
9. Schneeberger AG, Meyer DC, Yian EH. Coonrad-Morrey total elbow replacement for primary and revision surgery: a 2- to 7.5 year follow up study. J Shoulder Elbow Surg. 2007;16(3):S47–54.

Post-traumatic Arthritis of the Elbow

Matthew Binkley and Thomas R. Duquin

Incidence and Etiology

- Post-traumatic articular cartilage damage or residual articular joint incongruity alters load distribution across the elbow joint which can lead to degenerative changes and early arthritis [1].
- May involve isolated portions of the joint or entire joint.
- Rare but functionally debilitating disorder.

Clinical Presentation

- History regarding injury mechanism, type of fracture/dislocation, treatment including surgical approach, hardware, and complications.
- Symptoms either pain, stiffness, or instability.
- Pain at terminal motion may indicate impingement pain secondary to osteophyte formation or capsular contraction.
- Pain throughout motion indicates advanced degenerative changes which may be accompanied by night pain, effusions, and stiffness.

M. Binkley, MD (✉)
Department of Orthopedic Surgery, Erie County
Medical Center, Buffalo, NY, USA
e-mail: w104mtb@gmail.com

T.R. Duquin, MD
University at Buffalo,
Flint Entrance, Amherst, NY 14260, USA

- Pain at rest may indicate non-articular sources such as infection, cervical spine radiculopathy, or reflex sympathetic dystrophy.
- Examine the elbow for deformity, swelling, crepitus, range of motion, ligamentous stability, muscle strength, and ulnar nerve irritability.

Work-Up

- Dedicated elbow XR may demonstrate osteophyte formation, loose bodies, and joint space narrowing (Fig. 28.1).
- CT arthrography allows evaluation of cartilage and soft tissue pathology with CT recons helpful for visualizing osteophyte formation and complex deformity [2].
- MRI utility not generally required.
- EMG for assessing baseline nerve function if peripheral neuropathy is suspected.
- Infection labs with possible aspiration important to rule out septic arthritis especially if further surgery is planned.

Non-operative Treatment

- Goals of early treatment include maintaining range of motion and reducing activities that reduce stress across the elbow [3].
- Nonsteroidal anti-inflammatories, intra-articular corticosteroid injections, and activity modification are first-line temporizing measures.

© Springer International Publishing AG 2017
A.E.M. Eltorai et al. (eds.), *Orthopedic Surgery Clerkship*, DOI 10.1007/978-3-319-52567-9_28

Fig. 28.1
Post-traumatic
arthritis of the
elbow with
collapse of the
joint surfaces,
heterotopic
bone, and loose
bodies present

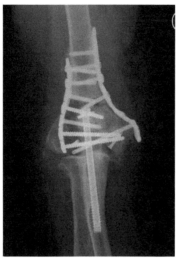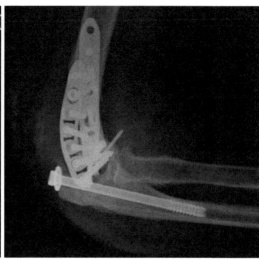

Operative Treatment

Stiffness and pain at terminal extension may benefit from arthroscopic or open joint debridement, whereas patients with pain throughout motion with advanced degenerative disease may benefit from joint resurfacing, interpositional arthroplasty, or joint arthroplasty.

Arthroscopy

- Indicated for loose body removal, osteophyte debridement, synovectomy, and capsular release.
- Technically demanding with risk to neurovascular structures.
- Improvement in elbow range of motion expected [4].
- Beware of prior surgeries, ulnar nerve subluxation, or previous transposition.
- Nerve palsy seen in 1–5% of patients with ulnar nerve most commonly.

Open Techniques

- Several surgical options described with goals of increasing range of motion and eliminating terminal pain
- Useful for earlier stages of arthritis

Interposition Arthroplasty

- Autograft or allograft used.
- In young, high-demand patients as alternative to total elbow arthroplasty.
- No postoperative weight-bearing restrictions after initial post-op phase.
- Contraindications include gross instability/deformity, active infection, and loss of elbow flexor power [3].
- Inadequate bone stock and pain at rest are associated with suboptimal results.

Total Elbow Arthroplasty

- Most definitive treatment for end-stage post-traumatic arthritis.
- Major complication rate associated with procedure with Schneeberger et al. reporting a major complication rate of 27% with most common complication involving mechanical failure [5].
- Failure associated with age <60 years at the time of surgery [6].
- May be the only option with significant bone loss, articular disruption, or prior treatment option failure.
- Implant longevity and patient age are important considerations.

- Reasonable range of motion and patient satisfaction expected.

Arthrodesis

- Rarely indicated due to limitations associated with procedure.
- Option in young patient who requires a strong, stable joint or as a last resort salvage procedure.
- Complications include non-union and fracture but are relatively uncommon.
- Many techniques described.

Isolated Radiocapitellar or Distal Humeral Joint Disease

- Isolated arthritis commonly results from malunion, non-union, or cartilage injury 1.
- Isolated radiocapitellar arthritis can present with lateral elbow pain and painful/limited forearm rotation.
- Treatment options for isolated radiocapitellar arthritis include radial head resection versus replacement, interposition arthroplasty, and

prosthetic replacement of the capitellum and/or radial head.
- Distal humerus hemiarthroplasty is an option for arthritis that involves primarily the distal humerus.

References

1. Wysocki R, Cohen M. Primary osteoarthritis and post-traumatic arthritis of the elbow. Hand Clin. 2011;27(2):131–7.. v.
2. Singson R, Feldman F, Roseberg Z. Elbow joint: assessment with double-contrast CT arthrography. Radiology. 1986;160(1):167–73.
3. Cheung E, Adams R, Morrey B. Primary osteoarthritis of the elbow: current treatment options. J Am Acad Orthop Surg. 2008;16(2):77–87.
4. Krishnan S, Harkins D, Pennington S, Harrison D, Burkhead W. Arthroscopic ulnohumeral arthroplasty for degenerative arthritis of the elbow in patients under fifty years of age. J Shoulder Elbow Surg. 2007;23(2):151–6.
5. Schneeberger A, Adams R, Morrey B. Semiconstrained total elbow replacement for the treatment of post-traumatic osteoarthritis. J Bone Joint Surg Am. 1997;79(8):1211–22.
6. Throckmorton T, Zarkadas P, Sanchez-Sotelo J, Morrey B. Failure patterns after linked semiconstrained total elbow arthroplasty for posttraumatic arthritis. J Bone Joint Surg Am. 2010;92(6):1432–41.

Cubital Tunnel Syndrome

29

Matt Binkley and Thomas R. Duquin

Incidence and Etiology

- The second most common nerve entrapment syndrome in the upper extremity after carpal tunnel syndrome.
- Five common sources of compression:
  - Medial intermuscular septum/arcade of Struthers
  - Medial epicondyle (sequelae of distal humerus fracture or osteophytes)
  - Osborne's ligament (cubital tunnel retinaculum, anconeus epitrochlearis muscle present in 11% of population)
  - Arcuate ligament (aponeurosis of flexor carpi ulnaris)
  - Deep flexor-pronator aponeurosis when the nerve exits the flexor carpi ulnaris
- External sources of compression include heterotopic ossification, osteophytes, malunions and nonunions, ganglion cysts, and tumors.
- Ulnar nerve subluxation and dislocation can be a source of ulnar neuropathy:

- Hypermobility is found in 20% of the population which may cause nerve irritation due to friction with the medial epicondyle [1].

Anatomy (Fig. 29.1)

- The ulnar nerve pierces the medial intermuscular septum approximately 8–10 cm above the medial epicondyle and descends along the medial head of the triceps.
- Cubital tunnel boundaries are formed by the flexor carpi ulnaris fascia and Osborne's

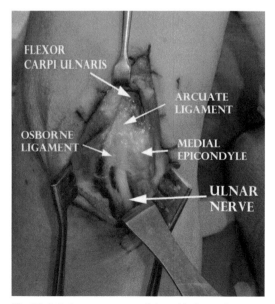

Fig. 29.1 Relevant anatomy of the cubital tunnel

M. Binkley, MD (✉)
Orthopedic Surgery, Erie County Medical Center, Buffalo, NY, USA
e-mail: w104mtb@gmail.com

T.R. Duquin, MD
University at Buffalo,
Flint Entrance, Amherst, NY 14260, USA

© Springer International Publishing AG 2017
A.E.M. Eltorai et al. (eds.), *Orthopedic Surgery Clerkship*, DOI 10.1007/978-3-319-52567-9_29

ligament on the roof, the MCL and elbow joint capsule on the floor, and the medial epicondyle and olecranon as the walls.

Clinical Presentation

- Symptoms can include medial elbow pain, numbness in the ring and small finger, and hand weakness.
- Initially symptoms are often positional with elbow flexion (sleeping, phone use).
- Examination:
  - Evaluate other sites of nerve compression (cervical spine, thoracic outlet).
  - Elbow range of motion and palpation of the ulnar nerve to assess for subluxation or external sources of compression. Elbow flexion test, direct cubital tunnel compression, and Tinel's examination.
  - Examination of the hand for atrophy, muscle weakness, and sensation:
    ○ Sensory changes in the ring and small finger. Preserved dorsal sensation may indicate compression at the wrist (Guyon's canal).
    ○ Muscle weakness is evaluated by:
      - Wartenberg sign (inability to adduct the small finger)
      - Froment's sign (flexion of the interphalangeal joint of the thumb to compensate for a weakened adductor pollicis)
      - Jeanne's sign (hyperextension of the metacarpophalangeal joint of the thumb)

Evaluation

- Radiographs of the elbow to evaluate for osteophytes and bone fragments.
- Electrodiagnostic studies can be helpful to confirm diagnosis and determine severity.
- MRI not typically useful for evaluating ulnar neuropathy unless a space-occupying mass is suspected as source of compression.

Non-operative Treatment

- Activity modification, avoiding prolonged elbow flexion, elbow pad, or extension splint
- Nonsteroidal anti-inflammatories

Operative Treatment [3]

- Goal of eliminating compression and restoring smooth excursion of the nerve.
- No reported differences in outcome between decompression and transposition.
- All surgical approaches should beware of the medial antebrachial cutaneous nerve during dissection.

In Situ Decompression (Fig. 29.2)

- Release of potential sites of compression from arcade of Struthers proximally to the deep flexor-pronator aponeurosis distally.

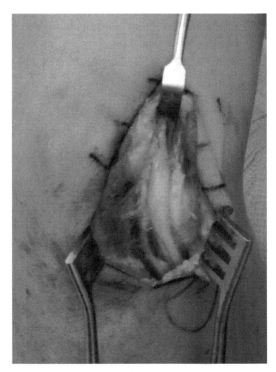

Fig. 29.2 The ulnar nerve after release with the distal aspect showing release of the flexor carpi ulnaris fascia

- Advantages include simplicity of procedure and lack of postoperative immobilization.
- Disadvantages include potential inadequacy of release and potential ulnar nerve subluxation.

Transposition

- Relieves traction and compression by placing nerve anterior to elbow motion axis
- No reported difference between subcutaneous and submuscular transposition

Subcutaneous Transposition
- Places the ulnar nerve superficial to the flexor-pronator origin.
- Fat sling can be helpful in preventing nerve posterior subluxation.
- Requires mobilization of the first motor branch for adequate nerve mobility.
- Attempt to preserve neve vascular supply.
- Risks include nerve irritation at medial intermuscular septum or edge of flexor carpi ulnaris tendon and vulnerability of nerve to trauma due to subcutaneous position.

Submuscular Transposition
- Detachment of the flexor-pronator mass with transposition to an anterior position under the muscle and reattachment of the flexor-pronator mass [4].
- Advantages include complete release of all sites of compression with protection of the nerve in a less vulnerable location.
- Disadvantages include longer postoperative immobilization, possible flexor-pronator weakness, and technical difficulty of procedure.

Medial Epicondylectomy

- Decompression of the ulnar nerve with osteotomy of the medial epicondyle.
- Avoid the origin of the medial collateral ligament and the joint surface.
- The flexor-pronator mass is removed and reattached to the periosteum with the elbow in extension [2].
- Disadvantages of procedure include risk of elbow instability, flexor-pronator muscle weakness, heterotopic ossification risk, and increased pain.

Postoperative complications of cubital tunnel release include incomplete decompression or perineural scarring, injury to the medial antebrachial cutaneous nerve, ulnar nerve subluxation, and potential medial collateral ligament injury [5].

References

1. Childress H. Recurrent ulnar-nerve dislocation at the elbow. Clin Orthop. 1975;108:168–73.
2. King T, Morgan F. Late results of removing the medial humeral epicondyle for traumatic ulnar neuritis. J Bone Joint Surg. 1959;41:51–5.
3. Taleisnik J, Szabo R. Compression neuropathies of the upper extremity. In: Chapman MW, Madiaon M, editors. Operative orthopedics, vol. 2. 2nd ed. Philadelphia: JB Lippincott; 1993. p. 1419–65.
4. Leffert R. Anterior submuscular transposition of the ulnar nerves by the Learmonth technique. J Hand Surg [Am]. 1982;7:147–55.
5. Rogers M, Bergfield T, Aulicino P. The failed ulnar nerve transposition: etiology and treatment. Clin Orthop Relat Res. 1991;269:193–200.

Radius and Ulna Fractures

30

Adam Martin and Hisham M. Awan

Introduction

- Forearm fractures typically result from high-energy injury, and a relatively large percentage are open fractures.
- The rotatory motion provided by the forearm is crucial to allowing objects to be manipulated by the hand; thus, loss of this motion can be clinically disabling.

Anatomy

Osteology

- The relatively straight ulna serves as an axis around which the radially bowed radius (Fig. 30.1) rotates to allow for pronation and supination.
  - The axis of rotation passes through the center of the radial head proximally and the fovea of the ulnar head distally.

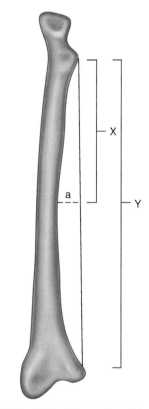

- a - maximum radial bow
- x/y*100 - location of radial bow
- average maximal bow is 15mm
- Location is 60% distal along length of radius

Fig. 30.1 Illustration of radial bow

A. Martin, MD • H.M. Awan, MD (✉)
Hand and Upper Extremity Center, The Ohio State University Wexner Medical Center,
Columbus, OH, USA
e-mail: hisham.awan@osumc.edu

© Springer International Publishing AG 2017
A.E.M. Eltorai et al. (eds.), *Orthopedic Surgery Clerkship*, DOI 10.1007/978-3-319-52567-9_30

Ligaments

- The proximal radioulnar joint (PRUJ) – stabilized by the annular ligament
- The interosseous membrane (IOM)
  - Occupies space between radius and ulna
  - Composed of five ligaments
    - Proximal oblique cord
    - Dorsal oblique accessory cord
    - Central band – key to stability during reconstruction
    - Accessory band
    - Distal oblique cord
- The distal radioulnar joint (DRUJ) – stabilized by the triangular fibrocartilage complex (TFCC)

Clinical Evaluation

History

- Important to obtain and document handedness, occupation, and mechanism of injury

Physical Exam

- Patients commonly present with gross deformity, pain, and swelling.
- A subjective and objective neurovascular exam is essential with assessment of anterior interosseous nerve (AIN), posterior interosseous nerve (PIN), and ulnar nerve function as well as radial and ulnar pulses.
- Carefully examine patient to assess for open wounds and signs of compartment syndrome, e.g., excruciating, unrelenting pain, tense forearm compartments, or significant pain with passive stretch of the digits

Radiographic Evaluation

- Anteroposterior (AP) and lateral views of forearm should be obtained.

- AP and lateral views of the wrist and elbow should also be obtained to rule out other associated fractures or dislocations.
  - Radial head must be aligned with the capitellum on all views of the elbow.

Classification

- Descriptive – closed vs open, displaced vs non-displaced, location, with or without comminution, or butterfly fragment

Treatment

Nonoperative Management

- Both-bone forearm fracture – if truly non-displaced (rare), then may be treated with well-molded, long-arm cast in neutral rotation
- Isolated ulna fracture – if non-displaced or displaced (<10° angulation in any plane or <50% displaced), may be treated with plaster immobilization in a sugar-tong splint
- Isolated radius fracture – if truly non-displaced, then may be treated with long-arm cast

Operative Management

- Open reduction internal fixation (ORIF) with compression plating (3.5 mm dynamic compression plate) with or without bone grafting is the procedure of choice for the majority of displaced forearm fractures.
  - Consider acute bone grafting if significant bone loss or comminution.
- Goals of surgery
  - Direct anatomic reduction, absolute stability, primary bone healing
  - Restore ulnar and radial length
  - Restore rotational alignment
  - Restore radial bow – most important variable in functional outcome

- Approaches
  - Volar Henry (radius) – safer and more extensile than dorsal approach
    ∘ Incision – from biceps tendon (proximally) to brachioradialis (BR) insertion (distally)
    ∘ Proximal interval – between BR and pronator teres (innervated by radial and median nerves, respectively)
    ∘ Distal interval – between BR and FCR (same internervous plane)
  - Dorsal Thompson (radius)– may be occasionally used for midshaft fractures
    ∘ Incision – from lateral epicondyle to Lister's tubercle
    ∘ Proximal interval – between extensor carpi radialis brevis (ERCB) and extensor digitorum communis (EDC); innervated by radial nerve proper and PIN, respectively
    ∘ Distal interval – between ERCB and EPL (same internervous plane)
  - Subcutaneous (ulna)
    ∘ Incision over subcutaneous border of ulna; interval between extensor carpi ulnaris (PIN) and flexor carpi ulnaris (ulnar nerve)

Complications

- Nonunion – rate less than 5% with dynamic compression plates
- Infection – less than 3%
  - Of note, open fractures may receive irrigation, debridement, and primary ORIF, except in severe injuries.

  - Treatment of infection includes surgical irrigation and debridement, wound cultures, and antibiotics.
- Neurovascular injury – uncommon
  - Nerve palsies may be observed for 3 months, with surgical exploration indicated for failure of return of nerve function.
  - Radial or ulnar artery injuries may be addressed with ligation, provided that the other vessel is patent.
- Compartment syndrome
  - Increased risk with high-energy crush injuries
  - Diagnosed clinically and treated with emergent fasciotomies
    ∘ May utilize compartment pressure measurements if patient is obtunded
- Radioulnar synostosis – uncommon (3–9%)
  - Increased risk with large crush injuries, closed head injuries, and single incision for fixation of both-bone forearm fractures
  - May require surgical excision if functionally limits forearm rotation

Suggested Readings

1. Egol KA, et al. Radius and ulna shaft. In: Handbook of fractures. 4th ed. Philadelphia: Lippincott Williams & Wilkins; 2010. p. 257–68.
2. Dodds SD, et al. Fractures and dislocations: forearm. In: Hammert WC, editor. ASSH manual of hand surgery. Phildelphia: Lippincott Williams & Wilkins; 2010. p. 255–63.
3. Means Jr KR, et al. Disorders of the forearm axis. In: Wolfe SW, et al., editors. Green's operative hand surgery. 6th ed. Philadelphia: Churchill Livingstone; 2010. p. 837–68.

Monteggia and Galeazzi Fractures

31

Adam Martin and Hisham M. Awan

Introduction

- Monteggia fractures and Monteggia variants are fractures of the proximal 1/3 ulna with concomitant proximal radioulnar joint (PRUJ) disruption (evident by radiocapitellar subluxation or dislocation).
- Galeazzi fractures are fractures of the radial shaft with concomitant dislocation of the distal radioulnar joint (DRUJ).
  - Typically involve distal 1/3 of radial shaft

Anatomy

Osteology

- The relatively straight ulna serves as an axis around which the radially bowed radius rotates to allow for pronation and supination.
  - The axis of rotation passes through the center of the radial head proximally and the fovea of the ulnar head distally

Ligaments

- Proximal radioulnar joint (PRUJ)
  - Stabilized by annular ligament
- Distal radioulnar joint (DRUJ)
  - Stabilized by triangular fibrocartilage complex (TFCC)
    ○ Components include:
    - A.1 – Palmar radioulnar ligament
    - A.2 – Articular disc
    - A.3 – Dorsal radioulnar ligament
    - A.4 – Meniscal homologue
    - A.5 – ECU subsheath

Clinical Evaluation

History

- Important to obtain and document handedness, occupation, and mechanism of injury

Physical Exam

- Patients commonly present with gross deformity, pain, and swelling.
- A subjective and objective neurovascular exam is essential with assessment of anterior interosseous nerve (AIN), posterior interosseous nerve (PIN), and ulnar nerve function as well as radial and ulnar pulses.
- Carefully examine patient to assess for open wounds and signs of compartment syndrome,

A. Martin, MD • H.M. Awan, MD (✉)
Hand and Upper Extremity Center,
The Ohio State University Wexner Medical Center,
Columbus, OH, USA
e-mail: hisham.awan@osumc.edu

© Springer International Publishing AG 2017
A.E.M. Eltorai et al. (eds.), *Orthopedic Surgery Clerkship*, DOI 10.1007/978-3-319-52567-9_31

e.g., excruciating, unrelenting pain, tense forearm compartments, or significant pain with passive stretch of the digits.

- Carefully examine DRUJ
  - Perform DRUJ shuck test in neutral and extremes of pronation/supination and compare to contralateral wrist.
    - "Shuck" joint by translating the ulna volarly and dorsally while stabilizing the distal radius.
    - There should be an equivalent amount of motion in neutral to contralateral wrist and firm endpoints at the extremes of supination and pronation.
    - In general, DRUJ is more stable in supination, whereas PRUJ is more stable in pronation.

Radiographic Evaluation
(Figs. 31.1 and 31.2)

- Anteroposterior (AP) and lateral views of forearm should be obtained.
- AP and lateral views of wrist and elbow should also be obtained to rule out other associated fractures or dislocations.
  - Line through radial shaft and head should bisect capitellum on all views of elbow.
  - Indications DRUJ disruption:
    - Ulnar styloid base fracture (not always reliable)
    - Widening of DRUJ space on AP view
    - Dislocation of ulna relative to the radius on true lateral view

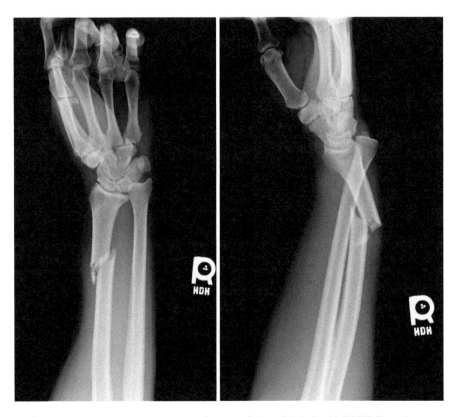

Figs. 31.1 and 31.2 AP and lateral X-rays showing fracture of the radial shaft with DRUJ disruption

Classification

- Galeazzi
  - Descriptive – closed vs open, location, with or without comminution
- Monteggia: Bado classification (Fig. 31.3)
  - Type I – anterior dislocation of radial head with associated anteriorly angulated fracture of the ulna diaphysis
  - Type II – posterior dislocation of radial head with associated posteriorly angulated fracture of the ulna diaphysis
  - Type III – lateral dislocation of radial head with associated fracture of the ulna metaphysic

- Type IV – anterior dislocation of radial head with fracture of both the radius and ulna within proximal third at the same level

Treatment

Nonoperative Management

- Monteggia and Galeazzi fractures – closed reduction and casting reserved for pediatric patients

Bado classification of monteggia fractures

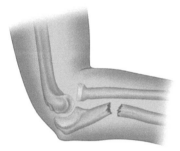

Type I

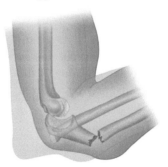

Type II

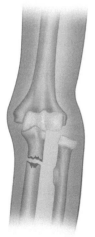

Type III

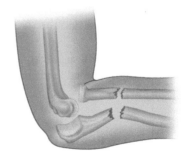

Type IV

Fig. 31.3 Bado classification of Monteggia fractures

Operative Management

- Monteggia fracture – open reduction internal fixation (ORIF) of ulna shaft with 3.5 mm dynamic compression plating (DCP) is the procedure of choice.
  - Radial head typically reduces and is stable (>90%) with reduction and stabilization of ulna.
    ◦ Failure radial head to reduce is usually due to nonanatomic reduction of ulna.
- Galeazzi fracture – ORIF with 3.5 mm DCP is treatment of choice.
  - The DRUJ should be assessed for stability after anatomic reduction and fixation of the radius.
    ◦ Fractures within 7.5 cm of the radio-carpal joint are more likely to be unstable.
  - If the DRUJ is still unstable, the forearm can be immobilized in mid-supination in splint for 4 weeks, or transfixation of the distal ulna to the radius may be achieved with smooth Kirschner wires.

Approaches

Volar Henry (Radius): Used for Galeazzi Fractures

- Incision – from brachioradialis (BR) insertion (distally) extending proximally in line with biceps tendon, centered over fracture site, utilizing the distal interval
- Distal interval – between BR and flexor carpi radialis (innervated by radial and median nerves, respectively)

Posterior Approach to Elbow: Used for Monteggia Fractures

- Lateral decubitus position with arm over padded support
- Midline posterior incision starting lateral to olecranon then gradually curving to midline as extend distally over proximal ulna

- Interval: between FCU and anconeus proximally (ulnar nerve and radial nerve); FCU and ECU (ulnar nerve and PIN) distally

Complications

- Nonunion – uncommon but may require bone grafting
- Neurovascular injury – most commonly associated with Bado II/III
  - Nerve palsies may be observed for 3 months, with surgical exploration indicated for failure of return of nerve function
  - Most commonly involve radial nerve/PIN or median nerve/AIN
- Compartment syndrome
  - Increased risk with high-energy crush injuries
  - Diagnosed clinically and treated with emergent fasciotomies
    ◦ May utilize compartment pressure measurements if patient is obtunded
- Radioulnar synostosis – uncommon (3–9%)
  - Increased risk with large crush injuries, closed head injuries, and single incision for fixation of both bone forearm fractures
  - May require surgical excision if functionally limits forearm rotation
- Radial head instability – uncommon
  - If dislocation occurs <6 weeks postoperatively with malreduction of ulna, then revision ORIF with an open reduction of radial head may be needed.
  - If dislocation occurs >6 weeks postoperatively, then consider radial head excision.

Suggested Readings

1. Egol KA, et al. Radius and ulna shaft. In: Handbook of fractures. 4th ed. Philadelphia: Lippincott Williams & Wilkins; 2010. p. 257–68.
2. Dodds SD, et al. Fractures and dislocations: forearm. In: Hammert WC, editor. ASSH manual of hand surgery. Phildelphia: Lippincott Williams & Wilkins; 2010. p. 255–63.

3. Means Jr KR, et al. Disorders of the forearm axis. In: Wolfe SW, et al., editors. Green's operative hand surgery. 6th ed. Philadelphia: Churchill Livingstone; 2010. p. 837–68.

4. Ring D, et al. Fractures of the proximal ulna. In: Wolfe SW, et al., editors. Green's operative hand surgery. 6th ed. Philadelphia: Churchill Livingstone; 2010. p. 821–36.

Distal Radius and Ulna Fractures

32

John Alexander and Hisham M. Awan

Distal Radius Fractures [1]

Anatomy

- Distal radius articulates with the carpus and serves as the origin of the volar and dorsal ligaments of the wrist.
- Articular surface consists of scaphoid and lunate fossae
- Sigmoid notch, a component of the distal radioulnar joint (DRUJ), forms a groove with which the ulnar head articulates with the radius.
- Average radiological parameters (Fig. 32.1):
  - Radial inclination: 23°
  - Radial height: 13 mm
  - Volar tilt: 11°

Presentation

- Epidemiology
  - Most common fracture seen in the emergency department
  - Incidence greater than 640,000 annually with a bimodal distribution
  - Represents a fragility fracture, thus patients should be evaluated for osteoporosis
- Mechanism
  - Fall on an outstretched hand
  - High-energy trauma
- Physical Exam
  - Evaluate for open wounds and associated injuries of the hand and upper extremity.
  - Evaluate and document a detailed neurovascular exam, particularly in open injuries.
  - Always evaluate for compartment syndrome, though this is rare in low-energy mechanisms.
  - Important to rule out concomitant acute carpal tunnel syndrome [2]
    - Occurs in 5.4–8.6% of all distal radius fractures
    - Presents with painful paresthesias
    - If worsened or no improvement in symptoms 24–48 h after closed reduction, requires carpal tunnel release and fracture fixation

Classification Systems
- No consensus regarding which classification system predicts should be utilized
- In general, tend to be based on articular involvement, number of fragments, and presence of an associated ulnar styloid fracture
- Fractures with eponyms

J. Alexander, MD • H.M. Awan, MD (✉)
Hand and Upper Extremity Center,
The Ohio State University Wexner Medical Center,
Columbus, OH, USA
e-mail: hisham.awan@osumc.edu

© Springer International Publishing AG 2017
A.E.M. Eltorai et al. (eds.), *Orthopedic Surgery Clerkship*, DOI 10.1007/978-3-319-52567-9_32

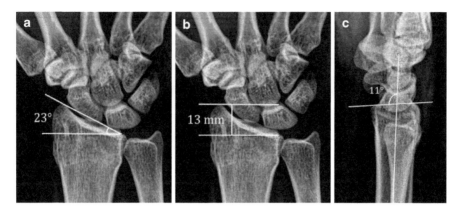

Fig. 32.1 Radiographic parameters of the distal radius. (**a**) Radial inclination as determined on the PA radiograph. (**b**) Radial height, also determined on PA radiograph. (**c**) Volar tilt determined on lateral radiographs

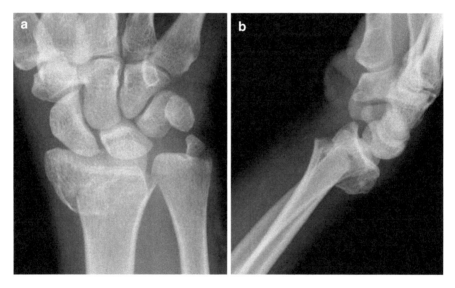

Fig. 32.2 PA (**a**) and lateral (**b**) radiographs of an extra-articular (Colles) distal radius fracture with associated ulnar styloid fracture. Note the apex volar deformity with dorsal tilt on the lateral view and shortening which is apparent on the PA view

- Colles' fracture (Fig. 32.2)
  - Extra-articular fracture with dorsal comminution, dorsal angulation, dorsal displacement, radial shortening, and an ulnar styloid fracture
- Smith's fracture
  - Volar displacement
- Barton's fracture
  - Displaced, unstable articular fracture with subluxation of the carpus along with the articular fragment
  - Can be volarly or dorsally displaced
- Chauffeur's fracture
  - Isolated radial styloid fracture, commonly associated with ligament injuries

given the force vector through the carpus
- Die punch
  - Depression of the dorsal aspect of the lunate fossa

Operative Indications

- Open fractures
- Fractures associated with acute carpal tunnel syndrome, compartment syndrome, or multiple injuries
- Current AAOS clinical practice guidelines [3]
  - Radial shortening >3 mm

- Dorsal tilt >10°
- Intra-articular displacement or step-off >2 mm

Non-operative Treatment

- If no reduction is required, can be treated with a splint or cast
- Closed reduction
  - Brachioradialis provides the major deforming force.
  - Perform reduction under hematoma block with finger traps, if available.
  - Apply a sugar-tong splint with the wrist in neutral to slight flexion, 20–30° ulnar deviation, and neutral pronation-supination.
  - Upon follow-up, convert to a short-arm cast for 4–6 weeks.
  - Follow with serial weekly radiographs early on to ensure maintenance of reduction.
- Effect of age on nonoperative management
  - With increasing age, the probability of maintenance of an acceptable reduction is decreased significantly [4].

- This increased incidence of malunion is of questionable importance as outcomes are similar to patients undergoing open reduction and internal fixation [5].
- Complications of nonoperative management
  - Extensor pollicis longus tendon rupture
    - Thought to be due to attritional rupture at a watershed area

Operative Techniques

- Goals of fixation
  - Articular congruity
  - Restoration of radial length, inclination, and volar tilt
  - Stable construct
- Closed reduction and percutaneous pinning (Fig. 32.3)
  - Various techniques available
  - Can be effective for extra-articular or simple intra-articular fractures
- External fixation
  - Utilizes ligamentotaxis to assist with fracture reduction

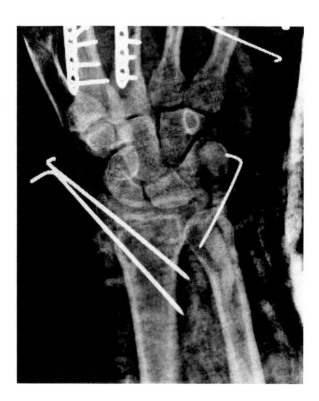

Fig. 32.3 PA radiograph of an extra-articular distal radius and ulnar styloid fractures after closed reduction and percutaneous pinning

- May be supplemented with K-wire stabilization
- Option when concurrent soft-tissue injury precludes the use of plate-screw constructs
• Open reduction and internal fixation
  - Can be performed with volar, dorsal, or fragment-specific implants.
  - Volar plating is associated with better early outcomes and allows for reliable restoration of volar tilt (Fig. 32.4).
  - Dorsal plating is associated with unacceptably high rates of extensor tendon irritation.
  - Postoperatively require splint immobilization with an early transition to removable splints.
  - Range of motion exercises can be initiated early than with nonoperative management.
• Complications with operative management [6]
  - Extensor tendon rupture/tenosynovitis
    • Most commonly involves extensor pollicis longus due to irrigation or injury to

the tendon from prominent screws or during drilling:
    (a) Thus recommend drilling unicortical for distal screws
    • Obtain a skyline view to more accurately assess for dorsal screw prominence.
  - Flexor tendon rupture
    • Higher risk when volar plates are positioned distal to the watershed line with an incidence of 2–12%
    • Flexor pollicis longus most commonly involved
  - Complex regional pain syndrome (CRPS) [7]
    • Occurs at a rate of 3–10% in patients undergoing volar plating.
    • Recent studies do not show a benefit with vitamin C supplementation for prevention of CRPS.
    • Difficult to treat and often requires referral to pain management specialists.

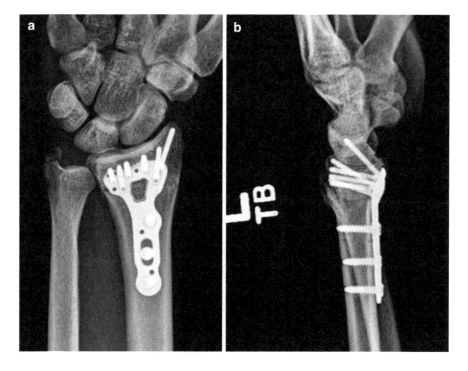

Fig. 32.4 PA and lateral postoperative radiographs after fixed-angle volar plate fixation of a distal radius fracture. Note the plate positioning proximal to the watershed line on the lateral view. More distal plate positioning may lead to plate prominence and irritation of the flexor tendons

Associated Injuries of the DRUJ

- Type I: stable
  - After fixation of the distal radius fracture, the DRUJ is stable.
  - Avulsion of the tip of the ulnar styloid or stable fractures of the ulnar neck.
  - No treatment required.
- Type II: unstable
  - Despite fixation, the DRUJ remains unstable.
  - Massive tear of the TFCC or ulnar styloid fracture below the TFCC attachment at the fovea
  - Treat with immobilization in supination, TFCC repair, fixation of ulnar styloid fragment, or pinning of the DRUJ
- Type III: comminuted articular injuries
  - Require reduction and fixation to achieve articular congruency of the sigmoid notch

Distal Ulna Fractures [1, 8]

Anatomy

- Serves as the center point about which the radius rotates.
  - Must remain stationary for this purpose
- Ulnar dome articulates with the proximal row of the carpus.
- Ulnar seat lies within the sigmoid notch of the distal radius.
- TFCC attaches to the ulnar head and stabilizes the DRUJ and the ulnocarpal joint.

Epidemiology

- Ulnar styloid fractures are frequently associated with distal radius fractures.
- In isolation, they are uncommon injuries.

Presentation

- Often related to direct trauma, as is seen with the classic "nightstick" fracture

Classification

- AO classification is the most frequently utilized system.

Treatment

- Isolated ulnar styloid
  - Commonly associated with distal radius fractures
  - When isolated, may be a sign of an injury to the TFCC or DRUJ
  - Treated nonoperatively, except when DRUJ instability is present
- Distal ulnar shaft/metaphysis
  - If displaced <50%, treat with short-arm casting
  - Operative indications
    - >50% displacement or 10° of angulation
      (a) Associated with a higher rate of nonunion and loss of pronation-supination
  - Operative approach
    - Direct approach similar to that utilized for mid-shaft ulna fractures.
    - Volar plating puts the ulnar neurovascular bundle at risk, but provides better soft tissue.
    - Hook plates are an option (Fig. 32.5).
- Salvage
  - Highly comminuted fractures may preclude operative fixation, necessitating salvage which studies have seen.
  - Options include:
    - Darrach
    - Sauvé-Kapandji
    - Ulnar head replacement
- Complications of operative management
  - Injury to dorsal sensory branch of the ulnar nerve
    - Emerges 1–4 cm proximal to the ulnar styloid
  - Symptomatic hardware
  - DRUJ arthrosis

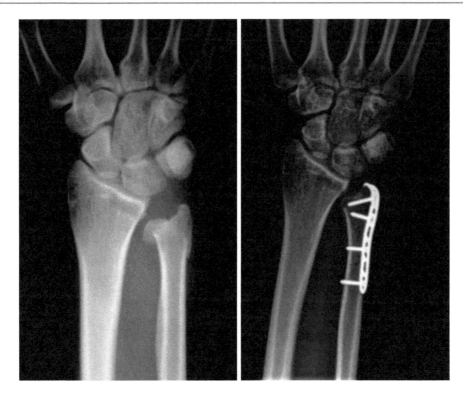

Fig. 32.5 Pre- and postoperative radiographs following open reduction and internal fixation of a comminuted distal ulna fracture with a hook plate (Used with permission from)

References

1. Wolfe SW. Distal radius fractures. Wolfe SW, Hotchkiss RN, Pederson WC, Kozin SH. Green's Operative Hand Surgery. 6th edition. Philadelphia: Churchill Livingstone; 2010. p. 561–638.
2. Niver GE, Ilyas AM. Carpal tunnel syndrome after distal radius fracture. Orthop Clin North Am. 2012;43:521–7.
3. Lichtman DM, Bindra RR, Boyer MI, et al. Treatment of distal radius fractures. J Am Acad Orthop Surg. 2010;18:180–9.
4. Beumer A, McQueen MM. Fractures of the distal radius in low-demand elderly patients: closed reduction of no value in 53 of 60 wrists. Acta Orthop Scand. 2003;74:98–100.
5. Arora R, Lutz M, Deml C, Krappinger D, Haug L, Gabl M. A prospective randomized trial comparing nonoperative treatment with volar locking plate fixation for displaced and unstable distal radial fractures in patients sixty-five years of age and older. J Bone Joint Surg Am. 2011;93:2146–53.
6. Berglund LM, Messer TM. Complications of volar plate fixation for managing distal radius fractures. J Am Acad Orthop Surg. 2009;17:369–77.
7. Ekrol I, Duckworth AD, Ralston SH, Court-Brown CM, McQueen MM. The influence of vitamin C on the outcome of distal radial fractures: a double-blind, randomized controlled trial. J Bone Joint Surg Am. 2014;96:1451–9.
8. Richards TA, Deal DN. Distal ulna fractures. J Hand Surg [Am]. 2014;39:385–91.

Carpal Tunnel Syndrome

33

Francisco A. Schwartz-Fernandes and Eildar Abyar

Introduction

- Entrapment neuropathy and compression of the median nerve in the carpal tunnel
- Most common compression neuropathy in upper extremity

Anatomy

- Floor: palmar radiocarpal ligament and the palmar ligament complex between the carpal bones
- Roof: 3 segments of flexor retinaculum
  - Proximal segment: deep investing fascia of the forearm
  - Transverse segment: inserts on the scaphoid tuberosity and part of the trapezium radially and on the pisiform and the hook of the hamate ulnarly
  - Distal segment: aponeurosis between the thenar and hypothenar muscles.

F.A. Schwartz-Fernandes
Department Orthopaedics and Sports Medicine, University of South Florida, Tampa, FL, USA

E. Abyar (✉)
Orthopedics, University of South Florida Morsani Center, Tampa, FL, USA
e-mail: eabyar@health.usf.edu

- Contains nine tendons along with the median nerve
  - Flexor pollicis longus
  - Four flexor digitorum superficialis
  - Four flexor digitorum profondus

Pathophysiology

- Nerve compression causes reduction in epineural blood flow.
  - Occurs with 20–30 mm Hg compression; intracarpal canal pressures in CTS routinely measure at least 33 mm Hg and often up to 110 mm Hg with wrist extension
- Edema in the epineurium and endoneurium (Fig. 33.1).
  - Occurs with continued or increased pressure and will increase endoneural fluid pressure fourfold and block axonal transport
- Injury to the capillary endothelium.
  - Protein leaks out into the tissues, which become more edematous, and a vicious cycle ensues
- More exudate and edema accumulate in the endoneurium, unable to diffuse across the perineurium. The perineurium resists and acts as a diffusion barrier creating in effect a "compartment syndrome" within the nerve.

© Springer International Publishing AG 2017
A.E.M. Eltorai et al. (eds.), *Orthopedic Surgery Clerkship*, DOI 10.1007/978-3-319-52567-9_33

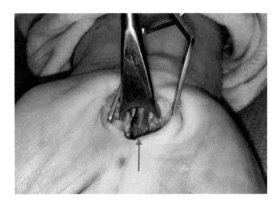

Fig. 33.1 Edema in the epineurium and endoneurium with injury to the capillary endothelium

Etiology

Trauma-Related Structural Changes

- Distal radius fracture
- Lunate dislocation
- Posttraumatic arthritis/osteophytes
- Edema
- Hemorrhage

Systemic Diseases

- Rheumatoid arthritis
- Diabetes mellitus
- Thyroid imbalance (especially hypothyroidism)
- Amyloidosis
- Hemophilia
- Alcoholism
- Raynaud's phenomenon
- Paget's disease
- Gout
- Chronic renal failure/hemodialysis

Anomalous Anatomic Structures

- Aberrant muscles (e.g., lumbricals, palmaris longus, palmaris profundus)
- Median artery thrombosis
- Enlarged persistent median artery

Hormonal Changes

- Pregnancy
- Menopause
- Acromegaly

Tumors/Neoplasms

- Lipoma
- Ganglion
- Multiple myeloma

Mechanical Overuse

- Vibrating machinery

Diagnosis

- Paresthesias in the distribution of the median nerve: radial 3–1/2 digits.
- Clumsiness and weakness in the affected hand, worse with activity.
- Night pain and paresthesia.
- Proximal radiation of pain or paresthesias to the elbow or even the shoulder.
- Thenar atrophy is a sign of advanced CTS of long-standing duration.
- Self-administered hand diagram.
  - The most specific test (76%) for carpal tunnel syndrome

Physical Examination

- Inspection: thenar atrophy in advanced CTS

Phalen's Test (Fig. 33.2)

- The test is done by having patient rest their elbows on the examination table with their forearms perpendicular to the floor and let their wrists drop into flexion with gravity assistance. Paresthesias in less than 60 s, test is positive.
- Paresthesias in less than 20 s in patients with advanced CTS.

Tinel's Sign

- Provocative test performed by tapping the median nerve over the volar carpal tunnel

Durkan's Test (Fig. 33.3)

- Carpal tunnel compression test.
- Most sensitive test.
- Pressing thumbs over the carpal tunnel and holding pressure for 30 s. Onset of pain or paresthesia in the median nerve distribution within 30 s is a positive test result.

Other Provocative Tests

Innervation-Density Tests
- Static two-point discrimination test:
  - Most commonly used innervation-density test.

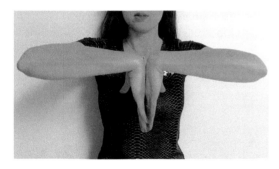

Fig. 33.2 Phalen's test

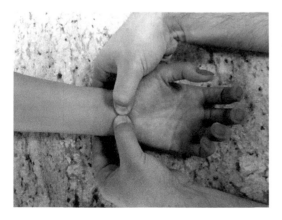

Fig. 33.3 Durkan's Test

- ◦ Performed by applying a force through two dull points placed at known distance apart (such as 5 mm) in the longitudinal axis of a digit without blanching the skin
  - Measures multiple overlapping of different sensory units and complex cortical integration.
  - The test is a good measure for assessing functional nerve regeneration after nerve repair.
- Threshold tests:
  - Semmes-Weinstein monofilament pressure testing:
    - ◦ Done by applying a monofilament perpendicularly to the palmar surface of a digit until it bends. Each given monofilament requires a certain known amount of applied force to bend. The subject is asked to localize verbally, without looking, which digit is being touched.
    - ◦ Most sensitive sensory test for detecting early carpal tunnel syndrome.
    - ◦ Measures a single nerve fiber innervating a receptor or group of receptors.
  - The tourniquet test:
    - ◦ Applying a tourniquet proximal to the elbow and inflating it to a pressure higher than the patient's systolic blood pressure.
    - ◦ If numbness and tingling in the median nerve distribution develop within 60 s, the test result is positive.

Imaging

- Rarely necessary for diagnosis

Electrodiagnostic Studies

Overview

- Not needed to establish diagnosis (diagnosis is clinical)
- Recommended if surgical management is being considered
- Most useful when trying to distinguish CTS from other conditions such as thoracic outlet syndrome or cervical radiculopathy

- Valuable when patient's secondary gain is suspected

Nerve Conduction Velocity Test (NCV)

- Increase latencies (slowing) of NCV: distal sensory latency of >3.2 ms, motor latencies >4.3 ms.
- Decreased conduction velocities less specific than latencies: velocity of <52 m/s is abnormal.

Electromyography (EMG)

- Technique for evaluating and recording the electrical activity produced by skeletal muscles and motor units
- Detail insertional and spontaneous activity
- Potential pathologic findings:
  - Increased insertional activity
  - Sharp waves
  - Fibrillations
  - Fasciculations
  - Complex repetitive discharges

Differential Diagnosis

- Cervical disk herniation
- Thoracic outlet syndrome
- Proximal compression of the median nerve
- Thenar atrophy from other causes: disuse, neuropathy, and pain due to first CMC arthritis
- De Quervain's tenosynovitis

Nonoperative Treatment

First Line

- Nonsteroidal anti-inflammatory drugs (NSAIDs)
- Activity modification (avoid aggravating activity)
- Initial trial of full-time splinting for 3–4 weeks followed by part-time night splinting for patients with nocturnal symptoms

Adjunctive Conservative Treatment

- Intracanal corticosteroid injection:
  - 80% have transient improvement of symptoms, of these 22% remain symptoms free at 1 year.
  - Good response to injection correlated with an excellent response to subsequent surgery.

Operative Treatment

Open Carpal Tunnel Release (Fig. 33.4)

- Division of the transverse carpal ligament under direct vision with an open procedure
- Indication:
  - Failure of nonoperative treatment
  - Acute CTS following ORIF of a distal radius fracture
- Outcome:
  - Pinch strength returns in 6 weeks
  - Grip strength returns in 12 weeks post-op

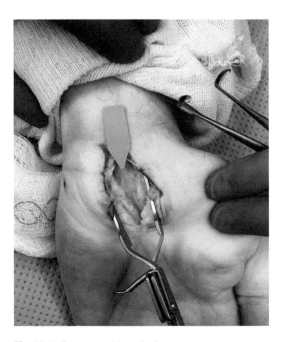

Fig. 33.4 Open carpal tunnel release

Complications

- Correlate with experience of surgeon
- Incomplete release
- Progressive thenar atrophy due to injury to a motor branch of the median nerve
- Endoscopic carpal tunnel release:
  - Endoscopic release of the transverse carpal ligament.
  - Advantage: accelerated rehabilitation.
  - Long-term results same as open CTR.
  - Complication: most common complication is incomplete release.
- Revision CTR for incomplete release:
  - Indication:
    - Failure to improve following primary surgery
    - Incomplete release
  - Outcome:
    - 25% complete relief, 50% partial relief, 25% no relief

Suggested Reading

1. English JH, Gwynne-Jones DP. Incidence of carpal tunnel syndrome requiring surgical decompression: a 10.5-year review of 2,309 patients. J Hand Surg [Am]. 2015. pii: S0363–5023(15)01030–8.
2. Jenkins PJ, Duckworth AD, Watts AC, McEachan JE. Corticosteroid injection for carpal tunnel syndrome: a 5-year survivorship analysis. Hand (NY). 2012;7(2):151–6.
3. Uchiyama S, Itsubo T, Nakamura K, Kato H, Yasutomi T, Momose T. Current concepts of carpal tunnel syndrome: pathophysiology, treatment, and evaluation. J Orthop Sci. 2010;15(1):1–13.
4. Keith MW, Masear V, Amadio PC, Andary M, Barth RW, Graham B, Chung K, Maupin K, Watters 3rd WC, Haralson 3rd RH, Turkelson CM, Wies JL, McGowan R. Treatment of carpal tunnel syndrome. J Am Acad Orthop Surg. 2009;17(6):397–405. Review.
5. El Miedany Y, Ashour S, Youssef S, Mehanna A, Meky FA. Clinical diagnosis of carpal tunnel syndrome: old tests-new concepts. Joint Bone Spine. 2008;75(4):451–7.
6. Aroori S, Spence RA. Carpal tunnel syndrome. Ulster Med J. 2008;77(1):6–17.
7. Keith MW, Masear V, Chung K, Maupin K, Andary M, Amadio PC, Barth RW, Watters 3rd WC, Goldberg MJ, Haralson 3rd RH, Turkelson CM, Wies JL. Diagnosis of carpal tunnel syndrome. J Am Acad Orthop Surg. 2009;17(6):389–96. Review.
8. Brown AR, Gelberman RH, Seiler JG, et al. Carpal tunnel release. J Bone Joint Surg Am. 1993;75:1265–75.
9. Kuschner SH, Ebramzadeh E, Johnson D, Brien WW, Sherman R. Tinel's sign and Phalen's test in carpal tunnel syndrome. Orthopedics. 1992;15(11): 1297–302.
10. Phalen GS. The carpal-tunnel syndrome. clinical evaluation of 598 hands. Clin Orthop. 1972;83: 29–40.

Kienbock's Disease (Lunatomalacia)

34

Francisco A. Schwartz-Fernandes
and James Vogler

Epidemiology

- Exact incidence is unknown.
  - It is estimated to occur in 2.5% of the population [1].
- Most common in dominant hand of males aged 18–40.
  - Ninety-five percent of patients report a history of manual labor in affected hand [2–4].

Anatomy

- In 80% of population, vascular supply of lunate is derived from dorsal and palmar sources.
  - Dorsal nutrient vessels derive from the dorsal radiocarpal arch.
  - Palmar nutrient vessels derive from palmar radiocarpal and intercarpal arches.
  - Three major intraosseal anastomotic patterns: I, X, and Y:
    - I present in 30% population.
    - X present in 10% population.
    - Y present in 60% population.

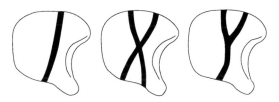

- In 20% of population, vascular supply of lunate is derived from palmar branches of palmar radiocarpal and intercarpal arches [5].
  - Higher risk for avascular necrosis during hyperextension injuries or dislocations [6]

Pathophysiology

- Acute fracture or stress fracturing may lead to segmental disruption of intraosseal blood supply and avascular necrosis [1, 6].
- Hulten [7] initially described an association between negative ulnar variance and increased incidence of lunatomalacia.
  - Wrist length discrepancy thought to increase shear forces on lunate leading to increased incidence of stress fracturing, disruption of intraosseal blood supply and avascular necrosis.
  - Validity of this finding is not well established in literature [8–15].
- Lunate morphology.
  - Based upon the presence (type I) or absence (type II) of a medial hamate facet
  - Type 1 lunate morphology higher incidence of advanced disease (>stage IIIA) and

F.A. Schwartz-Fernandes • J. Vogler (✉)
University of South Florida, 4202 East Fowler Ave,
Tampa, FL 33620, USA
e-mail: jvogler@mail.usf.edu

© Springer International Publishing AG 2017
A.E.M. Eltorai et al. (eds.), *Orthopedic Surgery Clerkship*, DOI 10.1007/978-3-319-52567-9_34

coronal fractures in patients with Kienbock's disease [31]

Clinical Presentation

- Unilateral, dorsal wrist pain aggravated by activity and relieved by rest
- Physical examination:
  - Dorsal wrist swelling (secondary to radio-carpal synovitis) with tenderness to palpation around dorsal aspect of lunate
  - Limited flexion/extension of wrist
  - Diminished grip strength as compared to contralateral side
  - Pain upon percussion of distal aspect of third metacarpal [4]

Natural History

- Few studies exist in literature regarding natural history of disease.
- Keith et al. 2004 [17]:
  - 8-year follow-up of 33 wrists with Kienbock's disease.
  - There is radiographic progression of disease, best measured by radioscaphoid angle.
  - There was no statistically significant difference in grip strength, wrist range of motion, or DASH scores at follow-up.

Imaging/Classification

Lichtman classification [16]	
Stage	Radiographic findings
I	Normal or linear/stress fracture on MRI/bone scan
II	Lunate sclerosis without collapse
IIIA	Lunate sclerosis and fragmentation without collapse Radioscaphoid angle >60°
IIIB	Lunate sclerosis and fragmentation with carpal collapse Radioscaphoid angle <60° Fixed scaphoid flexion
IV	Lunate sclerosis and fragmentation with or without collapse Radiocarpal or midcarpal arthritis

Stage I   Stage II   Stage IIIA

Stage IIIB   Stage IV

Treatment Based on Classification

Stage	Treatment options [18]
I	Splint immobilization
II or IIIA (negative ulnar variance)	Radial shortening osteotomy
II or IIIA (neutral or positive ulnar variance)	Capitate shortening osteotomy
IIIB	Scaphocapitate or scaphotrapeziotrapezoid arthrodesis Lunate excision and/or tendon interposition and intercarpal fusion if evidence of synovitis Nickel-titanium memory alloy arthrodesis
IV	Proximal row carpectomy (contraindicated if arthritic changes about head of capitate or lunate facet of radius) Total wrist arthrodesis

Technical Details

Radial Shortening Osteotomy

Biomechanics
- Lunate strain after radial shortening osteotomy decreased by 30% [19]
- Force transmission decreased by 45% following radial shortening osteotomy [20]

Outcome [21, 22]
- At 10-year follow-up, no evidence of radiographic progression on Lichtman classification
- Satisfactory clinical outcome in regard to pain, wrist flexion/extension, grip strength, and DASH scores

Complications
- Nonunion in 6% of patients [23–25]
- Joint incongruity or ulnar impaction if over-shortening occurs

Capitate Shortening Osteotomy

Biomechanics
- Force transmission across radiolunate joint decreased by 66% following capitate shortening osteotomy [20, 26, 27]

Outcome
- Excellent results with regard to patient satisfaction rate and grip strength. Grip strength is 80% contralateral side [27, 28].

Complications
- Nonunion

Scaphocapitate Arthrodesis

Biomechanics
- Force transmission across radiolunate joint decreased by 15% following scaphocapitate arthrodesis [20]

Outcome
- 5-year follow-up demonstrated 14°/11°/9° range of motion loss for wrist flexion/extension/ulnar deviation compared to contralateral side.
- Improvement in grip strength by 7 kg compared to preoperative studies.
- Satisfactory results with regard to pain [29].

Complications
- Carpal collapse
- Ulnar translocation of carpus [29]

Nickel-Titanium Memory Alloy Arthrodesis

Outcome
- 12-month follow-up demonstrated 12 kg grip strength improvement and 15° decrease in scapholunate angle.
- Satisfactory results with regard to pain [30].

Proximal Row Carpectomy

Outcome
- Grip strength 68% contralateral side
- No significant difference in wrist range of motion as compared to contralateral side
- Satisfactory results with regard to pain [32]

Complications
- Degenerative arthritis at capitate-radius articulation [32, 33]

References

1. Palmer A, Benoit M. Lunate fractures: kienböck's disease. In: Cooney W, Linscheid R, Dobyns J, editors. The wrist: diagnosis and operative treatment. Philadelphia: PA, Mosby; 1998. p. 431–73.
2. Taniguchi Y, Yoshida M, Iwasaki H, Otakara H, Iwata S. Kienböck's disease in elderly patients. J Hand Surg [Am]. 2003;28(5):779–83.
3. McMurtry RY, Youm Y, Flatt AE, Gillespie TE. Kinematics of the wrist: II. Clinical applications. J Bone Joint Surg Am. 1978;60(7):955–61.
4. Szabo RM, Greenspan A. Diagnosis and clinical findings of Kienböck's disease. Hand Clin. 1993;9(3):399–408.
5. Freedman DM, Botte MJ, Gelberman RH. Vascularity of the carpus. Clin Orthop Relat Res. 2001;383:47–59.
6. Gelberman RH, Bauman TD, Menon J, Akeson WH. The vascularity of the lunate bone and Kienböck's disease. J Hand Surg [Am]. 1980;5(3):272–8.
7. Hulten O. Uber Anatomische Variationen der Hand Gelenkknochen. Acta Radiol. 1928;9:155–69.
8. Mirabello SC, Rosenthal DI, Smith RJ. Correlation of clinical and radiographic findings in Kienböck's disease. J Hand Surg [Am]. 1987;12(6):1049–54.
9. Tsuge S, Nakamura R. Anatomical risk factors for Kienböck's disease. J Hand Surg [Br]. 1993;18(1):70–5.
10. Armistead RB, Linsheid RL, Dobyns JH, Beckenbaugh RD. Ulnar lengthening in the treatment of Kienböck's disease. J Bone Joint Surg Am. 1982;64(2):170–8.
11. Beckenbaugh RD, Schieves TC, Dobyns JH, Linsheid RL. Kienböck's disease: The natural history of Kienböck's disease and consideration of lunate fractures. Clin Orthop Relat Res. 1980;149:98–106.
12. Chen WS, Shih CH. Ulnar variance and Kienböck's disease: an investigation in Taiwan. Clin Orthop Relat Res. 1990;255:124–7.

13. Gelberman RH, Salaman PB, Jurist JM, Posch JL. Ulnar variance in Kienböck's disease. J Bone Joint Surg Am. 1975;57(5):674–6.
14. D'Hoore K, DeSmet L, Verellen K, Vral J, Fabry G. Negative ulnar variance is not a risk factor for Kienböck's disease. J Hand Surg [Am]. 1994;19(2):229–31.
15. Nakamura R, Imaeda T, Miura T. Radial shortening for Kienböck's disease: Factors affecting the operative result. J Hand Surg [Br]. 1990;15(1):40–5.
16. Lichtman DM, Mack GR, MacDonald RI, Gunther SF, Wilson JN. Kienböck's disease: the role of silicone replacement arthroplasty. J Bone Joint Surg Am. 1977;59(7):899–908.
17. Keith PP, Nuttall D, Trail I. Long-term outcome of nonsurgically managed Kienbock's disease. J Hand Surg [Am]. 2004;29(1):63–7.
18. Bozentka D, Beredjiklan P. Kienbock's Disease. Orthopedic Knowledge Online Journal. 2007;5(1):1–45.
19. Trumble T, Glisson RR, Seaver AV, Urbaniak JR. A biomechanical comparison of the methods for treating Kienböck's disease. J Hand Surg [Am]. 1986;11(1):88–93.
20. Horii E, Garcia-Elias M, Bishop AT, Cooney WP, Linscheid RL, Chao EY. Effect on force transmission across the carpus in procedures used to treat Kienböck's disease. J Hand Surg [Am]. 1990;15(3):393–400.
21. Matsui Y, Funakoshi T, Motomiya M, Urita A, Minami M, Iwasaki N. Radial shortening osteotomy for Kienbock disease: minimum 10-year follow-up. J Hand Surg [Am]. 2014;39(4):679–85.
22. Ebrahimzadeh MH, Moradi A, Vahedi E, Kachooei AR. Mid-term clinical outcome of radial shortening for kienbock disease. J Res Med Sci. 2015;20(2):146–9.
23. Quenzer DE, Dobyns JH, Linscheid RL, Trail IA, Vidal MA. Radial recession osteotomy for Kienböck's disease. J Hand Surg [Am]. 1997;22(3):386–95.
24. Weiss AP, Weiland A, Moore R. Radial shortening osteotomy for Kienböck's disease. J Bone Joint Surg Am. 1991;73:384–91.
25. Rock MG, Roth JH, Martin L. Radial shortening osteotomy for treatment of Kienböck's disease. J Hand Surg [Am]. 1991;16(3):454–60.
26. Viola RW, Piser PK, Bach AW, Hanel DP, Tencer AF. Biomechanical analysis of capitate shortening with capitate hamate fusion in the treatment of Kienböck's disease. J Hand Surg [Am]. 1998;23(3):395–401.
27. Hanel D, Hunt T. Capitate shortening osteotomy. Atlas Hand Clin. 1999;4(2):45–58.
28. Almquist EE. Capitate shortening in the treatment of Kienböck's disease. Hand Clin. 1993;9(3):505–12.
29. Rhee PC, Lin IC, Moran SL, Bishop AT, Shin AY. Scaphocapitate arthrodesis for Kienbock disease. J Hand Surg [Am]. 2015;40(4):745–51.
30. Xu Y, Li C, Zhou T, Su Y, He X, Fan X, et al. Treatment of aseptic necrosis of the lunate bone (Kienbock disease) using a nickel-titanium memory alloy arthrodesis concentrator: a series of 24 cases. Medicine (Baltimore). 2015;94(42):e1760.
31. Rhee PC, Jones DB, Moran SL, Shin AY. The effect of lunate morphology in Kienbock disease. J Hand Surg [Am]. 2015;40(4):738–44.
32. Chim H, Moran SL. Long-term outcomes of proximal row carpectomy: a systematic review of the literature. J Wrist Surg. 2012;1(2):141–8.
33. DiDonna ML, Kiefhaber T, Stern P. Proximal row carpectomy: Study with a minimum of ten years of followup. J Bone Joint Surg Am. 2004;86(11):2359–65.

De Quervain's Syndrome

35

Adam Martin and Hisham M. Awan

Introduction

- First described in 1895 by Fritz De Quervain, a Swiss general surgeon, when he reported on several patients who had painful, thickened first dorsal compartments.
- De Quervain's syndrome is a common cause of radial-sided wrist pain. It is defined as a stenosing tenosynovitis of the tendons in the first dorsal compartment of the wrist, namely, abductor pollicis longus (APL) and extensor pollicis brevis (EPB).

Anatomy

- The extensor tendons of the wrist are divided into six compartments based on synovial sheaths that extend from the overlying extensor retinaculum. The contents of each compartment from radial to ulnar, with their respective commonly associated pathology, are as follows:
  - I: APL, EPB – De Quervain's syndrome
  - II: ERCL, ECRB – Intersection syndrome
  - III: EPL – Chronic rupture in non-displaced distal radius fractures
  - IV: EIP, EDC – Middorsal wrist pain in piano players
  - V: EDM – Vaughn Jackson syndrome
  - VI: ECU – Snapping ECU syndrome
- First dorsal compartment
  - Contains APL and EPB which run through a rigid tunnel.
  - Base of tunnel is formed by a groove in the radial styloid, whereas roof to tunnel is formed by extensor retinaculum.
  - APL – larger, has multiple slips.
  - EPB – smaller, more dorsal, more distal muscle belly, and often contained within own subcompartment.

Pathophysiology

- Inflammation in the first dorsal compartment causes thickening of the overlying extensor retinaculum with resultant narrowing of the compartment. The narrowing then causes pain as the APL and EPB tendons become entrapped when moving through a confined space.
- De Quervain's syndrome is more common in women, particularly antepartum or postpartum, possibly due to increased fluid volume states or the combination of thumb abduction with wrist ulnar deviation when supporting a baby's head, respectively.

A. Martin, MD
Warren Alpert Medical School,
Brown University, Providence, RI, USA

H.M. Awan, MD (✉)
Hand and Upper Extremity Center,
The Ohio State University Wexner Medical Center,
Columbus, OH, USA
e-mail: hisham.awan@osumc.edu

© Springer International Publishing AG 2017
A.E.M. Eltorai et al. (eds.), *Orthopedic Surgery Clerkship*, DOI 10.1007/978-3-319-52567-9_35

- Repetitive motion (golfers, racquet sports, holding a baby's head), increased fluid volume, inflammatory disease, anatomic variations, and trauma have all been considered possible etiologies for this syndrome.

Clinical Evaluation

History

- Important to obtain and document handedness, occupation, and possible mechanism of injury.
- Patients commonly present with radial-sided wrist pain that is exacerbated by grasping and lifting objects.

Physical Exam

- Patients have tenderness to palpation over the first dorsal compartment, particularly in the area of the radial styloid. This differs from intersection syndrome in which tenderness is around 5 cm proximal to wrist joint.
- There are two common provocative maneuvers consistent with this syndrome.
  - Eichoff maneuver: commonly mistaken as Finkelstein's test
    ◦ Patient grasps thumb inside of a clenched fist, and ulnar deviates the wrist. A positive test will recreate the patient's pain.
  - Finkelstein maneuver
    ◦ Examiner grasps the patient's thumb and deviates the wrist ulnarly. Again, a positive test will reproduce the patient's pain.

Differential Diagnosis

- Radial styloid fracture – similar area of tenderness but provocative tests would be negative and would see fracture on radiographs.
- Scaphoid fracture – area of tenderness would be slightly distal in the anatomic snuffbox, provocative tests negative, and may see frac-

ture on radiographs depending on chronicity of fracture.
- Radioscaphoid arthritis – provocative tests negative and radiographs would reveal arthritic changes.
- Thumb carpometacarpal arthritis – provocative tests negative and radiographs would reveal arthritic changes.
- Intersection syndrome – tenderness 5 cm proximal to radiocarpal joint and pain with resisted wrist extension and thumb extension.

Radiographic Evaluation

- Anteroposterior (AP) and lateral views of wrist should be obtained to rule out differential diagnoses such as fractures.

Treatment

Nonoperative Management: First-Line Therapy

- Includes rest, NSAIDs, steroid injections, and removable thumb spica wrist splint
- Corticosteroid injection
  - Effective treatment option in 50–80% of patients but less effective in diabetes
  - Method:
    ◦ Palpate the first dorsal compartment tendons by placing them on stretch via thumb abduction and extension
    ◦ Clean injection site with alcohol swab, then inject lidocaine with corticosteroid into tendon sheath while keeping the needle parallel to tendons
  - Complications:
    ◦ Radial sensory neuritis, tendon attenuation, subcutaneous fat atrophy, and skin hypopigmentation

Operative Management

- Indicated when conservative management fails to provide relief

- Procedure:
  - Approximately 1 cm proximal to radial styloid, a 2-cm transverse skin incision is made over first dorsal compartment. Then use blunt longitudinal dissection to identify and protect branches of the superficial radial nerve. In general, if looking for a longitudinal structure, one should spread longitudinally in-line with that structure.
  - Incise compartment sheath on most dorsal edge to leave a palmar flap to prevent palmar subluxation of the tendons.
  - Identify both tendons, identify all tendon slips as it's common for APL to have multiple slips, and release all intervening septa.

  - ○ If gentle traction on a tendon results in passive extension of the thumb metacarpophalangeal joint, then EPB has been successfully identified.
  - Use a blunt retractor to elevate the tendons out of the tunnel to assess for complete decompression.
- Postoperative management
  - Apply bulky, soft sterile dressing. Patient may begin immediate thumb motion as tolerated.
- Complications
  - Inadequate release of the first dorsal compartment
  - Injury to superficial radial nerve branches
  - Complex regional pain syndrome
  - Palmar subluxation of APL or EPB

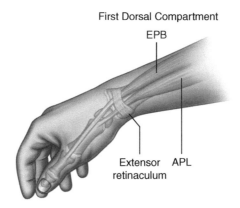

First Dorsal Compartment

EPB

Extensor   APL
retinaculum

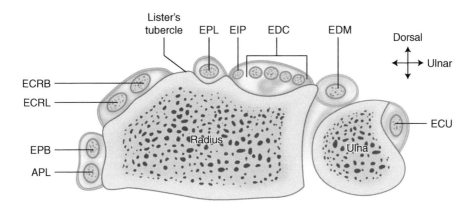

6 Extensor Compartments of the Wrist

Lister's
tubercle EPL EIP   EDC   EDM

Dorsal

Ulnar

ECRB

ECRL

ECU

EPB

APL

Radius

Ulna

References

1. Dodds SD, et al. Tendon. In: Hammert WC, editor. ASSH manual of hand surgery. Philadelphia: Lippincott Williams & Wilkins; 2010. p. 255–63. Print

2. Wolfe SW. Tendinopathy. In: Wolfe SW, et al., editors. Green's operative hand surgery. 6th ed. Philadelphia: Churchill Livingstone; 2010.

3. Brunton LM, et al. "Hand, upper extremity, and microvascular surgery". Review of orthopedics. 6th ed. Miller MD, et al. editor. Elsevier Saunders: 2012.

Dupuytren Disease (Contracture) 36

Steven R. Niedermeier and Hisham M. Awan

Dupuytren Disease (Contracture)

- *Anatomy* [1, 2]:
  - Disease of normal fascial bands in the hand that become pathologic nodules and cords (of collagen) creating flexion contractures.
  - Myofibroblasts and cytokines are implicated in this proliferative disorder.
  - *Spiral cord:*
    - ○ Responsible for proximal interphalangeal (PIP) joint contracture (most clinically relevant).
    - ○ Runs beneath the neurovascular bundle in the digits causing central and superficial displacement. This can place the neurovascular bundle at risk during surgical management.
  - *Central cord:*
    - ○ Causes metacarpal phalangeal (MCP) joint contracture
  - *Retrovascular cord:*
    - ○ Causes distal interphalangeal (DIP) joint contracture
    - ○ Can also displace neurovascular bundle

- *Staging:*
  - *Histopathologic staging (Luck)* [1, 2]:
    - ○ *Proliferative stage:* hypercellular (predominantly myofibroblasts)
    - ○ *Involutional stage:* transition from type I to type III collagen
    - ○ *Residual stage:* predominantly fibrocytes
  - *Clinical staging* [3]:
    - ○ *Phase I (early)*: skin changes, loss of normal architecture, and pitting of the skin
    - ○ *Phase II (intermediate):* presence of nodules and cords
    - ○ *Phase III (late):* joint and soft tissue contracture
- *Presentation* [1–3]:
  - *Epidemiology:*
    - ○ Northern European heritage.
    - ○ Incidence increases with age.
    - ○ Associated conditions: HIV, diabetes, and alcoholism.
  - *Mechanism:*
    - ○ Normal fascial bands become diseased cords. These cords shorten and cause soft tissue and joint contractures. Subsequent joint deformity and capsuloligamentous contracture lead to flexion contracture of the MCP and PIP joints.
  - *Physical exam:*
    - ○ Decreased range of motion (ROM) and flexion contracture.

S.R. Niedermeier, MD • H.M. Awan, MD (✉)
Hand and Upper Extremity Center,
The Ohio State University Wexner Medical Center,
Columbus, OH, USA
e-mail: hisham.awan@osumc.edu

© Springer International Publishing AG 2017
A.E.M. Eltorai et al. (eds.), *Orthopedic Surgery Clerkship*, DOI 10.1007/978-3-319-52567-9_36

- ○ Superficial palmar thickening and palpable cords.
- ○ Painful nodules.
- ○ Affect activities of daily living (ADLs).
- ○ Most commonly affect ring and small fingers.
- ○ *Hueston tabletop test*: patient places hand on table palm down to observe MCP or PIP contracture (Fig. 36.1).
- • *Surgical indications* [5]:
  - – Patients with MCP joint contractures of at least 30° and/or any PIP joint contractures with concomitant functional deficiency.
  - – Painful nodules are not a surgical indication.
- • *Nonoperative interventions* [3, 5]:
  - – Observation for patients with stable disease who have minimal contracture without affecting ADLs.
  - – Physical therapy, corticosteroid injections, and topical vitamin A and E have been found to be ineffective.
  - – Collagenase injections into diseased cords have proven efficacious when compared to placebo. However, high complication rates have been well documented with recurrence rates comparable to those seen in surgical interventions.
- • *Operative interventions* [5]:
  - – *Needle aponeurotomy* [6]:
    - ○ A needle is inserted percutaneously over the length of cord to incise it. This weakens the cord so that subsequent extension forces applied can rupture the cord.

- ○ Typically used in elderly patients with multiple comorbidities because it can allow for immediate increase in finger extension and can be done under local anesthesia.
- – *Palmar fasciectomy:*
  - ○ Region (subtotal) fasciectomy is the gold standard for surgical treatment of Dupuytren disease (Figs. 36.2 and 36.3).
  - ○ Dissection and excision of the involved diseased fascia.
  - ○ Multiple skin incision techniques can be utilized including Bruner, multiple V–Y advancement flaps, and a longitudinal incision closed with Z-plasties.
  - ○ *Postoperative care:* patient's hand and wrist are splinted with the MCP and PIP joints in extension. After 5–7 days, the splint is removed and early ROM is encouraged with night extension splinting with a removable brace.
- – *Radical (total) fasciectomy:*
  - ○ Dissection and excision of involved and uninvolved palmar and digital fascia
  - ○ Fallen out of favor due to no difference in recurrence rates when compared to other surgical options and high complication rate
- – *Open palm (McCash) technique:*
  - ○ A transverse incision is made over the distal palmar crease, which can be left open to heal via secondary intention or closed with delayed skin grafting.
  - ○ Useful in older patients, especially those prone to stiffness.

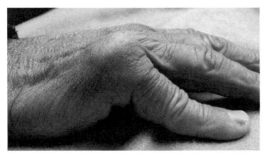

Fig. 36.1 Example of a left small finger MCP joint flexion contracture observed when performing the Hueston tabletop test [4]

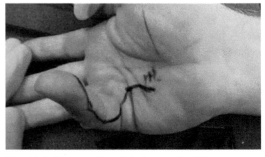

Fig. 36.2 Preoperative clinical example of Dupuytren disease causing a significant flexion contracture at the MCP joint of the right small finger

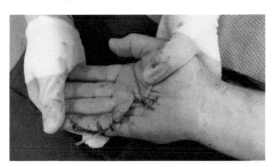

Fig. 36.3 Postoperative clinical example of a return to neutral extension of the right small finger MCP joint after a palmar fasciectomy with primary closure and a Penrose drain in place

– *Complications:*
  ◦ *Hematoma:*
    • Most common complication
    • Implicated in wound healing complications and skin necrosis
  ◦ *Recurrence:*
    • Reported up to 50% of cases. Recurrence has been implicated in level of dissection/excision during index procedure,

extent of disease on presentation; however, no correlation was found between incision type and recurrence.
  ◦ *Neurovascular injury:*
    • Can be avoided with careful dissection and identification of neurovascular structures

References

1. Black EM, Blazar PE. Dupuytren disease: an evolving understanding of an age-old disease. J Am Acad Orthop Surg. 2011;19(12):746–57.
2. Benson LS, Williams CS, Kahle M. Dupuytren's contracture. J Am Acad Orthop Surg. 1998;6(1):24–35.
3. Hammert WC, Calfee RP, Bozentka DJ, Boyer MI. ASSH manual of hand surgery. 1st ed. Philadelphia: Lippincott Williams & Wilkins; 2010 .Print
4. Kam CC, Kaplan TD. Injectable collagenase for the treatment of Dupuytren contracture: a critical analysis review. JBJS Rev. 2013;1(2):e5.
5. Desai SS, Hentz VR. The treatment of Dupuytren disease. J Hand Surg Am. 2011;36A:936–42.
6. Eaton C. Percutaneous fasciotomy for Dupuytren's contracture. J Hand Surg Am. 2011;36A:910–5.

Trigger Digit

37

Yoseph A. Rosenbaum and Hisham M. Awan

Overview

- Stenosing tenosynovitis, or trigger digit, is a common phenomenon.
- Affects women more than men.
- Occurs when tendons do not glide smoothly through their corresponding pulleys due to volume mismatch.
- Leads to symptoms of locking, catching, popping, or "triggering" of the involved digit during motion.
- Pediatric trigger thumb is a fundamentally different clinical entity:
  - Involves developmental growth differential between tendon and pulley

Anatomy

- System of cruciate and annular pulleys are thickenings of the fibro-osseous sheath.
- Closely adherent to metacarpals and phalanges.
- Maintain the biomechanical advantage for the flexor tendons and prevent bowstringing:

Y.A. Rosenbaum, MD • H.M. Awan, MD (✉)
Hand and Upper Extremity Center,
The Ohio State University Wexner Medical Center,
Columbus, OH, USA
e-mail: hisham.awan@osumc.edu

- "Bowstringing" is when tendons lacking the constraint of their corresponding pulleys drift away from the center of rotation of the joint they act upon and lose their mechanical advantage.
- FDS and FDP tendons pass through the more proximal pulleys before FDS splits at level of proximal phalangeal neck.
- A1 pulley at the level of the metacarpal head is most commonly involved.

Adult Trigger Finger

- The ring finger and thumb are most commonly affected.
- Most commonly involved in trigger finger is A1 pulley at volar aspect of metacarpal head:
  - Other potential sources of entrapment are rare but do exist:
    ° A3 pulley, seen with FDP enlargement
    ° Camper's chiasm (FDS decussation), seen in RA
- Trigger thumb involves the A1 pulley:
  - Mimickers include de Quervain's disease and EPL entrapment.
- Nearby pulleys are thought to be vital for preventing bowstringing:
  - A2 pulley in digits /A4
  - Oblique pulley in the thumb

© Springer International Publishing AG 2017
A.E.M. Eltorai et al. (eds.), *Orthopedic Surgery Clerkship*, DOI 10.1007/978-3-319-52567-9_37

Classification

- Patel and Moradia – 1997
  - Stage 1 – uneven movement and no clicking
  - Stage 2 – clicking present without locking
  - Stage 3 – locking present during active or passive motion
  - Stage 4 – locked and unable to be unlocked

Treatment

- Mainstay of initial treatment is splinting and/ or steroid injection for adults:
  - Steroid injections curative in anywhere from 60 to 90% of patients:
    ∘ Multiple injection techniques are described, with no difference in efficacy.
    ∘ Palmar (Fig. 37.1), webspace, and phalangeal approaches described.
  - Less effective in diabetic patients:
- If resistant to conservative therapy, it may be treated with surgical release.
- Surgical release can be done percutaneously or open:
  - Percutaneous: an 18-gauge needle is used to scrape against the pulley fibers (Fig. 37.2):

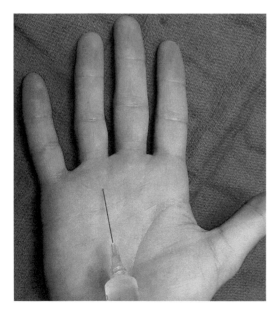

Fig. 37.1 The palmar proximal approach for steroid injections of the ring finger as administered in trigger finger

∘ Has a high initial learning curve
∘ Quick procedure and may be done in office under local anesthesia
∘ Not recommended for use in trigger thumbs
  - Open release (Figs. 37.3 and 37.4):
    ∘ Low complication rates but a somewhat high rate of patient dissatisfaction.
    ∘ May also be done wide awake with local anesthesia and no tourniquet (WALANT).
    ∘ A2 pulley must be avoided in surgical release to prevent bowstringing; however, up to 25% of it may be released safely.
    ∘ Oblique pulley in the thumb must be avoided to prevent bowstringing.
    ∘ Thumb trigger release carries elevated risk of radial > ulnar digital nerve injury.
- Pediatric trigger thumb is thought to be less responsive to conservative treatment and may lead to joint stiffness if ignored.

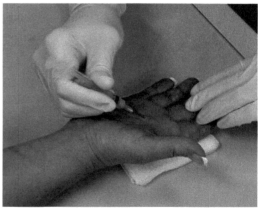

Fig. 37.2 Demonstrates a percutaneous trigger finger release being performed

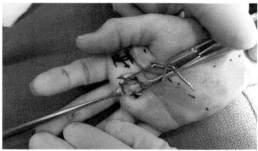

Fig. 37.3 Demonstrates an intraoperative look at the flexor tendon

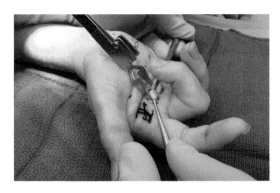

Fig. 37.4 Demonstrates the flexor tendons following complete release, being pulled through the incision and flexing the digit

- Is more often treated with early surgical release.
- Recent studies have demonstrated good response to conservative treatment:
  ◦ However, these studies are small and high level of investment is demanded of the parents.

Complications: Rare

- Stiffness

- Recurrence
- Pain
- Digital nerve injury
- Infection
- Tendon laceration
- Digital artery aneurysm

Suggested Readings

1. Bauer AS, Bae DS. Pediatric trigger digits. J Hand Surg Am. 2015;40(11):2304–9.
2. Patel MR, Moradia VJ. Percutaneous release of trigger digit with and without cortisone injection. J Hand Surg Am. 1997;22(1):150–5.
3. Chang J, Noland S, Adams JE, Mass DP, Seiler III JG, Taras JS, Trueblood A, Botte MJ, Kalainov DM, Johnson RC, Lauder AJ, Wolf JM. In: Hammert WC, editor. "Tendon." ASSH Manual of Hand Surgery. Philadelphia: Lippincott Williams & Wilkins; 2010. p. 93–110.
4. Wolfe SW. In: Wolfe SW, et al., editors. "Tendinopathy." green's operative hand surgery. 6th ed. Philadelphia: Churchill Livingstone; 2010.
5. Fahey JJ, Bollinger JA. Trigger-finger in adults and children. J Bone Joint Surg Am. 1954;36-A(6):1200–18.
6. Jung HJ, Lee JS, Song KS, Yang JJ. Conservative treatment of pediatric trigger thumb: Follow-up for over 4 years. J Hand Surg Eur Vol. 2012;37(3):2204.

Scaphoid Fractures

38

Andrew Campbell and Hisham M. Awan

Anatomy

- 80% cartilage – covered
- Limited vascularity:
  - Blood supply is retrograde from dorsal carpal branch of radial artery.
  - Limited hematoma and callus formation after fracture.
- Acts as a tie rod, linking the proximal and distal carpal rows, resulting in high forces across the bone

Demographics

- Most common carpal fracture (1–120/100,000)
- Low prevalence of true fractures among suspected fractures
- Majority in young adult males

A. Campbell, MD • H.M. Awan, MD (✉)
Hand Upper Extremty Center, The Ohio State
University Wexner Medical Center,
Columbus, OH, USA
e-mail: hisham.awan@osumc.edu

Presentation

- Mechanism:
  - Fall on extended, radially deviated wrist
    ○ Scaphoid levers on radioscaphocapitate ligament
  - Direct blow
- Snuffbox tenderness is classic.
- Pain may be subtle or non-specific:
  - Pain with thumb axial load, pinching the thumb and index finger, wrist pronation, and radial deviation

Imaging

- Radiography:
  - Often misses acute fracture.
  - Only 50% sensitive and 80% specific at detecting displacement.
  - High clinical suspicion should prompt serial radiographs or advanced imaging.
- Advanced imaging:
  - MRI
    ○ 98% sensitive, 99% specific
    ○ Detects concomitant ligamentous wrist injuries (e.g., scapholunate injuries)
  - CT
    ○ 94% sensitive, 96% specific
    ○ Useful for tracking fracture union

© Springer International Publishing AG 2017
A.E.M. Eltorai et al. (eds.), *Orthopedic Surgery Clerkship*, DOI 10.1007/978-3-319-52567-9_38

Classification

- By anatomy:
  - Waist (65%), proximal pole (25%), distal pole (10%)
- Stable:
  - Displaced <1 mm, normal intercarpal alignment, distal pole fractures
- Unstable:
  - Displaced >1 mm, comminuted, lateral intrascaphoid angle >35°, proximal pole fracture, perilunate fracture or dislocation

Treatment

Non-operative

- Indications:
  - Stable tubercle or distal pole fractures
  - Stable waist fractures (90–95% union rate with casting)

- Superiority of long- versus short-arm casting and thumb spica casting is inconclusive.
- Ultrasound bone stimulator may improve time to union.

Operative

- Indications:
  - Unstable (displaced, proximal pole)
  - Complex (open, perilunate, greater arc injury)
  - Polytrauma
  - Faster return to work or sport
- Treatment options:
  - Compression screws (see Figs. 38.1 and 38.2)

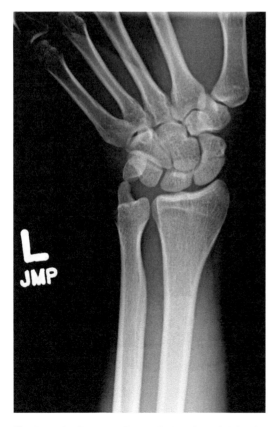

Fig. 38.1 Radiograph of a nondisplaced scaphoid waist fracture

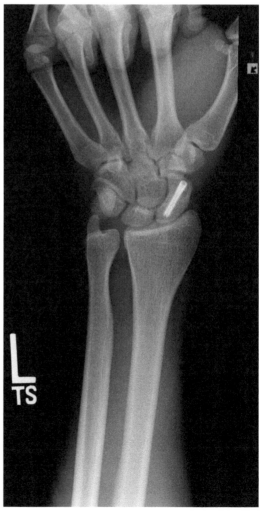

Fig. 38.2 Scaphoid fracture treated with percutaneous screw fixation

- – Central placement, longer, wider diameter more stable
- – Kirschner wire, plate, bioabsorbable implant fixation less common
- Approach:
  - – Open or percutaneous
  - – Dorsal or volar

Complications

- Delayed union/nonunion:
  - – More common after proximal pole fractures
  - – May require revision open reduction internal fixation with cancellous, corticocancellous, or vascularized bone grafting
- Avascular necrosis
- Humpback deformity
- Scaphoid nonunion advanced collapse (SNAC)

Suggested Readings

1. Doornberg JN, Buijze GA, Ham SJ, Ring D, Bhandari M, Poolman RW. Nonoperative treatment for acute scaphoid fractures: a systematic review and meta-analysis of randomized controlled trials. J Trauma. 2011;71(4):1073–81.
2. Geissler WB, Slade JF. Fractures of the Carpal Bones. In: Wolfe SW, Pederson WC, Hotchkiss RN, Kozen SH, editors. Green's Operative Hand Surgery. 6th ed. Philadelphia: Churchill Livingstone; 2010.
3. Hughes T. Scaphoid Fractures/Nonunions: ASSH Comprehensive Review Lecture. Presented at American Association of Hand Surgeons Annual Meeting, 10 January 2014, Kauai, Hawaii.
4. Temple CL, Ross DC, Bennett JD, Garvin GJ, King GJ, Faber KJ. Comparison of sagittal computed tomography and plain film radiography in scaphoid fracture model. J Hand Surg Am. 2005;30(3):534–42.
5. VanTassel DC, Owens BD, Wolf JM. Incidence estimates and demographics of scaphoid fracture in the US population. J Hand Surg Am. 2010;35A:1242–5.
6. Wolf JM, Dawson L, Mountcastle SB, Owens BD. The incidence of scaphoid fracture in a military population. Injury. 2009;40(12):1316–9.

Thumb Ulnar Collateral Ligament Injuries (Gamekeeper's and Skier's Thumb)

39

Andrew Campbell and Hisham M. Awan

Eponyms

- Gamekeeper's thumb: chronic thumb ulnar collateral ligament (UCL) injury
- Skier's thumb: acute thumb UCL injury

Anatomy

- UCL provides support against valgus stress and volar subluxation of the metacarpophalangeal (MCP) joint
- UCL composed of two bands
  - Proper collateral ligament
    - Taut in 30 degrees of flexion at MCP joint
  - Accessory collateral ligament
    - Taut when MCP joint in full extension
    - Inserts on the palmar plate

Presentation

- Mechanism
  - Hyperextension or hyperabduction at thumb MCP joint
- Pain over ulnar aspect of MCP joint
- Weak pinch/grip strength
- Palpable mass
  - Stener lesion – adductor aponeurosis interposed between torn UCL and MCP joint, preventing healing
- Laxity with valgus stress at MCP joint
  - Test proper collateral ligament at 30 degrees of MCP joint flexion.
  - Test accessory collateral ligament in full MCP joint extension.
  - Compare to the contralateral thumb.
  - Suspect complete tear if:
    - >35° opening with valgus stress
    - >20° variability between hands
  - Exam may require articular block to prevent guarding.

Imaging

- Radiography/fluoroscopy
  - Bony avulsion.
  - Volar subluxation.
  - Stress views may be helpful.
- MRI
  - Most sensitive and specific

A. Campbell, MD
Hand Upper Extremity Center, The Ohio State University Wexner Medical Center, Columbus, OH, USA

H.M. Awan, MD (✉)
Hand and Upper Extremities, The Ohio State University, 281 W. Lane Ave., Columbus 43210, OH, USA
e-mail: hisham.awan@osumc.edu

- Indicated only when examination is equivocal
- Ultrasound
  - Less expensive than MRI but operator dependent

Treatment

Nonoperative

- Indications
  - Acute, partial-thickness tear
  - Chronic tear
- Techniques
  - Immobilization in thumb spica splint for 4–6 weeks, followed by therapy with range of motion and strengthening exercises
- Variably successful in acute, full-thickness tears

Operative

- Indications
  - Acute, complete rupture.
  - Displaced avulsion fracture.
  - Stener lesion occurs in 64–88% of complete UCL ruptures.
- Techniques
  - Repair
    ° Indications

- Acute, complete UCL tears
- Displaced bony avulsion
  ° Considerations
  - UCL usually tears at insertion on proximal phalanx.
  ° Techniques
  - Suture, suture anchors
- Reconstruction
  ° Indications
  - Chronic injuries refractory to nonoperative management
  ° Techniques
  - Dynamic stabilization with tendon transfers — *Graft w/ Bone tunnels*
  - Adductor aponeurosis advancement
  - Static reconstruction with tendon autograft
- Arthrodesis
  ° Indication
  - Salvage for chronic UCL instability and painful MCPJ arthrosis

---

Suggested Reading

1. Rhee PC, et al. Management of thumb metacarpophalangeal joint ulnar collateral ligament injuries: current concepts review. JBJS. 2012;94:2005–12.
2. Merrell G, Slade JF. Dislocations and ligament injuries in the digits. In: Wolfe SW, et al. Green's operative hand surgery. 6th ed. Philadelphia: Churchill Livingstone; 2010.

Peri-lunate and Lunate Dislocations

40

Amy Speeckaert and Hisham M. Awan

Anatomy

- The carpus consists of a proximal and distal row of bones stabilized with both ligamentous connections and capsular attachments.
- Traumatic disruption of these ligaments and capsular attachments occurs in a well-described stepwise fashion defined by the *Mayfield classification* (Fig. 40.1).
- Mayfield *Stages I and II* produce *carpal instability*, while *Stage III* results in a *peri-lunate dislocation*, and *Stage IV* results in a *lunate dislocation*.
- In a lunate dislocation, the lunate remains attached to the carpus only by the *short radiolunate ligament*.

Classification

- Injuries that involve purely ligamentous injuries are called *lesser arc injuries.*

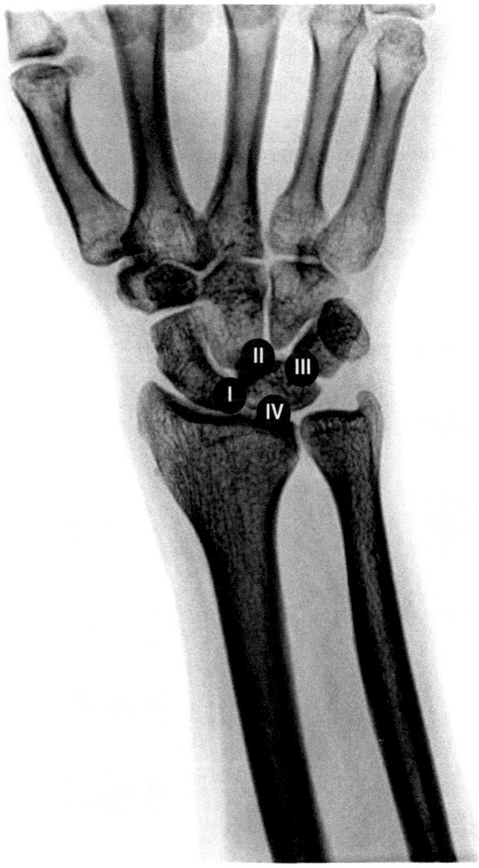

Fig. 40.1 Mayfield classification of peri-lunate dislocations. *Stage I*: Scapholunate ligament disruption. *Stage II*: Lunocapitate disruption. *Stage III*: Lunotriquetral disruption with peri-lunate dislocation. *Stage IV*: Long radiolunate disruption with lunate dislocation

A. Speeckaert, MD • H.M. Awan, MD (✉)
Hand and Upper Extremity Center, The Ohio State University Wexner Medical Center,
Columbus, OH, USA
e-mail: hisham.awan@osumc.edu

© Springer International Publishing AG 2017
A.E.M. Eltorai et al. (eds.), *Orthopedic Surgery Clerkship*, DOI 10.1007/978-3-319-52567-9_40

- Injuries that involve bony injury as well are termed *greater arc injuries* and are further classified by location of the associated fracture (*transradial styloid, trans-scaphoid, trans-capitate, or trans-triquetral peri-lunate fracture dislocations*)

Presentation and Diagnosis

- Timely diagnosis requires a heightened alert as these injuries, especially in the setting of high energy trauma or a fall from height, are commonly missed on initial presentation.
- Careful review of posteroanterior (PA) radiographs demonstrates disruption of *Gilula's arcs* and associated fractures in a greater arc injury (Fig. 40.2).
- Lateral film demonstrates incongruity of lunocapitate articulation in a peri-lunate dislocation ("*empty or spilled teacup appearance*") and a volarly displaced lunate in a lunate dislocation (Fig. 40.3).

- Most common pattern of dislocation is dorsal translation of the carpus with a volarly displaced lunate, although the opposite has been reported.
- A thorough neurovascular exam should be performed with attention to median nerve symptoms as an *acute carpal tunnel syndrome* may occur.

Treatment

Closed Reduction

- Initial treatment involves closed reduction and splinting and assessment of median nerve symptoms.
- Prolonged or worsening carpal tunnel symptoms at any point in time necessitate an urgent carpal tunnel release.
- Closed reduction of a peri-lunate dislocation is performed with adequate analgesia, axial traction, wrist extension, and a volarly directed force on the carpus.

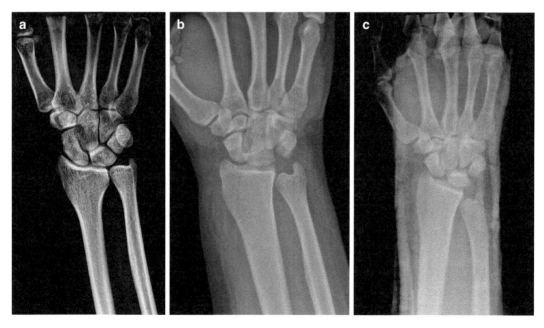

Fig. 40.2 (**a**) Normal appearance of Gilula's arcs in uninjured wrist. (**b**) Disruption of Gilula's arcs on PA radiograph with peri-lunate dislocation. (**c**) Restoration of Gilula's arcs following closed reduction of peri-lunate dislocation

- Closed reduction of a lunate dislocation is performed with adequate analgesia, axial traction, dorsally directed pressure on the lunate with a similar wrist extension, and volarly directed force on the carpus.
- If a concentric closed reduction is obtained, surgical intervention may be delayed until swelling is reduced.

Surgical Stabilization

- The algorithm for surgical intervention is controversial at best.
- In the setting of concentric reduction of the carpus, pinning with Kirschner wires (K-wires) alone is advocated by some.
- In the absence of concentric reduction, open reduction through a dorsal, volar, or combined approach is advocated with repair of the scapholunate ligament and pinning of the carpus with K-wires. Some also advocate repair of the lunotriquetral ligament and dorsal capsulodesis. A carpal tunnel release is performed by some even in the absence of symptoms to prevent delayed presentation of carpal tunnel syndrome.
- Associated fractures are treated simultaneously with a variety of implants including K-wires, screws, and plates (Fig. 40.3).

Postoperative Rehab

- The method of immobilization postoperatively varies from a short arm splint with the wrist in neutral position to long arm immobilization with the wrist in slight extension.
- Immobilization is typically carried out for 8–12 weeks, at which time K-wires are removed and gentle range of motion is initiated.

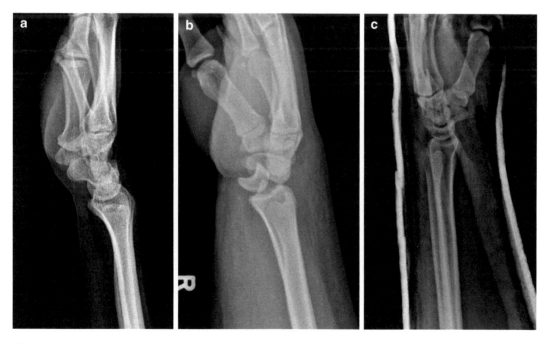

Fig. 40.3 (**a**) Normal appearance capitolunate articulation of lateral radiograph in uninjured wrist. (**b**) "Empty teacup" with capitolunate incongruity in a peri-lunate dislocation. (**c**) Restoration of capitolunate articulation following closed reduction of peri-lunate dislocation

Complications

- Chondrolysis, arthritis, transient lunate ischemia, carpal instability, delayed presentation of carpal tunnel syndrome, stiffness, and fracture nonunion have all been reported.
- Salvage procedures for arthritis, nonunion, and carpal instability are numerous and include partial or complete wrist fusions, proximal row carpectomy, and selective wrist sensory denervations.

Outcomes

- Studies demonstrate that restoration of anatomic carpal alignment is associated with improved outcomes.

- Despite best efforts, however, stiffness, pain, and weakness remain expected outcomes of these injuries.

Suggested Readings

1. Elfar JC, Stanbury SJ. Perilunate dislocation and perilunate fracture-dislocation. J Am Acad Orthop Surg. 2011;19:554–62.
2. Kozin SH. Perilunate injuries: diagnosis and treatment. J Am Acad Orthop Surg. 1998;6:114–20.
3. Lasanianos NG, Giannoudis PV. Greater arc injuries: Perilunate fracture-dislocations. In: Lasanianos NG, Kanakaris NK, Giannoudis PV, editors. Trauma and orthopedic classifications: a comprehensive overview. Greater arc injuries: perilunate fracture-dislocations. New York: Springer; 2015. p. 131–4.
4. Lasanianos NG, Giannoudis PV. Lesser arc injuries: perilunate dislocations. In: Lasanianos NG, Kanakaris NK, Giannoudis PV, editors. New York: Springer; 2015. p. 125–9.

First Metacarpal Base Fractures

41

Amy Speeckaert and Hisham M. Awan

Classification

- Extra-articular fractures
- Bennett fractures
- Rolando fractures

Extra-articular Fractures

Anatomy

- Extra-articular fractures at the base of the thumb metacarpal

Presentation and Diagnosis

- Result of an axially loaded and partially flexed thumb metacarpal.
- Pain and swelling about the base of the thumb.
- Three radiographic views of the thumb are diagnostic.

Treatment

- The thumb carpometacarpal joint is hypermobile, and therefore angular deformity of up to 30° is well tolerated by many.
- Stable fractures with up to 30° of angular deformity may be treated with immobilization of 4 to 6 weeks.
- Stable fractures with greater than 30° of angular deformity may undergo closed reduction and splinting for 6 weeks.
- Unstable or displaced fractures require closed versus open reduction and pinning versus internal fixation.

Postoperative Rehabilitation

- Fractures treated surgically require approximately 6 weeks of immobilization followed by gentle active and passive range of motion (ROM).

Outcomes

- Stiffness from immobilization is a common complication. Due to their extra-articular nature, however, these fractures can be expected to do well with little post-traumatic arthritis.

A. Speeckaert, MD • H.M. Awan, MD (✉)
Hand and Upper Extremity Center, The Ohio State
University Wexner Medical Center, Columbus, OH,
USA
e-mail: hisham.awan@osumc.edu

© Springer International Publishing AG 2017
A.E.M. Eltorai et al. (eds.), *Orthopedic Surgery Clerkship*, DOI 10.1007/978-3-319-52567-9_41

Bennett Fractures

Anatomy

- Intra-articular fracture at the base of the thumb metacarpal with stable volar-ulnar fragment known as the Bennett fragment.
- Bennett fragment does not displace due to the stabilizing force of the anterior oblique ligament which originates on the trapezium and inserts onto the base of the thumb metacarpal (Fig. 41.1).
- The metacarpal shaft displaces radially, proximally, and into a supinated position due to the pull of the adductor pollicis and the abductor pollicis longus.

Presentation and Diagnosis

- Result of an axially loaded and partially flexed thumb metacarpal.
- Pain and swelling about the base of the thumb.

- Three radiographic views of the thumb are diagnostic.
- A hyper-pronated thumb view best demonstrates the degree of fracture displacement.

Treatment

- Historically treated with immobilization, however often went on to develop symptomatic arthritis.
- Now often treated surgically with attempt at achieving a relative anatomic reduction of the base of the thumb metacarpal.
- Reduction may be achieved through both closed and open means.
- Manual reduction is achieved through axial traction, abduction, and pronation of the thumb, reducing the metacarpal to the stable Bennett fragment (Fig. 41.2).

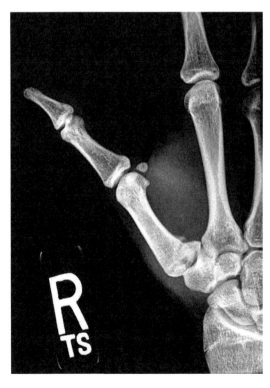

Fig. 41.1 Radiograph of a Bennett fracture, with the fragment clearly visible at the base of the thumb

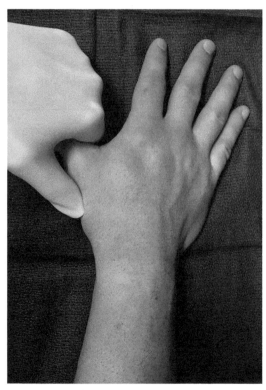

Fig. 41.2 Manual (closed) reduction of the fracture is accomplished with axial traction on the thumb and abduction and extension of the thumb metacarpal. The thumb is pronated to bring it in opposition with the non-displaced palmar fragment

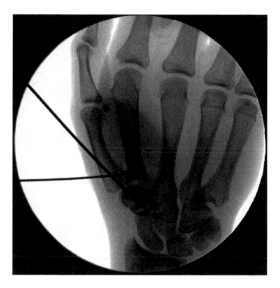

Fig. 41.3 Fluoroscopic view of pin fixation of the fracture. Pins are typically removed after four to six weeks

- Fixation may be achieved with pinning or, in the setting of a large Bennett fragment, screw fixation (Fig. 41.3).

Postoperative Rehabilitation

- Following closed or open reduction with pin fixation, patients are immobilized for approximately 6 weeks, followed by gentle active and passive ROM.
- Screw fixation may allow for earlier mobilization, depending on intraoperative stability as judged by the treating surgeon.

Outcomes

- Post-traumatic arthritis is an expected complication, both in the setting of anatomic and relative anatomic reductions. For this reason, many surgeons accept relative anatomic reductions.

Rolando Fractures

Anatomy

- Intra-articular fracture at the base of the thumb metacarpal with intra-articular

comminution. Despite comminution, a stable volar-ulnar fragment (Bennett fragment) is present and stabilized by the anterior oblique ligament.

Presentation and Diagnosis

- Result of an axially loaded and partially flexed thumb metacarpal.
- Pain and swelling about the base of the thumb.
- Three radiographic views of the thumb are diagnostic.

Treatment

- Nonoperative treatment reserved for low-demand, elderly patients or patients with stable fractures with severe comminution.
- Most Rolando fractures are treated surgically, with closed or open reduction and pinning or ORIF with plates and or screws.

Postoperative Rehabilitation

- Typically 6 weeks of immobilization followed by gentle active and passive ROM

Outcomes

Post-traumatic arthritis is a common and expected complication.

Suggested Reading

1. Giannoudis PV, Kanakaris NK. Open pelvic fractures. In:Lasanianos NG, Kanakaris NK, Giannoudis PV, editors. Green's Operative Hand Surgery, 6th edition. New York: Springer; 2011. p. 283–7.

Non-scaphoid Carpal Bone Fractures

42

Joseph Meyerson and Hisham M. Awan

General Anatomy

- Proximal carpal row (from radial to ulnar)
  - Scaphoid, lunate, triquetrum, and pisiform
- Distal carpal row (from radial to ulnar)
  - Trapezium, trapezoid, capitate, and hamate

Incidence of Fractures

- Carpal fractures account for approximately 8–19% of all hand fractures.
- The non-scaphoid carpal bones account for 30–40% of all carpal bone fractures.
- The incidence from highest to least in percentage of carpal bone fractures:
  - Triquetrum > trapezium > capitate > hamate > pisiform > lunate > trapezoid

J. Meyerson, MD
Department of Plastic Surgery,
The Ohio State University, Columbus, OH, USA

H.M. Awan, MD (✉)
Hand and Upper Extremity Center,
The Ohio State University Wexner Medical Center,
Columbus, OH, USA
e-mail: hisham.awan@osumc.edu

Triquetrum

- Incidence – 15–18% of all carpal bone fractures
  - Second most common carpal fracture after the scaphoid, often associated with perilunate fracture dislocation

Fracture Pattern

- Dorsal cortex (most common, 93% incidence)
- Body
- Volar cortex

Diagnosis

- History of fall on outstretched hand or axial load with point tenderness over ulnar wrist

Radiographs

- Standard films (posteroanterior (PA), lateral, and 45-degree pronated oblique) and radial wrist deviation
- CT scan for occult fractures and MRI scans for occult fractures and ligamentous injury

© Springer International Publishing AG 2017   183
A.E.M. Eltorai et al. (eds.), *Orthopedic Surgery Clerkship*, DOI 10.1007/978-3-319-52567-9_42

Treatment

- Immobilization of 4–6 weeks for nondisplaced dorsal cortex fracture or body fracture.
- Displaced, volar cortex fracture and associated LT ligament injury may require surgical fixation.

Complications

- Undiagnosed injury can lead to carpal instability and pisotriquetral arthritis.

Trapezium

- Incidence – 3–5% of all carpal bone fractures
  - Fractures often occur with fractures of the distal radius or first metacarpal, rarely isolated.

Fracture Pattern

- Palmar ridge
  - Type I – base of the bone
  - Type II – tip of the bone
- Body fracture
  - Vertical, horizontal, dorsoradial, and comminuted tuberosity

Diagnosis

- Present with point tenderness at the base of the thumb and a weakened, painful pinch
- Pain with resisted wrist flexion from flexor carpi radialis tendon proximity to the fracture

Radiographs: Standard Wrist Radiographs Often Not Adequate

- Bett's view (elbow raised, thumb extended/abducted, partially pronated) allows all articulations to be viewed with no bony overlap.

- Carpal tunnel view for assessment of palmar ridge.
- CT scan for occult and associated fractures.

Treatment

- Nondisplaced fractures of the ridge and body should be immobilized 4–6 weeks.
- Displaced or comminuted fractures of the body of the trapezium are best managed surgically.

Complications

- Carpal tunnel syndrome, flexor carpi radialis tendinitis and potential tendon rupture, first carpometacarpal arthritis, and decreased pinch strength

---

Capitate

- Incidence – 1–2% of all carpal bone fractures
  - Often associated with scaphoid fractures, rarely isolated

Diagnosis

- History of fall on to the palm with extended, ulnarly deviated hand
- Axial load through the third metacarpal

Radiographs

- Standard radiographs are sufficient for displaced fractures.
- CT scan or MRI for an isolated, nondisplaced fracture.

Treatment

- Nondisplaced fractures treated with 6–8 weeks of immobilization.
- Displaced fractures require operative fixation.

Complications

- Blood supply is via retrograde flow, making the proximal pole susceptible to avascular necrosis.
- High incidence of nonunion secondary to delay in diagnosis, carpal collapse, and arthritis are possible complications.

Hamate

- Incidence – 2% of all carpal bone fractures

Fracture Pattern

- Divided into those involving the body or hook (most common)

Diagnosis

- Hook fractures commonly involve an acute injury after a racquet sport injury.
- Direct compression forces of the handle against the hook.
- Body fractures are related to axial load on the fourth and fifth metacarpals.
- Present with pain at hypothenar eminence and pain with resisted flexion of fourth and fifth digits (which displaces the fracture) and may note ulnar nerve symptoms with proximity to Guyon's canal.

Radiographs

- Standard radiographs, carpal tunnel, and supinated oblique views are often sufficient.
- CT scan is most sensitive test.

Treatment

- Acute fractures of the hook and body may be treated with immobilization for 6 weeks.

- Chronic or delayed presentation of hook fractures treated with excision of fragment.
- Body fractures that are displaced can be treated and require operative fixation.

Complications

- Nonunion may occur secondary to poor blood supply to the distal fragment and continued fragment movement leading to AVN, flexor tendon rupture, and loss of grip strength.
- Operative repair has risk of ulnar nerve and artery injury.

Pisiform

- Incidence – less than 1% of carpal bone fractures

Diagnosis

- Pain over the hypothenar eminence after direct injury or forced hyperextension.
- Location of pisiform within the flexor carpi ulnaris tendon causes avulsion injury.

Radiographs

- Standard radiographs, reverse oblique with 45-degree supination, and carpal tunnel views.
- CT scan is often required for diagnosis.

Treatment

- Acute fractures, nondisplaced, can be immobilized.
- Pisiform excision for displaced fractures, chronic and symptomatic fractures, and comminuted or persistent ulnar nerve symptoms.

Complication

- Nonunion in missed or delayed diagnosis
- Injury to the ulnar nerve and artery during operative management

Trapezoid

- Incidence – less than 1% of all carpal fractures
  - Often seen with other fractures and CMC dislocation

Diagnosis

- Pain at the base of second metacarpal after axial load though the second metacarpal or forced flexion

Radiographs

- Standard radiographs may not diagnose the injury.
- CT scan should be obtained if there is a high suspicion for a trapezoid fracture.

Treatment

- Nondisplaced fractures can be treated with 4–6 weeks of immobilization.
- Displaced fractures can be fixed with operative intervention.

Complications

- Nonunion and subsequent osteoarthritis may result in CMC arthrodesis.
- Unilateral dorsal blood supply may make trapezoid prone to avascular necrosis.

Lunate

- Incidence – less than 1% of all carpal fractures
  - Acute fractures are rare; Kienbock's disease may alter numbers.

Diagnosis

- Pain in dorsal wrist, with history of injury with extended wrist in weight-bearing athletes

Radiographs

- Standard radiographs are diagnostic.
- CT scan can be obtained for subtle clinical findings.

Treatment

- Nondisplaced dorsal chip fractures can be treated with 4–6 weeks of immobilization.
- Displaced fractures, volar chip fractures, disruption of the scapholunate, and lunotriquetral ligaments require operative fixation.
- Chronic injury may lead to arthritis and collapse eventually requiring fusion or PRC.

Complications

- Nonunion, AVN leading to arthritis, and carpal instability

Suggested Readings

1. Vigler M, et al. Carpal fractures excluding the scaphoid. Hand Clin. 2006;22:501–16.
2. Urch EY, et al. Carpal fractures other than scaphoid. Clin Sports Med. 2015;34:51–67.
3. Geissler WB, Slade JF. Fractures of the carpal bones. In: Wolfe SW, et al., editors. Green's operative hand surgery. 6th ed. Philadelphia: Churchill Livingstone; 2011.
4. Garcia-Elias M. Carpal bone fractures (excluding scaphoid fractures). In: Watson HK, et al., editors. The wrist. Philadelphia: Lippincott Williams and Wilkins; 2001.

Boxer's Fractures

43

Yoseph A. Rosenbaum and Hisham M. Awan

Overview

- Fourth or fifth metacarpal neck fracture from a poorly delivered punch with clenched fist
  - Apex dorsal angulation from impact on flexed metacarpal head.
  - Maintained by the intrinsic muscle pull.
  - May have volar comminution.
  - Malunion is a potential complication.
  - Despite angulation, patients usually regain full range of motion and strength, and thus surgery is rarely indicated.

Evaluation

- Examine the skin for any puncture wounds (the so-called fight bite).
- Bite wounds may extend to the MPJ, creating a septic arthritis.
  - Skin, tendon, and joint capsule all pierced with hand in clenched position; when hand relaxes, these holes do not overlap, sealing in contamination.

Y.A. Rosenbaum, MD • H.M. Awan, MD (✉)
Hand and Upper Extremity Center, The Ohio State University Wexner Medical Center, Columbus, OH, USA
e-mail: hisham.awan@osumc.edu

- Determine if there is any angular deformity, pseudoclawing, or rotational deformity.
  - Pseudoclawing: MC neck flexion causes MPJ hyperextension and PIPJ flexion.
  - Rotational assessment: Closed fist; fingertips should cascade pointing to scaphoid.

Radiographs (Figs. 43.1 and 43.2)

- Hand AP, oblique, and lateral – lateral will demonstrate angulation.
- Tolerance for angulation depends which metacarpal is fractured:
  - Index and middle: 10–15°
  - Ring: 30–40
  - Small: 50–60 (up to 70° acceptable in some series)

Treatment: Most Treated Nonsurgically

- Nondisplaced and stable fractures can be treated in a cast or splint.
- Safe position for immobilization: Wrist extended 10–20°, MCPJ flexed to 70–90°, and IPs in full extension

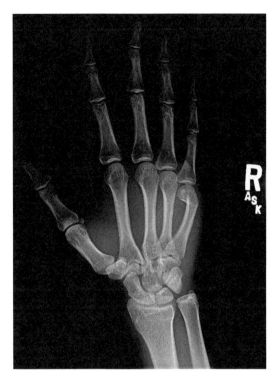

Fig. 43.1 Boxer's fracture X-ray oblique view

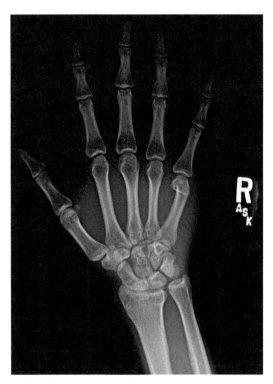

Fig. 43.2 Boxer's fracture X-ray AP view

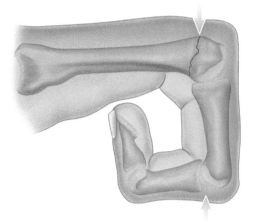

Fig. 43.3 Jahss maneuver – lateral view

- For displaced fractures, a closed reduction can be attempted.
- Jahss reduction maneuver (Fig. 43.3): MCP and IP joints flexed to 90°, pressure aimed dorsally transmitted through the flexed PIPJ, push fracture fragment back.
- Closed reduction may not alter long-term outcome.
- Irreducible, unacceptably angulated or rotated fractures require operative treatment.
  - CRPP vs. ORIF

Complications: Rare

- Stiffness
- Infection
- Malunion – usually well tolerated, even up to 70°
- Prominence of metacarpal head in the palm

Suggested Readings

1. Baltera RM, Hastings II H. Fractures and dislocations: hand. In: Hammert WC, editor. ASSH manual of hand surgery. Philadelphia: Lippincott Williams & Wilkins; 2010. p. 93–110.
2. Day CS, Stern PJ. Fractures of the metacarpals and phalanges. In: Wolfe SW, et al., editors. Green's operative hand surgery. 6th ed. Philadelphia: Churchill Livingstone; 2010.

Phalangeal Fractures

44

Yoseph A. Rosenbaum and Hisham M. Awan

Distal Phalanx

Shaft Fractures

- Different fracture patterns include transverse and longitudinal and can be stable or unstable.
- Nondisplaced fractures are typically stable and treated nonoperatively.
- Displaced fractures may have an associated nail bed laceration which should be repaired, and K-wire stabilization may be necessary for the fracture.
- When associated with nail bed laceration, these are technically open fractures.
- In immunocompetent hosts with intact circulations, antibiotics are not usually necessary.
- Irrigation and debridement are performed after the nail is removed; the nail bed laceration is repaired using absorbable suture.
- Replace the nail between the germinal matrix and eponychial fold to maintain growth of new nail thereafter.
- If the host is immunocompromised or the treatment was delayed 24 h, there is gross contamination, or if the patient has compromised circulation, a third-generation cephalosporin may be given.

Intra-articular Fractures

- Different fracture patterns include dorsal, volar, and physeal (pediatric).
- Small dorsal intra-articular fracture generally represents avulsion of the extensor tendon, also known as "mallet finger."
    - Acute treatment is in an extension splint for 6 weeks if there is no subluxation of the DIPJ.
    - If the DIPJ is unstable and subluxates, CRPP is indicated.
    - Chronic injuries may be treated electively with reconstruction.
- Larger dorsal fragments may need fixation if the joint becomes unstable.
- Small volar fragments typically represent an FDP (flexor tendon) avulsion or "jersey finger." It may be stabilized by K-wire fixation; however, it is important to remember that the flexor tendon may retract toward the palm.
- Physeal fractures to look out for are Seymour fractures (Fig. 44.1) (open distal phalanx physeal fracture with proximal nail fold incarceration).
- The distal phalanx is hyperflexed; the epiphyseal portion remains in extension, held by the EDC; and the distal fragment is pulled palmarly by the FDP and into flexion.
- These are open injuries with a nail bed laceration – an irrigation and debridement should be performed with nail bed repair.

Y.A. Rosenbaum, MD • H.M. Awan, MD (✉)
Hand and Upper Extremity Center, The Ohio State University Wexner Medical Center, Columbus, OH, USA
e-mail: hisham.awan@osumc.edu

© Springer International Publishing AG 2017
A.E.M. Eltorai et al. (eds.), *Orthopedic Surgery Clerkship*, DOI 10.1007/978-3-319-52567-9_44

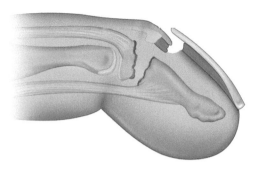

Fig. 44.1 Seymour fracture

Tuft Fractures

- Are either simple or comminuted.
- Typically secondary to a crush injury.
- May be associated with nail bed laceration which can be signified by subungual hematoma. Removing the nail and repairing the nail bed laceration with a fine absorbable suture will often result in an adequate fracture reduction.
- Subungual hematoma evacuation with a heated paper clip or ophthalmic electrocautery may be performed in cases where the nail is not removed, for pain relief.
- Brief immobilization period in a splint is the preferred treatment. Operative treatment is rarely indicated. Fractures may form a fibrous nonunion which is often asymptomatic and functionally acceptable.

Middle Phalanx

Articular Fractures

- Often unstable and may require CRPP or ORIF

Shaft Fractures

- With middle and proximal phalangeal fractures, stiffness becomes a possible complication, especially as the age of the patients increases.

- Stable, closed, nondisplaced diaphyseal fractures are typically treated with buddy taping for 3 weeks.
- Displaced fractures may angulate either apex dorsal or volar, depending on whether the fracture is proximal or distal to the FDS insertion, respectively.
- Indications for surgery include 10° or more of angulation and 2 mm shortening or rotational instability.
- CRPP or ORIF may be performed for displaced or unstable shaft fractures.
- Early range of motion is essential, as stiffness is common.

Proximal Phalanx

Articular Fractures

- Condylar
  - Unstable pattern, even when nondisplaced – CRPP vs. ORIF
- Neck
  - Nondisplaced or stable following closed reduction – splinting
  - Unstable CRPP vs. ORIF, may have entrapped volar plate which must be removed

Shaft Fractures

- Stable, nondisplaced fractures are treated nonoperatively with buddy taping or a forearm-based splint holding the wrist in the "safe" position:
  - 20–30° wrist extension
  - MCPJ flexed to 70–90°
  - IPs in full extension
- Displaced shaft fractures
  - Closed reduction and splinting if <10° angulation, no rotation, stable, and <2 mm shortening
  - Unstable or irreducible: CRPP vs. ORIF (Figs. 44.2, 44.3, 44.4, and 44.5)
    ° Tend toward apex volar angulation due to pull of intrinsic muscles

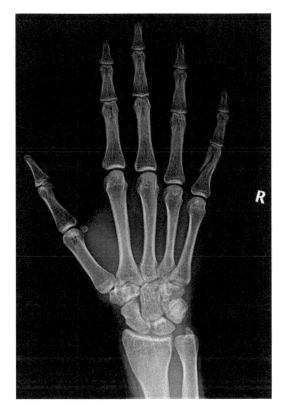

Fig. 44.2 Unstable proximal phalangeal fracture – AP view

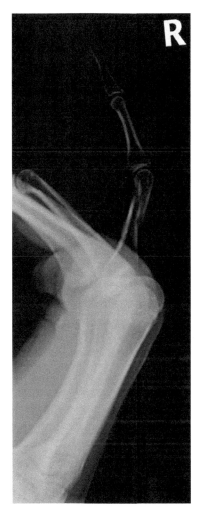

Fig. 44.3 Unstable proximal phalangeal fracture – lateral view

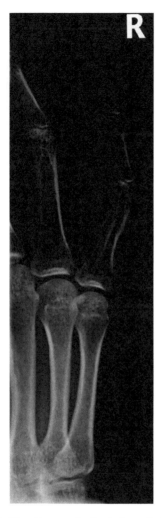

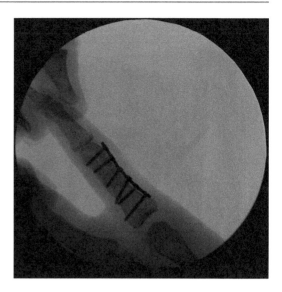

Fig. 44.5 Unstable proximal phalangeal fracture – ORIF

Suggested Readings

1. Baltera RM, Hastings II H. Fractures and dislocations: hand. In: Hammert WC, Boyer MI, Bozentka DJ, Calfee RP, editors. ASSH manual of hand surgery. Philadelphia: Lippincott Williams & Wilkins; 2010. p. 93–110.
2. Day CS, Stern PJ. Fractures of the Metacarpals and Phalanges. In: Wolfe SW, Pederson WC, Hotchkiss RN, Kozen SH. Green's operative hand surgery. 6th ed. Philadelphia: Churchill Livingstone; 2010. p. 239–90.

Fig. 44.4 Unstable proximal phalangeal fracture – oblique view

Phalangeal Dislocations

45

Yoseph A. Rosenbaum and Hisham M. Awan

Anatomical Considerations

Proximal Interphalangeal (PIP) Joint

- Ginglymus (hinge) joint, stabilized by a ligamentous "box."
- Does not tolerate prolonged immobilization well and tends to become very stiff.
- Stability imparted by bony contour, collateral ligaments, and volar plate.
- Also demonstrates up to 9° of supination due to condylar asymmetry.
- Collateral ligaments are divided into proper and accessory.
    - Proper insert on the volar one-third of the base of middle phalanx
    - Accessory insert on the volar plate
- Volar plate: thick fibrocartilaginous "floor" of the joint.
    - Thicker laterally and medially than centrally.
    - Blends into the volar periosteum of the middle phalanx centrally.
    - Thickenings laterally and medially called checkreins prevent hyperextension.

Distal Interphalangeal (DIP) Joint

- Similarly, volar plate may be interposed in dorsal dislocations.
- Less commonly encountered than PIP joint dislocations.
- FDP may be an obstacle to reduction attempts.
- Remember to consider nail bed injuries in distal phalangeal fractures.

Metacarpophalangeal (MCP or MP) Joint

- Volar plate ruptures may be interposed in dorsal dislocations.
- Mechanism is typically hyperextension with resulting dorsal dislocation.
- Volar dislocations are rare.
- Dorsal dislocations may cause the metacarpal head to buttonhole to the palm, called Kaplan's lesion.
- Juncturae tendinum join extensor tendons together and may become interposed in the dislocation, preventing reduction.

Dorsal Dislocations —

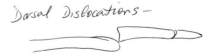

Y.A. Rosenbaum, MD • H.M. Awan, MD (✉)
Hand and Upper Extremity Center,
The Ohio State University Wexner Medical Center,
Columbus, OH, USA
e-mail: hisham.awan@osumc.edu

© Springer International Publishing AG 2017
A.E.M. Eltorai et al. (eds.), *Orthopedic Surgery Clerkship*, DOI 10.1007/978-3-319-52567-9_45

PIP Joint Injuries: Dorsal Dislocations

- More common than volar.
- Involves volar plate – if untreated – and leads to swan neck deformity.

Type I: Hyperextension Injury

- Partial or complete avulsion of volar plate
- Conservative treatment with buddy taping, early ROM

Type II: Pure Dorsal Dislocation

Simple Versus Complex
- In simple dislocation, P2 is adjacent to condyles of P1, whereas in complex, there is greater displacement proximally of P2 and bayonet apposition, with volar plate interposed between the phalanges (Fig. 45.1).
- Simple typically treated with closed reduction and buddy taping.
- Complex may require open approach to reduce and/or repair volar plate.

Type III: Fracture-Dislocation

Kiefhaber Modification of Hastings Classification
- Stable – less than 30% of articular base of middle phalanx fractured.
  - Treatment is splinting with dorsally based extension-block splint.

- Tenuous – 30–50% fractured, reduces with <30° flexion.
  - Treatment is splinting if stable reduction is obtainable with <40° flexion.
  - If unstable, it must be treated as unstable fracture (see below).
- Unstable – >50% articular involvement, or irreducible at 30° (Fig. 45.2).
  - Typically would fail conservative treatment
  - Surgical management – options
    ◦ Extension-block pinning
    ◦ Transarticular pinning
    ◦ ORIF
    ◦ Dynamic external fixation for comminuted fractures
    ◦ Volar plate arthroplasty
    ◦ Hemi-hamate arthroplasty
    ◦ Arthrodesis
- Obtain a true lateral image with superimposed condyles to evaluate reduction.
- Dorsal "V sign" indicates a subluxated joint which is not truly reduced (Fig. 45.3).

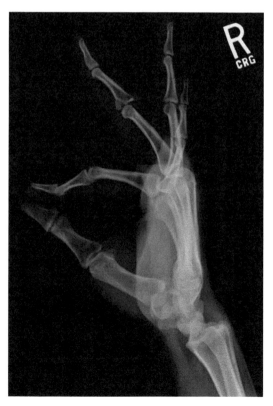

Fig. 45.2 Lateral X-ray of an unstable PIPJ dorsal fracture-dislocation

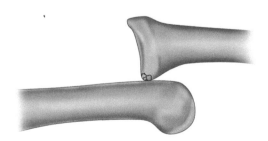

Fig. 45.1 Complex PIPJ dislocation

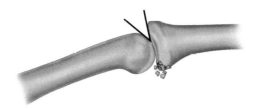

Fig. 45.3 Dorsal V sign

PIP Joint Injuries: Volar Dislocations

- Relatively uncommon.
- Involves central slip – if untreated – and leads to boutonniere deformity.
- Simple dislocation (no fracture).
  - Close reduction and splinting in extension 6–8 weeks.
  - Be sure to examine if there is extensor lag of PIP joint following reduction – this indicates injury to central slip which should be repaired.
- Complex dislocation (fracture-dislocation)
  - If there is <20% of articular base of middle phalanx fractured, <2 mm displacement, and stable reduction achieved, treatment is splinting in extension of 6–8 weeks.
  - If there is >20% involvement of articular surface or >2 mm displacement, or unstable, ORIF vs. CRPP is indicated.

PIP Joint Injuries: Rotatory Dislocations

- Relatively uncommon – condyle of P1 buttonholes between central slip and lateral band
- Not typically reducible by closed means
- Reduction technique – flex the MP and PIP joints to 90° to allow lateral bands to reduce dorsally
- Often require surgical intervention

DIP Joint Dislocations

- Closed reduction is generally adequate for these injuries.

- If stable closed reduction is achieved, splint in slight flexion for 2 weeks.
- If volar plate or FDP is interposed, they may require open reduction.
- Consider percutaneous pinning to stabilize nail bed repair if necessary.

MP Joint Dislocations

- Dorsal – simple vs. complex
  - In simple dislocation, there is no fracture or interposed volar plate.
    - May be treated conservatively with reduction and extension-block splint.
    - To reduce, flex wrist to relax flexor tendons.
    - Avoid axial traction which may drag the volar plate into the joint.
  - In complex dislocations, there is often skin dimpling which can help identify an interposed structure preventing reduction (most commonly the volar plate).
    - Often irreducible closed.
    - Require open reduction, via dorsal or volar approach.
    - Dorsal approach splits the sagittal band, but volar approach puts digital nerves at risk.
- Volar dislocations
  - These are uncommon.
  - Closed reduction should be attempted.
  - If it fails, open reduction via dorsal approach is recommended.

Suggested Readings

1. Baltera RM, Hastings II H. Fractures and dislocations: hand. In: Hammert, WC, Calfee, RP, Bozentka, DJ, Boyer, MI, editors. ASSH manual of hand surgery. Philadelphia: Lippincott Williams & Wilkins, 2010, p. 93–110.
2. Merrell G, Slade JF. Dislocations and ligament injuries in the digits. In: Wolfe SW, Pederson WC, Hotchkiss RN, Kozen SH, editors. Green's operative hand surgery. 6th ed. Philadelphia: Churchill Livingstone, 2010. p. 291–332.

Metacarpal Fractures

46

Yoseph A. Rosenbaum and Hisham M. Awan

Overview

- Very common fractures, typically from direct trauma.
  - Apex dorsal angulation from impact on flexed metacarpal head
    ° Maintained by the intrinsic muscle pull.
    ° Malunion and nonunion are potential complications.

Evaluation

- Examine the skin for any wounds.
- Determine if there is any angular deformity, pseudoclawing, or rotational deformity.
  - Pseudoclawing: MC neck flexion causes MPJ hyperextension and PIPJ flexion.
  - Rotational assessment: Closed fist, fingertips should cascade pointing to scaphoid.

Radiographic Evaluation and Treatment Options (Figs. 46.1, 46.2, and 46.3)

- Hand AP and lateral – lateral will demonstrate angulation.

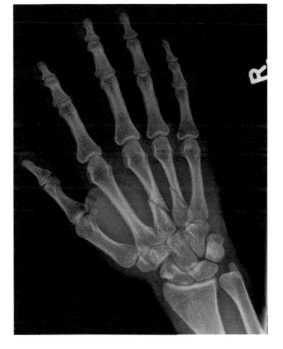

Fig. 46.1 Metacarpal fractures – AP view

- Tolerance for angulation depends on which metacarpal is fractured and location:
- Neck:
  - Index and middle: 10–15°
  - Ring: 30–40°
  - Small: 50–60°
- Shaft:
  - Index: 10°
  - Middle: 20°
  - Ring: 30°
  - Small: 40°

Y.A. Rosenbaum, MD • H.M. Awan, MD (✉)
Hand and Upper Extremity Center, The Ohio State University Wexner Medical Center, Columbus, OH, USA
e-mail: hisham.awan@osumc.edu

© Springer International Publishing AG 2017
A.E.M. Eltorai et al. (eds.), *Orthopedic Surgery Clerkship*, DOI 10.1007/978-3-319-52567-9_46

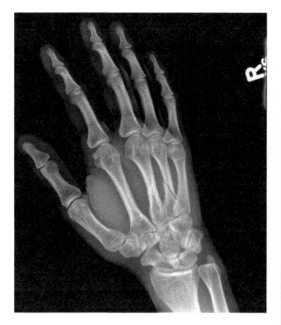

Fig. 46.2 Metacarpal fractures – oblique view

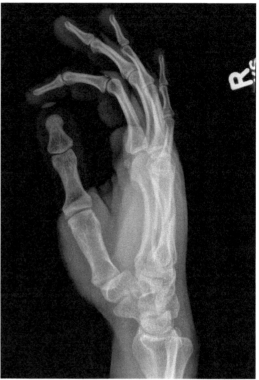

Fig. 46.3 Metacarpal fractures – lateral view

- Head:
  - No articular displacement is acceptable.
  - Require surgical fixation if any displacement is present.
  - Joint replacement is a salvage option if the head is severely comminuted.
- Base:
  - Extra-articular: treat along shaft guidelines.
  - Intra-articular: no degree of displacement is tolerated.
  - 30-degree pronated lateral view is necessary to rule out CMCJ dislocation of the fourth and fifth digits.
- No malrotation is tolerated.
- Shortening of up to 2–3 mm is tolerated.
  - Shortening is limited, especially in central digits, by the deep transverse metacarpal ligament.
- Thumb:
  - Extra-articular base fractures of the thumb metacarpal are more unstable than in the other metacarpals.

- Typical deformity is shortening, supination, and flexion due to pull of adductor pollicis and APL (Fig. 46.4).
- May be casted if angulation after reduction is stable at less than 30 degrees.
- Requires CRPP if unstable or irreducible.
- Rolando-type fracture is a T- or Y-shaped intra-articular metacarpal base fracture, which is unstable, and CRPP or ORIF is indicated.
- CMCJ fracture-dislocation typically displays pattern known as "Bennett fracture."
  - Small volar fragment remains attached to trapezium by the anterior oblique ligament.
  - Larger fragment is attached to APL and adductor pollicis and typically migrates proximally, dorsally, and radially.
  - These fractures are inherently unstable and usually require surgical treatment.

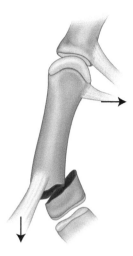

Fig. 46.4 Deforming forces involved in an extra-articular base of first metacarpal fracture

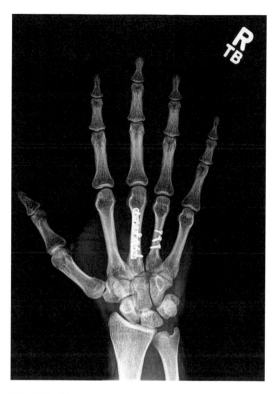

Fig. 46.5 Metacarpal ORIF – AP view

Treatment

- Nondisplaced and stable fractures are treated in a cast in the safe position:
    - 20–30° wrist extension
    - MCPJ flexed to 70–90°
    - IP's in full extension
- Unacceptably aligned fractures are treated with closed reduction and casting if stable.
    - Dorsal mold over the apex of the fracture to reduce the angulation
- Irreducible, unacceptably angulated or rotated fractures require operative treatment.
    - CRPP vs ORIF, occasionally external fixation or arthroplasty as indicated (Figs. 46.5 and 46.6)

Complications

- Stiffness
- Infection
- Malunion
- Nonunion
- Prominence of metacarpal head in the palm

CRPP - Closed Reduction + Percutaneous pinning

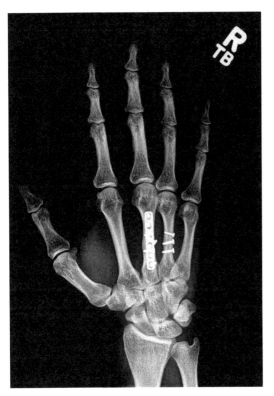

Fig. 46.6 Metacarpal ORIF – oblique view

Suggested Readings

1. Baltera RM, Hastings II H. Fractures and dislocations: hand. In: Hammert WC, editor. ASSH manual of hand surgery. Philadelphia: Lippincott Williams & Wilkins; 2010. p. 93–110.
2. Day CS, Stern PJ. Fractures of the metacarpals and phalanges. In: Wolfe SW, et al., editors. Green's operative hand surgery. 6th ed. Philadelphia: Churchill Livingstone; 2010.

Traumatic Upper Extremity Amputations

47

Margaret Jain and Erik White

Presentation

- Most frequently seen among young male laborers
- Fingertip amputations most common
- Long finger most commonly injured

Mechanism of Injury

- Crush: usually involves severe soft tissue injury
- Laceration: sharp injuries, may be suitable for amputation
- Avulsion
- Level of amputation is defined by level of bony injury

Factors Affecting Treatment:

- Viability of the amputated part: The indications for replantation of the extremity are addressed in the chapter on replantation. see Replantation – see 2-27.
- Extent of soft tissue injury-extensive soft tissue injury may require flap coverage or shortening of amputated limb with closure.

M. Jain (✉) • E. White, MD
Hand and Upper Extremity Surgery, University of Toledo School of Medicine, Toledo, OH, USA
e-mail: margaret.jain@utoledo.edu

- Exposed structures (tendon, bone, nerves).
- Size and geometry of skin deficit.
- Fingers involved:
  - Index finger is easily bypassed and long finger used for pinch activities.
  - Ulnar fingers are critical to grip strength.

Patient Factors:

- Hand dominance.
- Age – younger patients fare better with replantation surgery.
- Occupation, work status, and desire to return to work.
- Comorbidities that decrease success of microsurgical treatments:
  - Smoking and tobacco use
  - Vascular disease

Treatment by Injury Location

Goals of Amputation Surgery

- Maintain finger or limb length.
- Restore pain-free digital sensation.
- Provide well-padded, durable skin coverage.
- Prevent painful neuroma formation.
- Prevent nail deformities.
- Return patients to work and ADLs.

© Springer International Publishing AG 2017
A.E.M. Eltorai et al. (eds.), *Orthopedic Surgery Clerkship*, DOI 10.1007/978-3-319-52567-9_47

General Considerations:

- Sharp injuries require tetanus prophylaxis and should be treated as open fractures, with thorough irrigation of the stump and antibiotics.

Fingertip Amputations

- Amputations without exposed bone
  - Healing by secondary intention
    ° Ideal for transverse or dorsal oblique wounds <1 cm².
    ° Preserves some digital sensation.
    ° Dress wound with non-adherent dressing and monitor.
    ° Simple, low complication rate, and early return of function.
  - Primary closure: requires good-quality soft tissues and tension-free closure
  - Skin grafting
    ° No functional advantages over other treatments.
    ° Full-thickness grafts may come from the hypothenar eminence or any non-hair-bearing flexion crease.
    ° Split-thickness grafts may also be used.
- Fingertip amputations with exposed bone
  - Bone shortening and primary closure (revision amputation)

° Trim back exposed phalanx until there is adequate soft tissue for closure or to heal by secondary intention.
° Where possible, preserve the flexor and extensor tendon insertions.
° The digital nerves should be identified, cut, and allowed to retract proximally to prevent symptomatic neuromas.
° Nail bed must be resected back to the level of the bony injury to prevent a hook nail deformity.
° For injuries involving the germinal matrix, all nail matrix must be ablated to avoid the formation of nail "spikes" or "horns."
  - Flap coverage:
    ° Allows preservation of bone length.
    ° Always consider for thumb amputations.
    ° Flap types include local, regional, island, and distal flaps.
    ° V-Y advancement flaps (Fig. 47.1).
      - V–Y flap (Kleinert)
        • Transverse or dorsal oblique orientation
        • Contraindicated with volar soft tissue loss
        • Mobilizes volar soft tissue to cover distal finger
      - Lateral V–Y flap (Kutler)
        • Volar oblique or transverse-oriented amputations

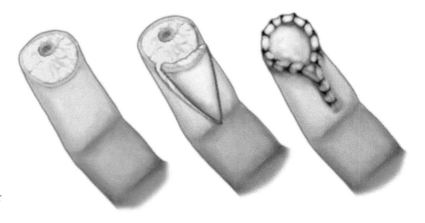

Fig. 47.1 V to Y flap for distal skin coverage

- Utilizes two triangular flaps from the midlateral fingertip to cover distal finger
- Moberg flap
  - Used to cover volar thumb defects <2 cm.
  - Two midaxial incisions allow mobilization of skin distally.
  - Remaining proximal defect is skin grafted.
- Cross finger flap (Fig. 47.2)
  - Used for volar soft tissue loss of any finger.
  - Borrows dorsal skin over neighboring middle phalanx to cover volar skin at injured digit.
  - Full-thickness skin graft is applied to donor site.
- Reverse cross finger flap used for dorsal soft tissue loss.
- Thenar flap (Fig. 47.3)
  - Used for volar or transverse amputation of index, long fingers
  - Flap of full-thickness skin from thenar area raised and sown to the defect of the flexed, injured finger
  - Flap divided at 10–14 days, donor site closed
  - Risks: IP joint flexion contractures, especially in older patients
- Island flaps
  - Regional flaps based on a neurovascular pedicle
  - Benefit: provide sensation, shorter immobilization time
  - Technically demanding

Fig. 47.2 Cross finger flap for volar distal skin coverage

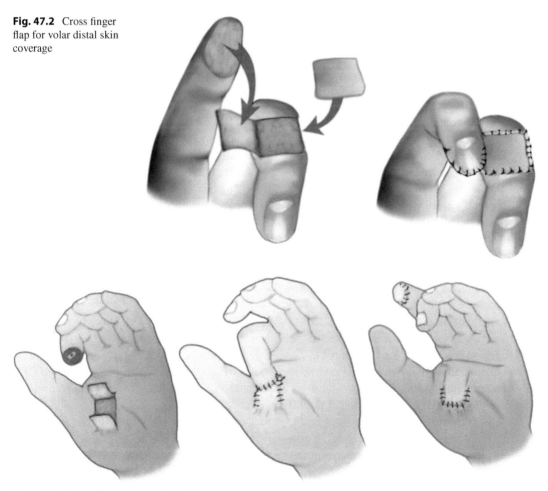

Fig. 47.3 Thenar flap for volar distal skin coverage

– Distant flaps (Groin, Arm flaps)
  • Used when regional flaps are not an option

Amputations Through the DIP Joint

• Treatment: shorten the phalanx, and close primarily.
• Remove articular cartilage and condyles of middle phalanx to contour the fingertip.
• Flexor and extensor tendons are cut and allowed to retract.
  – Tendons should not be sutured to one another or advanced, which may lead to quadriga (see below).
• Digital nerves identified, resected proximally, and buried away from scar to avoid painful neuroma.

Amputation Through the Middle Phalanx

• Amputations distal to FDS insertion
  – Shorten bone to allow primary closure of wound.
  – Preserving FDS insertion and central slip improves function allowing active PIP motion and improved grip.
  – If primary closure is not possible with FDS preservation, consider flap coverage.
• Amputations proximal to FDS insertion
  – If FDS is not retained, there is little functional advantage to maintaining length.
  – Bone shortening with primary closure should be performed.
• Amputations through the PIP joint
  – Treated in a similar manner to that of amputations through the DIP joint
• Amputation through proximal phalanx
  – Just proximal to PIP joint
    ◦ Allows 45 degrees of flexion at the MP joint (Intrinsic function).
    ◦ Remaining segment participates in gripping and keeps small objects from falling through the palm.
  – Near the MP joint

◦ Preservation of the metacarpal may pose functional problems; small objects may fall through the palm, especially with long, ring finger injury.
◦ Consider ray resection.

Proximal Limb Amputations

• Maintenance of limb length improves function.
• Amputations through the carpus.
  – Radiocarpal joint will allow some wrist motion and improved function.
• Wrist disarticulation.
  – Benefit: preserves DRUJ, which allows for improve pronation/supination
• Transradial (forearm) amputations.
  – The length of the forearm dictates remaining pronation/supination motion – more length correlations with more motion.
  – Flexor and extensor tendons are sutured to one another to provide coverage at the bone ends and to improve prosthesis function.
• Elbow disarticulation.
  – Allows for improved prosthetic fit around humeral condyles
• Transhumeral amputations and shoulder disarticulation.
  – Shoulder motion is preserved with distal amputations.
• Forequarter amputation.
  – Used primarily for tumor resection or severe trauma

Postoperative Management

• Bulky soft dressing, with non-adherent dressing applied, and wound check at 7–10 days.
• Splint may be used for protection.
• If no flap or graft is used, patients should start early motion to allow for early return of function.
• Desensitization training with occupational/hand therapy can be helpful.
• Prosthetic fitting should start as early as possible; earlier referral correlates with patient satisfaction, improved edema, and pain.

- Consider psychiatry referral to manage loss of limb.

Complications

- Cold sensitivity.
  - Very common with any amputation
  - Improves with time
  - Tx: keep finger warm to avoid
- Nail "spikes" or "horns" may result if any nail matrix is left after distal amputation.
- Flap necrosis.
- Phantom pain: rare in distal amputations.
- Joint contractures and stiffness.
- Painful neuroma formation.
  - Prevention is easier than treatment.
  - Resection can be considered; often, treatment improves but does not eliminate pain.
- Lumbrical plus finger.
  - The lumbrical muscles originate on FDP tendon.
  - After amputation, the FDP and lumbrical origin retract proximally, increasing tension in the lumbrical tendon.
  - When "lumbrical plus" finger occurs, attempted flexion of the FDP causes proximal pull of the lumbrical, causing paradoxical PIP joint extension.
  - Tx: lumbrical release.
- Quadregia effect
  - Caused by imbalance of flexor tendons after amputation.
  - FDP tendons have a single common muscle belly for all fingers.
  - If one FDP tendon is overlengthened after amputation, or advanced, the common muscle belly of the others loses mechanical advantage.
  - Result: loss of terminal flexion of non-amputated fingers.

References

1. Hammert WC, et al. Amputations. In: Hammert WC, Calfee RP, editors. ASSH manual of hand surgery. 2nd ed. American Society for Surgery of the Hand; 2015. E-book.
2. Jebson PLJ, Louis DS, Bagg M. Amputations. In: Wolfe SW, et al., editors. Green's operative hand surgery. 6th ed. Philadelphia: Churchill Livingstone; 2010.
3. Fitzgibbons P, Medvedev G. Functional and clinical outcomes of upper extremity amputation. J Am Acad Orthop Surg. 2015;23:751–60.

Tears of the Triangular Fibrocartilage Complex

48

Robert C. Matthias

Anatomy

- The six components of the triangular fibrocartilage complex (TFCC) include:
  - Central articular disk
  - Dorsal and volar radioulnar ligaments
  - Ulnar collateral ligament
  - Meniscus homologue
  - ECU subsheath
  - Ulnocarpal ligaments
- Function
  - Primary stabilizer of the DRUJ
- Vascular anatomy
  - TFCC vascular supply is from the ulnar and anterior interosseous arteries.
  - Perfusion
    ○ Periphery of TFCC is well perfused and amenable to repair.
    ○ Central portions of TFCC are poorly perfused and are not amenable to repair.

Injury Mechanism

- Acute injuries caused by extension-pronation force on an axially loaded wrist, dorsal rotation, or traction

R.C. Matthias, MD
University of Florida, Gainesville, FL, USA

- Chronic injuries result from either age-dependent attrition or ulnocarpal impaction syndrome.
- Ulnocarpal impaction syndrome:
  ○ Results from abutment of the distal ulna or TFCC against the ulnar carpus
    - Causes
      • Congenitally ulnar positive
      • Distal radius malunion
      • Radial head injury
      • Madelung deformity

Physical Exam

- Inspection may reveal ulnar prominence or volar sag/supination of the wrist.
- Palpation is performed with the elbow on the table, fingers to ceiling, and the forearm in neutral pronation/supination. The TFCC is located between the ECU and FCU just distal to ulnar styloid.
- Provocative maneuvers assist in the diagnosis and include the ulnocarpal impaction maneuver and the piano key test.
  - The ulnocarpal impaction maneuver is performed by ulnarly deviating the wrist, applying an axial load, and flexing and extending the wrist. Pain with or without a "click" is a positive test.
  - The piano key test is performed by applying a dorsal-to-volar load across DRUJ while

© Springer International Publishing AG 2017
A.E.M. Eltorai et al. (eds.), *Orthopedic Surgery Clerkship*, DOI 10.1007/978-3-319-52567-9_48

holding the ulna proximally. Evidence of DRUJ instability is a positive test.

Imaging

- Standard PA, lateral, and oblique X-ray views of the wrist are obtained. An ulnar variance view is performed as a PA wrist view in neutral pronation/supination with the elbow flexed 90° and the shoulder abducted 90°. A pronated power grip view may demonstrate dynamic ulnar positivity.
- A CT with axial imaging of both wrists through full pronation/supination is the best way to evaluate DRUJ subluxation.
- Arthrography was previously the gold standard of TFCC imaging but has been shown to have a high false-negative rate as it poorly evaluates noncommunicating TFCC defects.
- MRI is the current gold standard of evaluating TFCC as it has high sensitivity and specificity. The diagnostic significance of TFCC pathology on MRI, however, is unclear. In one study, up to 70% of asymptomatic patients less than 35 years old had positive findings of TFCC pathology on MRI. This correlates with a cadaver study assessing the prevalence of TFCC pathology. In this study of 180 cadaveric wrists, only 61% of cadavers of age 20–30 had normal-appearing TFCC. In cadavers over age 40, no specimens had a normal-appearing TFCC.
  - Ulnar impaction syndrome is well demonstrated on MRI with signal changes in the ulnar lunate (which have been confused with Kienbock's), radial triquetrum, and/or the radial ulnar head. Subchondral cysts may also be seen in these locations.

Classification

- Type 1 – Acute traumatic tears
  - 1A – Central TFCC perforation
  - 1B – Peripheral ulnar side TFCC tear (+/− ulna styloid fracture)
  - 1C – Distal TFCC disruption (disruption from distal ulnocarpal ligaments)
  - 1D – Radial TFCC disruption (+/− sigmoid notch fracture)
- Type 2 – Degenerative tears
  - 2A – TFCC wear
  - 2B – TFCC wear with lunate and/or ulnar chondromalacia
  - 2C – TFCC perforation with lunate and/or ulnar chondromalacia
  - 2D - TFCC perforation with lunate and/or ulnar chondromalacia with lunotriquetral ligament perforation
  - 2D + ulnocarpal arthritis

Treatment

- Acute tears of the TFCC can be treated nonoperatively only in the absence of DRUJ instability. Immobilization and injection are options and can be both diagnostic and therapeutic. In a study of nonoperative treatment for TFCC tears, 57% of patients improved after being treated for 1 month in a splint or cast. This study supports the fact that peripheral tears can heal and central tears can become asymptomatic. Importantly, no studies cite worsened outcome for delayed surgical treatment if the DRUJ is stable.
  - Operative treatment is utilized immediately in the setting of an unstable DRUJ or once nonoperative treatment has deemed to have failed with a stable DRUJ. Surgical treatment is specific to the type of tear based on the Palmer classification.
    ○ Type 1A tears are treated with arthroscopy and debridement with the goal of creating a stable rim while preserving the DRUJ ligaments. Studies have demonstrated success rates of 66–87%.
    ○ Type 1B tears are treated with either arthroscopic or open techniques.
      - The arthroscopic technique repairs the TFCC to the wrist capsule and can be accomplished through outside-in, inside-out, or all-inside techniques.
      - Open TFCC repair repairs the TFCC to fovea.

– Several studies have demonstrated no significant difference between arthroscopic and open repairs.

○ Type 1C tears are rarely diagnosed, symptomatic, or treated.

○ Type 1D tears rarely result in DRUJ instability and can be treated with either open or arthroscopic repair.

- Similar to acute TFCC tears, chronic tears can initially be treated nonoperatively with immobilization and/or injection. As the cause of the TFCC tears in this population is often related to ulnar positivity, surgical intervention may be necessary either in the form of an ulnar shortening osteotomy or wafer procedure.

– Ulnar shortening osteotomy (USO) is performed by removing a premeasured segment of ulna, reducing the remaining two ulnar fragments, and then stabilizing them with internal fixation. This can be done freehand or with one of several ulnar shortening osteotomy systems.

○ In multiple studies, patients experienced improved pain, functional scores, and high patient satisfaction.

○ Complications do occur and include nonunion (0–5%), symptomatic hardware, and DRUJ incongruity.

– The wafer procedure removes a portion of the distal ulna either arthroscopically or open and is particularly in a patient who is ulnar neutral.

○ Good to excellent results have been reported in several small studies.

○ Limitations and complications of the wafer procedure are that a limited amount of distal ulna can be removed; it is possible to remove too little or too much distal ulna, and DRUJ congruity or stability can be affected.

– Studies have compared ulnar shortening osteotomy with the wafer procedure, and the results have demonstrated similar pain relief and a similar complication rate. Most complications of ulnar shortening osteotomy were hardware related.

Type 2 Degenerative
2A   TFCC wear
2B   TFCC wear with lunate and/or ulnar chondromalacia
2C   TFCC perforation with lunate and/or ulnar chondromalacia
2D   TFCC perforation with lunate and/or ulnar chondromalacia with LTIOL perforation
2E   2D + ulnocarpal arthritis

Adapted from Palmer AK Triangular fibrocartilage complex lesions: a classification.J Hand Surg Am 1989 Jul: 14(4):594-606

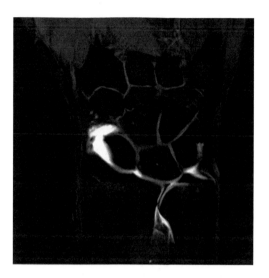

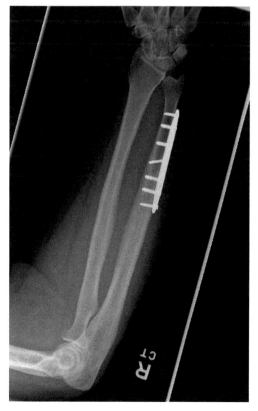

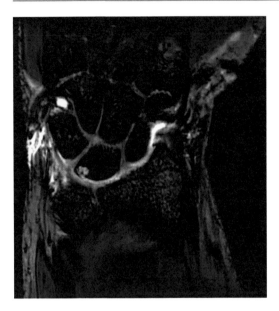

Suggested Reading

1. Kirschenbaum D, Sieler S, Solonick D, Loeb DM, Cody RP. Arthrography of the wrist. Assessment of the integrity of the ligaments in young asymptomatic adults. J Bone Joint Surg Am. 1995;77(8):1207–9.

2. Zanetti M, Linkous MD, Gilula LA, Hodler J. Characteristics of triangular fibrocartilage defects in symptomatic and contralateral asymptomatic wrists. Radiology. 2000;216:840–5.

3. Sugimoto H, Shinozaki T, Ohsawa T. Triangular fibrocartilage in asymptomatic subjects: investigation of abnormal MR signal intensity. Radiology. 1994;191(1):193–7.

4. Iordache SD, Rowan R, Garvin GJ, Osman S, Grewal R, Faber KJ. Prevalence of triangular fibrocartilage complex abnormalities on MRI scans of asymptomatic wrists. J Hand Surg [Am]. 2012;37(1):98–103.

5. Mikic ZD. Age changes in the triangular fibrocartilage of the wrist joint. J Anat. 1978;126(2):367–84.

6. Minami A, Ishikawa J, Suenaga N, Kasashima T. Clinical results of treatment of triangular fibrocartilage complex tears by arthroscopic debridement. J Hand Surg [Am]. 1996;21(3):406–11.

7. Miwa H, Hashizume H, Fujiwara K, Nishida K, Inoue H. Arthroscopic surgery for traumatic triangular fibrocartilage complex injury. J Orthop Sci. 2004;9(4):354–9.

8. Westkaemper JG, Mitsionis G, Giannakopoulos PN, Sotereanos DG. Wrist arthroscopy for the treatment of ligament and triangular fibrocartilage complex injuries. Arthroscopy. 1998;14(5):479–83.

9. Whipple TL, Geissler WB. Arthroscopic management of wrist triangular fibrocartilage complex injuries in the athlete. Orthopedics. 1993;16(9):1061–7.

10. Hulsizer D, Weiss AP, Akelman E. Ulna-shortening osteotomy after failed arthroscopic debridement of the triangular fibrocartilage complex. J Hand Surg [Am]. 1997;22(4):694–8.

11. Bernstein MA, Nagle DJ, Martinez A, Stogin Jr JM, Wiedrich TA. A comparison of combined arthroscopic triangular fibrocartilage complex debridement and arthroscopic wafer distal ulna resection versus arthroscopic triangular fibrocartilage complex debridement and ulnar shortening osteotomy for ulnocarpal abutment syndrome. Arthroscopy. 2004;20(4):392–401.

12. Corso SJ, Savoie FH, Geissler WB, Whipple TL, Jiminez W, Jenkins N. Arthroscopic repair of peripheral avulsions of the triangular fibrocartilage complex of the wrist: a multicenter study. Arthroscopy. 1997;13(1):78–84.

13. Degreef I, Welters H, Milants P, Van Ransbeeck H, De Smet L. Disability and function after arthroscopic repair of ulnar avulsions of the triangular fibrocartilage complex of the wrist. Acta Orthop Belg. 2005;71(3):289–93.

14. Estrella EP, Hung LK, Ho PC, Tse WL. Arthroscopic repair of triangular fibrocartilage complex tears. Arthroscopy. 2007;23(7):729–37. 737.e1.

15. Hermansdorfer JD, Kleinman WB. Management of chronic peripheral tears of thetriangular fibrocartilage complex. J Hand Surg [Am]. 1991;16A:340–6.

16. Iwasaki N, Nishida K, Motomiya M, Funakoshi T, Minami A. Arthroscopic-assisted repair of avulsed triangular fibrocartilage complex to the fovea of the ulnar head: a 2- to 4-year follow-up study. Arthroscopy. 2011;27(10):1371–8.

17. Anderson ML, Larson AN, Moran SL, Cooney WP, Amrami KK, Berger RA. Clinical comparison of arthroscopic versus open repair of triangular fibrocartilage complex tears. J Hand Surg [Am]. 2008;33(5):675–82.

18. Iwasaki N, Ishikawa J, Kato H, Minami M, Minami A. Factors affecting results of ulnar shortening for ulnar impaction syndrome. Clin Orthop Relat Res. 2007;465:215–9.

19. Moermans A, Degreef I, De Smet L. Ulnar shortening osteotomy for ulnar ideopathic impaction syndrome. Scand J Plast Reconstr Surg Hand Surg. 2007;41(6):310–4.

20. Fricker R, Pfeiffer KM, Troeger H. Ulnar shortening osteotomy in posttraumatic ulnar impaction syndrome. Arch Orthop Trauma Surg. 1996;115(3–4):158–61.

21. Feldon P, Terrono AL, Belsky MR. Wafer distal ulna resection for triangular fibrocartilage tears and/ or ulna impaction syndrome. J Hand Surg [Am]. 1992;17(4):731–7.

22. Tomaino MM. Results of the wafer procedure for ulnar impaction syndrome in the ulnar negative and neutral wrist. J Hand Surg (Br). 1999;24(6):671–5.

23. Constantine KJ, Tomaino MM, Herndon JH, Sotereanos DG. Comparison of ulnar shortening osteotomy and the wafer resection procedure as treatment

for ulnar impaction syndrome. J Hand Surg [Am]. 2000;25(1):55–60.

24. Bernstein MA, Nagle DJ, Martinez A, Stogin Jr JM, Wiedrich TA. A comparison of combined arthroscopic triangular fibrocartilage complex debridement and arthroscopic wafer distal ulna resection versus arthroscopic triangular fibrocartilage com-

plex debridement and ulnar shortening osteotomy for ulnocarpal abutment syndrome. Arthroscopy. 2004;20(4):392–401.

25. Bednar MD, Arnoczky SP, Weiland AJ. The microvasculature of the triangular fibrocartilage complex: Its clinical significance. J Hand Surg [Am]. 1991;16(6):1101–5.

Carpal Instability

49

Grant S. Buchanan and Alan Koester

The Carpal Rows

Ligamentous Anatomy of the Wrist

- Intrinsic – origins and insertions within the carpal bones
  - Avulse rather than rupture
  - Proximal carpal row – scapholunate interosseous ligament (SLIL) and lunotriquetral interosseous ligament (LTIL)
  - Distal carpal row – trapezium trapezoid, trapezium capitate, and capitohamate ligaments
  - Dorsal intercarpal – scaphotriquetral ligament
  - Palmar intercarpal – scaphoid trapezium trapezoid (STT) and triquetral hamate capitate ligaments
- Extrinsic – origins and insertions among carpal bones and forearm bones
  - Rupture rather than avulse
  - Volar – radioscaphocapitate, long radiolunate, short radiolunate, ulnolunate, ulnocapitate, and ulnotriquetralcapitate
  - Dorsal – dorsal radiotriquetral

Biomechanics

- Distal carpal row
  - Minimal interosseous motion – functions as one unit
  - Wrist flexion – distal row flexes and ulnarly deviates
  - Wrist extension – extends and shifts distal row radially
  - Wrist ulnar deviation – distal row flexes, shifts ulnarly, and pronates
  - Wrist radial deviation – distal row deviates radially and supinates
- Proximal carpal row
  - No tendon attachments, functions as intercalated segment, and motion directed by surrounding flexor and extensor tendons
  - Wrist flexion – proximal row flexes
  - Wrist extension – proximal row extends
  - Wrist radial and ulnar deviation – proximal row moves opposite to distal row
    - Ulnshifts radially
    - Radial deviation – proximal row flexes and shifts ulnarly

Carpal Instability

- Definition
  - Abnormal motion and load transfer in the wrist
- Types [1]

G.S. Buchanan, MD • A. Koester, MD (✉)
Department of Orthopaedic Surgery, Joan C. Edwards
School of Medicine, Marshall University,
Huntington, WV, USA
e-mail: buchanang@marshall.edu;
koestera@marshall.edu

© Springer International Publishing AG 2017
A.E.M. Eltorai et al. (eds.), *Orthopedic Surgery Clerkship*, DOI 10.1007/978-3-319-52567-9_49

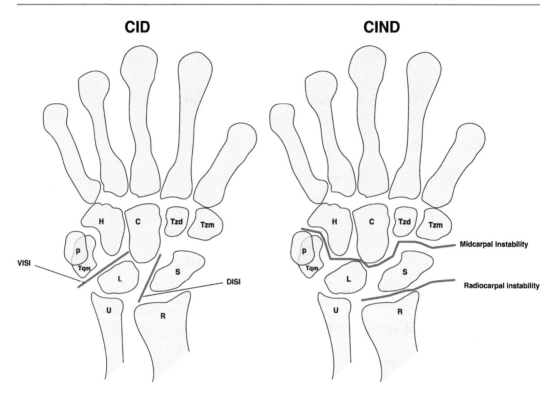

Fig. 49.1 *CID* vs. *CIND*. In CID, instability exists between carpal bones of a single row, between the scaphoid and the lunate in DISI or between the lunate and triquetrum in VISI. In CIND, the instability exists between carpal rows. Midcarpal instability occurs between the proximal and distal carpal rows, while radiocarpal instability occurs between the proximal carpal row and the radius

– Carpal instability dissociative (CID) – instability within proximal or distal row (dorsal or volar intercalated segment instability) (Fig. 49.1)
– Carpal instability nondissociative (CIND) – instability between rows and distal radius (Fig. 49.1)
– Carpal instability complex (CIC) – features of both CID and CIND, perilunate dislocations, and other carpal dislocations
– Carpal instability adaptive (CIA) – instability caused by distal radius malunion or Madelung deformity

Carpal Instability Dissociative (CID)

Scapholunate Ligament Injuries: Dorsal Intercalated Segment Instability (DISI)

- Mechanism of injury.
  - Direct force to wrist

  - Indirect force to wrist
- Abnormal scaphoid motion ultimately results in arthritis.
  - Scapholunate advanced collapse (SLAC) arthritis – proximal migration of capitate to space between scaphoid and lunate results in painful arthritis.
- History and physical exam.
  - Pain over dorsal SLIL.
  - Watson maneuver – apply pressure over scaphoid tubercle and perform radioulnar deviation [2].
    ◦ Dorsal pain over SL joint suggests partial tear.
    ◦ Audible clunk suggests complete tear.
    ◦ False positive in a third of patients – compare both wrists.
- Radiographs.
  - PA and lateral views, carpal series.
  - Static instability – radiographic intercarpal relationships do not change with manipulation or motion.

- Dynamic instability – radiographic intercarpal relationships change with manipulation or motion.
- Gilula's lines – three parallel arcs on PA view [3].
  - Arc of proximal articular surface of proximal row
  - Arc of distal articular surface of proximal row
  - Arc of proximal articular surface of distal row
  - Disruption of an arc suggests ligamentous injury or fracture
- Intercarpal angles – lateral view (Fig. 49.2).
  - Compare lines drawn perpendicular to contour of carpal bones, axial to radius.
  - Scapholunate angle – average 45°, <30° or >60° abnormal.
  - Radiolunate angle – average 0°, >15° dorsal or palmar abnormal.
  - >15° palmar – VISI
  - >15° dorsal – DISI
  - Deviation suggests SLIL or LTIL injury.
- Intercarpal distance – PA view.
  - >4 mm between scaphoid and lunate abnormal, suggests SLIL injury
- "Ring" sign on PA – distal pole of scaphoid in flexed position.
- "Clenched fist" PA view – capitate exerts pressure on scaphoid and lunate and may cause widening of SL interval (Terry Thomas sign) or increased SL angle.
- Early injury x-ray may be false negative.
- Arthrography.
  - Communication from midcarpal to radiocarpal joint indicates probable SLIL tear.
  - Former gold standard.
  - 91% sensitive, 88% specific, 83% positive predictive value, and 88% negative predictive value [4].

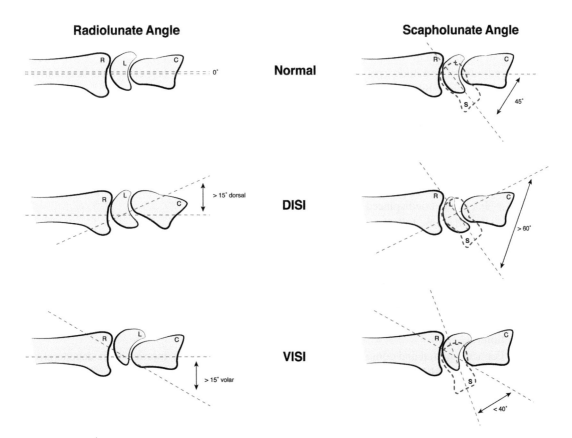

Fig. 49.2 Radiolunate and scapholunate angles demonstrate normal carpal anatomy, DISI, and VISI. The radiolunate angle is the angle between a *line* drawn through the axis of the radius and a *line* drawn perpendicular to the lunate. The scapholunate angle is the angle between a *line* drawn through the axis of the scaphoid and a *line* drawn perpendicular to the lunate. Radius (*R*), lunate (*L*), capitate (*C*), and scaphoid (*S*)

- – False positives in the elderly.
- Arthroscopy.
  - – Current gold standard.
  - – Allows direct inspection of SLIL and supporting extrinsic ligaments.
  - – Midcarpal view step-off or diastasis of SL joint indicates instability.
  - – Graded by Geissler classification [5].
    - ○ Grade I – attenuation or hemorrhage of interosseous ligament as seen from radiocarpal space. No incongruence of carpal alignment in midcarpal space.
    - ○ Grade II – attenuation or hemorrhage of interosseous ligament as seen from radiocarpal space. Incongruence or step-off of carpal space. There may be slight gap (less than width of probe) between carpal bones.
    - ○ Grade III – incongruence or step-off of carpal alignment as seen from both radiocarpal and midcarpal space. Probe may be passed through gap between carpal bones.
    - ○ Grade IV – incongruence or step-off of carpal alignment as seen from both radiocarpal and midcarpal space. There is gross instability with manipulation. 2.7 mm arthroscope may be passed through gap between carpal bones.
- Treatment.
  - – Nonoperative
    - ○ Splinting/casting with nonsteroidal anti-inflammatory drugs (NSAIDs)
      - – For acute, nondisplaced tears
      - – Provide close follow-up
  - – Closed reduction and pinning with K-wires [6]
    - ○ For acute instability
  - – Arthroscopic repair
    - ○ Debridement and electrothermal shrinkage or arthroscopic reduction and fixation [7]
    - ○ For acute partial and complete tears
  - – Open repair of SLIL
    - ○ If closed reduction and pinning are unsuccessful
    - ○ Only if enough ligament remains that can be repaired and no degenerative changes are present

- ○ Direct SLIL repair with dorsal radioscaphoid capsulodesis [8]
  - – Twenty-one patients all had improvement of grip strength, pain, and X-ray.
- – Ligament reconstruction
  - ○ If closed reduction is unsuccessful and ligament cannot be repaired.
  - ○ Contraindicated in patients with wrist degenerative joint disease.
  - ○ Four bone ligament reconstruction [9].
    - – Weave extensor carpi radialis brevis (ECRB) tendon through capitate, lunate, scaphoid, and radius.
    - – In a study of 36 cases of chronic complete SL separation, 86% returned to preinjury activity level [9].
  - ○ Bone-retinaculum-bone reconstruction [10].
  - ○ Complications – tendons grafts may become lax, and bone tunnels may cause fracture.
  - ○ Unpredictable outcome.
- – Dorsal capsulodesis
  - ○ Dorsal wrist capsule tethers scaphoid to prevent subluxation
  - ○ Blatt capsulodesis [11–13]
  - ○ Mayo capsulodesis [13]
  - ○ Szabo capsulodesis [14]
  - ○ Provides pain relief, decreases wrist motion, does not improve grip strength, and does not maintain carpal alignment [13, 14]
- – Tenodesis
  - ○ Tendon weave reestablishes SLIL and SL stability.
  - ○ Brunelli tenodesis [15].
    - – Slip of flexor carpi radialis (FCR) passed through bone tunnel in distal pole of scaphoid.
- – Arthrodesis
  - ○ For chronic injuries with degenerative changes
  - ○ Scaphoid trapezium trapezoid (STT) fusion [16]
  - ○ Four corner fusion
    - – Scaphoid excision and fusion of lunate, capitate, triquetrum, and hamate

– Satisfactory pain relief [17]
  ◦ Total wrist fusion
– Proximal row carpectomy
  ◦ Excision of the entire proximal carpal row
  ◦ Results in weakened, stiffened wrist [18]
  ◦ Poor outcome compared to other methods [18]
– Total wrist arthroplasty
  ◦ For advanced SLAC arthritis
  ◦ Satisfactory pain relief and function [19]

Lunotriquetral Ligament Injuries: Volar Intercalated Segment Instability (VISI)

- Volar intercalated segment instability (VISI) – loss of the LT and dorsal radiotriquetral ligaments allows the lunate to flex.
- History and physical exam.
  – Ulnar-sided wrist pain.
  – Tenderness at LT joint.
  – Radioulnar deviation may produce painful click.
  – LT ballottement [20].
    ◦ Pain and AP laxity with manipulation of pisotriquetral lunate joint
  – Shear (Kleinman) test [21].
    ◦ Dorsal pain with palmar loading of pisotriquetral joint
  – Compression test [22].
    ◦ Pain, crepitus, or abnormal motion with radial compression of the triquetrum
  – Rule out nondissociative carpal instability; presentation and exam can be similar.
- Radiographs.
  – Often normal
  – VISI deformity – triquetrum extends, scaphoid and lunate flex
  – Disruption of Gilula's lines [3]
  – Proximal migration of triquetrum, lunotriquetral overlap
  – SL angle <40° (Fig. 49.2)
  – Radiolunate angle >15° palmar (Fig. 49.2)
  – Capitolunate angle >10°

- Arthrography.
  – Communication at LT joint space
  – False positives in elderly patients
- Arthroscopy.
  – Gold standard
  – Instability graded by Geissler classification [5]
- Treatment.
  – Nonoperative
    ◦ Splint/cast immobilization and observation
  – LT ligament repair
    ◦ Reattach LTIL to site of avulsion (usually triquetrum) with sutures or suture anchors.
    ◦ Satisfactory results, better function, and pain relief than arthrodesis [23].
    ◦ 13.5% complication free at 5 years [23].
  – LT ligament reconstruction
    ◦ For chronic instability, degraded LT ligament, and highly functional patient
    ◦ Reconstruction with distal strip of extensor carpi ulnaris (ECU) tendon graft
    ◦ Satisfactory results, better function, and pain relief than arthrodesis [23]
    ◦ 68.6% complication free at 5 years [23]
  – LT arthrodesis
    ◦ <1% complication free at 5 years [23].
    ◦ Complications – 40.9% nonunion rate; ulnocarpal impingement required reoperation in 22.7% [23].
  – Proximal row carpectomy
    ◦ Salvage procedure for degenerative changes
    ◦ Excision of entire proximal carpal row [24]
  – Total wrist arthroplasty
    ◦ For advanced degenerative changes

Carpal Instability Nondissociative (CIND)

- Abnormal motion between proximal and distal carpal rows or proximal carpal row and radius. Normal stability among individual bones of proximal and distal carpal rows.

Radiocarpal Instability (Fig. 49.1)

- Incompetent radiocarpal ligaments
- Ulnar translocation of the carpus
- Four subcategories: palmar, dorsal, combined, and adaptive [25]
- Rare [26]
- Treatment involves reduction and restoration of ligaments [26]

Midcarpal Instability

- Disruption of reciprocal motion of proximal and distal rows (Fig. 49.1)
- Physical exam
  - Circumduction test – ulnar deviation and axial compression cause painful clunk.

Classification [27, 28]

- Palmar midcarpal instability – rupture of palmar midcarpal ligaments

- Medial – triquetral hamate capitate ligaments
- Lateral – scaphoid capitate trapezoid trapezium ligaments
  - Dorsal midcarpal instability – disruption of radiocapitate ligament
  - Combined dorsal and palmar instability – laxity of both midcarpal and radiocarpal ligaments
  - Extrinsic midcarpal instability – chronic dorsally angulated distal radius fracture malunion stretches volar carpal ligaments (form of CIA)

Treatment

- Nonoperative
  - Initial treatment for all patients: immobilization, rest, NSAIDs, and intra-articular corticosteroid injections [29]
- Operative
  - Arthroscopic thermal capsulorrhaphy [25]

- Soft tissue reconstruction [27, 29, 30]
- Arthrodesis [27]

Carpal Instability Complex (CIC)

- Combination of CID and CIND
- Five groups [31]
  - Dorsal perilunate dislocations
  - Dorsal perilunate fracture dislocations
  - Palmar perilunate fracture dislocations
  - Axial carpal dislocations
  - Isolated carpal dislocations

Perilunate Dislocations

- Carpus dislocates around lunate, which often remains bound to the radius by radiolunate ligaments.
- Dorsal perilunate dislocation – capitate dislocates dorsally.
- Palmar perilunate dislocation – capitate dislocates palmarly.
- Fractures may involve distal radius and carpal bones.
- History and physical exam.
  - High-energy trauma
  - Significant swelling, ecchymosis, and decreased range of motion
  - 25% acute carpal tunnel syndrome [31]

Radiographs

- Subtle findings, missed initially in 25% [31]
- Disrupted Gilula's lines and abnormal spacing among carpal bones on PA view
- Dislocated capitate or lunate on lateral view
- Mayfield classification [32]
  - Stage 1: Scapholunate disruption
  - Stage 2: Scapholunate and lunocapitate disruption
  - Stage 3: Scapholunate, lunocapitate, and lunotriquetral disruption
  - Stage 4: Volar dislocation of lunate, possible median nerve compression

Treatment

- Closed reduction
  - For acute injuries, non-definitive management
- Open reduction internal fixation (ORIF)
  - Reduce carpal bones and fix with K-wires and repair SLIL and LTIL.
  - Most reliable improvement in function and pain compared to other methods [33–35].
- Proximal row carpectomy
- Total wrist fusion

Axial Carpal Dislocations

- Severe trauma causes longitudinal split and displacement of the carpus [36].
- Uncommon, 1.4% of carpal fracture dislocations [36].
- Massive swelling and deformity.
- Associated with soft tissue injury, nerve injury, and other hand and forearm fractures.
- Classified by direction of instability; carpus is divided into two columns, ulnar and radial [37].
  - Axial-ulnar disruption – stable radial column and displaced ulnar column (includes metacarpals)
  - Axial-radial disruption – ulnar column stable and displaced radial column (includes metacarpals)
  - Combined axial-radial-ulnar disruptions

Treatment

- ORIF
- Debride devitalized tissue, reduce carpal bones and fix with K-wires, repair damaged neurovasculature and tendons, skin coverage with local or free flaps, and fasciotomy if concerned for compartment syndrome [37]

Isolated Carpal Bone Dislocation

- Rare, caused by direct or indirect force to focused area of wrist, and can involve any carpal bone. Removal of dislocated carpal bone is well tolerated except with lunate and scaphoid dislocation [28].

Carpal Instability Adaptive (CIA)

- Malpositioned carpus with distal radius malunion or Madelung deformity.
- Corrective osteotomy can resolve pain and instability from distal radius malunion [38, 39].

References

1. Cooney WP, Dobyns JH, Linscheid RL. Arthroscopy of the wrist: anatomy and classification of carpal instability. Arthroscopy J Arthrosc Relat Surg Off Publ Arthrosc Assoc N Am Int Arthrosc Assoc. 1990;6(2):133–40.
2. Watson HK, Ashmead DT, Makhlouf MV. Examination of the scaphoid. J Hand Surg. 1988;13(5):657–60.
3. Gilula LA. Carpal injuries: analytic approach and case exercises. AJR Am J Roentgenol. 1979;133(3):503–17.
4. Mahmood A, Fountain J, Vasireddy N, Waseem M. Wrist MRI arthrogram v wrist arthroscopy: what are we finding? Open Orthop J. 2012;6:194–8.
5. Geissler WB, Freeland AE, Savoie FH, McIntyre LW, Whipple TL. Intracarpal soft-tissue lesions associated with an intra-articular fracture of the distal end of the radius. J Bone Joint Surg Am. 1996;78(3):357–65.
6. Whipple TL. The role of arthroscopy in the treatment of scapholunate instability. Hand Clin. 1995;11(1):37–40.
7. Bednar JM. Acute scapholunate ligament injuries: arthroscopic treatment. Hand Clin. 2015;31(3):417–23.
8. Lavernia CJ, Cohen MS, Taleisnik J. Treatment of scapholunate dissociation by ligamentous repair and capsulodesis. J Hand Surg. 1992;17(2):354–9.
9. Almquist EE, Bach AW, Sack JT, Fuhs SE, Newman DM. Four-bone ligament reconstruction for treatment of chronic complete scapholunate separation. J Hand Surg. 1991;16(2):322–7.
10. Wolf JM, Weiss AP. Bone-retinaculum-bone reconstruction of scapholunate ligament injuries. Orthop Clin North Am. 2001;32(2):241–6. viii.

11. Blatt G. Capsulodesis in reconstructive hand surgery. Dorsal capsulodesis for the unstable scaphoid and volar capsulodesis following excision of the distal ulna. Hand Clin. 1987;3(1):81–102.

12. Deshmukh SC, Givissis P, Belloso D, Stanley JK, Trail IA. Blatt's capsulodesis for chronic scapholunate dissociation. J Hand Surg (Edinburgh, Scotland). 1999;24(2):215–20.

13. Moran SL, Cooney WP, Berger RA, Strickland J. Capsulodesis for the treatment of chronic scapholunate instability. J Hand Surg. 2005;30(1):16–23.

14. Szabo RM, Slater Jr RR, Palumbo CF, Gerlach T. Dorsal intercarpal ligament capsulodesis for chronic, static scapholunate dissociation: clinical results. J Hand Surg. 2002;27(6):978–84.

15. Brunelli GA, Brunelli GR. A new surgical technique for carpal instability with scapho-lunar dislocation. (Eleven cases). Annales de chirurgie de la main et du membre superieur : organe officiel des societes de chirurgie de la main Ann Hand Upper Limb Surg. 1995;14(4–5):207–13.

16. Watson HK, Ryu J, Akelman E. Limited triscaphoid intercarpal arthrodesis for rotatory subluxation of the scaphoid. J Bone Joint Surg Am. 1986;68(3):345–9.

17. Winkler FJ, Borisch N, Rath B, Grifka J, Heers G. Mid-term results after scaphoid excision and four-corner wrist arthrodesis using K-wires for advanced carpal collapse. Z Orthop Unfall. 2010;148(3):332–7.

18. Elfar JC, Stern PJ. Proximal row carpectomy for scapholunate dissociation. J Hand Surg Eur Vol. 2011;36(2):111–5.

19. Cooney W, Manuel J, Froelich J, Rizzo M. Total wrist replacement: a retrospective comparative study. J Wrist Surg. 2012;1(2):165–72.

20. Reagan DS, Linscheid RL, Dobyns JH. Lunotriquetral sprains. J Hand Surg. 1984;9(4):502–14.

21. Weiss LE, Taras JS, Sweet S, Osterman AL. Lunotriquetral injuries in the athlete. Hand Clin. 2000;16(3):433–8.

22. Beckenbaugh RD. Accurate evaluation and management of the painful wrist following injury. An approach to carpal instability. Orthop Clin North Am. 1984;15(2):289–306.

23. Shin AY, Weinstein LP, Berger RA, Bishop AT. Treatment of isolated injuries of the lunotriquetral ligament. A comparison of arthrodesis, ligament reconstruction and ligament repair. J Bone Joint Surg. 2001;83(7):1023–8.

24. Wall LB, Stern PJ. Proximal row carpectomy. Hand Clin. 2013;29(1):69–78.

25. Wolfe SW, Garcia-Elias M, Kitay A. Carpal instability nondissociative. J Am Acad Orthop Surg. 2012;20(9):575–85.

26. Dumontier C, Meyer zu Reckendorf G, Sautet A, Lenoble E, Saffar P, Allieu Y. Radiocarpal dislocations: classification and proposal for treatment. A review of twenty-seven cases. J Bone Joint Surg Am Vol. 2001;83-a(2):212–8.

27. Lichtman DM, Bruckner JD, Culp RW, Alexander CE. Palmar midcarpal instability: results of surgical reconstruction. J Hand Surg. 1993;18(2):307–15.

28. Shin AY, Moran SL. Carpal instability including dislocations. In: Core knowledge in orthopedics: hand, elbow, and shoulder. Elselvier; 2005. p. 139–76.

29. Wright TW, Dobyns JH, Linscheid RL, Macksoud W, Siegert J. Carpal instability non-dissociative. J Hand Surg (Edinburgh, Scotland). 1994;19(6):763–73.

30. Johnson RP, Carrera GF. Chronic capitolunate instability. J Bone Joint Surg Am. 1986;68(8):1164–76.

31. Herzberg G, Comtct JJ, Linschcid RL, Amadio PC, Cooney WP, Stalder J. Perilunate dislocations and fracture-dislocations: a multicenter study. J Hand Surg. 1993;18(5):768–79.

32. Kennedy SA, Allan CH. In brief: Mayfield et al. Classification: carpal dislocations and progressive perilunar instability. Clin Orthop Relat Res. 2012;470(4):1243–5.

33. Siegert JJ, Frassica FJ, Amadio PC. Treatment of chronic perilunate dislocations. J Hand Surg. 1988;13(2):206–12.

34. Inoue G, Shionoya K. Late treatment of unreduced perilunate dislocations. J Hand Surg (Edinburgh, Scotland). 1999;24(2):221–5.

35. Muppavarapu RC, Capo JT. Perilunate dislocations and fracture dislocations. Hand Clin. 2015;31(3):399–408.

36. Reinsmith LE, Garcia-Elias M, Gilula LA. Traumatic axial dislocation injuries of the wrist. Radiology. 2013;267(3):680–9.

37. Garcia-Elias M, Dobyns JH, Cooney 3rd WP, Linscheid RL. Traumatic axial dislocations of the carpus. J Hand Surg. 1989;14(3):446–57.

38. De Smet L, Verhaegen F, Degreef I. Carpal malalignment in malunion of the distal radius and the effect of corrective osteotomy. J Wrist Surg. 2014;3(3):166–70.

39. Taleisnik J, Watson HK. Midcarpal instability caused by malunited fractures of the distal radius. J Hand Surg. 1984;9(3):350–7.

Flexor Tendon Injuries of the Upper Extremity

50

Andrew Campbell and Kanu Goyal

Anatomy

Tendon Structure

- Composed of bundles of collagen fascicles surrounded by epitenon, a surface which is crucial for gliding

Tendon Nutritional Supply

- Arterial supply – vincula from digital arteries
- Synovial diffusion

Relationship of Flexor Digitorum Superficialis (FDS) and Flexor Digitorum Profundus (FDP)

- In the wrist and hand, FDS tendons lie superficial to FDP.
- At level of metacarpophalangeal (MCP) joints, within flexor sheath, FDS splits into two slips, and FDP becomes superficial.
- At Camper's chiasm, FDS slips rejoin and then insert on mid-middle phalanx.

A. Campbell, MD • K. Goyal, MD (✉)
Ohio State University Wexner Medical Center, Columbus, OH, USA
e-mail: kanu.goyal@osumc.edu

- FDP inserts on base of distal phalanx.
- Flexor tendon zones of injury (Fig. 50.1).

Phases of Tendon Wound Healing

- Hemostatic (immediate) – fibrin clot formation
- Inflammatory (days 1–7) – inflammatory cell migration and extracellular matrix deposition
- Proliferative (days 3–14) – fibroblast proliferation, vascular ingrowth along disorganized fibronectin scaffold
- Remodeling (day 10 onward) – linear organization of collagen fibers

Presentation

Mechanism

- Laceration or penetrating injury
  - Note position of finger when injury was sustained.
- Avulsion injury
  - Jersey finger – FDP avulsion from base of distal phalanx. Occurs due to forceful extension of distal interphalangeal (DIP) joint during FDP contraction.
- Loss of active flexion
  - Test FDS and FDP for each finger (Fig. 50.2).

© Springer International Publishing AG 2017
A.E.M. Eltorai et al. (eds.), *Orthopedic Surgery Clerkship*, DOI 10.1007/978-3-319-52567-9_50

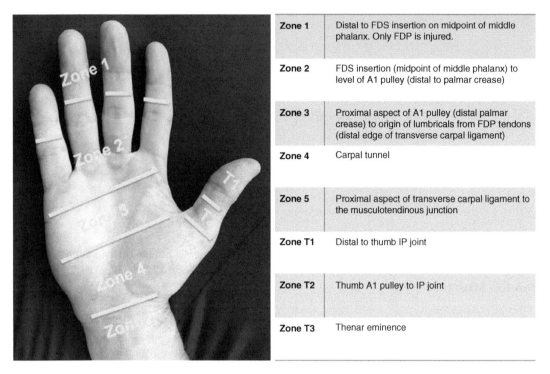

Zone 1	Distal to FDS insertion on midpoint of middle phalanx. Only FDP is injured.
Zone 2	FDS insertion (midpoint of middle phalanx) to level of A1 pulley (distal to palmar crease)
Zone 3	Proximal aspect of A1 pulley (distal palmar crease) to origin of lumbricals from FDP tendons (distal edge of transverse carpal ligament)
Zone 4	Carpal tunnel
Zone 5	Proximal aspect of transverse carpal ligament to the musculotendinous junction
Zone T1	Distal to thumb IP joint
Zone T2	Thumb A1 pulley to IP joint
Zone T3	Thenar eminence

Fig. 50.1 Flexor tendon zones of injury

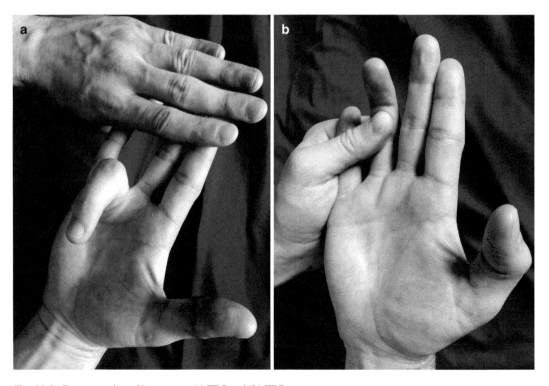

Fig. 50.2 Demonstration of how to test (**a**) FDS and (**b**) FDP

- Abnormal resting posture
  - Digit held in extended posture
- Abnormal digital cascade
  - Tenodesis effect – passive wrist extension normally causes flexion at MCP, PIP, and DIP joints.
  - Persistent extension at PIP or DIP joints during passive wrist extension is indicative of flexor tendon injury.
- Abnormal neurovascular exam
  - Concomitant neurovascular injuries are common. Document a thorough exam at the time of injury.
  - Assess perfusion to each digit (<2 s capillary refill is normal).
  - Assess two-point discrimination on radial and ulnar aspect of each digit (<6 mm is normal).

Treatment

Nonoperative Management with Wound Care and Early Range of Motion

- Indicated in partial lacerations <50% tendon width

Operative Management

- Lacerations <33% tendon width – debridement is often adequate to prevent triggering.
- Lacerations >50% width – flexor tendon repair indicated.
  - Optimal timing is within 3 weeks after injury.
- Emergency repair is indicated if digital perfusion is compromised, prompting exploration and possible microvascular repair.
  - Emergency department care
    ° Irrigate copiously and loosely close skin.
    ° Administer antibiotics and ensure tetanus is up to date.
    ° Apply a dorsal blocking splint.

- Treatment strategy depends on zone of injury (Fig. 50.1).
  - Zone I – tendon to bone repair if <1 cm of distal tendon stump is remaining, otherwise direct tendon repair
  - Zone II – direct tendon repair of FDP and FDS
    ° Historically poor results after tendon repair ("no man's land"), but results improving with modern rehab protocols.
  - Zone III – direct tendon repair
    ° Complicated by vicinity of tendons to digital nerves, superficial arch, and lumbrical muscles.
  - Zone IV – direct tendon repair
    ° Avoid violation of transverse carpal ligament (TCL). Repair TCL if it is lacerated unless median nerve is also injured; then, TCL must be completely released.
  - Zone V – direct tendon repair
    ° Often associated with neurovascular injury.
  - Thumb – repairs have higher re-rupture rate than fingers.
- Method of tendon repair depends on surgeon preference.
  - Core suture strength is related to suture material, caliber of suture, and most importantly the number of sutures crossing repair site.
  - Subsequent epitendinous suture improves gliding and increases repair strength.

Pearls

- Incorporate skin laceration into a Brunner incision.
- May require second incision proximally if tendon retracted into hand.
- Handle tendon atraumatically to prevent adhesion formation.
- If interposition graft is necessary, palmaris longus tendon is often used.
- Release pulleys as necessary to allow tendon glide without interference.

- Consider repairing one slip of FDS instead of both to decrease volume within flexor sheath.
- Wide-awake surgery allows the surgeon to test repair integrity and glide.
- Use a minimum of four core sutures with 3-0 or 4-0 tapered needle.

Postoperative Rehabilitation

Controlled Mobilization Postoperatively Is Key

- Tendon repairs weaken during first 3 weeks postop if immobilized.
- Tendons with repair site gap <3 mm begin developing increased tensile strength after week 3.
- Multiple early active and passive motion protocols have been described.

Complications

- Tendon adhesions – most common.
- Stiffness, joint contracture.

- Re-rupture – treatment is re-repair or two-stage tendon reconstruction:
- Two-stage reconstruction
  - Stage 1 – pulley reconstruction and placement of temporary silicone grafts (Hunter rod)
  - Stage 2 – 3 months later when the flexor sheath has reformed, the Hunter rods are removed, and a tendon graft is repaired to the distal phalanx.

References

1. Chang J, et al. Tendon. In: Hammert WC, editor. ASSH manual of hand surgery. Philadelphia: Lippincott Williams & Wilkins; 2010. p. 93–110.
2. Seiler III JG. Flexor tendon injury. In: Wolfe SW, et al., editors. Green's operative hand surgery. 6th ed. Philadelphia: Churchill Livingstone; 2010.
3. Gelberman RH, et al. The effect of gap formation at the repair site on the strength and excursion of intrasynovial flexor tendons. An experimental study on the early stages of tendon-healing in dogs. JBJS. 1999;81(7):975–82.
4. Kim HM, et al. Technical and biologic modifications for enhanced flexor tendon repair. J Hand Surg. 2010;35A:1031–7.

Extensor Tendon Injuries of the Upper Extremity

51

Erin F. Ransom and Nileshkumar M. Chaudhari

Anatomy

Muscles and Tendons

- Extensor digitorum communis (EDC)
  - Origin: Lateral epicondyle of humerus
  - Insertion: Extensor expansions of index, long, ring, and small fingers
  - Innervation: Posterior interosseous nerve (PIN)
  - Action: Extends fingers at MCP joints and extends the hand
- Extensor indicis proprius (EIP)
  - Origin: Posterior ulna
  - Insertion: Extensor expansion of the index finger ulnar to insertion of EDC
  - Innervation: PIN
  - Action: Extends the index finger at MCP joint
- Extensor digiti minimi (EDM)
  - Origin: Lateral epicondyle of humerus
  - Insertion: Extensor expansions of the small finger

  - Action: Extends the small finger at MCP joint
- Extensor pollicis longus (EPL)
  - Origin: Posterior surface of ulna
  - Insertion: Base of thumb distal phalanx
  - Innervation: PIN
  - Action: Extend thumb distal phalanx
- Abductor pollicis longus (APL)
  - Origin: Posterior ulna and radius
  - Insertion: Base of thumb metacarpal
  - Innervation: PIN
  - Action: Thumb abduction and extension at CMC joint
- Extensor pollicis brevis (EPB)
  - Origin: Posterior radius
  - Insertion: Base of thumb proximal phalanx
  - Innervation: PIN
  - Action: Thumb extension at MCP joint

Anatomy of the Extensor Mechanism

- EDC tendon splits into three portions proximal to the PIP joint.
  - Central portion becomes central slip that inserts on middle phalanx.
  - Each of the two lateral portions joins the intrinsic tendons of the lumbricals and interossei to form the lateral bands.

E.F. Ransom, MD (✉) • N.M. Chaudhari, MD
Division of Orthopaedic Surgery, Department of
Surgery, University of Alabama – Birmingham,
Birmingham, AL, USA
e-mail: efynan@uabmc.edu

© Springer International Publishing AG 2017
A.E.M. Eltorai et al. (eds.), *Orthopedic Surgery Clerkship*, DOI 10.1007/978-3-319-52567-9_51

- Lateral bands merge over the middle phalanx and continue dorsally over the DIP to insert into the distal phalanx.
- Triangular ligament and transverse retinacular ligaments hold lateral bands in place along the side of the PIP joint.
  - Triangular ligament prevents palmar subluxation during PIP flexion.
  - Transverse retinacular ligaments prevent dorsal subluxation during PIP extension.

Extensor Compartments

- First dorsal compartment: Contains EPB and APL
- Second dorsal compartment: Contains extensor carpi radialis longus and brevis
- Third dorsal compartment: Contains EPL
- Fourth dorsal compartment: Contains EIP, EDC, and PIN
- Fifth dorsal compartment: Contains EDM
- Sixth dorsal compartment: Contains ECU

Extensor Tendon Zone of Injury
(Fig. 51.1)

Other Structures

- Juncturae tendinae
  - Bands of tissue proximal to the MCP joint connecting the middle finger, ring finger, and small finger EDC tendons transversely.
  - Finger extension can be preserved if EDC tendon injured proximal to these bands.
- Sagittal bands
  - Sagittal bands keep extensor tendon in a central position at the MCP joint.

Presentation

Mechanism

- Laceration or crush injury
- Forced flexion of extended joint

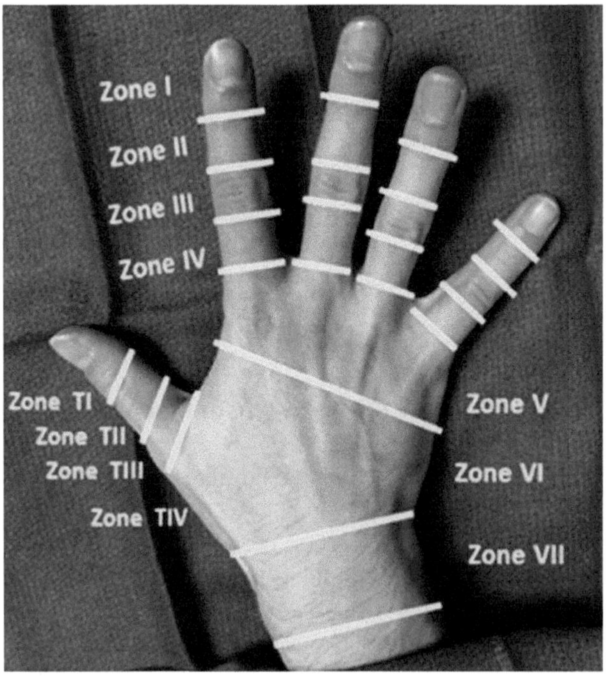

Zone I	Injury is distal to the DIP joint
Zone II	Injury is overlying the middle phalanx
Zone III	Injury is over the PIP joint
Zone IV	Injury is overlying the proximal phalanx
Zone V	Injury is over the MCP joint
Zone VI	Injury is over the metacarpal Most common zone of injury
Zone VII	Injury to the tendon and retinaculum over the wrist joint
Zone VIII	Injury to the muscle belly in the distal forearm
Zone TI	Injury is distal to the IP joint of the thumb
Zone TII	Injury is overlying the proximal phalanx of the thumb
Zone TIII	Injury is over the MCP joint of the thumb
Zone TIV	Injury is over the CMC joint of the thumb

Fig. 51.1 Image of the hand showing the different zones of extensor tendon injuries

- Zone I: Forced flexion of DIP joint → mallet finger
- Forced extension of flexed joint
  - Zone V: Forced extension leading to sagittal band rupture or "flea flicker injury"
  - Most common in the long finger
- Fight bite
  - Most common in Zone V

Loss of Active Extension

- Loss of active extension at the DIP joint
- Elson test
  - Best tested across table from patient.
  - Place PIP joint in flexion over a table at 90°.
  - Ask patient to extend while providing resistance over the middle phalanx.
  - If central slip intact → DIP supple.
  - If central slip injured → DIP rigid.

Neurovascular Exam

- Assess perfusion and two-point discrimination of each digit as discussed in the previous chapter.

Imaging

- Obtain AP and lateral of the digit to evaluate for bony avulsions.
- Obtain AP/lateral/oblique of the hand to evaluate for associated fractures.

Specific Injuries by Zone

- Zone I: Mallet finger
  - Soft tissue or bony avulsion of the terminal extensor tendon insertion
  - Can lead to swan neck deformity with DIP flexion and PIP hyperextension
- Zone III: Boutonniere deformity

- Rupture of central slip leads to palmar subluxation of the lateral bands.
- Lateral bands work to flex the PIP joint instead of extend.
- Leads to DIP extension with PIP flexion.
- Zone V
  - Fight bite
    - *Eikenella corrodens*
    - Important to treat with IV antibiotics, tetanus, and operative irrigation and debridement
  - Sagittal band rupture
    - Tendon subluxation ulnarly over the MCP joint when attempting extension

Treatment

Nonoperative Management

- Indications
  - Laceration with less than 50% of the tendon involved with maintained active extension against resistance
  - Acute mallet finger (<12 weeks)
  - Non-displaced bony mallet
  - Chronic mallet finger without joint stiffness
  - Closed central slip injury
  - Closed sagittal band rupture
- Technique
  - Extension splinting
    - DIP extension splinting for mallet finger does not need to include the PIP joint.
  - Timing
    - Full-time splinting for 6 weeks
    - Part-time splinting for 4–6 weeks

Operative Management

- Use any open wounds in incision planning.
- Immediate operative I and D for fight bite to MCP joint.
- Tendon repair.

- The number of crossing strands is most important with increasing strength per number of crossing strands.
- Four to six strands will allow for early active range of motion, but repairs distal to the PIP joint (Zones I–III) do not do well with early ROM.
- Extensor tendons are flat overlying the phalanges. Do not use a single core suture as it can lead to bunching.
- Weakest between postoperative days 6 and 12.
- Repair type by zone.
  - Zone I: Running suture that can incorporate the skin as well
  - Zone II: Running suture near the edge with cross-stitch dorsally
  - Zones III–V and Zones TII–III: Kessler suture in the thickest part of the tendon
  - Zones VI–VII: Same as Zones III–V but with circumferential cross-stitch as well
- Fixation of bony avulsion.
  - K-wire fixation
  - Screw fixation
- Tendon reconstruction.
  - Zones I–II: Spiral oblique retinacular ligament reconstruction where the flexor tendon sheath is connected to the terminal tendon stump to cause automatic DIP extension with active PIP extension
- Central slip reconstruction.
  - Terminal tendon tenotomy
    ∘ Creates a mallet finger that allows for DIP joint flexion and increases the tension at the PIP joint
    ∘ Must have full ROM of the PIP joint
    ∘ Tendon graft in figure of eight through the extensor mechanism
    ∘ Lateral band mobilization and relocation
    ∘ EIP to EPL tendon transfer

Postoperative Protocol

- Zones I–II: 6 weeks of immobilization
- Zones III–V: 4 weeks of immobilization with the wrist in extension, MCP slight flexion, and PIP extension

- Zones VI–VII: 4 weeks of immobilization with wrist and MCP joint extension with DIP and PIP joints free for active ROM

Complications

Adhesions

- Prevented with early protected ROM
- Treated with extensor tenolysis and early ROM
- Tendon rupture
  - Highest risk at 7–10 days post-op
- Swan neck deformity
  - Dorsal subluxation of the lateral bands causing DIP flexion and PIP hyperextension
- Boutonniere deformity
  - Volar subluxation of the lateral bands causing DIP extension and PIP flexion

References

1. Lin JD, Strauch RJ. Closed soft tissue extensor mechanism injuries (mallet, boutonniere, and sagittal band). J Hand Surg [Am]. 2014;39(5):1005–11.
2. Brunton LM, Chhabra AB. Hand, upper extremity, and microvascular surgery. In: Miller MD, et al., editors. Review of orthopedics. 6th ed. Philadelphia: Elsevier; 2012.
3. Seiler III JG. Extensor tendon injury. In: Wolfe SW, et al., editors. Green's operative hand surgery. 6th ed. Philadelphia: Churchill Livingstone; 2010.

Suggested Readings

1. Shewring DJ, Trickett RW, Subramanian KN, Hnyda R. The management of clenched fist 'fight bite' injuries of the hand. J Hand Surg Eur Vol. 2015;40(8):819–24.

Nerve Injury

52

Brooks W. Ficke and Nileshkumar M. Chaudhari

Anatomy

- Cell bodies are located in the spinal cord (lower motor neuron) or dorsal root ganglion (sensory neuron).
- A nerve fiber (axon, Schwann cell sheath, ± myelin sheath) is surrounded by endoneurium.
- A fascicle (several fibers) is surrounded by perineurium (strong connective tissue, resists stretch).
- A nerve (several bundles of fascicles) is surrounded by epineurium (looser, vascularized membrane, protects against compression).

Classification of Nerve Injuries (Modified Seddon Classification)

Nondegenerative Lesions

- Neurapraxia
  - Nerve anatomically intact but physiologically not functioning (conduction block)
  - Axons intact (do not degenerate), but may have focal demyelination
  - Good prognosis as long as inciting factor is removed

B.W. Ficke, MD (✉) N.M. Chaudhari, MD
Division of Orthopedic Surgery, University of
Alabama at Birmingham, Birmingham, AL, USA
e-mail: brooks.ficke@gmail.com

Degenerative Lesions (Undergo Wallerian Degeneration)

- Axonotmesis (axon cutting)
  - Axon ruptured, but Schwann cell basal lamina remains intact
- Neurotmesis (nerve cutting)
  - All nerve elements are cut.
  - Recovery only possible with nerve repair

Mechanism of Injury

- The tidy wound
  - Sharp object
  - The goal is primary repair.
- The untidy wound
  - Open fracture, penetrating missile or foreign body, and crush injury
  - Contamination and local tissue damage limit ability to acutely repair.
  - Compression/crush
    - Pressure leads to local ischemia.
    - Resultant edema impairs nerve function.
    - Crush injury can cause extensive damage and poor prognosis.
- The closed traction injury
  - Damage occurs to nerves with elongation of 12% or greater.
  - Axons may rupture even though the epineurium remains intact.
  - Extensive damage throughout the nerve leads to poorer prognosis.

© Springer International Publishing AG 2017
A.E.M. Eltorai et al. (eds.), *Orthopedic Surgery Clerkship*, DOI 10.1007/978-3-319-52567-9_52

Presentation

History

- Mechanism (including height of fall, speed of vehicle, type of weapon, etc.)
- Motor and sensory changes
- Other health issues

Physical Exam

- Any wound (including open fracture) along the course of a nonfunctioning nerve indicates nerve transection until proven otherwise
- Full motor exam for the relevant extremity
- Full sensory exam (remembering that dermatomes may be inconsistent)
- Tinel's sign
  - Helps identify the level of nerve injury
  - Tap lightly along the course of the relevant nerve, moving from distal to proximal
  - Patient reports pins and needles sensation radiating to the appropriate cutaneous distribution when the tapping approaches the zone of regenerating fibers
  - (+) Tinel's on day of injury likely represents axonotmesis
  - Can be used to trace recovery of a nerve as axons regrow
- Sympathetic paralysis (red warm dry skin, capillary pulsation) indicates interruption of axons
- Remember to obtain a vascular exam

Imaging

- X-rays can show displacement of bone fragments, fracture patterns associated with nerve injury (i.e., Holstein-Lewis distal humerus fractures), and subluxated or dislocated joints
- Nerve conduction velocity (NCV) and electromyography (EMG)
- Difficult to interpret acutely, often not used until 3–4 months post-injury

- Fibrillation potentials: signs of muscle denervation, generally indicate a degenerative lesion
- Positive sharp waves: signs of acute denervation
- Fasciculations, complex repetitive discharges: signs of chronic denervation
- Voluntary motor unit potential activity
  - Return indicates reinnervation
  - Often seen before clinical signs of recovery are present
- Indications of focal compression or demyelination
  - Increased latencies (slowing)
  - Decreased conduction velocities (<52 m/s)
  - Decreased amplitude of motor action potentials (MAP) and sensory nerve action potentials (SNAP)

Prognosis

- The most important factor is the amount and type of damage done at the time of injury.
- Patient's age (younger better)
- Level of the lesion (higher typically worse)
- Timing
  - Urgent repair (within approximately 24 h) leads to improved results over delayed repair.
  - Functional reinnervation can often be obtained up to 1 year out from injury.

Treatment

Nonoperative

- Indicated in cases of neurapraxia or axonotmesis
- Axons bud proximally and migrate ~1 mm/day
- Can use physical exam and serial EMG to monitor recovery

Operative

- Necessary for recovery in cases of neurotmesis
- General principles
  - Meticulous tissue handling is essential.
  - Resect damaged nerve tissue until recognizable nerve bundles are seen.
  - Avoid excessive mobilization (preserve nerve blood supply).
  - Tension-free repair is essential. Splinting can reduce tension and protect the repair.
  - A healthy tissue bed (no torn muscle, no exposed tendon, no arteries) is important for reducing scarring and postoperative pain.
- Suture repair
  - Small gaps requiring little mobilization
  - Epineural sutures provide general alignment and strength to the repair.
  - Fascicular repair (suture of individual fascicles) can be used in clean transections of large nerves, but has not demonstrated improved results over epineural repair.
- Interposition graft
  - When tension-free primary repair cannot be achieved (Fig. 52.1a)
  - Can use autograft (common donor sites: sural n., saphenous n., lateral antebrachial cutaneous n.) (Fig. 52.2) or allograft (Fig. 52.1b)
  - Individual nerve bundles can be grafted in certain situations (Fig. 52.2).
- Entubulation
  - Uses an artificial tube (collagen, silicone, or other material) to enclose the two nerve endings, creating a conduit for axonal regrowth along an interposed fibrin clot
  - Avoids donor site morbidity
  - Limit: 3 cm gap

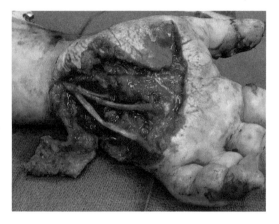

Fig. 52.2 Left segmental ulnar nerve injury treated with three sural nerve autograft segments

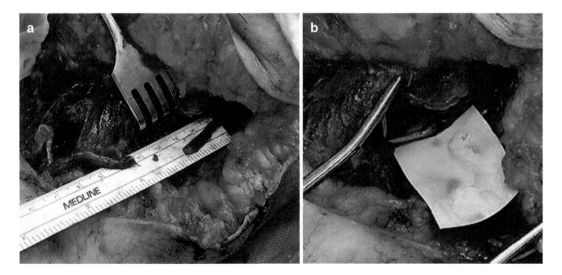

Fig. 52.1 Left radial nerve at the level of the elbow demonstrating a 2 cm gap (**a**) and showing repair with allograft (**b**)

- With long gaps, the fibrin clot becomes narrow in the center, preventing robust regrowth.
- Mostly used for small sensory nerves
- Nerve transfer
  - Sacrifices a nerve providing a less vital function to reinnervate a nerve and provide an essential function
  - A multitude of options are available.
- Muscular neurotization
  - A nerve avulsed from muscle can be reimplanted directly into muscle.
  - Does not achieve full function, but acceptable in some cases

Peripheral Neuromas

- Injured nerves make disorganized attempts at regeneration, sometimes creating a neuroma.

- Neuromas can be difficult to treat, and prevention is essential.
- Dozens of treatment options are available, including resection, wrapping, and implantation into muscle.

Suggested Readings

1. Birch R. Nerve repair. In: Wolfe SW, et al., editors. Green's Operative Hand Surgery. 6th ed. Philadelphia: Churchill Livingstone; 2010.
2. Boyd KU, Mackinnon SE. Nerve reconstruction. In: Weiss AP, editor. Textbook of Hand & Upper Extremity Surgery. Chicago: American Society for Surgery of the Hand; 2013.
3. Jabaley ME, Wegener EE. Acute repair. In: Weiss AP, editor. Textbook of Hand & Upper Extremity Surgery. Chicago: American Society for Surgery of the Hand; 2013.
4. Seddon HJ. Three types of nerve injury. Brain. 1943;66:237–88.

Upper Extremity Replantation

53

Dana Lycans, Jeffrey Kim, and Alan Koester

Introduction

Amputation
- Refers to the reattachment of a completely severed body part in which no soft tissue connection exists between the body part and the body itself.
- Most complete amputations are related to trauma (>90%) and involve the digits.
- This can occur from sharp or blunt dissection, avulsion-type injuries, or crush injuries.
- Males are four times more likely to have a complete amputation.

Evaluation and Early Management

- Length of time from injury is an important factor in considering whether or not to replant a body part.

D. Lycans, MD
Department of Orthopaedic Surgery, Marshall University/Cabell Huntington Hospital, Huntington, WV, USA
e-mail: Lycans42@gmail.com

J. Kim, MD
Department of Orthopaedic Surgery, Cabell Huntington Hospital/Marshall University School of Medicine, Huntington, WV, USA

A. Koester, MD (✉)
Department of Orthopaedic Surgery, Joan C. Edwards School of Medicine, Marshall University, Huntington, WV, USA
e-mail: koestera@marshall.edu

- Ischemia times differ for body parts (these times have been disputed in the literature with up to 96 h reported for digit ischemia times [2]).
- Digits: 12 h warm ischemia time, 24 h cold (if placed on ice).
- Hand and proximal to hand: 6 h warm ischemia time and 12 h for cold,
- Type and location of amputation (# of digits) should be noted. Condition of the stump and amputated digits should be assessed. Severely damaged or mangled digits are not good replantation candidates.
- Preservation of body part is done best by wrapping it in gauze moistened with lactated Ringer's solution. This should be placed in a plastic bag and placed on ice. Do not place digit in direct contact with ice.
- Stump should be wrapped in moist gauze as well.
- Associated injuries should be assessed and treated appropriately.
- Past medical history should be evaluated for psychiatric disorders and overall functional status. Expectations following replant should be thoroughly discussed prior to considering operative procedure.

Indications/Contraindications to Replantation

- Indications for replantation include amputation of:

© Springer International Publishing AG 2017
A.E.M. Eltorai et al. (eds.), *Orthopedic Surgery Clerkship*, DOI 10.1007/978-3-319-52567-9_53

– Thumb
– Multiple digits
– Metacarpal
– Wrist level/proximal to wrist
– Forearm
– Almost everything in children
– Individual digits distal to FDS insertion (Zone I)
– Contraindications for replantation include:
– Crushed or mangled parts, avulsions
– Segmental amputations

Other Severe Diseases or Injuries, Such as Polytrauma

• Severe arteriosclerosis.
• Prolonged ischemia time greater than those listed above (relative contraindication).
• Individual finger amputation in an adult proximal to the FDS insertion (Zone 2 – relative contraindication). This should still be a consideration in children.
• Amputations distal to the DIP joint can be difficult to replant due to tiny vascular structures that are difficult to find and anastomose.
• Advanced age.

Classification

• Generally described as incomplete or complete followed by description of level of the amputation and condition of the soft tissues.
• Ring avulsion injuries can be classified by the Urbaniak classification (below):
  – Class I: adequate circulation. Treated with standard bone and soft tissue procedures.
  – Class II: characterized by inadequate circulation requiring vascular repair.
  – Class III: involved a complete degloving or amputation. It may include concomitant phalangeal fractures. With this class, consider revision amputation of the digit or replantation depending on soft tissues.

Treatment

• Details of stump and amputated body part management discussed above. Goal is to get patient to the OR as soon as possible if deemed a candidate for replant.

Operative

• Operative microscope and microscopic instruments are used to achieve vascular and nerve repair.
• Rotating teams of surgeons and staff have been shown to have better outcomes.
• Can make bilateral mid-lateral incisions to isolate vessels and nerves in the stump and amputated part. Debride any gross contamination or dead tissues.
• Fasciotomies may be warranted to decrease risk of reperfusion injury on major limb replant.
• Operative sequence is important to make surgery go more smoothly and give good outcome.
• *The bone is usually stabilized first to provide structural support for soft tissue repair later in the procedure. This can be done with Kirschner wires or screws.*
• *Extensor tendons are commonly repaired next. This repair is often followed by flexor tendons. Some surgeons prefer to repair vascular structures first to allow for faster revascularization of the extremity.*
• *Arteries/veins are repaired next. Order of this repair is debatable.*
• For digit replantation, attempt to anastomose both arteries.
• For hand/forearm replantation, consider forming an arterial shunt.
• Before vascular anastomosis, give systemic heparin.
• Anastomose two veins for each artery (minimum three veins).
• Repairing veins prior to repairing arteries has potential for reperfusion toxins to be recirculated into the body.

- *Nerves are generally repaired next.*
- *The skin is always repaired last. Local flaps or skin grafts can be used. Avoid tight closure.*
- Finger order – thumb, long, ring, small, index.
- For multiple digit replant surgeries, using a structure-by-structure sequence rather than a digit-by-digit sequence can allow for shorter operative time.

Postoperative Care

Environment

- Warm room (at least 80°F (27°C)). Keep patient NPO for at least 24 h in case of need for return to the OR. When oral intake is begun, it is important to avoid intake of caffeine, chocolate, and nicotine as these can cause constriction of vessels and subsequent death of the digit.

Monitoring Replantation

- Skin temperature – most reliable indicator of adequate perfusion. Concerning if >2° drop in skin temp in <1 h or a temp below 30°C.
- Pulse oximetry should be monitored as well. If <94%, potential vascular compromise.
- Anticoagulation is a controversial topic. Use of some type of anticoagulation is generally recommended. This can be aspirin 325 mg daily, dipyridamole 50 mg three times daily, or dextran 40 (20 ml/h). Chlorpromazine can also be used as a vasodilator and to prevent vasospasm. Adequate hydration is also important.

Arterial Insufficiency

- Thrombosis secondary to vasospasm is the most common cause of early failure.
- Treat with:

- – *Loosening constricting bandages.*
- – *Put extremity in dependent position.*
- – *Heparinization (3000 to 5000 units).*
- – *Stellate ganglion blockade (spasm).*
- – *Early surgical exploration if others are not successful (if no improvement in 4–6 h).*
- – *Venous congestion should be treated with:*
- – *Elevation of extremity.*
- – *Leech application, which causes hirudin (anticoagulant) release.*
- – *If using leeches, should apply prophylaxis to prevent infection from Aeromonas hydrophila. This can be achieved with Bactrim and/or ciprofloxacin with newer data showing ceftriaxone is effective.*
- – *Heparin-soaked pledgets (if leeches not available).*

Complications

- Replantation failure is most frequently caused by arterial thrombosis (from vasospasm) within the first 12 h.
- Stiffness/flexor tendon adhesions can occur. Can treat with tenolysis. This is the most common secondary surgery performed for successful replantations.
- Myonecrosis can be a concern especially in replants proximal to the wrist.
- Myoglobinuria can cause renal failure and even lead to death. Important to monitor renal function following surgery.
- Reperfusion injury can occur after arterial repair. Thought to be caused by hypoxanthine conversion to xanthine which is caused by ischemia. Can give allopurinol as adjunctive therapy when this is a concern.
- Infection risk can be lowered by giving perioperative antibiotics.
- Cold intolerance usually diminishes within the first couple years following replantation.

References

1. Goldner RD, Urbaniak JR. Replantation. In: Wolfe SW, Hotchkiss RN, Pederson WC, et al., editors. Green's operative hand surgery. 6th ed. Philadelphia: Elsevier Churchill Livingstone; 2011. p. 1585–601.
2. Wolfe VM, Wang AA. Replantation of the upper extremity: current concepts. J Am Acad Orthop Surg. 2015;23(6):373–81.
3. Jobe MT. Microsurgery. In: Canale ST, Beaty JH, editors. Campbell's operative orthopedics. 12th ed. Philadelphia: Elsevier Churchill Livingstone; 2013. p. 3126–96.
4. Digit replantation/upper extremity reconstruction. In: Wheeless C III, editor. Wheeless' textbook of orthopedics. 14 May 2012. Web 16 July 2015.

54

Francisco A. Schwartz-Fernandes
and Nicolette Clark

Cubital Tunnel Syndrome

Introduction [1]

- Symptomatic ulnar nerve dysfunction at the level of the elbow
- Results from a combination of compression, traction, and friction
- Second most common peripheral nerve compression syndrome after carpal tunnel
- Four times more likely to present with advanced disease, i.e., muscle atrophy and diminished sensation

Anatomy [1]

- Roof of cubital tunnel formed by Osborne's ligament.
- Medial collateral ligament, elbow joint capsule, and olecranon form the floor.
- Most common site of compression is directly beneath Osborne's ligament.
- Other sites of compression:
  - Arcade of Struthers proximally
  - Medial epicondyle
  - Deep flexor pronator aponeurosis distally

- Intraneural pressure is lowest at 40–50° elbow flexion and increases dramatically when the elbow flexes past 90°.
- It is important to identify and protect branches of the medial antebrachial cutaneous nerve at the time of operative nerve decompression.

Presentation [1]

- Combination of history, physical exam, electromyogram and nerve conduction testing.
- Paresthesia in little finger and ulnar half of ring finger.
- Sensory disturbance on the dorsal ulnar hand confirms compression proximal to Guyon's canal.
- Weakness of various muscles occurs with advanced disease and may cause characteristic hand posture:
  - Interossei – Wartenberg sign
  - Adductor pollicis – Froment sign
  - Ulnar lumbrical muscles – claw hand deformity
- Clinical provocative testing includes:
  - Ulnar nerve percussion at the retrocondylar groove
  - Elbow flexion test
  - Stability of ulnar nerve assessed posterior to medial epicondyle
- Nerve conduction studies used to confirm clinical diagnosis:

F.A. Schwartz-Fernandes (✉) • N. Clark
Department Orthopaedics and Sports Medicine,
University of South Florida, Tampa, FL, USA
e-mail: schwartzfernandes@health.usf.edu

© Springer International Publishing AG 2017
A.E.M. Eltorai et al. (eds.), *Orthopedic Surgery Clerkship*, DOI 10.1007/978-3-319-52567-9_54

- Possible false negatives because of variable compression of fascicles
- Categorized as mild, moderate, or severe disease:
  - Common grading systems:
    ° McGowan
    ° Dellon
  - Mild disease patients report:
    ° Subjective sensory symptoms without objective loss of 2-point sensibility or muscular atrophy
      - McGowan and Dellon I
  - Moderate disease:
    ° Imparts weakness on pinch and grip without atrophy
      - McGowan 2A, Dellon 2
    ° Presence of atrophy and intrinsic muscle strength of only 3/5
      - McGowan 2B
  - Severe disease:
    ° Profound muscular atrophy and sensory disturbance
      - McGowan 3
    ° Weakness that inhibits active finger crossing
      - Dellon 3

Studies

Surgical Treatment Types [2]

- 2005 to 2012 study cohort 26,164 patients:
  - 80% underwent in situ decompression, increased throughout the study period
  - 16% underwent transposition
  - 4% underwent other surgical treatment
- Surgeon characteristics were associated with the type of procedure selected:
  - Case volume
  - Number of types of procedure performed

Comparison of Surgical Treatment [3]

- Extensive dissection is needed for nerve transposition and this may compromise its vascularity.
- A recent meta-analysis of four randomized trials showed no differences in motor nerve conduction velocities or clinical outcome scores

for either simple decompression or ulnar nerve transposition.
- Two out of the four studies excluded patients with nerve subluxation.
- The optimal surgical treatment is unclear.

Treatment [1]

Nonoperative

- Commonly prescribed nonsurgical measures
  - Discontinuing triceps strengthening exercises
  - Avoiding applying direct pressure to medial aspect of elbow on firm surfaces
  - Maintaining a resting elbow position of 45–50 degrees flexion
  - Using a nighttime elbow towel orthosis to prevent elbow flexion beyond 50°

Operative

- Commonly employed operative approaches:
  - Simple decompression
    ° Releasing fascial structures superficial to the ulnar nerve along the medial aspect of the elbow – can be performed endoscopically or open (Fig. 54.1)
  - Medial epicondylectomy
    ° Allows for anterior translation of ulnar nerve over the medial aspect of the elbow
    ° Limited nerve dissection required
  - Transpositions

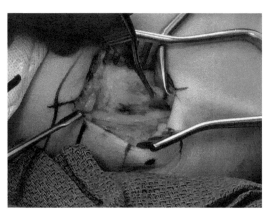

Fig. 54.1 Simple decompression of the cubital tunnel

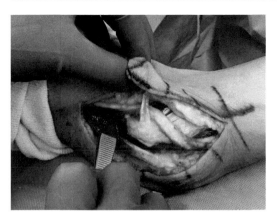

Fig. 54.2 Ulnar nerve transposition with sling

- ○ Place ulnar nerve anterior to ulnohu-
    meral axis of rotation.
- ○ Ulnar nerve is stabilized in its anterior
    position over the flexor pronator mass
    with either a fascial sling or subcutane-
    ous tissue (Fig. 54.2).

Complications

Surgical Failure [4]

- Incorrect diagnosis, incomplete decompression,
  persistent traction on the nerve, postoperative
  compression secondary to scar or new areas of
  compression, and recalcitrant advanced disease

Persistent or Recurrent Symptoms Can Lead to Revision Surgery

- Subcutaneous or submuscular transposition is
  recommended for revision.

Possible Symptomatic Complications

- Loss of elbow extension, smaller total arc of
  active elbow motion, residual ulnar nerve tenderness, weaker key pinch, increased 2-point
  discrimination in the ring and little fingers, a
  more frequent Wartenberg sign, and persistent
  claw posturing

Causes of Failed Surgery

- Incorrect diagnosis
- Improper release of ulnar nerve

Guyon's Canal Syndrome

Introduction

- Also called ulnar tunnel syndrome [5].
- Diagnosis can be difficult [5].
    - Paresthesias may be nonspecific or related
      to coexisting pathologies
    - Accuracy has increased with advances in
      electrodiagnosis
- True incidence and prevalence are not clear [5].
- Leading causes vary [5].
    - Ganglia, occupational neuritis, chronic
      repetitive trauma, and compression over
      hypothenar eminence [5]
    - Benign lesions, hook of hamate fractures,
      ulnar artery pathology, etc. [5]

Anatomy

- Guyon's canal is potential but not exclusive
  site for ulnar nerve compression [5].
    - Guyon's canal is a space at the base of the
      hypothenar eminence where the ulnar
      nerve bifurcates [5].
- Ulnar nerve continues into the forearm
  between the flexor carpi ulnaris and flexor
  digitorum profundus and innervates the flexor
  carpi ulnaris and flexor digitorum profundus
  of the ring and small fingers [5].
- Ulnar tunnel originates at the proximal edge
  of the palmar carpal ligament and extends
  distally to the fibrous arch of the hypothenar
  muscles at the level of the hook of the
  hamate [5].
    - The boundaries vary and cannot be distin-
      guished throughout the course.
    - Roof – palmar aponeurosis, palmaris
      brevis, and hypothenar fibroadipose
      tissue
    - Floor – flexor digitorum profundus ten-
      dons, transverse carpal ligament, pisoham-
      ate ligament, pisometacarpal ligament, and
      opponens digiti minimi

- Medial wall – flexor carpi ulnaris tendon, pisiform, and abductor digiti minimi
- Lateral wall – extrinsic flexor tendons, hook of hamate, and transverse carpal ligament
- Within the canal – ulnar nerve, ulnar artery, concomitant veins, and connective fatty tissue [5].
- Superficial branch innervates the palmaris brevis and provides sensation to the hypothenar eminence, small finger, and ulnar aspect of ring finger [5].
- Sites of compression [5]:
  - Zone I: begins from proximal edge of palmar carpal ligament and ends distally at bifurcation of the nerve [6].
    ◦ Manifests as motor weakness of all the ulnar-innervated intrinsic muscles and sensory deficits over hypothenar eminence and the small and ring fingers [5]
  - Zone II: from just distal to bifurcation to fibrous arch of hypothenar muscles [6].
    ◦ Manifests as motor weakness of ulnar-innervated intrinsic muscles with intact sensation along the nerve distribution [5]
  - Zone III: just distal to bifurcation and contains superficial branch of ulnar nerve [6].
    ◦ Manifests as sensory loss without hypothenar and interosseous weakness [5]
    ◦ Most commonly caused by anomalous muscles or thrombosis of ulnar artery [5]

Presentation

- Depends on anatomical zone of compression and may be purely motor, sensory, or both [5].
- Usually complaints of numbness and tingling in the small and ring fingers [5].
- Weakness of grip strength, ulnar-sided pain [5].
- Look for hypothenar or interossei wasting, clawing for inability to cross fingers, mass over dorsal, or volar wrist [5].
- Positive Phalen's test may be more accurate than positive Tinel sign [5].
- Objective sensory tests provide baseline information and severity [5].
  - Semmes-Weinstein monofilament test
  - 2-point discrimination test
- Vascular examination of the wrist can be useful [5].
  - Radial and ulnar pulses
  - Allen's test

- Radiographic views to rule out fracture [5].
- Electromyography and nerve conduction tests are used as confirmatory studies [5].

Treatment

Nonsurgical
- Protective braces [5]
- NSAIDS [5]
- Discontinuation of provocative activities [5]

Surgical
- Indicated in cases of a motor deficit, compressive lesion, or failure of conservative treatment [5]
- Standard treatment involves: [5]
  - Surgical exploration
  - Removal of lesion
  - Decompression of ulnar tunnel

Complications

- Mostly from surgery approach
- Injury to the motor or sensory ulnar nerve branches
- Injury to the ulnar artery and its branches

References

1. Boone S, Gelberman RH, Calfee RP. The management of cubital tunnel syndrome. J Hand Surg [Am] 2015;40:1897–904. PubMed PMID: 26243318.
2. Adkinson JM, Zhong L, Aliu O, Chung KC. Surgical treatment of cubital tunnel syndrome: trends and the influence of patient and surgeon characteristics. J Hand Surg [Am]. 2015; 40(9):1824–31. PubMed PMID: 26142079.
3. Kang HJ, Koh IH, Chun YM, Oh WT, Chung KH, Choi YR. Ulnar nerve stability-based surgery for cubital tunnel syndrome via a small incision: a comparison with classic anterior nerve transposition. J Orthop Surg Res. 2015; 10:121. PubMed PMID: 26243285.
4. Aleem AW, Krogue JD, Calfee RP. Outcomes of revision surgery for cubital tunnel syndrome. J Hand Surg [Am]. 2014;39(11):2141–9. PubMed PMID: 25169417.
5. Chen SH, Tsai TM. Ulnar tunnel syndrome. J Hand Surg [Am]. 2014; 39:571–9. PubMed PMID: 24559635.
6. Maroukis BL, Ogawa T, Rehim SA, Chung KC. Guyon canal: the evolution of clinical anatomy. J Hand Surg [Am]. 2015; 40:560–5. PubMed PMID: 25446410.

Degenerative Arthritis of the Hand

55

James L. McFadden
and Nileshkumar M. Chaudhari

Abbreviations

APL	Abductor pollicis longus
CMC	Carpometacarpal
DIP	Distal interphalangeal
FCR	Flexor carpi radialis
MC	Metacarpal
MCP	Metacarpophalangeal
NSAID	Nonsteroidal anti-inflammatory drug
IP	Interphalangeal
OA	Osteoarthritis
PE	Physical exam
PIP	Proximal interphalangeal
ROM	Range of motion

What Is Degenerative Arthritis?

- Degenerative arthritis = osteoarthritis (OA)
- Progressive joint disorder resulting in cartilage destruction and subchondral bony changes
- Can involve multiple joints but is not a systemic disease (unlike rheumatoid arthritis)

J.L. McFadden, MD (✉) • N.M. Chaudhari, MD
Orthopaedic Surgery, University of Alabama at
Birmingham, Birmingham, AL, USA
e-mail: jmcfadden@uabmc.edu; nchaudhari@uabmc.edu

Hand OA Epidemiology [1]

Prevalence

- The hand is the most common location of OA.
- Prevalence of radiographic hand OA: reported ranges from 29 to 76%.
- 80% of elderly people have evidence of hand OA on X-ray.

Factors Associated with Hand OA

- Increasing age, genetic predisposition, and sex (females affected greater than males).

Pathology of OA [2, 3]

Pathogenesis

- Hyaline cartilage composition: 80% H_2O.
  - Dry weight: 50% type II collagen, 20% proteoglycans
- In OA: ↑ H_2O, ↓ proteoglycans → collagen disruption, fibrillation, fissuring, and breakdown → eburnation/compensatory sclerosis of subchondral bone/osteophyte formation → bone destruction leads to cysts → chondrocytes release prostaglandins and proteolytic enzymes in an attempt at repair, which further increases the inflammatory environment.
- Soft tissue inflammation in periarticular ligaments and tendons is also observed.

Types

- Primary – idiopathic (unknown etiology) – majority of hand OA.
- Secondary – develops 2/2 trauma, congenital deformity, or another known cause.
- Nonerosive vs erosive subtypes: controversy exists as to whether erosive changes seen in OA constitute one end of a single disease spectrum vs an entirely different disease entity.

Presentation in the Hand [1, 4]

- While radiographic OA in the hand is prevalent, only about 8% of the population experience symptomatic hand OA.
- Symptoms include joint enlargement, pain, ↓ ROM/strength, and visible deformity.

Commonly Involved Hand Joints [1, 3, 4]

- DIP – most common digital joint affected by OA (54% of all hand OA)
  - Generally asymptomatic other than decreased ROM.
  - Bony enlargement can lead to nodule formation – Heberden's nodes (usually painless, but can lead to local soft tissue irritation, synovial fluid leakage, and mucous cyst formation that can be painful and cause nail deformity).
- PIP – third most common digital joint affected by OA (8% of all hand OA)
  - More symptomatic than DIP given increased ROM demands of PIP
  - Nodule formation – Bouchard's nodes (usually painless unless associated with mucous cyst development)
- First CMC – second most common digital joint affected by OA (20% of all hand OA)
  - Attenuation of the anterior oblique ligament ("beak ligament") contributes to first CMC OA by allowing dorsoradial subluxation, and adduction of first MC → can

lead to compensatory hyperextension deformity of first MCP joint.
  - If symptomatic: thenar eminence pain, decreased pinch strength, and ↓ ROM.
  - Specific PE tests: grind test, crank test, and relief with distraction of first CMC joint.

Radiographic Evaluation [2, 3, 5]

- X-ray findings: progressive joint space narrowing, osteophyte formation, joint malalignment, subchondral sclerosis, and cyst formation.
- Many different radiographic classification systems exist, but the Eaton and Littler classification for first CMC OA is the most commonly used:
  I. Normal to slightly widened joint space
  II. Joint space narrowing, osteophytes <2 mm
  III. Increased narrowing, osteophytes >2 mm
  IV. Pantrapezial arthritic changes
- MRI can show soft tissue involvement but is rarely necessary clinically.

Conservative Treatment [4, 6, 7]

- Activity modification, rest, and NSAIDs
- Joint immobilization with splints
- Hand therapy
- Corticosteroid injections – typically reserved for first CMC arthritis. Has been shown to be beneficial in early OA but has no significant effect on advanced OA.

Surgical Treatment [2, 3, 4]

Arthrodesis (Joint Fusion)

- Mainstay of operative treatment for painful DIP and PIP joints if preservation of ROM is not desired.
- Generally avoided in first CMC joint except for young laborers.
- Position of fusion is joint specific.

Arthroplasty (Joint Replacement)

- Traditionally higher complication rate compared to arthrodesis in IP joints but can preserve ROM (can be important for grasp in PIP joints).
- IP joint options: silicone or pyrocarbon implants exist (require competent collateral ligaments).
- First CMC arthroplasty:
  - Performed for advanced OA.
  - Typical procedure involves trapeziectomy, volar ligament reconstruction, and tendon interposition (usually with autograft portions of FCR or APL). Intervention for MCP hyperextension deformity may also be necessary if excessive.
  - Results: increases pinch strength, also associated with some subsidence/"settling" but no recorded clinical effect.

Arthroscopy

- Can be used in early stage OA of first CMC joint
- Allows for minimally invasive joint debridement, loose body removal, or hemitrapeziectomy
- Risk of injury to the superficial radial nerve does exist.

Mucous Cyst Excision

- Mucous cysts overlying Heberden and Bouchard's nodes can be painful (and at the DIP joint may cause nail deformities by interfering with the germinal matrix).
- Cyst excision and dorsal osteophyte excision = best outcome.
- Rotational flaps are sometimes required to provide soft tissue coverage following excision (cysts can communicate directly with the joint – poor coverage of these lesions after excision can place the patient at risk for developing a septic joint).

References

1. Kalichman L, Hernandez-Molina G. Hand osteoarthritis: an epidemiological perspective. Semin Arthritis Rheum. 2010;39(6):465–76.
2. Swanson AB, de Groot Swanson G. Osteoarthritis in the hand. Clin Rheum Dis. 1985;11(2):393–420.
3. Kaufmann RA, Logters TT, Verbruggen G, Windolf J, Goltz RJ. Osteoarthritis of the distal interphalangeal joint. J Hand Surg Am. 2010;35(12): 2117–25.
4. Bernstein RA. Arthritis of the thumb and digits: current concepts. Instr Course Lect. 2015;64:281–94.
5. Eaton RG, Littler JW. Ligament reconstruction for the painful thumb carpometacarpal joint. J Bone Joint Surg Am. 1973;55(8):1655–66.
6. Spaans AJ, van Minnen LP, Kon M, Schuurman AH, Schreuders AR, Vermeulen GM. Conservative treatment of thumb base osteoarthritis: a systematic review. J Hand Surg Am. 2015;40(1):16–21.
7. Beasely J. Osteoarthritis and rheumatoid arthritis: conservative therapeutic management. J Hand Ther. 2012;25(2):163–71.

Inflammatory Arthritis of the Hand

56

Jonathan Ludwig and Nileshkumar Chaudhari

Types of Inflammatory Arthritis

Rheumatoid Arthritis (RA)

- Most common inflammatory arthritis
- Hand and wrist are most commonly affected joints
- Affects ~1% of US population, 3:1 females to males
- Systemic disease with strong genetic component
- *T cell*-mediated autoimmune response
- Rheumatoid factor – IgM antibody targeting Fc portion of IgG
  - Scleroderma
  - Systemic lupus erythematosus
  - Psoriatic arthritis

Effects of RA

- RA is a disease of *synovial tissue*

J. Ludwig, MD (✉) • N. Chaudhari, MD
Orthopedic Surgery, University of Alabama at
Birmingham Hospital, Birmingham, AL, USA
e-mail: jonathan.a.ludwig@gmail.com;
nchaudhari@uabmc.edu

- All secondary effects of RA are due to local effect of diseased synovium [2]:
  - Deformity
  - Tendon rupture
  - Joint destruction
- Cartilage is degraded via poorly understood enzymatic reaction

Medical Management of RA

- Three drug classes:
  - Nonsteroidal anti-inflammatory drugs (NSAIDs):
    - Decrease pain and inflammation
    - Do not alter course of disease
  - Corticosteroids:
    - More effective than NSAIDs
    - Multiple adverse side effects:
      - Weight gain
      - Increased susceptibility to infection
      - Osteoporosis
      - Diabetes
  - Disease-modifying antirheumatic drugs (DMARDs):
    - Dramatically alter course of disease
    - Reduce symptoms, slow radiographic disease progression
    - Have significantly decreased rates of surgery for RA

© Springer International Publishing AG 2017

245

A.E.M. Eltorai et al. (eds.), *Orthopedic Surgery Clerkship*, DOI 10.1007/978-3-319-52567-9_56

- Subgroups of DMARDs:
  - Nonbiologic – methotrexate, sulfasalazine, and hydroxychloroquine
  - Biologic:
    - TNF inhibitors – etanercept, infliximab, and adalimumab
    - IL-1 receptor antagonists – anakinra

Surgical Management of the RA Hand

- Dictated by individual patient-specific conditions
- Better outcomes if surgery is performed before fixed deformity develops
- Surgical priorities:
  - Relieve pain
  - Improve function
  - Prevent loss of function
  - Improve appearance

- Types of surgery performed on the RA hand:
  - Synovectomy
  - Tenosynovectomy
  - Tendon repair/realignment
  - Arthroplasty
  - Arthrodesis

Characteristic Pathology of the RA Hand

- Wrist (radiocarpal) arthritis:
  - Synovectomy in early disease
  - Fusion or arthroplasty for advanced disease (Fig. 56.1)
- Distal radioulnar joint dorsal dislocation (caput ulna):
  - Distal ulna resection (Darrach procedure)
  - Distal ulna pseudoarthrosis (Sauve-Kapandji procedure)

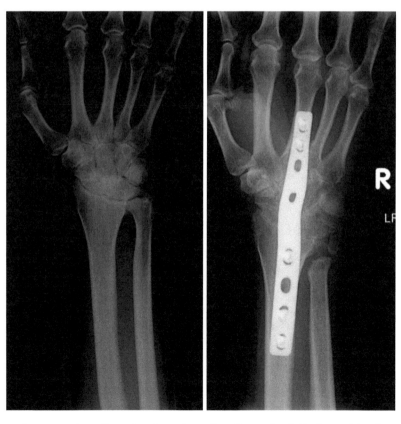

Fig. 56.1 Pre- and postoperative radiographs of a patient with radiocarpal arthritis due to RA, who underwent total wrist fusion (Image courtesy Dr. Nilesh Chaudhari, University of Alabama at Birmingham)

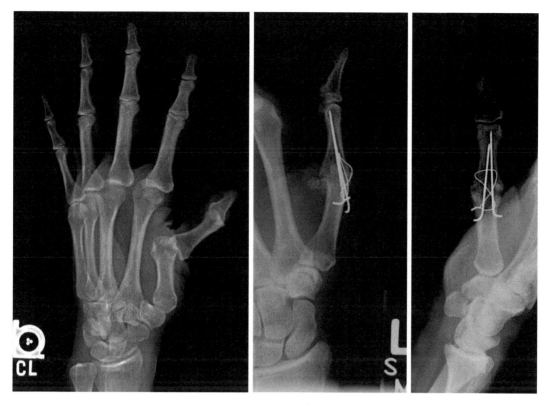

Fig. 56.2 Pre- and postoperative radiographs of a patient with thumb MCP joint subluxation due to SLE, who underwent MCP fusion. Fusion of the MCP is preferred in the thumb to provide a stable base for opposition (Image courtesy Dr. Nilesh Chaudhari, University of Alabama at Birmingham)

- Ulnar deviation and volar subluxation at metacarpophalangeal (MCP) joints:
  - Develop due to MCP synovitis causing stretching of sagittal band and collateral ligaments with ulnar subluxation of extrinsic tendons
  - Early disease – soft-tissue procedures (synovectomy, extensor tendon centralization, cross-intrinsic transfer)
  - Chronic deformity or joint destruction – MCP arthroplasty or arthrodesis (Fig. 56.2)
- Boutonniere deformity:
  - Develops due to proximal interphalangeal (PIP) joint synovitis
  - PIP arthroplasty or fusion
- Swan neck deformity:
  - Can be caused by disruption of extensor mechanism at MCP, PIP, or DIP.
  - Treatment depends on underlying cause of deformity.

- Extensor tendon rupture:
  - Tendon repair
  - Tendon transfer
  - Correction of bony deformity causing tendon abrasion
- Flexor pollicis longus (FPL) rupture:
  - FPL abraded on scaphoid osteophyte
  - FDS to FPL transfer

References

1. Chung KC, Pushman AG. Current concepts in management of the rheumatoid hand. J Hand Surg Am. 2011;36A:737–47.
2. Feldon P, Terrono AL, Nalebuff EA, Millender LH. Rheumatoid arthritis and other connective tissue diseases. In: Wolfe SW, et al., editors. Green's operative hand surgery. 6th ed. Philadelphia: Churchill Livingstone; 2010.

Chronic Regional Pain Syndrome

57

Joseph J. King

Definition

- Chronic regional pain syndrome is a term to describe a constellation of signs and symptoms including pain disproportional to an inciting event combined with sensory, vasomotor, sudomotor, and motor/ trophic changes.
- Older terminology: reflex sympathetic dystrophy, shoulder-hand syndrome, causalgia, and algodystrophy.
- Types:
  - Type 1: No direct nerve injury (about 90% of cases)
  - Type 2: Following a direct nerve injury (about 10% of cases)

Pathophysiology

- The theory is that multiple pathologic mechanisms are responsible for the disease leading to variable signs and symptoms.
  - Some form of nerve injury/trigger
    ○ Any surgery or injury can be considered a potential inciting event.

- Repetitive stimulation and sensitization of the peripheral nervous system lead to central nervous system sensitization.
  - Acute phase theory: accompanied by vasodilation and fluid extravasation
    ○ Inflammatory mediated
      - Warmth, erythema, and edema
    ○ Sympathetic nervous system dysfunction.
    ○ Decreased sweating and failure to vasoconstrict to cold stimuli.
  - Chronic (cold) phase theory: accompanied by vasoconstriction and sweating
    ○ Theorized because cold exacerbates pain and sympathetic blockade alleviates pain.
- Autoimmune theory
  - Autoantibodies against autonomic neurons

Epidemiology

- Affects females more commonly than males (reported 2.3–5:1)
- Less severe clinical course seen in older patients

Signs and Symptoms

- Variable initial clinical presentation after neurologic insult and variable subsequent clinical course.

J.J. King, MD
Orthopaedics and Rehabiliation, UF Health Shands
Hospital, Gainesville, FL, USA
e-mail: kingjj@ortho.ufl.edu

Acute or Warm Stage

- Exaggerated pain:
  - Hyperalgesia – increased sensitivity to pain.
  - Allodynia – pain with stimuli that do not normally cause pain.
  - Quality of pain is burning, tearing, stinging, aching, or throbbing.
  - Pain is worse with cold weather, movement, and stress.
  - One third of patients have sympathetically mediated pain.
- Vasomotor dysfunction
  - Warmth, erythema/skin color changes, and/or limb edema
- Sudomotor
  - Decreased sweating
- Motor changes
  - Weakness, dystonia, and/or tremors

Intermediate or Dystrophic Stage

- Increased pain
- Sensory dysfunction
- Continued vasomotor dysfunction
- Trophic changes:
  - Glossy or thickened skin
  - Thickened or striated nails
  - Hair growth changes (increased or decreased)

Third or Chronic Stage (Cold, Atrophic)

- Vasomotor dysfunction
  - Decreased blood flow
- Motor/tropic changes
  - Skin thinning, muscle atrophy, and joint stiffness/contractures
- Bone demineralization

Diagnosis

- *Clinical diagnosis is based on the signs and symptoms* (see diagnostic criteria in Tables 57.1 and 57.2).

Table 57.1 International society for the study of pain Orlando criteria

1. The presence of an inciting event or immobilization
2. Continuing pain, allodynia, or hyperalgesia in which the pain is disproportionate to the inciting event
3. Edema, skin blood flow changes, and abnormal sudomotor activity in the affected area at some point in the clinical course
4. Excludes the existence of other conditions that may account for the amount of pain or dysfunction

Table 57.2 Budapest clinical diagnostic criteria

The following criteria must be met:
1. Continued pain disproportionate to any inciting event
2. At least *one symptom* in three of the four categories:
Sensory (hyperesthesia, allodynia)
Vasomotor (temperature or skin color changes)
Sudomotor (report edema, sweat changes/asymmetry)
Motor/trophic (report decreased motion, motor dysfunction, or trophic changes involving the hair, nails, or skin)
3. At least *one sign* at the time of evaluation in at least two categories:
Sensory (hyperalgesia to pinprick, allodynia)
Vasomotor (temperature or skin color asymmetry)
Sudomotor (edema or sweat changes/asymmetry)
Motor/trophic (decreased ROM, motor dysfunction, or trophic changes involving the hair, nails, or skin)
4. No other diagnosis can better explain the signs and symptoms

- Average patient sees four physicians prior to the diagnosis.
- Ice test: placing ice on the affected limb causes an increase in burning pain.
- EMG/NCS can rule out other neurologic disorders.

Imaging [1, 2]

- Imaging is supplemental to diagnosis as CRPS is a clinical diagnosis.

- Can be used to rule out other causes of pain
- Radiographs may reveal osteopenia in chronic CRPS.
- MRI may show soft tissue or marrow edema associated with CRPS but is often nonspecific.
- Infrared thermography allows color mapping of the affected and unaffected limbs for comparison.
  - One degree Celsius temperature difference is considered significant.
- Triple-phase bone scan: increased tracer uptake in bone (third phase) is associated with the acute phase (increased blood flow and bone turnover).

Treatment Options

- *Multidisciplinary approach* recommended due to several pathologic mechanisms with initiation of treatment as soon as possible [2].

Physical Therapy/Occupational Therapy

- The goal is to overcome the fear of pain and for functional rehabilitation.
- Incremental program to accomplish these goals:
  - Desensitization with contrast bath, texture therapy, and stress loading
  - Increase range of motion
  - Increase strength
- Edema control.
- Mirror-box therapy has been shown to decrease neuropathic pain.

Psychological Therapy

- Treats the emotional burden of chronic pain
- Cognitive-behavioral therapy
- Teaches biofeedback and relaxation skills

Pharmacologic Therapy [2]

***Pharmacologic therapy is used when the pain severity is limiting functional rehabilitation.

- Oral corticosteroids (prednisone)
  - Some success reported in the acute phase
- NSAIDs
  - Utilized clinically, but no studies have proven efficacy
- Antioxidants:
  - Vitamin C
    - Several studies reported that vitamin C administration after distal radius fracture decreased CRPS incidence (studies are conflicting).
  - Topical dimethyl sulfoxide (DMSO) and N-acetylcysteine.
- Gabapentin or pregabalin.
- Ketamine (NDMA receptor blocker)
  - Possible reversal of central nervous system sensitization
  - Subanesthetic intravenous infusions, ketamine comas, and topical ketamine
- Sympathetic blockers (help sympathetic-mediated pain)
  - Phenoxybenzamine, phentolamine, and topical clonidine
- Opioid therapy is not recommended in CRPS.

Procedural Interventions

- Stellate ganglion (primary sympathetic ganglion) blockade
  - Diagnosis and treatment of sympathetic-mediated pain
- Brachial plexus block
- Spinal cord stimulator in the epidural space
- Intrathecal baclofen
- Sympathectomy of the sympathetic trunks or stellate ganglion
  - Chemical, radio-frequency, or open surgical technique

Prevention

Distal Radius Fractures

- Vitamin C (500 mg daily for 6 weeks)
  1. Studies Are Conflicting but Low Risk for Complications and Inexpensive [3, 4]

Surgery on Limb Previously Affected by CRPS

- Preoperative stellate ganglion or brachial plexus blockade
- Multimodal anesthesia

References

1. Bailey J, et al. Imaging and clinical evidence of sensorimotor problems in CRPS: utilizing novel treatment approaches. J Neuroimmune Pharmacol. 2013;8:564–75.

2. Cristo PJ, Wilhelmi BG. Complex regional pain syndrome. In: Nicholson GP, editor. Orthopedic knowledge update: shoulder and elbow. Rosemont: American Academy of Orthopedic Surgeons; 2013 . Print.

3. Ekroi I, et al. The influence of vitamin C on the outcome of distal radius fractures. J Bone Joint Surg Am. 2014;96(17):1451–9.

4. Malay S, Chung KC. Testing the validity of preventing chronic regional pain syndrome with vitamin C after distal radius fracture. J Hand Surg Am. 2014;39(11):2251–7.

Upper Extremity Infections

58

Martin Skie

General

Incidence

- Trauma – penetrating injuries, abrasions, nail biting, etc.
- Bite wounds – human or animal
- Other causes

Treatment Principles

- Early – within 48 h of onset of symptoms
  - Oral or IV antibiotics
  - Elevation
  - Splints
- Late
  - Surgical debridement.
  - Intraoperative cultures.
  - Leave wounds open.
  - Maintain coverage of joints, tendons, and nerves.

Organisms

- *Staphylococcus aureus* and *Streptococcus* species are most frequent.
- Significant increase in community-acquired MRSA.

Common Soft Tissue Infections

Cellulitis

- Superficial soft tissue (skin) infection
- Oral/IV antibiotics
- Elevation

Felon

- Infection of the fingertip pulp (Fig. 58.1)
- Compartmentalized by vertical fibrous septa in the soft tissue
- Usually requires open debridement to release the septa

M. Skie, MD
Orthopedic Surgery, University of Toledo Medical
Center, Toledo, OH, USA
e-mail: martin.skie@utoledo.edu

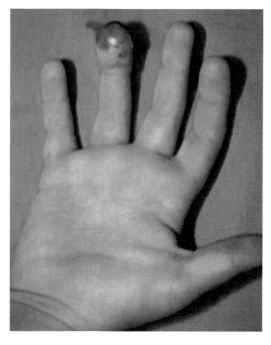

Fig. 58.1 Infection of the soft tissue pulp of the fingertip (felon)

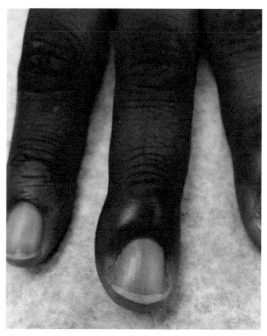

Fig. 58.2 Paronychia infection involving the lateral nail fold and eponychium (proximal nail fold)

Paronychia/Eponychia

- Infection of the nail folds (Fig. 58.2)
- Usually respond to oral antibiotics
- May require removal of nail plate to evacuate infection

Onychomycosis

- Fungal infection of the nail plate and nail bed
- Requires topical or oral antifungal medication until normal nail has grown out (3 months)

Flexor Tendon Infections

- Infection of the flexor tendon sheath of the finger (Fig. 58.3)
- Can cause interruption of tendon nutrition and resultant tendon necrosis
- Kanavel's signs:
  - Fusiform swelling of the digit
  - Tenderness along the flexor
  - Finger rest in a flexed posture

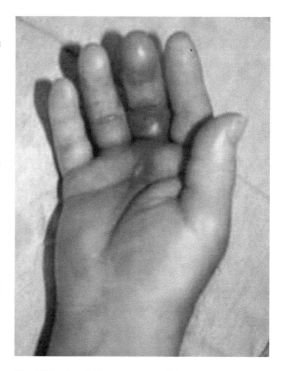

Fig. 58.3 Septic flexor tenosynovitis

Bite Wounds

Human Bites

- Often result of punching injury (Fig. 58.4)
- *Staph*, *Strep*, and *Eikenella* (classically, but not recent studies)

Animal Bites

- Dog bites
  - Tearing-type wounds, less frequently cause infection
- Cat bites
  - Puncture-type wounds with deeper inoculation of bacteria
  - *Staph*, *Strep*, and *Pasteurella*
- Treat both human and animal bite with amoxicillin/clavulanate.

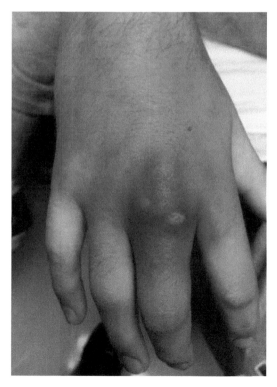

Fig. 58.4 Bite wound with cellulitis resulting from a punching injury

Osteomyelitis

- Not common in the hand:
  - Most frequently from open fractures
  - Postsurgical
  - Spread from adjacent soft tissue infection, usually in immunocompromised patients

Atypical Infections

- Rare infections require good history and suspicion.
- *Mycobacterium marinum* most common in the hand.
- Culture in Lowenstein-Jensen gel, 30°C, 6–8 weeks

Necrotizing Fasciitis

- Rapidly spreading infection along fascial planes
- Group A Strep, polymicrobial, *Clostridium*
- Requires high index of suspicion, aggressive surgical debridement
- Amputation and mortality rates above 20%

Immunocompromised Patients

- Insulin-dependent diabetics, HIV, organ transplants, and chronic steroid use
- Need to treat aggressively:
  - Polymicrobial infections.
  - Gram-negative bacteria are frequent.
  - Rapid spread along tendon sheaths and through palmar spaces.
- Treatment with IV antibiotics and surgical debridement

Suggested Reading

1. Babovic N, Cayci C, Carlsen B. Cat bite infection of the hand: assessment of morbidity and predictors of severe infection. J Hand Surg. 2014;39A:268–90.
2. Capo J. Infections. In: Chung K, Murry P, editors. Hand surgery update. American Society for Surgery of the Hand: Rosemont; 2012.

3. Draeger R, Bynum Jr D. Flexor tendon sheath infections of the hand. J. Am. Acad. Orthop. Surg. 2012;20:373–82.
4. Henry M. Septic flexor tenosynovitis. J Hand Surg. 2011;36A:322–3.
5. Jalil A, Barlaan P, Fung B, Ip J. Hand infections in diabetic patients. Hand Surg. 2011;16:307–12.
6. Kozin S, Bishop A. Atypical mycobacterium infections of the upper extremity. J Hand Surg. 1994;19A: 480–7.
7. McDonald L, Bavaro M, Hofmeister E, Kroonen L. Hand infections. J Hand Surg. 2011;36A:1403–12.
8. O'Malley M, Fowler J, Ilyas A. Community-acquired methicillin-resistant Staphylococcus aureus infection: prevalence and timeliness of treatment. J Hand Surg. 2009;34A:504–8.
9. Sharma K, Rao K, Hobson M. Space of Parona infections: experience in management and outcomes in a regional hand centre. J. Plast. Reconstr. Aesthet. Surg. 2013;66:968–72.

Part III

Lower Extremity

Hip Fractures

59

Brock Johnson and Thomas Gill

Femoral Neck Fractures

Background [2, 4]

- Incidence 63.3 per 100,000 females, 27.7 per 100,000 males.
- Bimodal distribution, average age 72
  - Majority low-energy mechanism in elderly
  - Smaller subset of high-energy mechanism in younger patients
- Incidence is increasing due to aging population.
- Mortality ~25% at 1 year.
  - Loss of independence in ~50%

Risk Factors [2, 4]

- Female gender
- Age
- Medical comorbidities
- Low estrogen levels
- Prior/frequent falls
- Prior fractures
- Tobacco and alcohol use
- Caucasian race

Orthopedic Surgery Clerkship: A Quick Reference Guide for Senior Medical Students Springer, 2016

B. Johnson, MD (✉) • T. Gill, MD
Department of Orthopedic Surgery, Marshall University/Cabell Huntington Hospital, Huntington, WV 25705, USA
e-mail: johnsonbr@marshall.edu

Anatomic Considerations [4]

- Synovial ball-and-socket joint:
  - The head and neck are intracapsular structures, bathed in synovial fluid.
    - No periosteum and thus no callus formation
      - Healing relies on endosteal bone formation, and thus anatomic reduction is necessary.
- Neck-shaft angle ~$130° \pm 7°$.
- Neck anteversion $10° \pm 7°$ relative to shaft.
- Calcar femorale: vertically oriented dense area of strong bone from posteromedial shaft running toward posterior femoral neck.
- Femoral neck has tenuous blood supply which is easily disrupted in displaced fractures.
  - Capsular vessels (main contributor in adults)
    - Branches from medial and lateral femoral circumflex arteries:
      - Circumflex arteries form anastomosis at the base of femoral neck.
      - Lateral circumflex is the main contributor.
    - Capsular arteries penetrate capsule and become retinacular arteries which supply the femoral head:
  - Intramedullary vessels
  - Foveal artery through ligamentum teres (insignificant contributor in adults)

Classification

Garden Classification: Based on Displacement (Figs. 59.1 and 59.2) [2]

- Type I: incomplete, valgus impacted
- Type II: complete, nondisplaced
- Type III: complete, <50% displaced
- Type IV: complete, >50% displaced:
  - Garden system has most utility when dealing with low-energy fragility-type fractures.
  - Treatment implications: nondisplaced fractures (types I and II) may be treated with percutaneous screw fixation; displaced fractures (types III and IV) generally require arthroplasty (elderly patients) or ORIF (younger patients).

Pauwel Classification: Based on Angle of Fracture Line Relative to Horizontal

- Type I: <30°
- Type II: 30°–50°
- Type III: >50°
  - Pauwel system has most utility when dealing higher-energy fractures.
  - Prognostic implications: steeper-angled fracture lines (i.e., higher Pauwel type) experience greater shear forces and thus greater instability.

Stress Fractures [2]

- Seen in patients participating in cyclic-loading impact activities and in osteopenic/osteoporotic patients
- Tension sided
  - Most require operative fixation
- Compression sided
  - May be treated with period of nonweight bearing

Presentation/Evaluation

Impacted and Stress Fractures [4]

- May have groin pain or pain referred to the medial thigh and knee
- No obvious gross deformity
- Painful percussion over greater trochanter, minor pain with ROM, worse at extremes of motion

Displaced Fractures [4]

- Severe pain in entire hip region, often worse in groin area
- Inability to bear weight on affected extremity
- Leg held in abduction and external rotation, shortened compared to contralateral
- *Imaging*
- Plain film X-ray
  - AP and cross table lateral of affected hip.
  - AP pelvis.
  - Traction internal rotation view may be helpful for defining fracture type.
- CT
  - May be helpful in defining displacement and comminution especially in higher-energy injuries
- MRI
  - Rule out occult and stress fractures
- Bone scan
  - Rule out occult and stress fractures

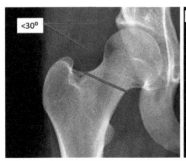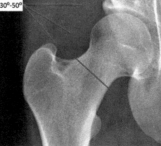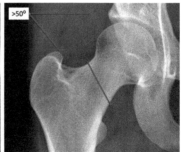

Fig. 59.1 Valgus-impacted nondisplaced femoral neck fracture [2]

Treatment Considerations

Basic Principles [3]

- Early mobilization is the goal to reduce decubitus complications.
- Surgical fixation should occur as soon as patient is medically optimized.
  - In elderly patients, surgery within 48 h of hospital admission is associated with better outcomes and decreased mortality at 1 year.
- The presence or lack of displacement is the main consideration when determining treatment options.
- In younger patients, emergent fixation is indicated to limit vascular insult.
  - Anatomic reduction is crucial in this population.

Nonoperative Treatment [3]

- Reserved for certain nonambulatory patients and patients at too high risk for surgery

- Extended bed rest leads to high rates of complications including pneumonia, DVT, UTI, and decubitus ulcers.
- Compression-sided stress fractures [3]
  - Period of nonweight bearing, patients generally able to remain relatively mobile with assistive devices

Open Reduction Internal Fixation [3]

- Displaced fractures in young patients
  - Evacuate hematoma
  - May insert K wires to act as joysticks to aid reduction
  - Cannulated screws vs. sliding hip screw
    - Sliding hip screw is biomechanically stronger than cannulated screws in especially in more vertical fracture patterns.

Cannulated Screws (Fig. 59.3) [3, 4]

- May be used in ORIF of displaced fractures or percutaneously in nondisplaced fractures

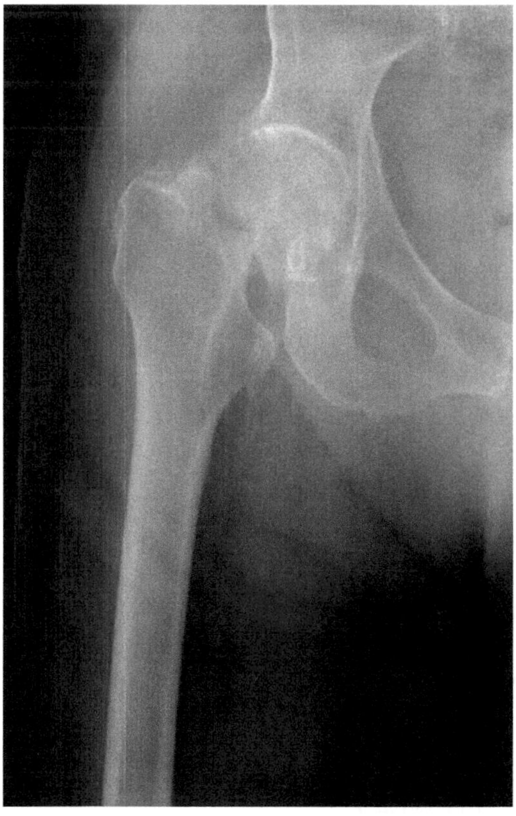

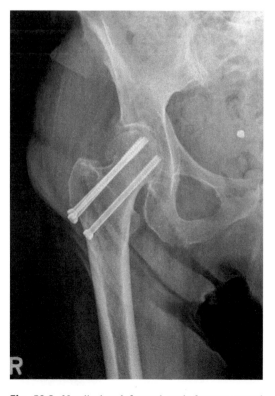

Fig. 59.2 Displaced femoral neck fracture

Fig. 59.3 Nondisplaced femoral neck fracture treated with percutaneous cannulated screws

- Inverted triangle configuration.
  - ○ Inferior screw along calcar (posterior to midline)
  - ○ Superior anterior screw
  - ○ Superior posterior screw
- Start point at or above lesser trochanter to avoid stress riser.
- Goal is large screw spread.
- Screws should not be convergent.

Sliding Hip Screw [1, 3]

- More vertical fracture patterns in younger patients.
- May use additional cannulated screw for rotational stability.
- This construct is more commonly used for intertrochanteric fractures.

Arthroplasty (Fig. 59.4) [3]

- Hemiarthroplasty
  - Displaced fractures in elderly, less physiologically demanding patients

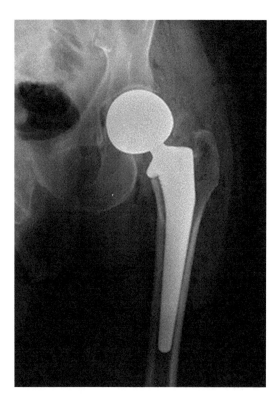

Fig. 59.4 Displaced femoral neck fracture treated with hemiarthroplasty

- Total hip arthroplasty [3]
  - Displaced fractures in elderly, more active patients
  - May offer higher functional scores and lower reoperation rates compared to hemiarthroplasty
  - Higher dislocation rate than hemiarthroplasty

Complications

Avascular Necrosis [4]

- 10% of nondisplaced fractures, up to 45% of displaced fractures.
  - Increased risk with initial displacement and nonanatomic reduction
- If symptomatic, treat with arthroplasty in older patients.
  - Consider core decompression, osteotomy, vascularized graft, or arthroplasty in younger patients

Nonunion [4]

- 5% of nondisplaced fractures, up to 25% displaced fractures.
- No radiographic union at 12 months.
- Symptoms include groin/buttock pain, painful weight bearing, and pain with hip extension.
- Treatment in elderly is arthroplasty; younger patients may benefit from proximal femoral osteotomy.
- Prosthetic dislocation.
- Total hip arthroplasty after femoral neck fracture has approximately 10% dislocation rate.
  - About seven times higher than hemiarthroplasty

Intertrochanteric Femur Fractures

Background [2, 4]

- Defined as extracapsular proximal fractures located between the greater and lesser trochanters
- Incidence 63 per 100,000 females, 34 per 100,000 males
  - Similar to femoral neck fractures, there is a bimodal distribution of low-energy mecha-

nisms in the elderly and higher-energy injuries in the elderly.

- Risk factors [2, 4]
  - History of fragility fractures
  - Old age
  - Female gender
  - Increased dependence with activities of daily living
  - Mortality at 1 year ~20–30%

Anatomic Considerations [4]

- Located between greater and lesser trochanters with occasional subtrochanteric extension
- Extracapsular, dense cancellous bone with rich blood supply
  - Avascular necrosis and nonunion less of a concern than femoral neck fractures
- Calcar femorale: vertically oriented dense area of strong bone from posteromedial shaft running toward posterior femoral neck
  - Posteromedial bony contact acts as buttress to collapse, which is important for determining stability.
- Deforming forces
  - Hip abductors displace the greater trochanter proximal and lateral.
  - Iliopsoas displaces the lesser trochanter proximal and medial.
  - Hip flexors, extensors, and adductors displace the distal fragment proximal.

Classification

- Based on characteristics that contribute to stability vs. instability [2]
  - Implications for treatment options
  - Stable fracture patterns (Fig. 59.5)
    - Characteristics that will resist medial compressive forces once reduced
      - Intact posteromedial cortex
      - Minimal comminution
      - Normal obliquity
  - Unstable fracture patterns (Fig. 59.6) [2]
    - Factors that contribute to varus collapse or distal fragment (shaft) migration proximally and medially

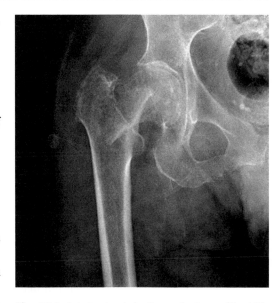

Fig. 59.5 Intertrochanteric femur fracture with stable fracture pattern

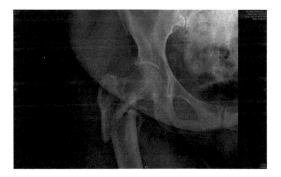

Fig. 59.6 Unstable intertrochanteric femur fracture. Note the reverse obliquity

- Posteromedial comminution
- Lateral wall comminution
- Subtrochanteric extension
- Reverse obliquity

Presentation/Evaluation [4]

- Buttock/hip/groin pain
- Affected extremity shortened and externally rotated

Imaging
- Plain film X-ray
  - AP and cross table lateral of the hip.

- AP pelvis.
- Full-length femur.
- Traction/internal rotation hip films may be helpful to determine fracture characteristics.
• MRI/CT/bone scan
  - MRI study of choice for occult fractures not seen on plain film
  - CT or bone scan if contraindications to MRI

Treatment Considerations

Basic Principles [3]
• Similar to femoral neck fractures, early mobilization and fixation within 48 h if medically optimized is the goal.
• AVN and nonunion is less of a concern than with femoral neck fractures.
• Fixation method is generally guided by determination of stability.

Nonoperative Treatment [3]
• Reserved for certain nonambulatory patients and those deemed too high risk for surgery
  - Extended bed rest leads to high rates of complications including pneumonia, DVT, UTI, and decubitus ulcers.

Sliding Hip Screw (Fig. 59.7) [1, 3]
• Indicated for stable fracture patterns.
  - If utilized in unstable patterns, this may lead to collapse, femoral shaft medialization, and limb shortening.
• Requires open approach.
• Allows for controlled, dynamic interfragmentary compression.
• Screw should be placed within 1 cm of subchondral (calcar) bone to provide buttress support to the construct.
• Device must match patient's neck-shaft angle.
• Tip-to-apex distance >25 mm shown to be predictive of screw cutout/hardware failure.

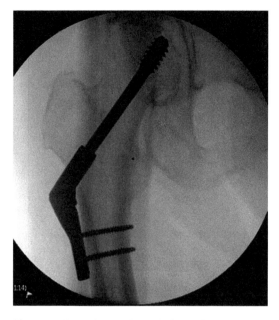

Fig. 59.7 Stable intertrochanteric femur fracture treated with sliding hip screw

  - Calculated sum of screw tip distance to apex of femoral head on AP and lateral radiographs

Cephalomedullary Nail (Fig. 59.8) [3]
• Indicated for both stable and unstable fracture patterns
• Construct consisting of intramedullary nail with screw or blade component which interdigitates with the nail and extends into the femoral neck
• Allows for percutaneous approach
• Available in short or long nail designs

Arthroplasty [3]
• Generally reserved for revision procedures in patients with failed fixation using the above devices.
  - Calcar-replacing implant may be necessary.
• Primary treatment with arthroplasty in unstable fracture patterns has shown good outcomes in limited case series.
• Possible early return to full weight bearing.
• Increased intraoperative blood loss and tissue dissection.

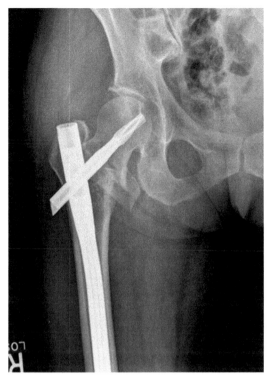

Fig. 59.8 Intertrochanteric femur fracture treated with cephalomedullary nail

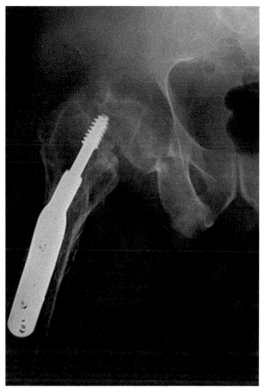

Fig. 59.9 Example of failed fixation with sliding hip screw

Complications [4]

Hardware Failure/Cutout (Fig. 59.9)
- Most common complication
- Tip-to-apex distance >45 mm associated with 60% failure rate
- Treatment
  - Young patients: corrective osteotomy vs. revision ORIF
  - Elderly patients: arthroplasty

Nonunion
- Rare, incidence <2%
- Treatment: revision ORIF with bone grafting vs. arthroplasty

Malunion
- Varus and rotational deformities most common
- Treatment: corrective osteotomies if symptomatic

References

1. Baumgaertner MR, Curtin SL, Lindskog DM, Keggi JM. The value of the tip-apex distance in predicting failure of fixation of peritrochanteric fractures of the hip. J Bone Joint Surg Am. 1995;77(7):1058–64.
2. Egol KA, Koval KJ, Zuckerman JD, Koval KJ. Handbook of fractures. Philadelphia: Wolters Kluwer/Lippincott Williams & Wilkins Health; 2010.
3. Roberts KC, Brox WT. AAOS clinical practice guideline: management of hip fractures in the elderly. J Am Acad Orthop Surg. 2015;23:138–40.
4. Rockwood CA, Green DP, Bucholz RW. Rockwood and green fractures in adults, vol. vol. 2. 7th ed. New York: J. B. Lippincott; 1991.

Hip Dislocations

60

Jeffery Kim, Charles Bishop, Dana Lycans, and James B. Day

Overview

- Usually due to high-energy mechanism
  - Motor vehicle accidents, falls, automobile vs pedestrian, industrial accidents, and athletic injuries [1]
- High incidence of associated injuries
- Anatomy
  - Hip joint is an inherently stable joint due to bony anatomy and soft tissue constraints and usually requires significant force to dislocate.

Classification

Simple

- Hip dislocation without associated fractures

Complex

- Hip dislocation with associated fractures of the acetabulum or proximal femur

Anatomic Classification

- Posterior dislocation – most common [1]
  - Mechanism due to axial load on femur with hip flexed and adducted.
  - Position of the hip during trauma determines associated acetabulum fracture.

    ○ Increased flexion and adduction more commonly associated with simple dislocation
  - Associated injuries:
    ○ Posterior wall acetabulum fracture
    ○ Femoral head fractures
    ○ Sciatic nerve injury
    ○ Ipsilateral knee injuries
- Anterior dislocation
  - Mechanism due to axial load with the hip abducted and external rotated.

Orthopedic Surgery Clerkship: A Quick Reference Guide for Senior Medical Students
Springer, 2016

J. Kim, MD
Department of Orthopaedic Surgery, Cabell Huntington Hospital/Marshall University School of Medicine, Huntington, WU, USA

C. Bishop, MD
Department of Orthopaedics, Marshall University School of Medicine, Huntington, WU, USA

D. Lycans, MD
Orthopaedic Resident, Marshall University/Cabell Huntington Hospital, Huntington, WU, USA

J.B. Day, MD, PhD (✉)
Director of Orthopaedic Trauma, Department of Orthopaedics, Joan C. Edwards School of Medicine, Marshall University, Huntington, WU, USA

© Springer International Publishing AG 2017
A.E.M. Eltorai et al. (eds.), *Orthopedic Surgery Clerkship*, DOI 10.1007/978-3-319-52567-9_60

- Position of the hip determines dislocation.
  - ○ Extended hip results in a superior dislocation (pubic).
  - ○ Flexed hip results in an inferior dislocation (obturator).
- Associated injuries
  - ○ Femoral head impaction
  - ○ Chondral injuries

Presentation

Symptoms

- Pain
- Unable to weight bear
- Deformity of lower extremity

Physical Exam

- High-energy traumatic mechanism
  - Follow Standard Advanced Trauma Life Support (ATLS) protocol
  - High incidence of associated injuries
- Must perform meticulous neurovascular exam
- Hip exam
  - Posterior dislocation
    - ○ The hip/leg in slight flexion, adduction, and internal rotation

- Anterior dislocation
  - ○ The hip/leg in slight flexion, abduction, and external rotation
- Knee exam
  - Associated with ipsilateral knee injury
  - Must examine for associated injury and/or instability

Imaging

Radiographs

- Anteroposterior (AP) pelvis
  - Disruption of Shenton's line
- AP and cross table lateral hip
  - Determine direction of dislocation
- Look for femoral neck fracture prior to attempting closed reduction

Computed tomography (CT) scan

- Postreduction CT scan of the pelvis must be performed for all traumatic hip dislocations to look for associated bony injuries (Fig. 60.1).
  - Femoral head fractures
  - Acetabulum fractures
  - Loose bodies – intra-articular fragments
  - Joint incongruity

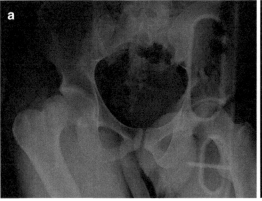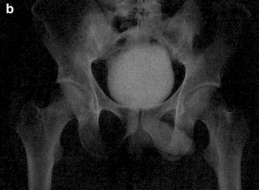

Fig. 60.1 AP pelvis of right posterior hip dislocation (**a**) and AP pelvis postreduction (**b**)

MRI

- Routine use not currently supported in acute setting
- Can be useful to evaluate for soft tissue, labrum, cartilage, and femoral head vascularity (AVN)

Treatment

Nonoperative

- Emergent closed reduction within 6 h
- Indications
  - Acute anterior and posterior hip dislocations (Fig. 60.2)
- Contraindications
  - Ipsilateral femoral neck fracture that precludes using the lower extremity to manipulate the hip and risk displacement
- Closed reduction technique
  - Allis maneuver [1–3]
  - Must have adequate sedation and muscle relaxation
  - Assess hip stability after reduction

- Treatment
  - Protected weight bearing for 4–6 weeks for simple dislocations

Operative

- Open reduction with or without debridement
  - Indications
    - Irreducible hip dislocation
    - Incongruent reduction with incarcerated fragments
    - Incongruent reduction with soft tissue interposition
    - Delayed presentation
  - Should be performed urgently
- Open reduction internal fixation
  - Indications – associated fractures
    - Acetabulum fracture (Figs. 60.3 and 60.4)
    - Femoral head fracture
    - Femoral neck fracture
      - Non-displaced should be stabilized prior to reduction.
- Technique
  - Posterior dislocation
    - Kocher-Langenbeck approach

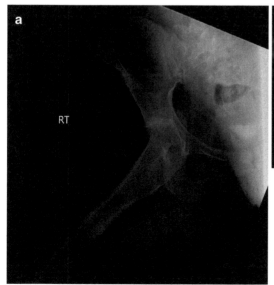
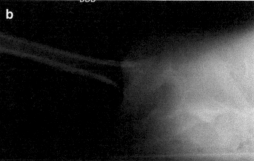

Fig. 60.2 Right anterior hip dislocation. AP right hip (**a**) and lateral right hip (**b**)

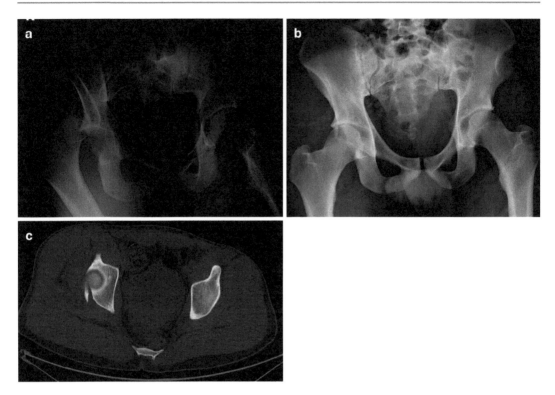

Fig. 60.3 AP pelvis of right hip dislocation (**a**), AP pelvis postreduction (**b**), postreduction CT scan showing complex fracture-dislocation with associated posterior wall acetabulum fracture (**c**)

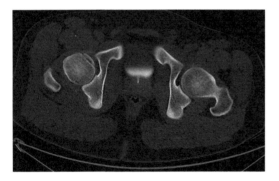

Fig. 60.4 Postreduction CT scan showing associated femoral head fracture

    – Anterior dislocation
       ◦ Smith-Petersen approach
       ◦ Watson-Jones approach
• Hip arthroscopy
    – Relative indications as alternative to open arthrotomy for a simple dislocation with a nonconcentric reduction
       ◦ Can potentially remove intra-articular fragments
       ◦ Can evaluate intra-articular injuries to capsule, labrum, and cartilage

Complications

- Post-traumatic arthritis – most common complication
  - Up to 20% for simple dislocations [3]
  - Increased for complex dislocations
- Avascular necrosis (AVN)
  - 1.7–40% incidence [1]
  - Increased risk with increased time to reduction
- Neurologic injury (sciatic nerve palsy)
  - 10–15% incidence [3] – most commonly affecting peroneal branch
  - Associated with increased time to reduction
- Heterotopic ossification – most common after posterior fracture-dislocation
- Recurrent dislocations

References

1. Rockwood CA, Green DP, Heckman JD, Bucholz RW. Rockwood and green's fractures in adults. Philadelphia: Lippincott Williams & Wilkins; 2001.
2. Browner BD, Green NE. Skeletal trauma. Edinburgh: Saunders; 2008.
3. Foulk DM, Mullis BH. Hip dislocation: evaluation and management. J Am Acad Orthop Surg. 2010;18: 199–209.

Osteoarthritis of the Hip and Knee

61

Nicole Meschbach, Daniel J. Gehling, and Andrew H. Glassman

Introduction

Definition [2–4]

- Osteoarthritis (OA) is a degenerative disease of a synovial joint that includes bone loss and progressive articular cartilage loss and may be determined radiographically in conjunction with clinical examination.
- When symptomatic, OA is generally defined by the presence of pain, aching, or stiffness in a joint with concomitant radiographic characteristics.
- Etiology is multifactorial involving both systemic and local factors.

Epidemiology [2, 4]

- Most common joint disorder in the United States
- 10%–15% in both genders 34–44 years old
- Increases to 50% in 65–74-year-olds

Risk Factors [2, 4]

- Age
- Obesity
- Prior trauma
- Joint laxity
- Female gender
- Muscle weakness
- Bone density
- Malalignment
- Dysplasia

Pathology [2]

- Synovium and capsule
  - Increasing inflammation, increased cytokines, articular cartilage damage, and thickening of capsule and synovium
- Articular cartilage
  - Initial damage to the tangential zone below the articular surface
  - Disorganized collagen, loss of proteoglycans, swelling, hypertrophic repair, generalized loss of cellularity, and formation of fibrocartilage

N. Meschbach
Warren Alpert Medical School, Brown University, Providence, Rhode Island, USA

D.J. Gehling (✉)
Department of Orthopaedic Surgery, University of Toledo – Health Science Campus, Toledo, OH, USA
e-mail: daniel.gehling@utoledo.edu

A.H. Glassman, MD, MS
Orthopaedic Surgery, The Ohio State University Wexner Medical Center, Columbus, OH, USA
e-mail: andrew.glassman@osumc.edu

© Springer International Publishing AG 2017
A.E.M. Eltorai et al. (eds.), *Orthopedic Surgery Clerkship*, DOI 10.1007/978-3-319-52567-9_61

- Bone
  - Subchondral bone remodeling, bony edema, generation of fibrocartilage, and bone cyst formation

Physical Exam and Clinical Evaluation [2–4]

- Joint pain, often worse in the morning
- Swelling
- Stiffness
- Decreased range of motion, crepitus with motion
- Malalignment, joint deformity
- Joint effusion

Other Factors to Consider and Evaluate [2, 3]

- Inflammatory arthritis
- Referred pain from the spine
- Ipsilateral joint arthritis
- Ankle/foot deformity
- Vascular disease (arterial or venous)
- Soft tissue disorders
- Neoplasm
- Neuropathy
- Stress fractures, insufficiency fracture, osteonecrosis, or symptomatic metabolic bone disease

Imaging [3]

- Joint space narrowing, osteophytes, subchondral cysts, and sclerosis

- Knee
  - Standing AP of bilateral knees
  - PA view in 30° of flexion (Rosenberg view)
  - View of bilateral patellae (Merchant view)
  - Lateral view of the affected knee

- Hip
  - Standing AP of the pelvis
  - Lateral view of the affected hip

Nonsurgical Treatment of Symptomatic Osteoarthritis [1, 3, 4]

Activity

- Activity modification
- Quad strengthening
- Weight loss
  - Patients who are overweight (BMI >25) should be encouraged to lose weight (a minimum of 5% of body weight).
- Encourage participation in low-impact aerobic fitness exercises

Medications

- Glucosamine and/or chondroitin sulfate or hydrochloride
  - Should not be prescribed for patients with symptomatic knee OA
- NSAIDs
  - Oral and topical, COX-2 inhibitors
  - Consider adding gastroprotective agent in patients >60 years old and those at risk of GI bleed
- Tylenol
  - Not to exceed 4 g per day
  - Consider in patients >60 years old and those at risk of GI bleed
- Intra-articular injections
  - Corticosteroid injection
    ◦ Short-term pain relief
    ◦ May delay surgical intervention 3–7 months due to immunosuppressive effects and infection risk
  - Hyaluronic acid (viscosupplementation) injection
    ◦ Inconclusive evidence to suggest for or against its use

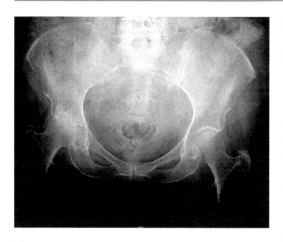

Fig. 61.1 Right hip osteoarthritis. Note the destruction of joint space compared with the left hip, where the joint space is preserved

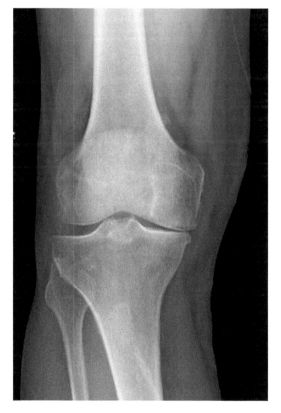

Fig. 61.2 Right knee osteoarthritis. Note the narrowing of the medial joint space

Bracing

• Inconclusive evidence for the use of valgus- or varus-directing force for patients with medial or lateral compartment OA, respectively

Surgical Treatment of Symptomatic Osteoarthritis [1, 3]

• CPGs recommend against performing arthroscopy with debridement or lavage for the treatment of symptomatic OA.
• In patients who have symptomatic arthritis and primary symptoms of a torn meniscus and/or loose body, arthroscopic partial meniscectomy or loose body removal is an option.
• Realignment osteotomy.
• After exhausting all conservative measures, perform arthroplasty.

References

1. Brown GA. AAOS clinical practice guideline: treatment of osteoarthritis of the knee: evidence-based guideline, 2nd edition. J Am Acad Orthop Surg. 2013;21(9):577–9. doi:10.5435/JAAOS-21-09-577.
2. Einhorn TA, O'Keefe RJ, Buckwalter JA. Orthopedic basic science: foundations of clinical practice. 3rd ed. American Academy of Orthopedic Surgeons: Rosemont; 2007.
3. Yates Jr AJ, McGrory BJ, Starz TW, Vincent KR, McCardel B, Golightly YM. AAOS appropriate use criteria: optimizing the non-arthroplasty management of osteoarthritis of the knee. J Am Acad Orthop Surg. 2014;22(4):261–7. doi:10.5435/JAAOS-22-04-261.
4. Zhang Y, Jordan J. Epidemiology of osteoarthritis. Clin Geriatr Med. 2010;26(3):355–69.

Avascular Necrosis

62

John Alexander, Richard Boe, and Joel Mayerson

Avascular Necrosis

Definition

- Avascular necrosis, also referred to as osteo-necrosis, is the death of cells within bone due to lack of circulation.

Pathophysiology [1]

- Subchondral ischemia of the bone develops from a variety of mechanisms (Fig. 62.1):
  - Vascular disruption
    - ○ Trauma is the most common cause of avascular necrosis (often seen in fracture/dislocations).
  - Extravascular compression or constriction, either arterial inflow or venous outflow
    - ○ Associated with corticosteroid use, alcohol intake, and Gaucher disease.
    - ○ Increased intramedullary pressure leads to decreased perfusion.

J. Alexander, MD • J. Mayerson
Department of Orthopaedics, The Ohio State
University Medical Center, Columbus, OH, USA
e-mail: john.alexander@osumc.edu;
joel.mayerson@osumc.edu

R. Boe (✉)
Department of Orthopaedics, Marshall University
Medical Center, Huntingston, WV, USA
e-mail: richiebie@gmail.com

- Corticosteroids and alcohol → lipocyte hypertrophy
- Gaucher → disease accumulation of glucocerebroside
  - Intravascular occlusion
    - ○ Associated with sickle cell anemia, fat emboli, or other acquired or congenital coagulation abnormalities.
    Low flow or obstructed flow leads to increased rate of vascular obstruction.
- Direct cellular toxicity.
  - Seen with certain medications, radiation, or oxidative stresses
- Altered mesenchymal stem cell differentiation.

Histologic Changes

- Osteocyte necrosis occurs early in the process.
  - Within hours of anoxic event, histologically observed within 24–72 hours
- Early (second week) – death of various cell lines including hematopoietic, endothelial, and adipocytes.
- Lysosomes released by adipocytes lead to acidification of the osseous environment and increase in water content which is manifested by interstitial marrow edema (observed on MRI).
- Capillary revascularization leads to resorption of bone and limited bone formation.

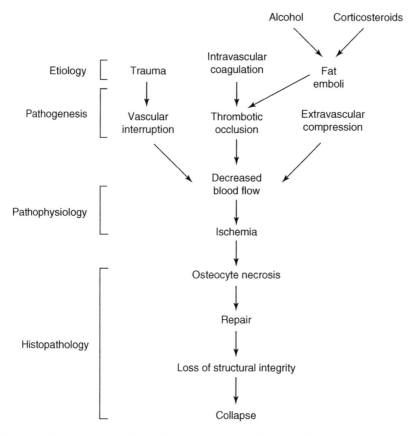

Fig. 62.1 Diagram depicting the various insults that may lead to altered vascular flow and the development of avascular necrosis. Used with permission from Shah et al. [1]

- In subchondral bone, the process is not equal → loss of subchondral support, fracture, and articular incongruity.

Radiographic Changes (Fig. 62.2)

- Plain radiographs
  - Normal in early stages
  - Later stages, develop cystic changes that progress to sclerosis with subchondral collapse
- Nuclear bone scans
  - Nonspecific, but can detect early-stage disease (increased bone remodeling)
  - MRI more sensitive for detecting AVN
- Magnetic resonance imaging
  - MRI is 99% sensitive and specific for avascular necrosis.
  - Early on demonstrating increased marrow edema and later can identify the border between dead and living bone.

Presentation

- Early – commonly asymptomatic.
- With disease progression, patients often develop a deep pain, and later mechanical symptoms develop due to articular incongruity.

Classification and Staging

- Ficat and Arlet
  - *Stage I*: normal
  - *Stage II*: sclerotic or cystic lesions
    ∘ *A:* no crescent sign
    ∘ *B:* subchondral collapse (crescent sign) without flattening of the femoral head
  - *Stage III*: subchondral collapse or flattening of the femoral head on plain radiographs
  - *Stage IV*: osteoarthritis with decreased joint space with articular collapse

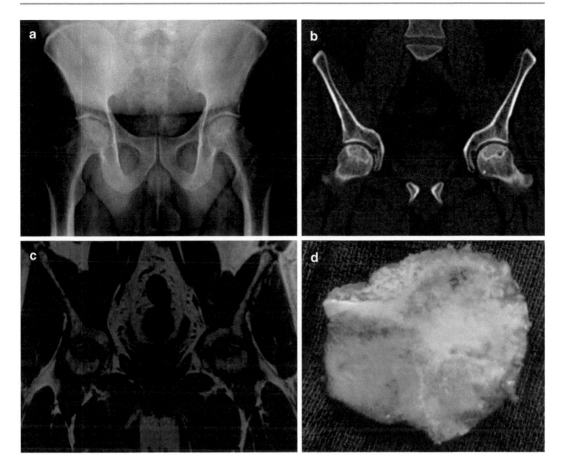

Fig. 62.2 (**a**) AP pelvis XR imaging demonstrating bilateral femoral head avascular necrosis with subchondral collapse. Representative cross-sectional coronal CT (**b**) and T1 MRI (**c**) images demonstrating further detail of the anterior-superior subchondral collapse. Associated cross-sectional gross pathology demonstrating subchondral collapse (**d**)

Femoral Head [2]

- Epidemiology
  - Commonly secondary to trauma (femoral neck fracture or hip dislocation).
  - In children, it can also be idiopathic as is the case with Legg-Calve-Perthes or iatrogenic secondary to excessive abduction with a Pavlik harness.
  - Corticosteroids account for 10–30% of cases of femoral head AVN.
    - Chronic steroid use is associated with a 4–7% rate of avascular necrosis.
  - Excessive alcohol use is associated with 10–40% of cases of femoral head AVN.
- Treatment
  - Nonoperative
    - Observation for small asymptomatic lesions.
    - Some recent studies have shown benefit of extracorporeal shock wave therapy.
    - Treatment of the underlying condition may slow progression.
  - Operative
    - Core decompression
      - Beneficial when performed in early stages with 70% not requiring additional surgeries, effective at providing pain relief and preventing radiographic progression
      - May be combined with various bone grafting adjuncts
    - Vascularized bone grafting
      - Vascularized fibular or iliac crest grafts are anastomosed to the ascending branch of the lateral femoral circumflex artery and vein and Introductionduced into the core decompression tract.

- Studies have shown promising results with improved outcomes compared to core decompression alone.
- Associated with donor site morbidity in 20% of patients.
  ○ Total hip arthroplasty
    - Collapse leads to progressive degenerative changes associated with debilitating pain necessitating total joint replacement.
    - Patients tend to be younger and are associated with higher rates of dislocation and revision than similarly aged patients with osteoarthritis.
- Prognosis
  - Long-term studies show that the majority of asymptomatic lesions become symptomatic with collapse.
    ○ The rate of collapse is proportional to the size of the lesion.

Knee [3]

- Second most common site of AVN
- Three types:
  - Secondary
  - Spontaneous
  - Postarthroscopic
- Secondary
  - Bilateral in >80% of cases and >90% of patients have involvement of other joints
  - Associated with corticosteroid use and alcohol abuse.
  - Treatment
    ○ Majority of patients do not respond to nonoperative management.
    ○ Early stages can be treated with core decompression or osteochondral grafts.
    ○ When subchondral collapse is present, total knee arthroplasty is the standard.
- Spontaneous
  - Most commonly affects the medial femoral condylar epiphysis and is most commonly unilateral
  - Affects women more frequently than men (3:1) and older patients

- Thought to be secondary to subchondral insufficiency fractures or other trauma
- Treatment
  ○ Protected weightbearing and NSAIDs lead to clinical improvement in >89% of patients with early disease.
  ○ Osteochondral grafts and core decompression are an option for patients with refractory symptoms.
  ○ Unicompartmental arthroplasty is an option for patients with osteoarthritis, given the tendency to affect only the medial femoral condyle.
- Postarthroscopic [4]
  - Most commonly affects the medial femoral condyle followed by the lateral femoral condyle, rarely can affect the tibial plateaus and the patella.
  - True incidence is unknown, but likely very low.
  - Iatrogenic occult damage to the cartilage or menisci alters biomechanics of the knee → subchondral fracture.
  - Treatment is the same as for spontaneous osteonecrosis of the knee.

Humeral Head [5]

- Epidemiology
  - Incidence is similar to AVN of the knee and etiologies similar to AVN of the hip.
  - Untreated will lead to glenohumeral arthritis.
- Presentation
  - Shoulder pain worse with overhead activities
- Treatment (Fig. 62.3)
  - Core decompression has demonstrated promising outcomes with improved pain and function and decreased need for arthroplasty for stage I–III disease.
  - Arthroscopic debridement can improve mechanical symptoms.
  - Stage IV AVN with humeral head collapse is managed with hemiarthroplasty with total shoulder arthroplasty being reserved for patients with glenoid degeneration.

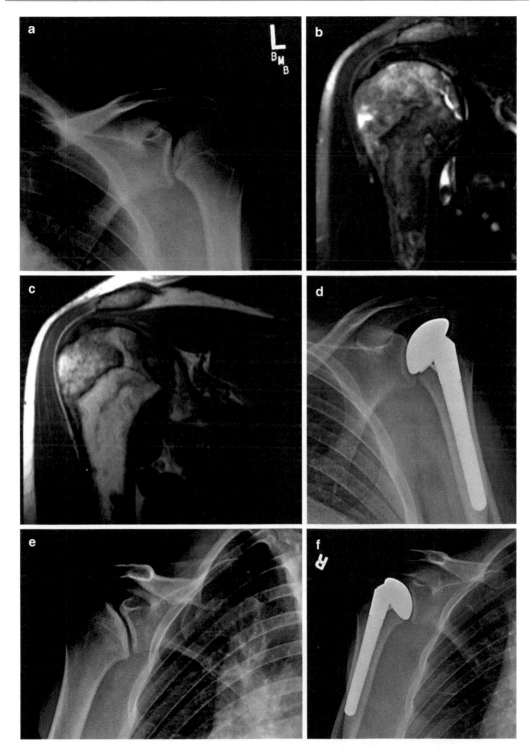

Fig. 62.3 Representative preoperative AP (**a**, **e**) radiographs, PA T2 (**b**) and T1 (**c**) coronal MRI imaging, and postoperative radiographs (**d**, **f**) after hemiarthroplasty in an adult male with bilateral humeral head AVN secondary to high-dose steroids for T-cell lymphoma

- When epiphyseal bone stock is adequate, humeral head resurfacing may be an option.
  - Lacks long-term outcome studies to support its use in patients with AVN

Talus [6]

- Common after talar neck fractures, with Hawkins type III fractures associated with a 90% incidence of AVN
- May also be secondary to systemic conditions as with AVN of the femoral head (Figs. 62.4 and 62.5)
- Hawkins sign
  - Subchondral lucency seen at 6 weeks due to revascularization
- Treatment
  - Nonoperative management with limited weightbearing and activity modification.
  - No consensus exists on the gold standard for operative intervention.

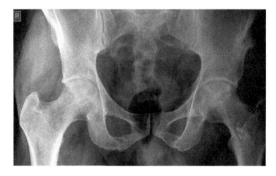

Fig. 62.4 Hip osteonecrosis, stage 2 of left femoral head

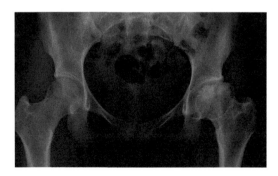

Fig. 62.5 Hip osteonecrosis stage 5

Lunate

- AVN of the lunate is called Kienbock's disease.
- Likely multifactorial in etiology.

Scaphoid [7]

- Most commonly secondary to scaphoid fractures due to the retrograde blood supply of the scaphoid.
  - Higher incidence with proximal fractures
  - Leads to the development of scaphoid nonunion advanced collapse (SNAC)
- Idiopathic form is called Preiser's disease.

Navicular

- Most commonly due to trauma; when idiopathic, they are referred to as Kohler's disease (pediatric) and Muller-Weiss disease (adults).
- Kohler's disease.
  - Presents between ages 2–9 years of age.
  - May be a normal variant.
  - Treats nonsurgically with casting.
  - Prognosis is excellent with studies showing all patients asymptomatic at long-term follow-up.
- Adults
  - Most commonly secondary to trauma, but can be due to Muller-Weiss disease
  - Treat with either bone-block midfoot fusion or triple arthrodesis

Freiberg's Disease

- AVN of the second metatarsal head
- Classically affects girls during their growth spurt
- Most respond favorably to conservative treatment

References

1. Shah KN, Racine J, Jones LC, Aaron RK. Pathophysiology and risk factors for osteonecrosis. Curr Rev Muscoskelet Med. 2015;8:201–9.
2. Zalavras CG, Lieberman JR. Osteonecrosis of the femoral head: evaluation and treatment. J Am Acad Orthop Surg. 2014;22:455–64.

3. Mont MA, Marker DR, Zywiel MG, Carrino JA. Osteonecrosis of the knee and related conditions. J Am Acad Orthop Surg. 2011;19:482–94.
4. Pape D, Seil R, Anagnostakos K, Kohn D. Postarthroscopic osteonecrosis of the knee. Arthroscopy. 2007;23:428–38.
5. Harreld KL, Marker DR, Wiesler ER, Shafiq B, Mont MA. Osteonecrosis of the humeral head. J Am Acad Orthop Surg. 2009;17:345–55.
6. DiGiovanni CW, Patel A, Calfee R, Nickisch F. Osteonecrosis in the foot. J Am Acad Orthop Surg. 2007;15:208–17.
7. Wolfe SW, Pederson WC, Hotchkiss RN, Kozin SH. Green's operative hand surgery: 2-volume set, 6e (Operative Hand Surgery (Green's)). Churchill Livingstone. 2010:2392.

Total Hip Arthroplasty

63

Karl Balch and Andrew H. Glassman

Overview

- Total hip arthroplasty (THA): For management of hip arthritis when conservative measures (NSAIDs, physical therapy) have failed. THA is primarily a pain-relieving operation and one of the most effective operations for improving quality of life in all of medicine.
- THA is composed of three components: femoral, acetabular, and the bearing surface.

Femoral Component: Cementless and Cemented

- Cementless – Relies on bony ingrowth or on-growth (osseointegration) to the surface of implant.
  - Requires initial mechanical stability and close contact with host bone. Majority of THA is cementless.
  - Best for younger patients or patients with good bone stock.
  - Proximally or extensively porous coated – defines area available for bony fixation. Can be identified by surface texture on implant.

K. Balch, MD (✉) • A.H. Glassman, MD, MS
Orthopaedic Surgery, The Ohio State University
Wexner Medical Center, Columbus, OH, USA
e-mail: karlbalch@gmail.com;
andrew.glassman@osumc.edu

- Cemented – Cement acts as grout to stabilize component.
  - Best when cement can interdigitate with porous osteoporotic bone

Acetabular Component

- Cementless – Cemented acetabular components have higher failure rate, so cementless fixation of acetabular components is dominant. Can be hemispherical or elliptical shaped and can be used with adjunct screw fixation

Bearing Surfaces (Femoral Head on Cup Liner)

- Femoral head material is commonly metal (cobalt chrome) or ceramic.
- Acetabular cup liner can be metal, polyethylene, or ceramic.
- The couple of head with liner are defined as:
  - Metal on polyethylene (MOP): Low cost, long track record of success. Gold standard.
  - Metal on metal (MOM): Lower wear rate than metal on poly, more expensive, and creates metal ions/particles in serum/urine. Complications – formation of pseudotumor (deep fluid collection) and failures led to recalls and lawsuits.

© Springer International Publishing AG 2017   285
A.E.M. Eltorai et al. (eds.), *Orthopedic Surgery Clerkship*, DOI 10.1007/978-3-319-52567-9_63

- Ceramic on ceramic (COC): Best wear properties, low friction, and high cost compared to poly on metal. Brittle material can fracture (rare) or cause squeaking.
- Ceramic on poly (COP): Hybrid ceramic and poly coupling combine strengths and weaknesses of both materials.

Approaches: Direct Anterior, Anterolateral, Direct Lateral, and Posterior/Posterolateral Approach

Direct Anterior (Smith-Petersen)

- Increasing prevalence, studies reporting lower dislocation rate, and quicker early rehab/recovery equivalent long term. Good exposure of acetabulum. More difficult femoral exposure. Minimally extensile. Studies report higher femur fracture rate.
  - Interval: Superficially, tensor fasciae latae (TFL) and sartorius; deep, rectus femoris and gluteus medius.
  - Pearls: Lateral femoral cutaneous nerve must be protected at the level of fascia in initial approach in the interval. Can cause painful neuroma/or lateral thigh paresthesia. The ascending branch of lateral femoral circumflex artery is in interval and should be identified and ligated to prevent bleeding and improve visualization.

Anterolateral (Watson-Jones)

- Infrequently used as violates abductors →Trendelenburg gait. Reported lower dislocation rate
  - Interval: Superficial – TFL and gluteus medius. Deep,– trochanteric osteotomy or partial abductor release
  - Pearls: Management of abductors (achieving union of trochanteric osteotomy) or abductor repair after release defines recovery. Must avoid compression femoral nerve with medial retraction

Direct Lateral (Hardinge)

- No true interval (muscle splitting), lowest dislocation rate of approaches, and access to anterior and posterior hip without osteotomy. Violates abductor mechanism
  - Interval: Superficial splits gluteus medius proximally and vastus lateralis distally (centers on vastus ridge).
  - Pearls: Best for patients at high risk for dislocation, i.e., Parkinson's, limited mental status/dementia, and noncompliance as these patients may not be able to comply with hip precautions. Superior gluteal nerve runs between gluteus medius and minimus 3–5 cm above the greater trochanter.

Posterolateral

- Most common approach. Is extensile for revisions, obese patients requiring larger exposure or dealing with complications such as periprosthetic fractures. Good femoral and acetabular exposure. Reported higher dislocation rate
  - Interval: No internervous plane, intermuscular plane through gluteus maximus muscle split proximally. Piriformis is the "lighthouse" to the hip and will direct to the short external rotators and level of release to get into the joint.
  - Pearls: Repair of short external rotators released during approach and posterior hip precautions important for preventing postop dislocation. Protect sciatic nerve during approach. Sciatic nerve most commonly travels under piriformis and is located on the posterior surface of quadratus femoris during approach.

Ideal Positioning of Components

- Cup placed in $45 \pm 10°$ of abduction and $20 \pm 10°$ of anteversion. Overly vertical cup predisposes to dislocation and loads a small area of poly leading to rapid wear and failure. Overly horizontal cup leads to impingement. Poor version can increase impingement or dislocation risk. Medial border of cup should lie close to the radiographic tear drop (depth). Femoral component should be placed in 10–15° of anteversion.

Postoperative

Hip Precautions

- Prevent dislocation post-op. Limited motions vary by approach. Anterior approaches – avoid extension; extreme external rotation; and adduction past midline. Posterior approaches – avoid extreme internal rotation, hip flexion beyond 90°, and adduction past midline

Anticoagulation

- Risk of DVT/PE elevated postoperatively so anticoagulation needed to prevent thrombosis. Multiple options and widely debated in the literature. Established orthopedic guidelines have recommended one of the following: acetylsalicylic acid (aspirin) and sequential compression devices (SCDs), enoxaparin, or warfarin for anticoagulation. Research into newer medications (such as direct thrombin inhibitors) for anticoagulation is ongoing.

Complications

- Dislocation, periprosthetic fracture, periprosthetic joint infection, leg length inequality, nerve injury, thromboembolic disease, heterotopic ossification, late loosening, wear problems, or premature failure of components

Dislocation

- Stability of THA affected by components selected, position, soft tissue tension, and control/function

- Components: Large femoral heads – reduce impingement/increase arc of motion and increase jump distance (translation prior to dislocation). Cup design can partially mitigate risk through using a lateralizing liner or elevated rim liner.
- Position: Idealized cup position (see above) improves stability. Posterior approaches should favor anteversion, and anterior approaches should favor retroversion slightly.
- Soft tissue tension: Restoration of offset (distance from femoral head center of rotation to axis femur). Increased offset increases tension; decreased offset leads to instability and weak abductors.
- Control/function: Any pathology of the nervous system or inability to control muscles through voluntary or involuntary means increases risk of dislocation (dementia, stroke, Parkinson's, alcoholism, etc.).

Periprosthetic Fracture

- Vancouver classification widely employed. Defines fracture and guides treatment
  - Periprosthetic infection: 0.3–1.3% complication rate. Chronicity of infection guides treatment. Aspiration and culture gold standard for diagnosis. Synovial WBC >1100 cells/mL and/or PMNs >64%. Current gold standard of management requires explantation and two-stage exchange with an antibiotic spacer targeted to culture results.

Revision

- Indications: Loosening, instability, infection, malalignment, poly wear, fracture, and component failure. Discussion of revision classifications and components is beyond the scope of this review.

General Tips for Medical Students

- Anatomy, Anatomy, Anatomy: In the operating room, anatomy will always be a primary focus for questions. Asking ahead of time to know which approach the surgeon uses will allow you to review the anatomy in detail prior to going in the OR. Medical students will frequently be helping to retract, across the table, or holding the leg, so you will not always have a good view of the surgical field but that won't stop residents and attending surgeons from asking you anatomy questions based on the approach.

- As with any rotation, know your patients! Keeping track of postoperative labs, vitals, anticoagulation, and other protocols will help you understand your patients better. Getting in early and gathering info on the patients before the resident shows up and giving them a sheet summarizing the patients on the floor will help you stand out and make a valuable contribution to the team. Ask a resident or attending surgeon to go over how to read x-rays systematically when evaluating pre- and post-op patients.

External Snapping Hip

64

Anne Marie Chicorelli

Overview

- Earliest type of snapping hip described [1]

Anatomy

- Posterior thickening of the iliotibial band and an anterior thickening of fibers of the gluteus maximus.
- Fibers snap on the greater trochanter with flexion and extension of the hip.

Classification of Snapping Hip

- External snapping hip
- Internal snapping hip: iliopsoas tendon snapping over the iliopectineal eminence or femoral head
- Intra-articular snapping hip: intra-articular pathology causing mechanical symptoms

Evaluation

- Patient reported symptoms of pain or snapping over greater trochanter.

- May be reproducible in office by patient.
- If symptomatic, associated with pain over greater trochanter.
- Flexion/extension of the hip elicits pain and/or snapping.
- Pain is from resultant bursitis and/or gluteus medius tendinosis.

Imaging

- AP pelvis
- Dynamic ultrasound
- MRI to diagnose tendon tears, bursitis, and tendinosis

Treatment

Nonoperative Treatment

- Physical therapy: stretching
- NSAIDS
- Steroid injections of the greater trochanter bursae

Operative Treatment After Failure of Conservative Treatment

- Indications: pain and snapping over the area of the greater trochanter with flexion/extension

A.M. Chicorelli, DO, MPH
Orthopaedics and Sports Medicine, The Ohio State University Wexner Medical Center,
Wooster, OH, USA
e-mail: anne.chicorelli@osumc.edu

© Springer International Publishing AG 2017
A.E.M. Eltorai et al. (eds.), *Orthopedic Surgery Clerkship*, DOI 10.1007/978-3-319-52567-9_64

of the hip after failure of conservative treatment
- Contraindications: severe hip osteoarthritis, infection
- Open iliotibial band release and bursectomy:
  - Z-plasty
  - Star release
- Arthroscopic iliotibial band release and bursectomy:
  - Patient positioning: lateral or supine on radiolucent table (unless concomitant intra-articular arthroscopy then placed on hip arthroscopy distraction table)
  - Portal placement:
    ○ Greater trochanter landmark delineated by spinal needle on x-ray.
    ○ Infiltrate space under iliotibial band with 50 ml saline.
    ○ Inferior trochanteric portal using the cannula under the skin directed proximally.
    ○ Develop working space bluntly and then place 30° arthroscope into the cannula.
    ○ Proximal trochanteric portal created under direct visualization with spinal needle to ensure adequate angle for iliotibial band release.
    ○ Shave/ablation device placed in proximal portal.

○ Create vertical retrograde cut with ablation device on iliotibial band extending between portals and maintain hemostasis.
○ Superior and inferior flaps resected to create defect and transverse posterior cut and superior and posterior flaps resected with shaver resulting in star-shaped pattern.
○ The greater trochanteric bursae visualized and resected with shaver; abductor tendons evaluated for tears.

Complications

- Incomplete release of posterior iliotibial band
- Scarring of previous iliotibial band tendon release
- Hematoma
- Continued pain

Reference

1. Binnie JF. Snapping hip (Hanche a resort; Schnellend Hefte). Ann Surg. 1913;58:5966.

Femoral Shaft Fractures

65

LeeAnne Torres, Dana Lycans, and Akshay Goel

Introduction

- Incidence is 1–1.3/10000 people per year [1]

Bimodal Age Distribution [1]

Younger Population
- Peaks around 20–30 years of age.
- Usually high-energy trauma. Motor vehicle collision is most common cause.
- Associated with high morbidity and mortality.

Older Population
- Peaks around 60–70 years of age.
- Low-energy trauma.
- Can be pathological.
- Higher incidence of periprosthetic femur fractures.
- Up to 50% of patients have associated injuries including ipsilateral femoral neck fracture,

bilateral femur fractures, patellar fractures, tibial fractures, acetabular fractures, pelvic ring injuries, and ligamentous/meniscal injuries of the knee.

Anatomy [1–3]

- The femur is the strongest and longest bone with an anterior bow.
- Medial cortex under compression and lateral cortex under tension.
- Surrounded by muscular attachments: leads to significant displacement after fracture:
  - Linea aspera – middle third of the posterior femur
  - Compressive strut to accommodate anterior bow:
    - Attachment site for the vastus medialis, vastus lateralis, adductor longus, biceps femoris, adductor brevis, and adductor magnus
  - Musculature (divided into three compartments):
    - Anterior compartment (femoral nerve) – iliopsoas, sartorius, quadriceps femoris, and pectineus
    - Posterior compartment (sciatic nerve) – biceps femoris, semitendinosus, semimembranosus, and portion of adductor magnus

L. Torres, MD • D. Lycans, MD
Department of Orthopaedic Surgery, Marshall University/Cabell Huntington Hospital, Huntington, WV, USA
e-mail: Torresl@live.marshall.edu; Lycans42@gmail.com

A. Goel, MD (✉)
Department of Orthopaedics, Three Rivers Medical Center, Louisa, KY, USA
e-mail: akshaypgimer@gmail.com

© Springer International Publishing AG 2017
A.E.M. Eltorai et al. (eds.), *Orthopedic Surgery Clerkship*, DOI 10.1007/978-3-319-52567-9_65

○ Medial/adductor compartment (obturator nerve) – gracilis, adductor longus, adductor brevis, adductor magnus, and obturator externus
– Deforming forces result in the proximal segment going into abduction and flexion from the pull of the hip abductors and iliopsoas. The distal segment goes into varus and extension from the force that the hip adductors and gastrocnemius exert [3].

Classification: Based on Fracture Pattern and Comminution [1–3]

Winquist and Hansen (Fig. 65.1)

Type 0	No comminution
Type I	Minimal comminution
Type II	Some comminution with at least 50% cortical contact
Type III	Comminution with minimal cortical contact
Type IV	Segmental comminution with no cortical contact

Vascular Supply [1]

- Profunda femoris artery injury often associated with hemorrhage rather than ischemia due to rich muscular collaterals in the thigh
- Superficial femoral artery damage usually leads to distal ischemia
- Average blood loss into the thigh: 1200 mL

Clinical Evaluation [5]

- ATLS should be initiated.
- Symptoms: trauma, painful thigh, and inability to ambulate.
- Physical exam: shortening of the thigh, swelling, deformity, and tenderness.

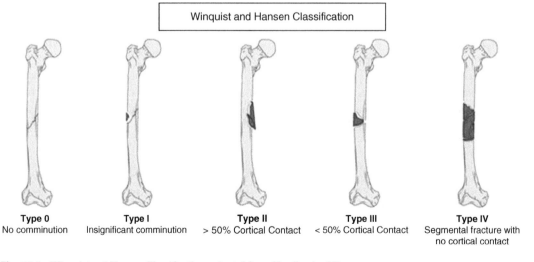

Winquist and Hansen Classification

| Type 0 | Type I | Type II | Type III | Type IV |
| No comminution | Insignificant comminution | > 50% Cortical Contact | < 50% Cortical Contact | Segmental fracture with no cortical contact |

Fig. 65.1 Winquist and Hansen Classification, adapted from Handbook of Fractures

- Always check for open fractures.
- Examine distal neurologic and vascular integrity.
- Identify compartment syndrome of the thigh and calf.
- Examination for concomitant injuries – Knee ligaments, ipsilateral femoral neck, lumbar spine, pulmonary injury, and head injuries.

Imaging [5]

- Radiographs (Figs. 65.2 and 65.3).
  - AP and lateral views (femur, hip, and knee)
  - AP pelvis

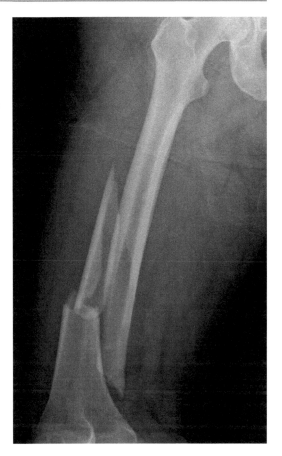

Fig. 65.3 Lateral view of a comminuted femur shaft fracture

- CT should be considered to rule out associated femoral neck or acetabulum fracture.

Treatment

Nonoperative [1, 2]

- Skeletal traction can be used for temporary stabilization while awaiting definitive surgery.
- Safe pin placement: medial to lateral in extracapsular location of the distal femur or lateral to medial at the proximal tibia.
- Associated knee ligament injury precludes use of tibial traction pin.

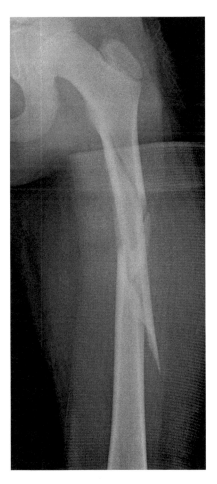

Fig. 65.2 AP view of a comminuted mid-shaft pediatric femur shaft fracture with open physis

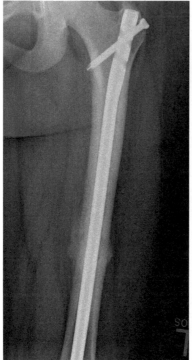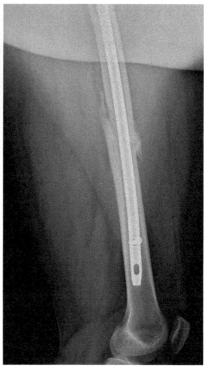

Fig. 65.4 AP and lateral views of a femur mid shaft fracture showing fixation with piriformis entry antegrade femoral nail

Operative Fixation of Femoral Shaft Fractures Is Mainstay of Treatment [1, 3]

- Early fixation (within 24 h of injury) is associated with better outcomes.

Antegrade Reamed Intramedullary Nail (IMN) (Figs. 65.4 and 65.5) [6]
- Treatment of choice
- High union rates and low complications
- Can be done in supine or lateral position
- Fracture table or radiolucent bed
- Entry point: trochanteric tip or piriformis fossa
- Piriformis entry point:
  - Advantages: entry point collinear with the femoral shaft and reduced risk of varus malalignment
  - Disadvantages: technically challenging and risk of iatrogenic fracture of proximal femur
- Trochanteric entry point:

  - Advantages: technically easier especially obese patients
  - Disadvantages: risk of varus malalignment

Retrograde IM Nailing [6]
- Insertion through intercondylar entry portal in the knee just above notch (Blumensaat's line)
- Supine position radiolucent bed
- Indications:
  - Ipsilateral acetabular fracture
  - Ipsilateral femoral neck fracture
  - Ipsilateral tibia shaft fracture
  - Fracture line extending to the distal femur
  - Morbid obesity
  - Pregnant females
  - Bilateral femur shaft fractures

Plate Fixation (Fig. 65.6) [5]
- Indicated in fractures with extremely narrow canal where IMN is difficult, ipsilateral femoral neck fracture (can also use retrograde nail),

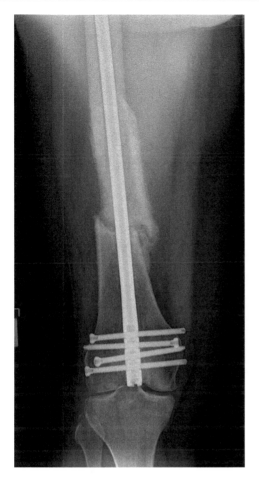

Fig. 65.5 AP view of a distal femur shaft fracture showing fixation with a retrograde femoral nail

fractures near metaphyseal-diaphyseal junction, periprosthetic femur fractures, and open physes

External Fixation [11]
- Indicated in damage control situations (polytrauma patients with injuries precluding immediate fixation)
- Usually convert to IM nail within 2 weeks

Complications [1, 5, 6]

Malunion [10]

- Angular malunion more common in proximal femur fractures.
- Rotational malunion, especially external rotation, remains the concern in mid-diaphyseal fractures.

- Always examine rotation symmetry after fracture fixation before exiting operating room.
- Symptomatic malunion requires osteotomy.

Nonunion [9]

- Low rates of nonunion <10%
- Higher in open fractures , segmental fractures, and bone loss
- Treatment options:
  - Exchange nailing: union rates range from 53 to 95%
  - Dynamization
  - Plating with bone graft

Leg Length Discrepancy

- More common in comminuted fractures (up to 43%).
- Intraoperatively use radiopaque ruler to compare length to uninjured side.
- After fixation leg lengths should be compared before exiting operating room.

Infection

- Low rates (1–3.8%)
- Attempt nail retention with serial debridements and antibiotics in early phase until fracture union
- Nail removal indicated when this fails
- Options include antibiotic cement nails or external fixation
- Heterotopic ossification (25% incidence): proximally or within the quadriceps
- Neurovascular injury including the pudendal nerve and femoral artery and nerve
- Weakness of the quadriceps and hip abductors

Special Situations

Multitrauma Patients [1, 7, 6]

- Timing of IMN is controversial especially in patients with pulmonary compromise.

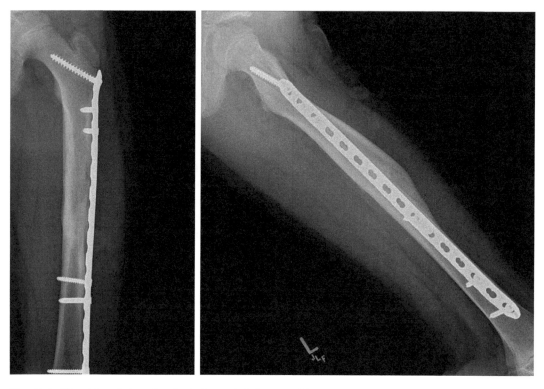

Fig. 65.6 AP and lateral view of pediatric femur shaft fracture with open physis managed using femoral plating

- Stable patients: best treated with early definitive care (IM nailing).
- Unstable or "in extremis": treated with principals of damage control orthopedics (temporary external fixator).
- Borderline patients: treatment is controversial. Period of aggressive resuscitation prior to definite fixation is beneficial. Early reamed IM nailing is safe if patient is adequately resuscitated.

Ipsilateral Femoral Shaft and Hip Fractures (Femoral Neck or Intertrochanteric) [8, 6]

- Present in 2–9% of all shaft fractures
- Requires high index of suspicion (20–50% missed)
- Often minimally displaced
- Diagnosis requires fine cut CT pelvis, internal rotation hip radiographs
- Neck fractures are usually Pauwels C

- Anatomical reduction and fixation of neck takes precedence over shaft fracture
- Treatment options:
  - Separate implants for both fractures: retrograde IMN or plate construct for shaft fracture and cannulated screw or sliding hip screw for proximal femur fracture
  - Single implant fixation using antegrade IMN with reconstruction screw

Open Fractures [6]

- High morbidity and mortality
- Generally Gustilo and Anderson type III due to high-energy mechanism
- Higher rate of complications: infection, segmental bone loss, nonunion, and delayed union

Treatment

- Intravenous antibiotics initiated in ER and continued until wound closure

- Urgent aggressive debridement
- Immediate IM nailing can be done in most cases:
  - Consider provisional fixation with external fixator with serial debridement at 24–48 h intervals in highly contaminated wounds.
  - Can use adjunctive treatment like vacuum-assisted closure if large wounds present.
- In cases of significant bone loss, consider placement of antibiotic bead spacer

Gunshot Injuries
- Low-velocity wounds (less than 2000 feet per second) do not require extensive debridements:
  - Can be treated with standard fixation and perioperative antibiotics
- High velocity (greater than 2000 feet per second) wounds and shotgun injuries:
  - Require extensive debridements.
  - Consider provisional fixation with external fixation.
  - Definite fixation with nail or plate once wound is clean.

Periprosthetic Femoral Shaft Fractures [5]
- Fractures around hip prosthesis:
  - If prosthesis is loose, it needs to be revised.
  - If prosthesis is well fixed, treat with internal fixation using cerclage wires and plate.
    - Consider cabled strut allografts
- Femoral fractures near total knee prosthesis:
  - Retrograde IMN can be used if femoral component is "open box" or PCL-sparing implant
  - Locking plates

References

1. Smith RM, Giannoudis PV. Femoral shaft fractures. In: Browner BD, et al., editors. Skeletal trauma: basic science, management, and reconstruction. 4th ed. Philadelphia: Elsevier; 2009.
2. Egol KA, Koval KJ, Zuckerman JD. Femoral shaft. In: Handbook of fractures. 4th ed. Philadelphia: Lippincott Williams & Wilkins; 2010.
3. Nork S. Femoral shaft fractures. In: Bucholz RW, et al., editors. Rockwood and Green's fractures in adults. 7th ed. Philadelphia: Wolters Kluver/Lippincott Williams & Wilkins; 2010.
4. Norris BL, Nowotarski PJ. Femoral shaft fractures. In: Stannard JP, et al., editors. Surgical treatment of orthopedic trauma. New York: Thieme; 2007. p. 611–32. Print
5. Decoster BS, Figueiredo FCS. Femoral shaft fractures. OKOJ. 2008;6(3).
6. Ricci WM, Gallagher B, Haidukewych GJ. Intramedullary nailing of femoral shaft fractures: current concepts. J Am Acad Orthop Surg. 2009;17:296–305.
7. Pape HC, Rixen D, Morley J, et al. Impact of method of initial stabilization for femoral shaft fractures in patient with multiple injuries at risk for complications (borderline patients). Ann Surg. 2007;246(3):491–9.
8. Wolinsky PR, Johnson KD. Ipsilateral femoral neck and shaft fractures. Clin Orthop Relat Res. 1995;318:81–90.
9. Hak DJ, Lee SS, Goulet JA. Success of exchange reamed intramedullary nailing for femoral shaft nonunion or delayed union. J Orthop Trauma. 2000;14:178–82.
10. Ricci WM, Bellabarba C, Lewis R, et al. Angular malalignment after intramedullary nailing of femoral shaft fractures. J Orthop Trauma. 2001;15:90–5.
11. Scalea TM, Boswell SA, Scott JD, Mitchell KA, Kramer ME, Pollak AN. External fixation as a bridge to intramedullary nailing for patient with multiple injuries and with femur fractures: damage control orthopedics. J Trauma. 2000;48:613–23.

Knee Ligament Injuries

66

Aristides I. Cruz Jr.

Anterior Cruciate Ligament (ACL) [1, 2]

Anatomy/Biomechanics

- Primary restraint to anterior translation of the tibia relative to the femur
- Secondary restraint to tibial rotation
- Anteromedial (AM) bundle:
  - More isometric
  - Tight in flexion
- Posterolateral (PL) bundle:
  - Tight in extension
  - Contributes primarily to rotational stability

Diagnosis

History

- Contact or noncontact sports injury
- Pivoting knee injury
- "Pop" followed by knee effusion (swelling)

Physical Exam

- Anterior drawer
- Lachman exam:

  - Anteriorly directed force on the tibia with the knee flexed 30°
  - Grading:
    - I = 3–5 mm translation
    - II = 6–10 mm
    - III > 10 mm:
      - A = Firm endpoint
      - B = Soft endpoint
- Pivot shift exam:
  - Valgus force as the knee is brought from extension into flexion.
  - In extension, the tibia subluxated anteriorly and reduces at 20–30° of flexion as IT band transitions from knee extensor to flexor thus reducing the tibia.

Imaging

- X-ray:
  - "Segond fracture," avulsion fracture off the anterolateral proximal tibia; classically associated with ACL rupture
- MRI: definitive diagnosis

Treatment

Nonoperative

- Low-demand patients
- Primarily consists of activity/lifestyle modification
- PT to emphasize hamstring strength
- ACL specific bracing with activity

A.I. Cruz, Jr., MD
Assistant Professor of Orthopaedics, Warren Alpert Medical School at Brown University, Rhode Island Hospital/Hasbro Children's Hospital, Providence, RI, USA
e-mail: aristides_cruz@brown.edu

© Springer International Publishing AG 2017
A.E.M. Eltorai et al. (eds.), *Orthopedic Surgery Clerkship*, DOI 10.1007/978-3-319-52567-9_66

Operative

- Active, high-demand patients.
- Failed nonoperative treatment (persistent knee instability).
- Reconstruction is current gold standard (as opposed to repair).

Surgical Options

- Single vs. double bundle:
  - Double bundle may better reproduce knee kinematics [3].
  - No clear difference in clinical outcomes between single and double bundle.
- Graft choice:
  - Hamstring (semitendinosus, gracilis):
    - Smaller patients yield smaller grafts:
      - Graft size <8 mm associated with higher risk of failure [4]
    - No bone-bone healing
  - Bone-patellar tendon-bone:
    - Longest history of use
    - "Gold standard"
    - Bone-bone healing
    - Donor-site morbidity (anterior knee pain)
    - Complication – patella fracture
  - Quadriceps tendon
- Allograft vs. autograft [5]:
  - Autograft:
    - Pro: patient's own tissue, no risk of disease transmission, and faster graft incorporation
    - Cons: donor-site morbidity
  - Allograft:
    - Pro: no donor-site morbidity and can select graft size.
    - Cons: slower graft incorporation, theoretic risk of disease transmission, and irradiated allograft may be associated with higher failure rates.
- Femoral tunnel drilling:
  - Transtibial:
    - More "traditional" technique
    - Femoral tunnel location accessed via the tibial tunnel
  - Independent tunnel:
    - May allow for more "anatomic" femoral tunnel placement by allowing more oblique drill trajectory

- Requires knee hyperflexion to prevent posterior wall "blowout"
  - Retrograde or "outside-in" drilling:
    - Requires specialized instrumentation
    - Allows independent femoral tunnel drilling without need for knee hyperflexion

Rehab/Injury Prevention [6]

- Neuromuscular training/jump training
- Jump landing in valgus and relative extension implicated in increased risk of injury
- Address relative hamstring weakness

Complications

- Re-rupture:
  - Most common cause – tunnel malposition
- Loss of motion/arthrofibrosis:
  - Delay surgery until patients regain motion and swelling from acute injury controlled
- Tunnel osteolysis
- Fixation failure
- "Cyclops" lesion:
  - Due to fibroproliferative tissue within the intercondylar notch
  - Blocks extension
  - Treat with arthroscopic debridement
- Posttraumatic arthritis:
  - May be associated with concomitant meniscal pathology

Posterior Cruciate Ligament (PCL) [7, 8]

Anatomy/Biomechanics

- Anterolateral (AL) bundle:
  - Tight in flexion
- Posteromedial (PM) bundle:
  - Tight in extension
- Meniscofemoral ligaments:

– Originate from posterior horn lateral meniscus and insert onto PCL
– Anterior, ligament of Humphrey; posterior, ligament of Wrisberg

Diagnosis

History

• Posteriorly directed blow to the flexed knee (i.e., "dashboard" injury)
• Knee hyperflexion injury with the plantar-flexed foot

Physical Exam

• Posterior drawer test:
  – Grading:
    ○ I = 1–5 mm translation
    ○ II = 6–10 mm
    ○ III > 10 mm
• Posterior sag sign:
  – With the knee at 90° flexion, the tibia lies posterior relative to the femoral condyles compared to contralateral side.
• Quadriceps active test:
  – With the knee flexed at 90°, the tibia subluxated posteriorly relative to the femur; resisted activation of the quadriceps reduces the tibia anteriorly.
• Dial test:
  – See section below (posterolateral corner injuries).

Imaging

• X-ray:
  – May show avulsion fracture off posterior tibial insertion
  – Posterior drawer stress test → posterior subluxation of the tibia
• MRI

Treatment [9]

Nonoperative

• Most isolated PCL tears (Grade I–II)
• Rehab to concentrate on quadriceps strengthening

Operative

• Isolated Grade III tears with persistent functional instability
• Multi-ligament knee injury

Surgical Options

• Tibial avulsion fracture → direct repair
• Reconstruction options:
  – Transtibial technique:
    ○ Beware of "killer turn":
      – PCL graft is passed from anterior to posterior through tibial tunnel; graft then passed from posterior to anterior into femoral tunnel.
      – May cause attenuation of graft tissue.
  – Tibial inlay technique:
    ○ Avoids "killer turn":
      – Tibial portion of graft seated into the socket in posterior aspect of the tibia
  – Graft choice:
    ○ Allograft vs. autograft:
      – Same inherent issues as above.
      – Allograft affords more graft options especially during multi-ligament knee reconstruction.

Medial Collateral Ligament (MCL) [10]

Anatomy/Biomechanics

• Superficial MCL:
  – Primary restraint to valgus stress of the knee
• Deep MCL:
  – Secondary restraint to valgus stress.
  – Attaches to the medial meniscus.
  – Posterior fibers blend with the posteromedial capsule and the posterior oblique ligament (POL).

Diagnosis

History

• Commonly associated with ACL rupture

Physical Exam

- Tenderness along medial aspect of the knee.
- Valgus stress testing at 30° knee flexion isolates superficial MCL.
- Grading:
  - I = 1–4 mm medial joint line gapping
  - II = 5–9 mm
  - III ≥ 10 mm
- Valgus stress at 0° knee flexion indicates posteromedial capsule or cruciate ligament injury.

Imaging

- X-ray:
  - Rule out bony injury.
  - Valgus stress test may show medial joint line gapping.
- MRI:
  - Can characterize sprain vs. partial vs. complete tear

Treatment

Nonoperative

- Primary treatment in both isolated and combined ACL injury
- NSAIDs, rest, physical therapy, and bracing (to resist valgus)

Operative treatment

- Relative indications:
  - Acute repair in Grade III (complete) injuries
  - Multi-ligament knee injury
- Reconstruction indicated in chronic injuries with persistent functional instability

---

Posterolateral Corner (PLC) [11, 12]

Anatomy/Biomechanics [13]

- PLC structures consist of static and dynamic structures:
  - Static:
    - Lateral collateral ligament (LCL)
    - Popliteus tendon
    - Popliteofibular ligament (PFL)
    - Lateral capsule
    - Arcuate ligament
    - Fabellofibular ligament
  - Dynamic:
    - Biceps femoris
    - Popliteus muscle
    - Iliotibial band
    - Lateral head of gastrocnemius
- PLC resists external rotation, varus, and posterior translation.

Diagnosis

History

- Acute injuries:
  - Be suspicious with high-energy injury mechanisms and multi-ligamentous knee injury (i.e., knee dislocation).

Physical Exam

- Varus thrust with gait exam
- Varus stress at 30° knee flexion:
  - Grading:
    - I = 0–5 mm lateral joint line gapping
    - II = 6–10 mm
    - III > 10 mm
- Varus laxity at 0° (LCL + cruciate injury)
- Dial test:
  - Tests for isolated PLC vs. PLC + PCL injury.
  - External rotation of tibia at 30° and 90° of knee flexion.
  - Positive test is >10° of side-to-side difference:
    - + test @ 30° and 90° flexion → PLC + PCL injury
    - + test @ 30° flexion only → isolated PLC injury
- Reverse pivot shift:
  - Valgus/external rotation force as the knee is brought from flexion into extension.
  - In flexion, the tibia subluxated posteriorly and reduces at approximately 20–30° of flexion as IT band transitions from knee flexor to extensor.

Imaging

- X-rays:
  - Avulsion fracture off the fibula ("arcuate fracture") represents bony avulsion of lateral ligamentous complex.
- MRI:
  - Imaging of choice

Treatment

Nonoperative

- Isolated PLC Grade I/II injuries
- Knee immobilizer with protected weight-bearing ×2 weeks followed by progressive rehab

Operative

- PLC repair:
  - Indicated only in acute injuries (within 2 weeks from injury)
  - Fibular avulsion → ORIF
- PLC reconstruction:
  - Grade III injury
  - Chronic injuries
  - Correct varus malalignment (if present) with high tibial osteotomy in chronic injuries
- Reconstruction techniques:
  - Multiple described
  - Goal: reconstruct LCL and PFL
- Acute multi-ligament knee injury:
  - Staged reconstruction:
    - Repair/reconstruct PLC early (within 2 weeks of injury).
    - Reconstruct PLC prior to ACL.

Complications

- Knee stiffness/arthrofibrosis
- Missed PLC injury:
  - Unrecognized PLC injury may lead to failed ACL reconstruction.
- Peroneal nerve injury

References

1. Beynnon BD, Johnson RJ, Abate JA, Fleming BC, Nichols CE. Treatment of anterior cruciate ligament injuries, part I. Am J Sports Med. 2005;33(10):1579–602.
2. Beynnon BD, Johnson RJ, Abate JA, Fleming BC, Nichols CE. Treatment of anterior cruciate ligament injuries, part 2. Am J Sports Med. 2005;33(11):1751–67.
3. Kopf S, Musahl V, Bignozzi S, Irrgang JJ, Zaffagnini S, Fu FH. In vivo kinematic evaluation of anatomic double-bundle anterior cruciate ligament reconstruction. Am J Sports Med. 2014;42(9):2172–7.
4. Mariscalco MW, Flanigan DC, Mitchell J, et al. The influence of hamstring autograft size on patient-reported outcomes and risk of revision after anterior cruciate ligament reconstruction: a Multicenter Orthopedic Outcomes Network (MOON) Cohort Study. Arthroscopy. 2013;29(12):1948–53.
5. Kaeding CC, Pedroza AD, Reinke EK, Huston LJ, Consortium M, Spindler KP. Risk factors and predictors of subsequent ACL injury in either knee after ACL reconstruction: prospective analysis of 2488 primary ACL reconstructions from the MOON cohort. Am J Sports Med. 2015;43(7):1583–90.
6. Donnell-Fink LA, Klara K, Collins JE, et al. Effectiveness of knee injury and anterior cruciate ligament tear prevention programs: a meta-analysis. PLoS One. 2015;10(12):e0144063.
7. Sekiya JK, Whiddon DR, Zehms CT, Miller MD. A clinically relevant assessment of posterior cruciate ligament and posterolateral corner injuries. Evaluation of isolated and combined deficiency. J Bone Joint Surg Am. 2008;90(8):1621–7.
8. Lee BK, Nam SW. Rupture of posterior cruciate ligament: diagnosis and treatment principles. Knee Surg Relat Res. 2011;23(3):135–41.
9. Montgomery SR, Johnson JS, McAllister DR, Petrigliano FA. Surgical management of PCL injuries: indications, techniques, and outcomes. Curr Rev Muscoskelet Med. 2013;6(2):115–23.
10. Roach CJ, Haley CA, Cameron KL, Pallis M, Svoboda SJ, Owens BD. The epidemiology of medial collateral ligament sprains in young athletes. Am J Sports Med. 2014;42(5):1103–9.
11. Ranawat A, Baker 3rd CL, Henry S, Harner CD. Posterolateral corner injury of the knee: evaluation and management. J Am Acad Orthop Surg. 2008;16(9):506–18.
12. LaPrade RF, Wentorf F. Diagnosis and treatment of posterolateral knee injuries. Clin Orthop Relat Res. 2002;402:110–21.
13. LaPrade RF, Bollom TS, Wentorf FA, Wills NJ, Meister K. Mechanical properties of the posterolateral structures of the knee. Am J Sports Med. 2005;33(9):1386–91.

Meniscal Tear

67

Jonathan Gillig and Albert Pearsall

Anatomy and Basic Science

Function

- To disperse the load transmitted through the knee joint by increasing the contact surface area:
  - Knee extension – up to 50% of joint reactive force absorbed
  - Knee flexion – up to 90% of joint reactive force absorbed
- Deepens the surface area of the joint – provides stability
- Peripheral boarders attached to joint capsule and provides proprioception
- Assists in joint lubrication and assists with cartilage nutrition

Histology

- Fibrocartilage disks composed of collagen (95%), fibrochondrocytes, water, proteoglycans (1%), glycoproteins (1%), and elastin (0.6%)

J. Gillig, MD • A. Pearsall, MD (✉)
Department of Orthopaedic Surgery, University of South Alabama, 1601 Center Street, #N-3160, Mobile, AL 36604, USA
e-mail: jgillig@health.southalabama.edu; apearsal@health.southalabama.edu

- Collagen components – type 1 (90%), types 2, 3, 5, and 6 (5–10%)
- Cellular function – synthesizes extracellular matrix and limited anaerobic metabolism

Layers

- Superficial – radially oriented fibers, woven in meshwork
- Surface layer – random fiber orientation
- Middle layer – fibers circumferential to disperse hoop stress and radial to hold the circumferential together

Vascular Supply

- Superior and inferior medial and lateral geniculate arteries:
  - Branch circumferentially to form a plexus
- Supply peripheral meniscus (medial has improved supply).
- Central meniscus has limited nutrient supply – provided by synovial fluid.
- Fibrochondrocyte primarily responsible for healing.
- Three zones:
  - Red zone – 3 mm from the joint capsule (best chance of healing)

© Springer International Publishing AG 2017
A.E.M. Eltorai et al. (eds.), *Orthopedic Surgery Clerkship*, DOI 10.1007/978-3-319-52567-9_67

- Red-white zone – 3–5 mm from the joint capsule
- White zone – >5 mm from the joint capsule (most tears do not heal)

Innervation

- Peripheral two-third:
  - Type 1 and 2 nerve endings
  - Anterior < posterior horn concentration
  - Limited in meniscal body

Medial Meniscus

- C-shaped, broader posteriorly than anteriorly.
- Anterior horn attaches to the tibial intercondylar area anterior to the ACL.
- Posterior horn attaches to the tibial intercondylar area anterior to the PCL.
- Medially attaches to the tibial collateral ligament.

Lateral Meniscus

- Nearly circular and smaller/more mobile.
- Tethered to the medial meniscus through the transverse ligament.
- Popliteus tendon separates the lateral meniscus from the fibular collateral ligament.
- Attached to the PCL and the medial femoral condyle by the posterior meniscofemoral ligament

Injury

Epidemiology

- Tears are present in 32% of painful/symptomatic knees and 23% of asymptomatic knees.
- Meniscal tears are the most common indication for knee surgery.
- Risk increases in ACL-deficient knees.
- Medial and lateral tears occur in equal frequency.

- Lateral tears more common in traumatic setting and concurrent with acute ACL tears:
  - Longitudinal and transverse tears most common.
  - Mechanism of injury is usually rotation of the flexed knee as it begins extension.
  - Discoid menisci have increased tear rates.
- Degenerative tears occur most commonly occur in the posterior horn of the medial meniscus:
  - Horizontal cleavage tears, flap tears, and complex tears.
  - Partial thickness tears involve inferior surface of the meniscus more commonly than the superior surface.

Patterns of Injury

- Longitudinal:
  - Very common with ACL tears, repair when peripheral
- Radial:
  - High-energy tears perpendicular to the long axis of the meniscus
- Horizontal:
  - More common in the elderly as degenerative changes make the meniscus less mobile
  - Associated with meniscal cysts which are found more common on the lateral side
- Oblique:
  - May cause mechanical locking symptoms
- Bucket handle:
  - Subtype of longitudinal tear that may displace into the intercondylar notch
  - Can progress to pedunculated if one side detaches

Presentation and Physical Exam

Symptoms

- Knee pain – can be generalized or localized to affected side.
- Mechanical symptoms mostly occur with longitudinal tears and bucket handle lesions:
  - Not pathognomonic for meniscal tear
- Knee effusion – can be after acute event or recurrent with activity.
- Sensation of the leg giving away.

Physical Exam Maneuvers (Sensitivity, Specificity)

- Apley grind test (97%, 87%):
  - Patient lies prone with the knee flexed to 90°.
  - Examiner places own knee across the patient's posterior thigh.
  - Tibia compressed onto the knee joint while externally rotated
  - Pain with External rotation = medial meniscus; internal rotation = lateral meniscus
- Joint line tenderness (83%, 83%)
- McMurray (61%, 84%):
  - Knee flexed to 90° with the foot in one hand and the other hand at joint line.
  - Induce varus stress with one hand pushing medial side of the knee laterally.
  - Use the second hand to rotate the leg externally.
  - If pain or click is felt, test is positive for medial meniscal tear.
  - Similar signs with valgus stress indicate lateral meniscal tear.
- Thessaly test (75%, 87%) – dynamic test of joint loading:
  - Patient stands on one knee with the examiner holding arms for support.
  - Patient flexes weight-bearing knee to 5° and rotates body internally and externally three times.
  - Procedure then repeated with the knee in 20° of flexion.
  - Joint line discomfort, locking, or catching indicate positive test.

Diagnostic Studies

- Radiographs – likely normal in meniscal pathology
- MRI – most sensitive test:
  - High rate of false positives.
  - Grade III signal indicates a tear.
  - Parameniscal cyst – fluid collection that indicates concurrent tear.
  - Double PCL sign – indicates bucket handle pathology.

Treatment

Nonoperative

- Indications – first-line treatment for degenerative tears:
  - Incomplete tears, <5 mm peripheral tear, and no other pathology
- Management – activity modification, rest, NSAIDs, and rehabilitation

Operative

Partial Meniscectomy
- Indications – irreparable tears with no healing potential
- Occurs in the white zone of the meniscus
- Outcomes – >80% satisfaction and function at follow-up:
  - 50% have radiographic changes (osteophytes, flattening, joint space narrowing) postoperatively.
  - Improved outcomes:
    - ° Age <40, normal alignment, minimal arthritis, and single tear
  - Causes slight increase in joint laxity.
  - Medial partial meniscectomy has better results than lateral.
- Total meniscectomy – historical procedure as meniscus thought to have been inconsequential:
  - 20% progression to arthritic lesions.
  - 70% have radiographic changes within 3 years of surgery.
  - 100% arthritis at 20 years.
  - Severity directly correlated to amount removed.

Meniscal Repair
- Indications – peripheral tear in the red zone:
  - Rim width – distance from the tear to the blood supply (i.e., peripheral junction with capsule)
  - Improved healing potential:
    - ° Lower rim width
    - ° Vertical or longitudinal tears
    - ° 1–4 cm in length

○ Acute repair with ACL reconstruction concurrently
• Outcomes – 70–95% success rate, highest with ACL reconstruction:
  – 30% success rate with untreated ACL deficiency.
  – Healing occurs by fibrocartilaginous scar at 10 weeks.
  – Maturation occurs for several months following repair.

Meniscal Transplant
• Indications – young patient (< 50 years) with near total meniscectomy.
• Contraindications – instability, obesity, malalignment, significant arthritis, inflammatory arthritis, chondrosis, and immunodeficiency.
• Weight-bearing with patient in full extension for first 6 weeks.
• Gradually increase flexion between 6 and 12 weeks.
• Requires 8–12 months for full graft maturation.
• Return to full activity in 6–9 months.
• A 10-year follow-up demonstrates improved pain and function:
  – Lateral and medial survival of 70% and 74%, respectively
  – Poor results if advanced cartilage degeneration has begun

• Re-tears, extrusion, and progressive radiographic changes common

Complications

• Saphenous neuropathy (7%)
• Arthrofibrosis (6%)
• Sterile effusion (2%)
• DVT (1.2–4.9%)
• Peroneal Neuropathy (1%)
• Infection (0.23–0.42%)

References

1. McCulloch, Patrick. Meniscal pathology. In: Orthobullets. N.p., 13 Sept. 2015. Web. 1 Nov; 2015.
2. Miller MD. In: Hart JA, editor. Review of orthopedics. Philadelphia: Saunders/Elsevier; 2008. Print
3. Moore KL, Agur AMR. Basic sciences. In: Essential clinical anatomy. Philadelphia: Lippincott Williams & Wilkins; 2007. p. 42–3. Print
4. Smith BE, Thacker D, Crewesmith A, Hall M. Special tests for assessing meniscal tears within the knee: a systematic review and meta-analysis. Evid Based Med Evidence Based Medicine. 2015;20(3):88–97. Web
5. Thompson JC, Netter FH. Netter's concise orthopedic anatomy. Philadelphia: Saunders Elsevier; 2010. p. 384–5. Print
6. Wiesel, Sam W. Part 1: sports medicine. In: Operative techniques in orthopedic surgery. 2nd ed. vol. 1. N.p.: n.p; n.d. p. 276–330. Print.

Extensor Mechanism Injuries: Quadriceps and Patellar Tendon Ruptures

68

David C. Flanigan, Joshua Troyer,
Joshua S. Everhart, John W. Uribe, Eric Wherley,
and Gautam P. Yagnik

Anatomy

- The quadriceps tendon is formed from muscle bellies of rectus femoris, vastus medialis, vastus lateralis, and vastus intermedius and inserts on proximal aspect of patella:
  - Trilaminar structure
  - Supplied by medial, lateral, and peripatellar vascular arcades
  - Vulnerable to injury at watershed area, 1–2 cm proximal to superior pole of patella
- The patellar tendon originates at the distal aspect of the patella and inserts at the anterior tibial tuberosity:
  - Considered tendon instead of ligament as patella is sesamoid bone
  - Supplied by geniculate arteries
  - Site of rupture most commonly in proximal portion of tendon
- Fascia from the vastus passes anterior to the patella forming prepatellar fascia and also forms medial and lateral retinaculum contributing to patellar stability.

Epidemiology

- Knee extensor tendon injuries are relatively rare occurrences:
  - Patellar fractures 2–3× as common as tendon rupture
  - Quadriceps tendon rupture more common than patellar tendon rupture
- Age:
  - Quadriceps tendon ruptures more common after 45, most frequently seen in sixth and seventh decades of life.
  - Patellar tendon ruptures occur in younger patients in twenties and thirties.
- 8:1 male to female ratio.
- Risk factors:
  - Intra-articular injections – history of injections in 20–33% of ruptures
  - Steroid use
  - Rheumatoid arthritis
  - Connective tissue disorders
  - Diabetes

D.C. Flanigan (✉) • J. Troyer • J.S. Everhart
Department of Orthopaedics, The Ohio State
University Wexner Medical Center,
Columbus, OH, USA
e-mail: David.Flanigan@osumc.edu

J.W. Uribe
Department of Orthopedic Surgery, Herbert Wertheim
College of Medicine at Florida International
University, Coral Gables, FL, USA

E. Wherley
Herbert Wertheim College of Medicine at Florida
International University, Miami, FL, USA

G.P. Yagnik
Department of Orthopedics, West Kendall Baptist
Hospital, Miami, FL, USA

© Springer International Publishing AG 2017
A.E.M. Eltorai et al. (eds.), *Orthopedic Surgery Clerkship*, DOI 10.1007/978-3-319-52567-9_68

- Chronic renal failure
- Hyperthyroidism
- Gout
- Bilateral tears may occur up to 12% of time and are associated with delay in diagnosis due to misdiagnosis as neurologic problem.

Presentation

- Commonly due to indirect trauma:
  - Sudden contraction of quadriceps muscle on flexed knee most commonly to avoid fall:
    - Eccentric loading disrupts extensor mechanism.
- History of pain prior to rupture indicates presence of tendinopathy.
- Patellar tendon rupture in younger patients more likely to be due to direct trauma.

Exam

- Diagnostic triad:
  - Acute onset of pain
  - Inability to actively extend knee:
    - Intact retinaculum and IT tract may preserve some extension.
    - Inability to perform straight leg raise.
  - Palpable gap at rupture site:
    - Presence of hemarthrosis may obscure this finding; these injuries often have significant effusions.
- Note findings of displaced patella, superiorly in patellar tendon rupture and inferiorly in quadriceps rupture (Fig. 68.1).
- Aspiration of effusion and lidocaine injection:
  - May be helpful in distinguishing between partial and complete ruptures

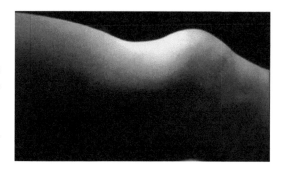

Fig. 68.1 Quadriceps tendon gap (Reprinted with permission from Maffulli et al. [1])

Imaging

- AP and lateral X-ray:
  - Patella baja – quadriceps tendon ruptures (Fig. 68.2).
  - Patella alta – patella tendon ruptures (Fig. 68.3):
    - Insall-Salvati method can be used to determine patella baja or alta:
      - Measure length ratio of patellar tendon to patella
      - Normal tendon/patella ratio = 0.8–1.2
      - Patella baja <0.8
      - Patella alta >1.2
  - Note anterior or posterior patella rotation in lateral view.
  - Look for possible avulsion fracture.
- MRI:
  - May be used to determine extent of tear
  - Considered gold standard
  - Used for preoperative planning
- Ultrasound:
  - Can be used in cases of diagnostic uncertainty
  - Caution-operator dependent

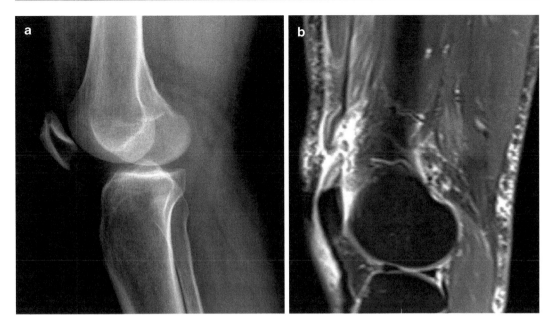

Fig. 68.2 (a) Lateral X-ray image demonstrating patella baja. (b) T2-weighted sagittal MRI image of same knee demonstrating complete rupture of quadriceps tendon

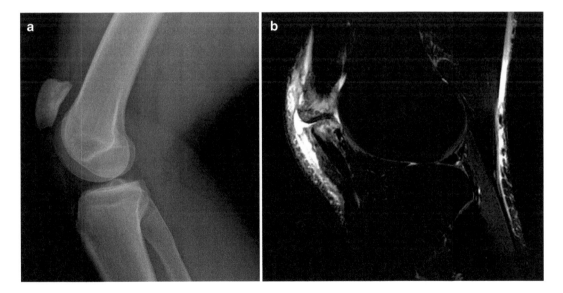

Fig. 68.3 (a) Lateral X-ray image demonstrating patella alta. (b) T2-weighted sagittal MRI image of same knee demonstrating complete rupture of patellar tendon

Treatment

- Partial rupture:
  - May be managed nonoperatively with knee immobilization
- If >50% of the tendon is torn, consider surgical repair.

- Complete rupture should be repaired within 7–14 days:
  - Due to tendon retraction proximally with delay as little as 2 weeks
- Technique for acute repair:
  - Transosseous repair:
    ○ Midline anterior knee incision.

○ Two–three longitudinal drill holes in patella (Fig. 68.4).
○ Ethibond or FiberWire suture through tendon using Krackow or Becker technique with possible use of fascial strips for reinforcement (Fig. 68.5).
○ Pass suture through drill holes and tie on opposite pole of the patella with knee in full extension.
○ Repair retinaculum.

– Suture anchor repair:
  ○ Midline anterior knee incision
  ○ Two–three anchors placed at superior or inferior pole of patella
  ○ Suture passed through torn tendon and tied with knee placed in extension
• Techniques for chronic repair:
  – Multiple techniques described.
  – V-Y advancement flap is the most common.
  – Allograft augmentation.

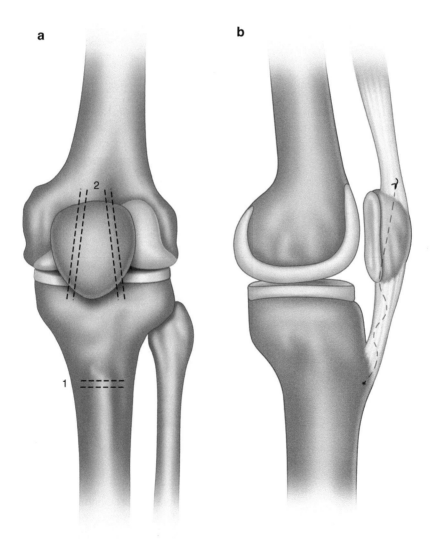

Fig. 68.4 Patellar tendon repair. (**a**) Route of the burr channels (*1, 2*) in the Mersilene loop tendon repair operation. (**b**) Suturing of the ruptured tendon (Reprinted with permission from Persson et al. [13])

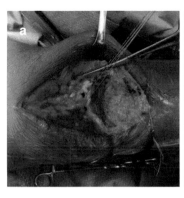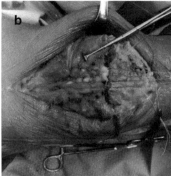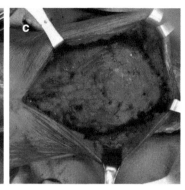

Fig. 68.5 Repair of complete re-rupture of quadriceps tendon. (**a**) Quadriceps tendon rupture identified with Krakow stitch completed. (**b**) Reduction of quadriceps tendon after release performed to identify anchor sites. (**c**) Completed repair including repair of medial and lateral retinaculum

Postoperative Rehabilitation

- Four–six weeks' immobilization
  - Knee immobilizer or range of motion knee brace.
  - Some centers utilize early passive ROM.
- Crutch walking for 6–8 weeks

Complications

- Stiffness:
  - More common in patella tendon ruptures.
  - Consider early passive ROM or CPM to minimize stiffness.
- Extensor lag:
  - More common in quadriceps tendon rupture repairs.
  - Consider delaying motion or prolonging period of immobilization in quad repairs.
- Quadriceps muscle weakness reported at 25–67% decrease noted in many studies.
- Tendon re-rupture is a concern given tendinopathy often present prior to injury.
- Rare serious complications also include DVT and PE from immobilization.
- Wound complications are rare.

References

1. Maffulli N, Via AG, Oliva F. Reconstruction of neglected tears of the extensor apparatus of the knee. Sports Inj. doi:10.1007/978-3-642-36801-1_132-1.

Suggested Reading

1. Saragaglia D, Pison A, Rubens-Duval B. Acute and old ruptures of the extensor apparatus of the knee in adults (excluding knee replacement). Orthop Traumatol Surg Res. 2013;99(1 Suppl):S67–76.
2. Siwek CW, Rao JP. Ruptures of the extensor mechanism of the knee joint. J Bone Joint Surg Am. 1981;63(6):932–7.
3. Miller MD, Thompson SR, Hart J. Review of orthopedics. 6th ed. Philadelphia: Elsevier, 2012.
4. Ilan DI, Tejwani N, Keschner M, Leibman M. Quadriceps tendon rupture. J Am Acad Orthop Surg. 2003;11(3):192–200.
5. Lee D, Stinner D, Mir H. Quadriceps and patellar tendon ruptures. J Knee Surg. 2013;26(5):301–8. doi:10.1055/s-0033-1353989.
6. Matava MJ. Patellar tendon ruptures. J Am Acad Orthop Surg. 1996;4(6):287–96.
7. McMahon PJ, Kaplan LD, Popkin CA (2014) Chapter 3. Sports medicine. In: Skinner HB, McMahon PJ, editors. Current diagnosis & treatment in orthopedics. 5th ed. New York: McGraw-Hill Medical, 2014.
8. Pang J, Shen S, Pan WR, Jones IR, Rozen WM, Taylor GI. The arterial supply of the patellar tendon: anatomical study with clinical implications for knee surgery. Clin Anat. 2009;22(3):371–6.
9. Perfitt JS, Petrie MJ, Blundell CM, Davies MB. Acute quadriceps tendon rupture: a pragmatic approach to diagnostic imaging. Eur J Orthop Surg Traumatol. 2014;24(7):1237–41.
10. Petersen W, Stein V, Tillmann B. Blood supply of the quadriceps tendon. Unfallchirurg. 1999;102(7):543–7.
11. Ristic V, Maljanovic M, Popov I, Harhaji V, Milankov V. Quadriceps tendon injuries. Med Pregl. 2013;66(3–4):121–5.
12. Persson K, Merkow RL, Templeman DC, Sieber J, Gustilo RB. Patellar tendon rupture. Description of a simplified operative method for a current therapeutic problem. Arch Orthop Trauma Surg. 1992;112(1):47–9.

Tibial Plateau Fractures

69

Patrick Bergin and Tracye J. Lawyer

Introduction/Overview [1]

- Fractures of the tibial plateau involve the articular surface of the proximal tibia.
- Imaging studies need to be of good quality to demonstrate the location of the fracture, the fracture pattern, and the degree of displacement.
- Assessing associated soft tissue injuries around the knee is critically important.
- Certain fractures have a high risk of limb-threatening complications such as compartment syndrome.

Anatomy [2]

- The medial and lateral tibial plateaus are the articular surfaces of the medial and lateral tibial condyles which articulate with the medial and lateral femoral condyles.
- The medial plateau is the larger of the two and is concave. The lateral plateau is smaller and higher than the medial and is convex.
- The articular surfaces of the tibia slope approximately 10° from anterior to posterior.
- The tibial tubercle is located on the anterior tibial crest 2–3 cm below the anterior joint line

and provides attachment for the patellar tendon.
- The iliotibial band inserts on the lateral tibial flare into a prominence known as Gerdy's tubercle.
- The fibular head is prominent along the posterolateral aspect of the tibial condyle and serves as a site of attachment for the fibular collateral ligament and biceps tendon.
- The proximal tibiofibular joint is a true synovial joint and can communicate with the knee joint.
- The outer portion of each plateau is covered by the meniscus. The meniscotibial ligaments attach these structures to the tibia. The lateral meniscus covers a much larger portion of the articular surface than the medial.

Mechanism of Injury [1]

- The magnitude, type, and direction of forces that injure the knee dictate the fracture pattern. The greater the energy absorbed by the proximal tibia, the more severe is the fracture, and the more fragments are displaced and comminuted.
- The energy of the fracture results from a combination of forces applied and quality of the bone.
- Injuries to the plateaus occur as a result of a force directed medially or laterally, an axial

P. Bergin, MD (✉) • T.J. Lawyer, MD, PhD
Department of Orthopaedic Surgery, University of
Mississippi Medical Center, Jackson, MS, USA
e-mail: PBergin@umc.edu

© Springer International Publishing AG 2017
A.E.M. Eltorai et al. (eds.), *Orthopedic Surgery Clerkship*, DOI 10.1007/978-3-319-52567-9_69

compressive force, or both an axial force and a force from the side.

- In elderly patients, simple falls lead to lateral fracture patterns. Split-depression fractures of the lateral plateau are most common because with age the dense cancellous bone becomes osteopenic and cannot withstand compressive forces as well.
- Higher speed injuries in younger patients can cause split fractures or rim avulsion fractures associated with knee ligament injuries. These pure split fractures are more common in younger patients because the strong subchondral bone of the tibial condyle is able to withstand the compressive force of the femoral condyle, but the shear component of the load produces a split in the condyle.
- Motor vehicle accidents and falls from heights often produce more severe patterns which may involve both condyles and have a high risk for associated neurovascular injuries, compartment syndrome, and open fractures.
- Tibial plateau fractures most often occur with the leg in a weightbearing position, so axial load typically contributes to some component of the injuring force.

Associated Injuries [2]

- Tibial plateau fractures have typical local soft tissue injuries that are important to recognize because they may influence fracture management and prognosis.
- The force that produces medial and lateral plateau fracture may lead to associated collateral ligament injuries. There are also frequent associated intra-articular soft tissue injuries to both the cruciate ligaments and the menisci.
- Fractures of the lateral plateau are rarely associated with arterial or nerve lesions.
- Fractures of the medial plateau are associated with much greater violence often represent a knee dislocation and are frequently associated with lesions of the peroneal nerve or the popliteal vessels. The arterial injuries are typically a small intimal tear which may enlarge or initiate clotting.

- Tibial plateau fractures, particularly if they extend into the diaphysis, may be associated with acute compartment syndrome because of hemorrhage and edema of the involved compartments.
- Severe contusions of the skin envelope surrounding the proximal tibia occur with high-energy injuries. Even in the absence of open fractures, the contused soft tissue may be in jeopardy because of instability of underlying fractures, severe swelling, or poorly timed surgical procedure.
- Fractures of the proximal tibia may become complicated by wound sloughs, infections, and osteomyelitis.

Classification [1]

- The most widely used and accepted classification of tibial plateau fractures in North America is that proposed by Schatzker.
- The six fracture categories indicate increasing severity but also a worse prognosis:
  - Type I: pure wedge or split fracture of the lateral plateau. It occurs in young patients in whom the strong cancellous bone of the plateau resists depression; therefore, there is no associated articular depression. If displaced, this fracture is frequently associated with a peripheral tear of the lateral meniscus.
  - Type II: split-depression fracture of the lateral tibial plateau. It usually occurs in older patients where the cancellous bone is usually weaker because of some osteoporosis and does not resist depression as it does in the younger population.
  - Type III: pure depression fracture of the lateral plateau. The depression may involve any portion of the articular surface but is usually located centrally or laterally. Lateral and posterior peripheral depressions are usually associated with a greater incidence of joint instability than the central depressions.
  - Type IV: fracture of the medial tibial plateau that may be split or split-depression fracture.

The medial plateau resists fracture more than the lateral, and, therefore, its fractures are usually the result of a much greater force. This type of fracture actually represents a dislocation of the knee that has been realigned prior to the radiograph. It is not the fracture of the medial plateau that gives this injury its bad prognosis but the associated soft tissue injuries, such as the peroneal nerve, the popliteal artery, and the cruciate and lateral collateral ligaments. Because of associated popliteal artery injuries, Doppler arterial pressure and sometimes arteriography should be done to evaluate arterial integrity and to identify limb-threatening popliteal artery thrombosis.

- Type V: bicondylar fracture that involves a split of the lateral and medial plateaus and is usually the result of a pure axial load applied to the extended knee. The prognosis depends on whether the fracture line involves the articular surfaces or begins in the intercondylar area and bypasses the articular surfaces as it exits in the metaphysis.
- Type VI: combined articular surface fractures with a metaphyseal fracture that separates the tibial condylar components from the diaphysis or diaphyseal-metaphyseal disassociation.

History and Physical Exam [1]

- The mechanism of injury provides clues to the fracture pattern. This information has an important bearing on associated soft tissue injuries, such as fracture blisters, arterial injury, and compartment syndrome.
- The physical examination of the knee and the leg is critically important to diagnose associated injuries and complications, plan for surgical treatment, and decide optimal timing for interventions.
- Physical examination is the most accurate means of evaluating the neurologic status of the extremity and assessing the vascular status including the presence or absence of a major tear of the collateral ligaments.

- Fullness or tenseness of any compartment in the leg and severe pain with on passive stretch of the muscles in the specific compartment are indications of a compartment syndrome.
- Pedal pulses must be assessed early with quantitative assessment of the ankle-brachial index (ABI). An abnormal pulse or ABI is ground for arteriography or vascular surgery consultation.

Imaging [2]

- The diagnosis of a tibial plateau fracture is typically made on plain radiographs. Anteroposterior (AP), lateral, and AP views in the plane of the plateau (10–15-degree caudal view) are the standard examinations. The caudal view provides a better view of the articular surface and helps assess displacement and depression better than the standard AP view.
- CT scans are routinely obtained for most tibial plateau fractures. They provide excellent detail of the fracture pathoanatomy and serve as a critically important aid to preoperative planning for operative approaches and fixation techniques.
- CT typically demonstrates more articular displacement and comminution than is apparent on plain films.
- CT also helps with surgical planning and leads to more reliability in classifying the fracture and deciding on a treatment plan.
- MRI assesses the location of fracture lines and the degree of articular displacement and also identifies occult fracture areas better than plain films and has been found to be equivalent to traditional two-dimensional CT.
- MRI provides additional information about injuries to the soft tissue structures of the knee; however, whether MRI should be a routine part of evaluating tibial plateau fracture is controversial.

Overview Fracture Management [1]

- The goals of treatment of any intra-articular fracture are to preserve joint mobility, joint stability, articular surface congruence, and axial alignment, to provide freedom from pain, and to prevent posttraumatic arthritis.

- The primary factors that ultimately determine the prognosis of proximal tibial plateau injuries are the degree of articular depression, the extent and separation of the condylar fracture line, the degree of diaphyseal-metaphyseal comminution and dissociation, and the integrity of the soft tissue envelope.

- When the soft tissues are significantly compromised, immediate exposure for internal stable fixation is risky; thus the concept of staged fixation has now gained favor.

- Overall limb realignment and stabilization, important for soft tissue healing, can be achieved with an external fixator that initially spans the zone of injury. During this period of soft tissue recovery, external fixation is available to splint the fracture and its surrounding soft tissues as well as maintain a general ligamentotaxis reduction of the major metaphyseal and diaphyseal fracture components.

- When the soft tissues have recovered sufficiently to allow for a secondary procedure, delayed fixation can be accomplished through a safe operative corridor of healthy soft tissue.

Nonoperative Treatment [2]

- Nonoperative treatment is indicated for many tibial plateau fractures. Fractures that occur after a low-energy injury are usually incomplete or nondisplaced.

- Another relative indication for nonoperative treatment is the presence of significant cardiovascular, pulmonary, neurologic, or metabolic compromise.

- Nonoperative treatment of these injuries does require early motion and subsequent prevention of displacement. This is prevented by controlling motion with a hinged knee brace, and weightbearing is prohibited.

- Frequent clinical and radiographs follow-up is required early in the course of treatment to guard against unrecognized loss of metaphyseal reduction. The goal is to achieve at least 90 degrees of flexion by 4 weeks after injury.

Surgical Treatment [1]

- An open fracture should be operated on immediately, as should a fracture associated with an acute compartment syndrome or arterial occlusion. All other tibial plateau fractures should be evaluated individually.

- The isolated complex tibia plateau fracture is not a life-threatening injury, and adequate time should be taken to evaluate the fracture thoroughly. The timing of surgery for these injuries depends primarily on the soft tissue conditions.

- Operative treatment is indicated for displaced unstable tibial plateau, almost all bicondylar and shaft-dissociated patterns fractures. For the lateral patterns, the presence of a split fragment, a depression affecting over half of the lateral articular surface, a fibular head fracture, and valgus alignment are all strong indications for surgery.

- The treatment techniques that result in the most favorable patient outcomes depend on the patient and the fracture pattern. In planning to operatively treat a tibial plateau fracture, the fracture pattern will dictate the operative approach, the technique of reducing the fracture, and the appropriate use of internal or external fixation devices.

- Accurately reducing the displaced articular surface is an important aspect of treating displaced plateau fractures. Many surgeons prefer to directly access the fracture reduction through a joint arthrotomy. In lateral side patterns, the meniscus can either be incised anteriorly or elevated with a submeniscal arthrotomy (Fig. 69.1).

- Plates and screws are the most frequent implants used to stabilize tibial plateau fractures. The simplest implants are lag screws used to compress simple fracture lines in isolation or in conjunction with other fixation devices.

- Plates serve different functions depending on the fracture pattern and where they are anatomically placed. A common plate application is for the anterolateral proximal tibia where it is used as a buttress and to substitute for the damaged lateral cortex that occurs with lateral split-depression fractures.

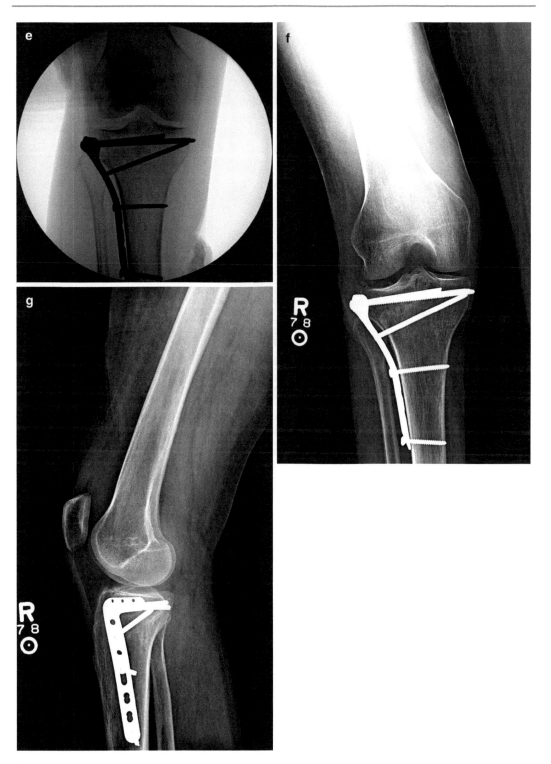

Fig. 69.1 (**a**, **b**) Show a displaced intra-articular tibial plateau fracture with significant lateral-sided depression. (**c**) Shows the use of a femoral distractor on the lateral side of the knee with isolation of the articular depression. (**d**) Shows reconstruction of the articular step-off using a bone tamp. (**e**) Is the final result after exchange of temporary K-wires for a laterally based plate. (**f**, **g**) Are final X-rays showing healing of the plateau fracture

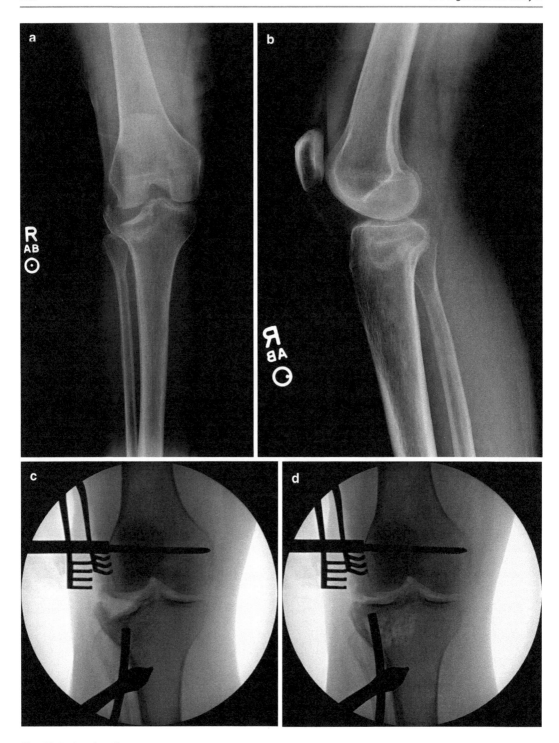

Fig. 69.1 (continued)

- Posteromedial plates serve a different mechanical function than anterolateral plates. In the area, the plate must function as an antiglide device to resist shearing forces.
- In some bicondylar patterns, the fracture needs to be fixed on two sides based on the characteristics of the medial side injury. When dual plates are planned to treat a tibial plateau fracture, the most important factor is the associated soft tissue injury.
- The optimal postoperative program should minimize complications and loss of reduction of the fracture and maximize knee motion while speeding recovery and return to function. A period of non-weightbearing is necessary to minimize the chances of displacing the reduced fracture. The duration depends on the fracture pattern and the strength of the fixation, but it usually takes 6–12 weeks to heal.
- Complications include loss of reduction, wound breakdown and infection, knee stiffness, prominent or painful hardware, nonunion, malunion, and posttraumatic arthritis.

References

1. Bucholz, et al. Rockwood and green's fractures adults. 7th ed. Philadelphia: Lippincott Williams & Wilkins; 2010.
2. Browner, et al. Skeletal trauma: basic science, management and reconstruction. 3rd ed. Philadelphia: Saunders; 2003.

Distal Femoral Fractures

70

Patrick Bergin and Tracye J. Lawyer

Introduction/Overview [1]

- The surgical goals of treatment for distal femoral fractures are anatomic reduction of the articular surface; restoration of limb alignment, length, and rotation; and stable fixation that allows for early mobilization.
- Internal fixation of the distal femur can be very difficult secondary to thin cortices, a wide medullary canal, osteopenia, and fracture comminution.

Anatomy [1]

- The distal end of the femur encompasses the lower third of the femur. The supracondylar or metaphyseal area of the distal portion of the femur is the transition zone between the distal diaphysis and the femoral articular condyles.
- At the diaphyseal-metaphyseal junction, the metaphysis flares especially on the medial

side to provide a platform for the condylar weight-bearing surface of the knee joint.

- Anteriorly between these condyles is a smooth articular depression for the patella called the trochlear groove. Posteriorly between the condyles is the intercondyloid notch.
- The powerful muscles of the distal part of the thigh produce characteristic bony deformities with fractures. The muscle pull of the quadriceps and posterior hamstrings produce shortening of the femur. As the shaft overrides anteriorly and the gastrocnemius muscle pulls posteriorly, the condyles are displaced and angulated posteriorly. Varus angulation occurs at the fracture site as a result of the strong pull of the adductor muscles.
- In fractures with intercondylar extension, soft tissue attachments to the respective femoral condyles tend to produce splaying and rotational malalignment of the condyles that contributes to joint incongruity.

Mechanism of Injury [1]

- The mechanism of injury in most supracondylar femur fractures is axial loading with varus, valgus, or rotational forces.

P. Bergin, MD (✉) • T.J. Lawyer, MD, PhD
Department of Orthopaedic Surgery, University of
Mississippi Medical Center, Jackson, MS, USA
e-mail: PBergin@umc.edu

- In younger patients, these fractures typically occur after high-energy trauma related to motor vehicle or motorcycle accidents. In these patients, there may be considerable fracture displacement, comminution, open wounds, and associated injuries.
- In elderly patients, these fractures frequently occur after a minor slip or fall on a flexed knee, leading to fragility fractures through the compromised bone.

Associated Injuries [2]

- In patients injured as the result of a high-energy mechanism, ipsilateral hip and femoral shaft fractures are fairly common. Approximately 50% of these patients have diaphyseal fracture extension of the distal femur fracture.
- Ipsilateral injuries to the tibia, ankle, and foot are common.
- Although the femoral and popliteal arteries are in close proximity to the distal femur, vascular injury is less common than in patients with a knee dislocation.

History and Physical Examination [1]

- Assessment must include careful scrutiny of the hip joint above the fracture and the knee joint below the fracture. If vascularity is a concern, then Doppler pulse pressure readings can be obtained.
- Clinical examination usually reveals tenderness, fracture crepitus with thigh swelling, limb deformity, shortening, and external rotation.
- The skin should be examined for bruising, contusion, or open fracture.
- A careful neurovascular examination including the presence or absence of distal pulses, as

well as sensorimotor assessment, should be performed and documented. If there are differences in distal pulses between the injured and noninjured sides, then ankle-brachial index should be obtained.

Imaging [2]

- AP and lateral radiographs of the knee and distal femur are routinely obtained and are usually sufficient for diagnosis.
- In most patients, X-rays of the pelvis, ipsilateral hip, and femoral shaft are necessary to rule out associated injuries.
- Comparison radiographs of the noninjured extremity help the surgeon with preoperative planning.
- CT scans with axial, coronal, and sagittal reconstruction of the distal femur are an important adjunct to plain radiographs and are recommended with most displaced fractures.

Classification [1]

- There is no universally accepted method of classification for supracondylar femur fractures. All classifications distinguish among extra-articular, intra-articular, and isolated condylar fractures.
- Fractures are further subdivided according to the degree and direction of displacement, amount of comminution, and involvement of joint surfaces.
- For a classification system to have clinical significance, it must be able to allow for adequate documentation of all fractures so that a common language is possible when discussing injuries, be simple enough that it is user-friendly, help the surgeon in clinical decision-making so that the correct treatment option can be selected for a particular fracture, and

provide prognostic information detailing the results that can be expected for a particular fracture.

Management [2]

- It is essential to follow the goals of operative management of periarticular fractures which include anatomic reconstitution of the articular surface; reduction of the metaphyseal component of the fracture to the diaphysis; restoration of normal axial alignment, length, and rotation; stable internal fixation; fracture healing; and early motion and functional rehabilitation of the limb.
- Nonoperative treatment is reserved for patients with nondisplaced fractures and those who are not surgical candidates because of significant medical comorbidities.
- Nonoperative treatment of a displaced distal femur fracture includes closed reduction with skeletal traction with or without subsequent cast-bracing. This method requires confinement to bed, is time-consuming and expensive, and is not well tolerated by elderly patients.

Operative Treatment [2]

- Operative treatment is generally carried out with either a combination of plates and screws or retrograde intramedullary nails.
- Early on distal femur fractures were most commonly treated with an anatomically con-

toured but angular unstable distal femur plate. High complication rates were reported which included infection, nonunion, delayed union, malunion, and knee stiffness.
- More recently, locked plating systems have been developed in which screws are inserted that lock into the plate forming a fixed-angle construct.
- Retrograde intramedullary nails have been used to treat selected distal femur fractures. The intramedullary nail is a load-sharing device compared with a plate. It has the potential to stabilize complex fracture with less soft tissue dissection, and it can be inserted quickly in a polytrauma patient.
- External fixation can be used for temporary stabilization of severely injured patients or when a delay to surgical repair of more than 36 hours is anticipated which is called damage control orthopedics. The advantages of external fixation include rapid application, minimal soft tissue dissection, and the ability to maintain length, access wound, and mobilize the patient.
- Once the patient and the soft tissues have improved, definitive internal fixation should be undertaken.
- Anatomic articular reconstruction with reconstitution of the length, rotation, and alignment of the metaphyseal component is critical to a quality outcome (Fig. 70.1).
- Complications include malalignment/malunion, nonunion, infection, knee stiffness, hardware problems, and posttraumatic arthritis.

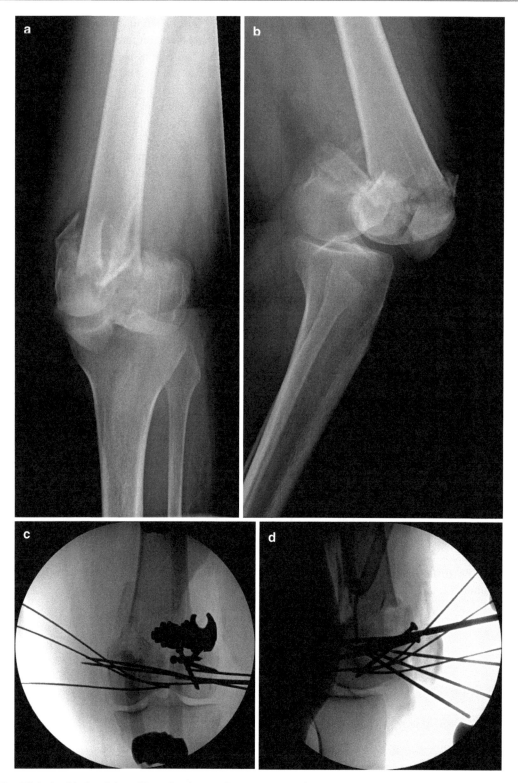

Fig. 70.1 (**a**, **b**) Are injury films showing an intra-articular distal femur fracture. (**c**, **d**) Show reconstruction of the articular surface initially using K-wires and small fragment screws. Once the articular surface is rebuilt, an external fixator is used to restore the length, rotation, and alignment of the metaphyseal block. (**e**, **f**) Show the final result after submuscular plating of the femoral fracture. (**g**) Shows the final result after healing of the injury

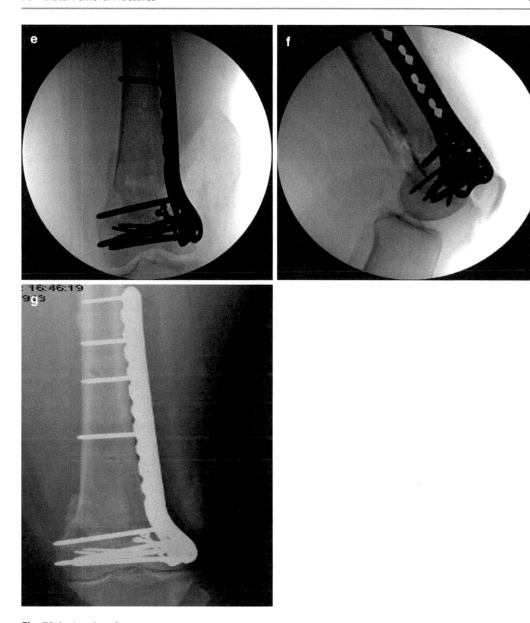

Fig. 70.1 (continued)

References

1. Bucholz, et al. Rockwood and green's fractures adults. 7th ed. Philadelphia: Lippincott Williams & Wilkins; 2010.

2. Browner, et al. Skeletal trauma: basic science, management and reconstruction. 3rd ed. Philadelphia: Saunders; 2003.

Patella Fractures

Patrick Bergin and Tracye J. Lawyer

Overview

- Before the beginning of the twentieth century, treatment of patella fractures consisted of nonoperative methods which included extension splinting and rest. However, results were poor and associated with high rates of residual pain, nonunion, and permanent disability.
- Operative treatment over extension splinting was advised in order to improve fracture reduction, maintain reduction until union, reestablish soft tissue continuity, and restore functional integrity of the knee joint.
- Currently, three forms of operative treatment for displaced patella fractures are most commonly used which include open reduction internal fixation with a tension band wiring technique, partial patellectomy, or total patellectomy.
- The goals of surgical treatment are restoration of the articular surface of the patella, maximum preservation of the patella, and preservation of the functional integrity and strength of the extensor mechanism.

Anatomy

- The patella lies deep to the fascia lata and the tendinous fibers of the rectus femoris.
- The quadriceps muscle complex is composed of four separate muscles, the rectus femoris, vastus medialis, vastus lateralis, and vastus intermedius.
- The patellofemoral ligaments, deep transverse fibers that are palpable thickenings of the joint capsule connecting the patella with the femoral epicondyles, complete the retinaculum.
- The lateral aspect of the vastus lateralis and iliotibial tract both contribute to the thicker lateral patellar retinaculum.
- The patellar tendon is flat and strong and inserts on onto the tibial tubercle; it is derived primarily from the fibers of the rectus femoris.
- The fascial expansions of the iliotibial tract and the patellar retinaculum blend into the patellar tendon as it inserts onto the anterior surface of the tibia.
- The anterior surface of the patella is covered with an extraosseous arterial ring derived mainly from branches of the geniculate arteries. The patellar tendon receives its blood supply from two sources: the infrapatellar fat pad supplies the deep surface of the patellar tendon, and the anterior surface of the tendon is supplied by the retinaculum, which receives its supply from the inferior medial geniculate artery and the recurrent tibial artery.

P. Bergin (✉) • T.J. Lawyer
Department of Orthopaedic Surgery, University of
Mississippi Medical Center, Jackson, MS, USA
e-mail: PBergin@umc.edu

© Springer International Publishing AG 2017
A.E.M. Eltorai et al. (eds.), *Orthopedic Surgery Clerkship*, DOI 10.1007/978-3-319-52567-9_71

Extensor Mechanism Biomechanics

- The principal function of the extensor mechanism of the knee is to maintain the erect position in humans, which includes ambulation, rising from a chair, and ascending or descending stairs.
- The force necessary for knee extension is directly dependent on the perpendicular distance between the patellar tendon and the knee flexion axis or moment arm.
- Twice as much torque is needed to extend the knee, the final 15° as to bring it from a fully flexed position to 15°. The knee requires a moment arm that increases during extension so that it can maintain a constant level of torque.
- As the knee begins extension from the fully flexed position, the patella functions primarily as a link between the quadriceps and the patellar tendon. This linking function allows for generation of torque from the quadriceps muscle to the tibia.
- From 45° of flexion to full extension, the patella acts to displace the quadriceps – patellar tendon complex away from the axis of knee rotation. This action increases the effective moment arm of the quadriceps mechanism and increases the torque needed to gain the last 15° of knee extension. Thus, after a patellectomy, this moment arm is decreased, and the extensor force is effectively diminished.

Mechanism of Injury

- The patella is prone to injury from a direct blow as a consequence of its anterior location and thin overlying soft tissue envelope. Direct injuries may be low energy, such as a fall from standing, or high energy, such as a dashboard injury in a motor vehicle accident.
- Comminuted fractures are often a result of high-energy, direct injuries.
- Indirect injury can occur secondary to the large forces generated through the extensor mechanism and typically result from forceful contraction of the quadriceps with the knee in a flexed position.
- Indirect injuries frequently cause a greater degree of retinacular disruption compared with direct injuries, and active knee extension is compromised in most cases.
- The majority of patellar fractures have a transverse fracture pattern resulting from excessive tensile forces the extensor mechanism.
- Vertical fractures are typically the result of a direct blow to a partially flexed knee and may be non-displaced if the retinaculum and extensor mechanisms are intact.
- Comminuted stellate fractures are typically the result of a direct blow with impaction against the femoral condyles and can be associated with substantial injury to both the femoral and patellar chondral surfaces (Fig. 71.1).

History and Physical Examination

- Patient history usually includes a direct blow to the patella, a fall from standing height, or a near fall with forceful contraction of the quadriceps on a partially flexed knee.
- Complaints of anterior knee pain, swelling, and difficulty ambulating after a fall are common and may reflect an injury to the extensor mechanism.
- On physical exam, displaced patella fractures typically present with an acute hemarthroses and a tender, palpable defect between the fracture fragments.
- Competence of the extensor mechanism must be assessed by asking the patient to perform a straight leg raise or extend a partially flexed knee against gravity. Aspiration of the hemarthroses followed by injection of a local anesthetic into the joint may be helpful.
- An inability to extend the knee suggests a discontinuity in the extensor mechanism. With a patellar fracture, such inability implies a tear to both the medial and lateral quadriceps expansion.
- The patient's ability to extend the knee does not rule out a patella fracture but suggests that the continuity of the extensor mechanism is maintained by the intact retinacular sleeve.

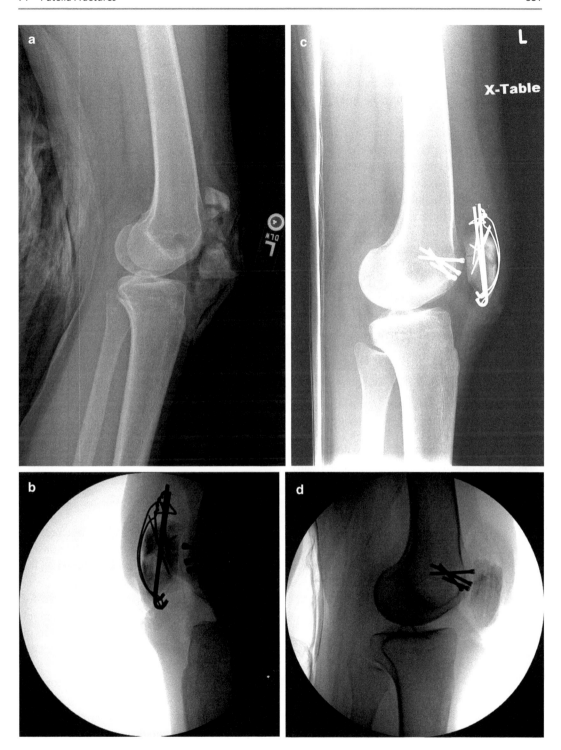

Fig. 71.1 (a) Shows a comminuted displaced patella fracture. (b) Shows intraoperative films with a stable articular surface being recreated to allow a tension band technique to work. (c) Shows postoperative studies with relatively long K-wires with this technique that can cause soft tissue irritation. (d) Shows a healed patella after removal of K-wires that were causing soft tissue irritation

Imaging

- Plain radiography, anteroposterior (AP), and lateral view are sufficient to confirm the diagnosis of a patellar fracture or injury to the extensor mechanism.
- Views of the contralateral knee are helpful for comparison and may prevent the erroneous diagnosis of a normal variant as a fracture.
- A bipartite or tripartite patella can often be mistaken for a fracture in the setting of a trauma history. These anatomic variants reflect incomplete fusion of two or more ossification centers. The opposing edges are usually smooth and corticated on plain radiographs.
- The most common bipartite is located in the superolateral aspect of the patella and is not associated with any pain, tenderness, or functional compromise of the extensor mechanism on physical exam.
- The lateral radiograph view is critical to define facture pattern and associated extensor mechanism disruption.
- With the knee flexed 90°, the proximal patellar pole normally rests at or below the level of the anterior cortex of the femur. With the knee flexed 30°, the inferior patellar pole normally projects to the level of Blumensaat line. The loss of the relationship suggests extensor mechanism disruption.
- CT scanning is rarely necessary in the evaluation and treatment of isolated patellar fractures. While CT allows for improved evaluation of articular congruity and fracture comminution, it rarely provides additional information that will alter the treatment plan.

Classification

- The three major categories of patella fractures are transverse, stellate, and vertical. Comminuted transverse fractures often have retinacular disruption, whereas stellate patellar fractures are associated with an intact retinaculum.

- Stellate fractures of the patella are the result of a direct compressive blow that forces the bone against the femoral condyles. Damage to the articular cartilage of the femoral condyles and osteochondral fragments may occur and must be ruled out.
- Transverse fractures of the patella are the result of a tensile stress applied to the extensor mechanism.
- Vertical fractures may be caused by different mechanisms. The fracture may be missed on standard radiographs, and therefore an axial view may be necessary to make the diagnosis. Because the fracture fragments are minimally displaced and the patellar retinaculum remains intact, these fractures are best treated nonoperatively.
- Polar fractures of the patella are transverse fractures occurring either proximal or distal to the patella equator. Proximal or basal pole fractures imply avulsion of the quadriceps mechanism from the patella. Distal or apical pole fractures are bony avulsions of the proximal patellar tendon. These fractures are almost always associated with loss of knee extension.

Nonoperative Treatment

- The management of patellar fractures is largely based on the fracture classification and physical exam with particular attention on the integrity of the extensor mechanism.
- Nonoperative treatment may be indicated for patellar fractures with less than 3 mm of fragment displacement or less than 2 mm of articular incongruity in which the extensor mechanism remains intact.
- Acute nonoperative treatment usually consists of 4–6 weeks of extension splinting or bracing. A long leg cylinder cast may be preferred if patient is not compliant or unreliable.
- Straight leg raises and isometric quadriceps exercises are initiated early in the cast or brace to minimize atrophy.

Operative Treatment

- Operative treatment is indicated for patellar fractures with greater than mm of fragment displacement or greater than 2 mm of articular incongruity, osteochondral fractures with associated intraarticular loose bodies, and/or compromised extensor mechanism with loss of active knee extension.
- For a displaced non-comminuted transverse patellar fractures, open reduction internal fixation using a modified anterior tension band technique is the treatment of choice.
- The principle of the tension band wire fixation for patellar fractures is to convert the tensile forces generated from the quadriceps complex at the anterior cortical surface of the patella into compressive forces at the articular surface (Fig. 71.1).
- When comminution of the distal pole or a fragment of the patella is extensive and cannot be stabilized with internal fixation, a partial patellectomy should be performed.
- A total patellectomy is occasionally performed for highly displaced, comminuted fractures in which stable fixation cannot be achieved and when no large fragments can be retained; however, the retention of even on fragment is necessary to maintain a lever arm.
- Complications of operative intervention include infection, hardware failure, symptomatic hardware, delayed union and malunion, and loss of knee motion.

Suggested Reading

1. Bucholz, et al. Rockwood and green's fractures adults. 7th ed. Philadelphia: Lippincott Williams & Wilkins; 2010.
2. Browner, et al. Skeletal trauma: basic science, management and reconstruction. 3rd ed. Philadelphia: Saunders; 2003.

Patella Dislocation

72

David Flanigan, Benjamin Leger-St. Jean,
and Alex C. DiBartola

Anatomy

- Patella articulates with the intercondylar groove of the distal femur.
- Dynamic restraints – vastus medialis obliquus (VMO) and vastus lateralis, extensor mechanism.
- Static restraints – medial patellofemoral ligament (MPFL), congruency of osseous anatomy, and retinaculum.
- Q angle – the angle formed between the ASIS, center of patella, and tibial tubercle (Fig. 72.1) should be approximately 15° or less.

Risk Factors

- Previous patellar dislocation
- Ligamentous laxity or collagen disorders (i.e., Ehlers-Danlos)
- Patella alta
- Increased Q angle (i.e., genu valgum, excessive femoral anteversion)
- Lateral femoral condylar hypoplasia or trochlear dysplasia

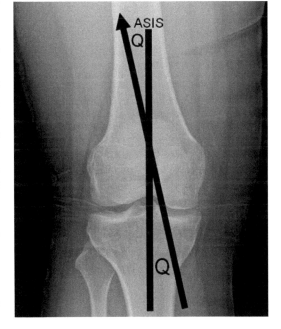

Fig. 72.1 The Q angle is defined as the angle formed by a line drawn from the tibial tuberosity to the center of the patella and a second line drawn from the ASIS to the center of the patella

- Atrophy/atony of the VMO
- Lateral patellar tilt
- Tight lateral retinaculum, iliotibial band, or vastus lateralis
- Excessive tibial torsion
- Pes planus

D. Flanigan (✉) • B. Leger-St. Jean, MD
A.C. DiBartola
Department of Orthopaedics, The Ohio State
University Wexner Medical Center,
Columbus, OH, USA
e-mail: david.flanigan@osumc.edu

© Springer International Publishing AG 2017
A.E.M. Eltorai et al. (eds.), *Orthopedic Surgery Clerkship*, DOI 10.1007/978-3-319-52567-9_72

Mechanism

- Often a noncontact twisting injury with the foot planted and externally rotated, the patella dislocates laterally.
- Can also be caused by a direct blow to the medial patella.
- MPFL acts as a checkrein to dislocation in the first 30° of flexion; this tissue inevitably attenuates/tears with instability.

Presentation

- Patients have acute, intense pain with deformity of the knee.
- Often associated with an acute hemarthrosis.
- Dislocation often spontaneously reduces with reflexive contraction of the extensor.
- Mechanism in response to the injury.

Physical Exam

- Inspect for deformity.
- Palpate for an effusion and tenderness over the MPFL.
- Check for lateral translation of the patella with the knee extended (measured in quadrants); patients often have apprehension when examining this.
- Evaluate Q angle and lower extremity alignment.
- Check for a "J" sign – patella tracks with excessive lateral translation as patient terminally extends the knee, and the patella disengages from the trochlea.

Imaging

Weight-Bearing Plain Radiographs of the Knee

- Evaluates reduction of the joint and can help detect loose bodies (Fig. 72.2)
- Can assess patella alta on the lateral view (Insall-Salvati ratio, Caton-Deschamps, etc.) (Fig. 72.3)
- Lateral view and sunrise view can evaluate lateral condylar hypoplasia or trochlear dysplasia

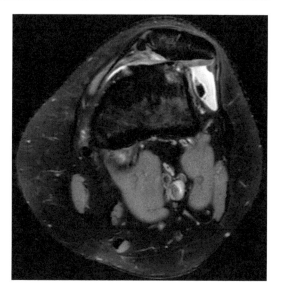

Fig. 72.2 Loose bodies and chondral defect after recurrent patellar instability

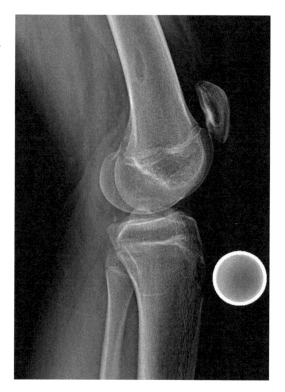

Fig. 72.3 Patient with patella alta and Blumensaat's line intersecting the inferior pole of the patella

CT Scan

- Can accurately evaluate the patient's tibial tubercle- trochlear groove (TT-TG) distance –

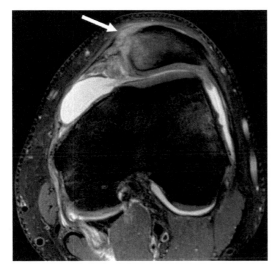

Fig. 72.4 Following a lateral patellar dislocation, a classic pattern of marrow edema (bone bruising) can be seen on the medial aspect of the patella and the anterolateral distal femur. Also, disruption of the MPFL insertion off of the medial patella (*white arrow*) is seen

the distance from the tibial tubercle to the trochlear groove as evaluated on axial images. This distance should be <20 mm.

MRI

- Gold standard to detect osteochondral injuries or loose bodies in the knee (Fig. 72.2).
- Can evaluate the MPFL in detail.
- Classic pattern is bone bruise of the medial patella and non-weight-bearing portion of lateral femoral condyle.
- Anterolateral aspect of distal femur. MPFL tears off of the medial femoral condyle (Fig. 72.4).

Treatment

Nonoperative: Generally for First-Time Dislocators Without Osteochondral Defects

- Immobilization, rest, ice, physical therapy, and bracing
- Focus on core strengthening and biomechanics of the VMO – closed chain short arc quadriceps activity.
- Approximately 50% of nonoperative group will have a recurrence.

Operative: Generally for Repeat Dislocators or Acute Dislocations with Osteochondral Injuries

- Arthroscopic removal or fixation of the fragment
- MPFL repair – falling out of favor
- MPFL reconstruction with autograft hamstrings or allograft:
  - Femoral origin of the MPFL is Schöttle's point (Fig. 72.5)
    - On perfect lateral of the distal femur the point just anterior to the posterior femoral cortex and just proximal to Blumensaat's line
- Fulkerson osteotomy – anterior and medialization of the tibial tubercle:
  - Indicated for a TT-TG >20 mm
- Tibial tubercle distalization – for patella alta:
  - Isolated lateral lengthening
  - Rarely indicated but can be done for lateral patellar tilt
- Trochleoplasty – open or arthroscopic groove deepening procedure

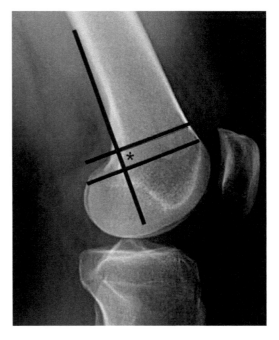

Fig. 72.5 Schöttle's point lies between a line drawn along the posterior femoral cortex and two perpendicular lines drawn through the posterior most point on Blumensaat's line and the point where the femoral condyles meet the posterior femoral cortex

Complications

- Recurrent dislocation
- Patellofemoral arthritis
- Medial dislocation – an iatrogenic complication

Suggested Reading

1. Bollier M, Fulkerson JP. The role of trochlear dysplasia in patellofemoral instability. J Am Acad Orthop Surg. 2011;19(1):8–16.
2. Colvin AC, West RV. Patellar instability. J Bone Joint Surg Am. 2008;90(12):2751–62.
3. Fithian DC, Paxton EW, Cohen AB. Indications in the treatment of patellar instability. J Knee Surg. 2004;17(1):47–56.
4. Fulkerson JP. Diagnosis and treatment of patients with patellofemoral pain. Am J Sports Med. 2002;30(3):447–56.
5. Lewallen LW, McIntosh AL, Dahm DL. Predictors of recurrent instability after acute patellofemoral dislocation in pediatric and adolescent patients. Am J Sports Med. 2013;41(3):575–81.
6. Schöttle PB, Fucentese SF, Romero J. Clinical and radiological outcome of medial patellofemoral ligament reconstruction with a semitendinosus autograft for patella instability. Knee Surg Sports Traumatol Arthrosc. 2005;13(7):516–21.

Total Knee Arthroplasty

Karl Balch and Andrew H. Glassman

Overview

- TKA (total knee arthroplasty): For management of knee arthritis when conservative measures (NSAIDs, physical therapy, injections of corticosteroid ± viscosupplementation, and off-loader bracing) have failed. TKA is primarily a pain-relieving operation.

TKA Components

- Most TKA consists of femoral, tibial, and polyethylene components (tibial/patella).

TKA Design Concepts

Designs are generally categorized by level of constraint. Constraint refers to the ability of a prosthesis to stabilize the knee substituting for loss of ligament stability or bone. This can be in anterior/posterior, flexion/extension, or varus/valgus planes. Increasing constraint of components grants greater stability at the cost

of longevity of the implant. Highly constrained implants put higher forces across the components leading to faster wear and failure. There are four major categories of constraint.

Cruciate Retaining (CR) Knee

- Least constrained design. Resects ACL and retains native PCL. Depends on native ligaments to provide stability. No box cut in the femur. Theoretically increased longevity due to low constraint, improved proprioception with native PCL and tissue, and risk of PCL rupture and instability. If PCL rupture occurs, it needs to revise femoral component to make box cut to accommodate polyethylene post for posterior-stabilized (PS) design.

Posterior-Stabilized (PS) Knee

- Resects ACL/PCL and cuts femoral cam/box to accommodate tibial polyethylene post during flexion. Provides partial constraint anterior to posterior (AP) substituting for PCL. Resection of PCL provides easier exposure and is easier to balance compared to CR knees. Unique complications associated with PS design:
  - Cam jump "jumping the post": If PS knee is loose in flexion or can hyperextend, then polyethylene post can escape the femoral

K. Balch, MD • A.H. Glassman, MD, MS (✉)
Orthopaedic Surgery, The Ohio State University
Wexner Medical Center, Columbus, OH, USA
e-mail: karlbalch@gmail.com;
andrew.glassman@osumc.edu

© Springer International Publishing AG 2017
A.E.M. Eltorai et al. (eds.), *Orthopedic Surgery Clerkship*, DOI 10.1007/978-3-319-52567-9_73

box and dislocate. Requires initial reduction and eventual revision to provide appropriate flexion/extension balancing to prevent further dislocation.

- Patellar clunk: Fibrous tissue (nodule) superior to the patella (on quad tendon undersurface) gets caught in femoral box in the trochlea. Creates catching or popping sensation when extending the knee from a flexed position. Usually engages at roughly 40°. Risk factors are a small patellar component or valgus knee. Treat with open or arthroscopic resection of fibrous nodule.
- Polyethylene post wear: Tibial post provides an additional wear surface.

Constrained Non-hinged Knee

- A deeper femoral box and larger polyethylene post provide even greater constraint/stability. Provides partial (AP), varus/valgus, and some rotational stability. Used for knees with LCL or MCL deficiency, bone loss, or flexion gap laxity. Increased constraint means more rapid wear and loosening. Used in revisions/more severe tissue loss/deformity.

Constrained Hinged Knee

- Highest level of constraint has linked femoral and tibial components (hinge). Used for most global ligamentous laxity, severe deformity, revisions, or oncologic procedures with significant bone loss. High level of constraint significantly reduces longevity of implant.

Approaches for TKA

Medial parapatellar approach through midline incision in the skin is most common approach for TKA. If multiple incisions from prior surgery, use the most lateral as medial blood supply to tissue flaps.

Minimally Invasive Approaches

- Midvastus/subvastus approaches attempt to preserve extensor mechanism. Both are more limited exposure and should be avoided in obese patients or revisions.

Extensile Approaches/Exposure

- Quadriceps snip: Oblique 45° angle cut into the vastus lateralis from proximal end of medial parapatellar approach. Increases exposure and no long-term difference in rehabilitation or postoperative protocols/weight bearing/activity
- Tibial tubercle osteotomy: Allows greater exposure than quadriceps snip. Docs not disrupt the quad like in a V-Y turndown but does have risk of tibial tubercle avulsion after repair and nonunion of osteotomy and often requires changing post-op protocol for weight bearing/rehabilitation
- V-Y turndown: Normal medial parapatellar incision that proximally extends obliquely down the vastus lateralis tendon from proximal to distal. Provides excellent exposure and preserves patellar tendon/tibial tubercle but disrupts post-op rehab and has a risk of extensor lag and disruption of the quad mechanism

TKA Alignment

- Normal anatomy: Distal femur 5–7° of valgus, proximal tibia 2–3° of varus. Try to establish mechanical alignment of zero.
  - Mechanical axis femur: Line connecting center femoral head to the intercondylar notch
  - Mechanical axis tibia: Center of the proximal tibia to center of the ankle.
  - Anatomic axis femur/tibia: Line bisects the medullary canal of the femur/tibia.
  - Q angle: Angle between ASIS to center of the patella and the axis of the patellar tendon to tibial tuberosity. Increased Q angle produces lateral force on the patella/maltracking. If severe enough, it can cause pain/dislocation. Patellar maltracking is

one of most common complications of TKA.

- NEVER internally rotate femoral or tibial components. Increases Q angle!
- DO NOT medialize femoral component or place patellar component lateral.

TKA Balancing (Need to Balance Coronal and Sagittal Planes)

Coronal Balancing

- Varus deformity most common in TKA. Typically tight medial side with lax lateral side. To correct resect osteophytes, meniscus, deep MCL, and capsular attachments. If still unbalanced, then release posteromedial corner (posterior along proximal tibia), superficial MCL (distal to deep portion), and PCL release that can assist in balancing.
- Valgus deformity less common in TKA. Tight laterally and lax medially. Resect osteophytes, meniscus, lateral capsule, and IT band. IT band can be released with Z-plasty, off of Gerdy's, or via "pie-crusting" (puncture hole) technique. Next can release popliteus (if tight in flexion) or lastly LCL if planning to use constrained prosthesis.

Sagittal Balancing: Balance Components in Flexion and Extension

- Modifying the tibia (via tibial cut or poly thickness) affects both flexion and extension gap. Distal femur cut affects extension gap, and femoral component size affects flexion gap.
- Tight in flexion and extension: Cut more tibia.
- Loose in flexion and extension: Thicker poly or thicker tibial metal component.
- Tight in flexion only: Decrease size femoral component, release PCL, resect posterior slope tibia, and resect more posterior femoral condyle and posterior capsular release.

- Loose in flexion only: Increase femoral component size and augment posterior femur.
- Tight in extension only: Cut more distal femur and release more posterior capsule.
- Loose in extension only: Augment distal femur.
- Combination tight/loose in flexion/extension: Use mix of the balancing techniques above.
- Anticoagulation: Risk of DVT/PE elevated postoperatively so anticoagulation is needed to prevent thrombosis. Multiple options and widely debated in the literature. Established orthopedic guidelines have recommended one of the following: acetylsalicylic acid (aspirin) and sequential compression devices (SCDs), enoxaparin, or warfarin for anticoagulation. Research into newer medications (such as direct thrombin inhibitors) for anticoagulation is ongoing.

Complications of TKA

Patellar maltracking, arthrofibrosis/stiffness, periprosthetic infection, wound complications, periprosthetic fracture, heterotopic ossification, instability/poorly balanced, nerve injury, thromboembolic disease, late loosening, wear problems, or premature failure of components.

Patellar Maltracking

- Most common reason for revision following TKA. Ensure appropriate imaging lateral and merchant (sunrise) x-rays to assess patellar component. See Q angle section above for discussion of technical considerations to avoid maltracking.

Stiffness/Arthrofibrosis

- Flexion <90°. If identified within the first 12 weeks post-op, can perform manipulation under anesthesia (MUA) to improve ROM. Caution with MUA as overly aggressive manipulation can lead to fracture or failure of the extensor mechanism.

Periprosthetic Infection

- Chronicity of infection guides treatment. Aspiration and culture gold standard for diagnosis. Synovial WBC > 1100 cells/mL and/or PMNs >64%. Current gold standard of management requires explantation and two-stage exchange with an antibiotic spacer targeted to culture results. In limited cases where infection is acute (less than 4 weeks post-op), can attempt irrigation and debridement with polyethylene exchange and retention of components.

Poorly Balanced/Unstable TKA

- Flexion/extension, varus/valgus, global instability. Responsible for up to 20% of revisions. See balancing section above for technical considerations to properly balance a TKA.

Nerve Injury

- Peroneal nerve is most commonly injured. Pre-op risk factors include valgus knee or flexion deformity. Fifty percent improve over time; after 3 months of nerve disruption, get EMG.

Revision

- Indications: Patellofemoral maltracking, loosening (tibial > femoral), poorly balanced, instability, infection, poly wear, fracture, and component failure. Further discussion of revision beyond the scope of this review.

General Tips for Medical Students

- TKA surgery has a large number of steps done quickly with extensive instrumentation. Find out what type of implant your team will be using, and typically you can get access to free technique guides online for the specific components and instrumentation you will be using. This allows you to familiarize yourself with the steps and the specific components you will see in the case. Repetition will breed familiarity. Knowing how to properly balance a TKA is critical.
- As with any rotation, know your patients! Keeping track of postoperative labs, vitals, anticoagulation, and other protocols will help you understand your patients better. Getting in early and gathering info on the patients before the resident shows up and giving them a sheet summarizing the patients on the floor will help you stand out and make a valuable contribution to the team. Ask a resident or attending surgeon to review how to systematically evaluate pre- and post-op imaging for TKA.

Patellofemoral Pain Syndrome

Ryan J. McNeilan and Grant L. Jones

Anatomy

- The patellofemoral joint consists of the bony patella and the trochlear groove of the distal femur.
- Joint stability is conferred by patella-trochlea congruence, medial and lateral retinacular structures, and medial patellofemoral (MPFL) and patellomeniscal ligaments.

Patella

- Largest sesamoid in the human body.
- Cartilage surface up to 6 mm thickness.

Trochlea

- Concavity of the anterior distal femur.
- Dysplasia resulting in loss of the concavity is implicated in patellar instability.
- In the normal knee, the patella glides smoothly, fully engaging the trochlea at approximately 30° of flexion with the joint contact surface moving more distally on the femur and proximally on the patella with increasing degrees of flexion.

Presentation

- Patellofemoral pain syndrome (PFPS) is characterized by insidious onset diffuse pain originating from the anterior knee, most commonly along the medial aspect of the patella but lateral and retro-patellar discomfort may be present.
- Reproducible pain with running, ascending and descending stairs, squatting, and prolonged sitting.
- Common source of knee discomfort in young, active athletes, especially runners.
- More common in females.
- Diagnosis of exclusion; patellar tendinitis/tendinosis, patellar instability, and patellofemoral arthritis are alternative sources of anterior knee pain.
- Clinical diagnosis – radiographic demonstration of severe patellofemoral arthritis or patellar tendinitis/tendinosis excludes the diagnosis.
- Physical exam should include assessment of hip abductor, hip external rotation, quadriceps, and hamstring strength, static and dynamic knee alignment, and patella tracking through flexion/extension.

R.J. McNeilan (✉) • G.L. Jones
Department of Orthopaedics, The Ohio State
University Wexner Medical Center,
Columbus, OH, USA
e-mail: ryan.mcneilan@osumc.edu;
grant.jones@osumc.edu

© Springer International Publishing AG 2017
A.E.M. Eltorai et al. (eds.), *Orthopedic Surgery Clerkship*, DOI 10.1007/978-3-319-52567-9_74

Pathophysiology

- Likely multifactorial:
  - Patellar maltracking [1, 2]:
    ○ Lateralization and lateral tilt:
      - Relative weakness and delayed activation of vastus medialis obliquus
  - Hip muscular strength deficits [3–5]:
    ○ Hip abduction and hip external rotation weakness
  - Dynamic knee valgus malalignment:
    ○ Static Q-angle measure may also contribute but data remains equivocal
  - Altered foot mechanics [6]:
    ○ Pronated foot type, increased forefoot abduction, and rear foot eversion

Treatment

Nonoperative

- Mainstay of treatment

Multimodal Approach

- Pharmacologic
- Limited short-term benefit with Naprosyn in a database review [7]

Tape/Bracing

- Medially directed taping and bracing have demonstrated decreased pain and increased VMO function in PFPS patients [8], though some data suggests this may be related to placebo effect.
- Orthotics for correction of pes plano valgus.

Physical Therapy

- Individualized multimodal approach addressing deficiencies in hip, quadriceps, hamstring, and trunk strength while addressing deficiencies in dynamic knee control is likely best.

Operative

- No role for operative intervention.
- Prospective randomized trial comparing arthroscopy with therapy showed no positive effect over therapy alone [9].

Outcomes

- Multimodal treatment strategies produce positive short- and long-term results [10]:
  - 73% were pain-free and the remaining 27% had less pain than pretreatment.
  - 82% resumed sport.
  - Patellofemoral pain recurred in 7%.

References

1. Draper CE, Besier TF, Santos JM, Jennings F, Fredericson M, Gold GE, Beaupre GS, Delp SL. Using real-time MRI to quantify altered joint kinematics in subjects with patellofemoral pain and to evaluate the effects of a patellar brace or sleeve on joint motion. J Orthop Res. 2009;27(5):571–7.
2. Wilson NA, Press JM, Koh JL, Hendrix RW, Zhang LQ. In vivo noninvasive evaluation of abnormal patellar tracking during squatting in patients with patellofemoral pain. J Bone Joint Surg Am. 2009;91(3): 558–66.
3. Ireland ML, Willson JD, Ballantyne BT, et al. Hip strength in females with and without patellofemoral pain. J Orthop Sports Phys Ther. 2003;33:671–6.
4. Cichanowski HR, Schmitt JS, Johnson RJ, et al. Hip strength in collegiate femal atheletes with patellofemoral pain. Med Sci Sports Exerc. 2007;39:1227–32.
5. Robinson RL, Nee RJ. Analysis of hip strength in females seeking physical therapy treatment for unilateral patellofemoral pain syndrome. J Orthop Sports Phys Ther. 2007;37:232–8.
6. Barton CJ, Bonanno D, Levinger P, Menz HB. Foot and ankle characterisstics in patellofemoral pain syndrome: a case control and reliability study. J Orthop Sports Phys Ther. 2010;40(5):286–96.
7. Heintjes E, Berer MY, Bierma-Zeinstra SM, Bernsen RM, Verhaar JA, Koes BW. Pharmacotherapy for patellofemoral pain syndrome. Cochrane Database Syst Rev. 2004;(3):CD003470.

8. Petersen W, Ellermann A, Gosele-Koppenburg A, Best R, Rembitzki IV, Bruggemann GP, Liebau C. Patellofemoral pain syndrome. Knee Surg Sports Traumatol Arthrosc. 2014;22:2264–74.

9. Kettunen JA, Jarilainen A, Sandelin J, Schlenzka D, Hietaniemi K, Seitsalo S, Malmivaara A, Kujala UM. Knee arthroscopy and exercise versus exercise only for chronic patellofemoral pain syndrome: a randomized controlled trial. BMC Med. 2007;13(5):38–45.

10. Keays SL, Mason M, Newcombe PA. Three-year outcome after a 1-month physiotherapy program of local and individualized global treatment for patellofemoral pain followed by self-management. Clin J Sport Med. 2016;26(3):190–8.

Iliotibial Band Syndrome

75

Anne Marie Chicorelli

Anatomy

- ITB is a fibrous band of tissue that originates from the anterior superior iliac spine region, courses laterally, and inserts on the lateral tibia at Gerdys tubercle.
- It is formed from a coalescence of fascial elements from the tensor fascia lata as well as the gluteus maximus and minimus at the level of the greater trochanter.
- At knee flexion less than 30°, the band passes anterior to the knee axis and works as an extensor.
- At knee flexion beyond 30°, the band passes posterior to the axis of the knee and works as a flexor.

Risk Factors

- Leg length discrepancy
- Increased forefoot varus
- Increased Q-angles

A.M. Chicorelli, DO, MPH
Orthopaedics and Sports Medicine, The Ohio State
University Wexner Medical Center,
Wooster, OH, USA
e-mail: anne.chicorelli@osumc.edu

- Excessive running in the same direction on a tract, downhill running, and running long distances

Differential Diagnosis

- Hamstring strain
- Lateral meniscus pathology
- Lateral collateral ligament sprain

Evaluation

- Patient reported symptoms of pain or snapping over lateral knee while running or cycling.
- If symptomatic, associated with pain over ITB/lateral femoral condyle.
- Noble's and Ober's tests on physical exam aid in diagnosis.
- Pain aggravated with single-leg squat.
- Pain is from resultant bursitis and/or gluteus medius tendinosis.

Imaging

- AP/lateral X-ray of the knee to exclude other diagnoses

© Springer International Publishing AG 2017   347
A.E.M. Eltorai et al. (eds.), *Orthopedic Surgery Clerkship*, DOI 10.1007/978-3-319-52567-9_75

- MRI to diagnose meniscus tears, bursitis, and tendinosis

Treatment

Nonoperative Treatment

- Physical therapy – stretching of ITB/TFL/hip external rotators, strengthening hip external rotators, and adjusting stride length
- Orthoses
- NSAIDs
- Activity modification
- Steroid injections if conservative treatment fails at site of maximal pain

Operative Treatment After Failure of Conservative Treatment

- Indications: continued pain over the lateral femoral condyle with flexion/extension of the knee after failure of conservative treatment
- Contraindications: severe knee osteoarthritis and infection
- Iliotibial band lengthening:
  - Percutaneous release:
    - Open release
    - ITB Z-lengthening
    - Arthroscopic technique
  - Open release:
    - Patient positioning – lateral or supine on table with tourniquet around the upper thigh
    - Open release (usually perform concomitant knee arthroscopy to visualize intraarticular pathology first):
      - Preoperatively, the site of maximal tenderness is demarcated with pen.

- Arthroscopy performed under standard technique after tourniquet elevated.
- Knee is then flexed to 30° and move to open procedure.
- Mark out our incision over lateral femoral condyle approximately 3 cm in length.
- Skin knife down to the level of the subcutaneous tissue then dissection down to the level of the ITB, paying careful attention to protect neurovascular structures.
- Then use 15 blades to make small stab incisions in the ITB, pie crust technique.
- Resect small posterior triangular portion of ITB at site of LFC impingement approximately 2 cm length and 1.5 width.
- Range knee to ensure adequate release/resection of ITB.
- Irrigation of incision and hemostatic closure.

Complications

- Incomplete release of posterior iliotibial band
- Scarring of previous iliotibial band tendon release
- Hematoma
- Continued pain

Suggested Reading

1. Renne JW. The iliotibial band friction syndrome. J Bone Joint Surg Am. 1975;57:1110–1.

Tibial and Fibular Fracture

76

Grant S. Buchanan and Franklin D. Shuler

Overview

- The tibia is the most commonly fractured long bone in the body. It is typically injured by low-energy trauma in the elderly and high-energy trauma in the young. Due to its subcutaneous location, a thorough physical examination is needed to assess for soft tissue injuries and open fractures. Tibia fractures can cause an increase in intracompartmental swelling leading to compartment syndrome (see Chaps. 1, 2, 3, 4, and 5) [1].

Anatomy

Compartments

Anterior
- Muscles – tibialis anterior, extensor hallucis longus, and extensor digitorum longus
- Function – dorsiflexion of the foot and ankle
- Neurovascular – deep peroneal nerve and anterior tibial artery/vein

Lateral
- Muscles – peroneus brevis and peroneus longus
- Function – plantarflexion and eversion of the foot
- Neurovascular – superficial peroneal nerve

Deep Posterior
- Muscles – tibialis posterior, flexor hallucis longus, and flexor digitorum longus
- Function – plantarflexion and inversion of the foot
- Neurovascular – peroneal artery/vein, posterior tibial artery/vein, and tibial nerve

Superficial Posterior
- Muscles – soleus and gastrocnemius (medial and lateral heads)
- Function – plantarflexion of the foot and ankle
- Neurovascular – medial sural nerve

Classification

Open Fractures: Gustilo-Anderson System [2]

- Grade I – wound <1 cm, simple fracture with minimal comminution, minimal contamination, and minimal soft tissue injury
- Grade II – wound 1–10 cm, moderate comminution, moderate contamination, and moderate soft tissue injury

G.S. Buchanan, MD • F.D. Shuler, MD, PhD (✉)
Department of Orthopaedic Surgery, Joan C. Edwards
School of Medicine, Marshall University,
Huntington, WV, USA
e-mail: buchanang@marshall.edu;
shulerf@marshall.edu

© Springer International Publishing AG 2017
A.E.M. Eltorai et al. (eds.), *Orthopedic Surgery Clerkship*, DOI 10.1007/978-3-319-52567-9_76

- Grade III (A–C) – wound >10 cm, high-energy trauma, severe soft tissue injury, severe comminution or segmental fractures, and periosteal stripping:
  - Adequate tissue for local coverage
  - Requiring rotational or free flap for soft tissue coverage
  - Vascular injury requiring repair

Soft Tissue Injury: Tscherne Classification [3]

- Grade 0 – minimal soft tissue damage, indirect trauma, and simple fracture
- Grade 1 – superficial abrasion/contusion and mild fracture
- Grade 2 – deep abrasion, skin/muscle contusion, direct trauma, and severe fracture
- Grade 3 – crush injury, extensive injury to skin/muscle, compartment syndrome, and closed degloving

Orthopedic Trauma Association Classification [4]

- Type 42 (Fig. 76.1):
  - A – simple
  - B – wedge
  - C – complex

Evaluation

History

- Trauma, pain, and inability to bear weight

Physical Exam

- Deformity, open wound, and abrasion/contusion
- Signs of compartment syndrome [5]:
  - Pain with passive stretch is the most sensitive finding.

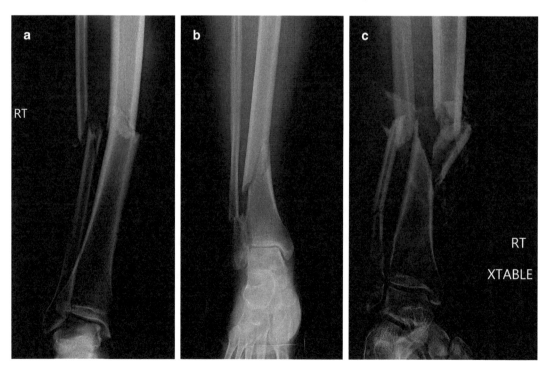

Fig. 76.1 AP radiographs of the tibia demonstrating a simple fracture pattern (**a**), a wedge pattern (**b**), and a complex pattern (**c**)

- The five "P's" are late findings: pain, pallor, paresthesia, pulselessness, and paralysis.
- Deep posterior and anterior compartments are most commonly involved.
- Intracompartmental pressure readings within 5 cm of the fracture site are beneficial in obtunded patients or when clinical examination findings equivocal.
- Intracompartmental pressure within 30 mmHg of diastolic blood pressure is diagnostic.
- Emergent surgical release is needed to minimize the risk of irreversible muscle and nerve damage (see Chaps. 1, 2, 3, 4, and 5).

Imaging

- AP and lateral radiographs of the full tibia, knee, and ankle
- CT – for suspicion of proximal or distal intraarticular extension or posterior malleolar involvement

Treatment

Nonoperative

- Closed reduction and long-leg casting
- Acceptable alignment parameters for closed management [6]:
  - <10° varus/valgus
  - <5° pro-/recurvatum, rotation
  - <1 cm shortening
  - <50% displacement
- Conversion to functional bracing by 4–6 weeks with patient to begin weight-bearing by 6 weeks to decrease risk of nonunion
- Contraindications [7]:
  - Open fracture, comminuted/unstable fracture, intact fibula (risk of varus malunion/nonunion), and associated ipsilateral fracture

Operative

External Fixation

- Useful for temporary stabilization, open fractures, or poor soft tissue quality
- High incidence of pin site infections
- Controversial whether there is a significant difference in fracture union, infection, or complications when compared to intramedullary nailing for open tibial fractures [8]

Plate Fixation

- Useful for very proximal or distal diaphyseal fractures that cannot be treated with an intramedullary nail.
- Care must be taken to preserve soft tissue and blood supply.
- Controversy regarding superiority over intramedullary nailing [9].

Intramedullary Nailing

- Most common form of fixation for unstable tibia fractures.
- Provides adequate stability without compromising soft tissue.
- Over 90% union [10].
- Impact of reaming remains controversial [11, 12].
- Anterior knee pain is common (47%) [13]:
  - Theories for this include proximal nail protrusion, division of the patellar tendon during approach, and fat pad fibrosis causing impingement.
  - Hardware removal may provide relief [14, 15].

Complications

Open Fracture

- Requires irrigation and debridement and early antibiotic administration.
- Do not place tourniquets on damaged extremities; direct pressure with sterile saline sponges preferred.

- Make sure that tetanus is up to date.
- Antibiotics depend on fracture classification and are usually given for 24 h after wound closure:
  - Gustilo Type I and II – first-generation cephalosporin (clindamycin or vancomycin if allergic).
  - Gustilo Type III – first-generation cephalosporin plus aminoglycoside.
  - Farm injury – add penicillin G for anaerobe coverage (*Clostridium*).

Compartment Syndrome

- Treat with urgent four-compartment fasciotomy (see Chaps. 1, 2, 3, 4, and 5)

Malunion

- Most commonly valgus and procurvatum (apex anterior)

Nonunion

- Treatment methods include exchange nailing, dynamization, and bone grafting, with emerging use of biologics.

Isolated Fibular Shaft Fractures

- The fibula is a non-weight-bearing bone, but it does contribute to ankle stability.
- Often result from direct lateral blow or torsional injury.
- Most can be treated conservatively:
  - Maisonneuve fracture – external rotation injury resulting in proximal third fibula fracture, syndesmosis disruption, medial malleolus fracture, and disruption of deep deltoid ligament:
    ○ Typically requires surgical intervention to reestablish ankle stability

References

1. Shuler F, Obremskey WT. Tibial shaft fractures. Surgical treatment of orthopedic trauma. New York: Thieme Medical Publisher; 2007. p. 742–66.
2. Gustilo RB, Anderson JT. Prevention of infection in the treatment of one thousand and twenty-five open fractures of long bones: retrospective and prospective analyses. J Bone Joint Surg Am. 1976;58(4):453–8.
3. Tscherne H, Oestern HJ. A new classification of soft-tissue damage in open and closed fractures (author's transl). Unfallheilkunde. 1982;85(3):111–5.
4. Marsh JL, Slongo TF, Agel J, Broderick JS, Creevey W, DeCoster TA, et al. Fracture and dislocation classification compendium – 2007: Orthopedic Trauma Association classification, database and outcomes committee. J Orthop Trauma. 2007;21(10 Suppl):S1–133.
5. Frink M, Hildebrand F, Krettek C, Brand J, Hankemeier S. Compartment syndrome of the lower leg and foot. Clin Orthop Relat Res. 2010;468(4):940–50.
6. Lindsey RW, Blair SR. Closed tibial-shaft fractures: which ones benefit from surgical treatment? J Am Acad Orthop Surg. 1996;4(1):35–43.
7. Anglen J. Tibial shaft fractures. Core knowledge in orthopedics. 1st ed. Mosby; 2007. p. 326–46.
8. Hutchinson AJP, Frampton AE, Bhattacharya R. Operative fixation for complex tibial fractures. Ann R Coll Surg Engl. 2012;94(1):34–8.
9. He GC, Wang HS, Wang QF, Chen ZH, Cai XH. Effect of minimally invasive percutaneous plates versus interlocking intramedullary nailing in tibial shaft treatment for fractures in adults: a meta-analysis. Clinics (Sao Paulo). 2014;69(4):234–40.
10. Zelle BA, Boni G. Safe surgical technique: intramedullary nail fixation of tibial shaft fractures. Patient Saf Surg. 2015;9:40.
11. Shao Y, Zou H, Chen S, Shan J. Meta-analysis of reamed versus unreamed intramedullary nailing for open tibial fractures. J Orthop Surg Res. 2014;9:74.
12. Duan X, Al-Qwbani M, Zeng Y, Zhang W, Xiang Z. Intramedullary nailing for tibial shaft fractures in adults. Cochrane Database Syst Rev. 2012;(1):Cd008241.
13. Katsoulis E, Court-Brown C, Giannoudis PV. Incidence and aetiology of anterior knee pain after intramedullary nailing of the femur and tibia. J Bone Joint Surg. 2006;88(5):576–80.
14. Court-Brown CM, Gustilo T, Shaw AD. Knee pain after intramedullary tibial nailing: its incidence, etiology, and outcome. J Orthop Trauma. 1997;11(2):103–5.
15. Keating JF, Orfaly R, O'Brien PJ. Knee pain after tibial nailing. J Orthop Trauma. 1997;11(1):10–3.

Stress Fractures

77

Michael J. Chambers

Epidemiology

- Typically seen in military cadets, athletes, and elderly
- Incidence:
  - 3–6% in male military cadets and athletes
  - 9–10% in female military cadets and athletes
  - 20% in runners
- 95% of stress fractures are in the lower extremity:
  - 49.1% in tibia
  - 25.3% in tarsals
  - 8.8% in metatarsals
  - Bilateral 16.6%

Pathogenesis

Overuse Injuries

- Excessive repetitive, submaximal loads that cause imbalance of bone formation and resorption
  - Microdamage vs repair processes

M.J. Chambers, MD
Marshall University Orthopaedics, King's Daughters
Medical Center, Ashland, KY, USA
e-mail: chambersm@marshall.edu

- Abrupt change in duration, intensity, frequency, or type of physical activity without adequate periods of rest

Risk Factors

Extrinsic Factors
- Training regiment
- Type of activity
- Equipment:
  - Running surfaces
  - Footwear
- Diet

Intrinsic Factors
- Metabolic state:
  - Nutritional deficiencies:
    - Low levels of 25-hydroxy vitamin D
  - Sleep deprivation
  - Metabolic disorders
  - Collagen abnormalities
  - Female athlete triad:
    - Osteopenia, eating disorder, and amenorrhea
- Anatomic alignment:
  - Limb-length discrepancy
  - Subtalar pronation
- Bone structure
- Bone vascularity:
  - Watershed area (areas of poor blood supply)

© Springer International Publishing AG 2017
A.E.M. Eltorai et al. (eds.), *Orthopedic Surgery Clerkship*, DOI 10.1007/978-3-319-52567-9_77

History

- Change in activity
- Insidious onset of pain over a period of days to weeks
- Aggravated by activity

Physical Exam

- Bony tenderness to palpation
- Pain with ROM in nonpalpable areas

Differential Diagnosis

- Periostitis
- Infection
- Avulsion injuries
- Muscle strain
- Bursitis
- Neoplasm
- Exertional compartment syndrome
- Nerve entrapment

Imaging

Radiographs

- Initial radiographic assessment
- Initially: subtle radiolucency or poor definition of the cortex
- Later: thickening and sclerosis of the endosteum and periosteal bone formation (Fig. 77.1)
- Sensitivity 12–56%, specificity 88–96%

Technetium-99M-labeled Diphosphonate Bone Scan

- Tracer uptake at areas of bone remodeling
- Sensitivity 50–97%, specificity 33–98%

MRI

- T2 sequence (Fig. 77.2)

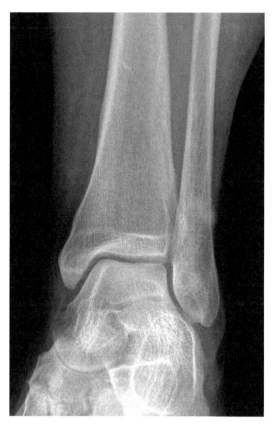

Fig. 77.1 X-ray of lateral malleolus stress fracture with periosteal bone formation

- Endosteal marrow edema and periosteal edema
- Hypointense fracture line
- Sensitivity 68–99%, specificity 4–97%

Ultrasound

- Evaluate outer surface cortex for step-off, hypoechoic band, periosteal reaction, and hyperechoic callus.
- Tenderness to transducer.
- Sensitivity 43–99%, specificity 13–79%.

CT

- Rarely indicated
- More accurate evaluation of osseous anatomy
- Sensitivity 32–38%, specificity 88–98%

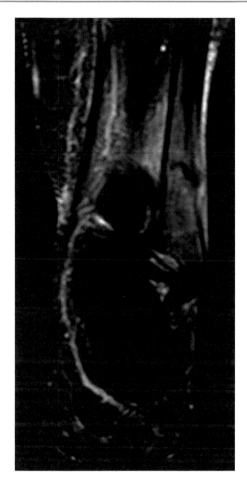

Fig. 77.2 MRI of lateral malleolus stress fracture

Single-Photon Emission Computed Tomography (SPECT)

- Most sensitive for sacral and pars stress fractures

High-Risk Stress Fractures

- High risk of nonunion, fracture completion, and displacement

Characteristics

- Area of increased stress
- Tension side of the bone
- Watershed area

Femoral Neck

- Tension side (superior cortex)
- High complication rate:
  - Complete and displace
  - Varus deformity and osteonecrosis
- Treatment: cannulated screw fixation

Tibia

- Tension side (anterior cortex)
- Dreaded black line
- High risk of completion and nonunion
- Treatment: intramedullary nail or tension band plating

Medial Malleolus

- Secondary to impingement on the talus
- Treatment: immobilization vs open reduction internal fixation

Navicular

- Central 1/3
- Area of maximum shear stress
- Treatment: immobilization vs screw fixation

Fifth Metatarsal

- Just distal to metaphyseal-diaphyseal junction
- Treatment immobilization and strict nonweight-bearing vs intramedullary screw fixation

Great Toe Sesamoids

- Medial more likely than lateral
- Repeated dorsiflexion of great toe
- Differentiate from bipartite sesamoid
- Treatment: nonweight-bearing cast extended to the tip of the toes vs open reduction internal fixation vs sesamoid excision and reconstruction of flexor hallucis brevis

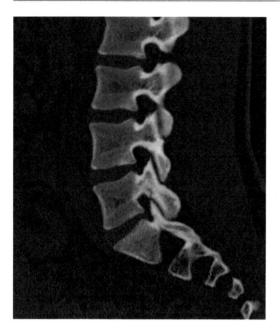

Fig. 77.3 L5 pars interarticularis defect

Pars Interarticularis

- Low back pain in athlete
- Gymnasts, divers, and football lineman
- Most common L5
- 85–90%
- If not treated can lead to pars defect (Fig. 77.3) and spondylotic spondylolisthesis

Low-Risk Stress Fractures

- Low risk of nonunion, malunion, and fracture completion

Characteristics

- Compression side of bone
- Lower area of stress
- Adequate blood supply

Upper extremity

- Throwing sports, tennis, swimming, and rowing

- Clavicle, scapula, humerus, olecranon, ulna, radius, metacarpals, and ribs
- Treatment: activity modification and rest vs immobilization

Lower extremity

Pelvis
- Sacrum, pubic rami, symphysis pubis (osteitis pubis), and sacroiliac joint
- Elderly, runners, military recruits, and weight lifters

Femur
- Neck, shaft, supracondylar region, condylar region, and compression side of femoral neck

Tibia
- Posteromedial cortex (compression side)

Fibula
- Proximal: due to muscle traction and torsional forces:
  - R/O proximal tibiofibular joint instability
- Distal: most commonly just proximal to inferior tibiofibular ligament:
  - Distance runners on hard surfaces

Calcaneus
- Long-distance runners, osteoporotic people, and military recruits
- Differential diagnosis: Achilles tendinitis, retrocalcaneal bursitis, and plantar fasciitis

Metatarsals
- Second, third, and fourth metatarsals:
  - Second metatarsal neck most common
- Ballet dancers base of second metatarsal and metatarsal heads
- Metatarsal shaft:
  - Military personnel from marching "march foot"
  - Also seen in distance runners, ballet dancers, and after dorsal malunion after first metatarsal osteotomy

Suggested Readings

1. Boden BP, Osbahr DC. High-risk stress fractures: evaluation and treatment. J Am Acad Orthop Surg. 2000;8(6):344–53.
2. Boden BP, Osbahr DC, Jimenez C. Low-risk stress fractures. Am J Sports Med. 2001;29(1):100–11.
3. McCormack RG, Lopez CA. Commonly encountered fractures in sports medicine. In: Miller MD, Thompson SR, editors. DeLee & Drez's orthopedic sports medicine. 4th ed. Philadelphia: Elsevier Health Sciences; 2014.
4. Shindle MK, Endo Y, Warren RF, Lane JM, Helfet DL, Schwartz EN, Ellis SJ. Stress fractures about the tibia, foot, and ankle. J Am Acad Orthop Surg. 2012;20(3):167–76.
5. Wright AA, Hegedus EJ, Lenchik L, Kuhn KJ, Santiago L, Smoliga JM. Diagnostic accuracy of various imaging modalities for suspected lower extremity stress fractures: a systematic review with evidence-based recommendations for clinical practice. Am J Sports Med. 2016;44(1):255–63.

Metatarsalgia

Tonya W. An, Alexander Kish, Matthew Varacallo,
Amiethab A. Aiyer, and Ettore Vulcano

Definition

- Pain and inflammation in the forefoot region, involving the metatarsals (MT) or associated joints [1]
- A symptom rather than a discrete condition:
  - Metatarsalgia (i.e., central metatarsalgia): pathology of second through fourth MT
  - Transfer metatarsalgia: pathology of the great toe transfers abnormal forces over to lesser toes:
    - Hallux rigidus: degenerative disease of the first metatarsal-phalangeal (MTP) joint
    - Hallux valgus (i.e., bunion deformity): MT varus with valgus of the phalanx:

T.W. An
Orthopedics Cedars-Sinai Medical Center,
Los Angeles, CA, USA

A. Kish
Orthopaedic Surgery, University of Mayland Medical
Center, Baltimore, MD, USA

M. Varacallo
Department of Orthopaedic Surgery, Hahnemann
University Hospital, Philadelphia, PA, USA

A.A. Aiyer
Department of Orthopaedic Surgery,
University of Miami, Miami, FL, USA

E. Vulcano (✉)
Orthopedics, Mount Sinai Health System,
New York, NY, USA
e-mail: ettorevulcano@hotmail.com

- Can also physically deform second toe
- Iatrogenic: following reconstructive procedures to correct hallux valgus [2]

Pathophysiology

- Repetitive loading of the forefoot during gait, especially during the midstance phase (from heel rise to toe off) [1]
- Frequently an overuse injury associated with increased or abnormal stresses on forefoot

Causes [1, 3]

Primary: Related to the Anatomic Configuration of the MT

- Insufficiency of first ray (i.e., transfer metatarsalgia): excessive force is transferred to lesser toes (Fig. 78.1).
- Disproportionately long second MT: exposed to higher pressures during gait
- Excessively plantar-flexed MT
- Cavus foot: forefoot deformity with increased declination of MT
- Soft tissue imbalances:
  - Hammertoe deformity—flexion deformity at PIP, with DIP extension and neutral or extended MTP joint:

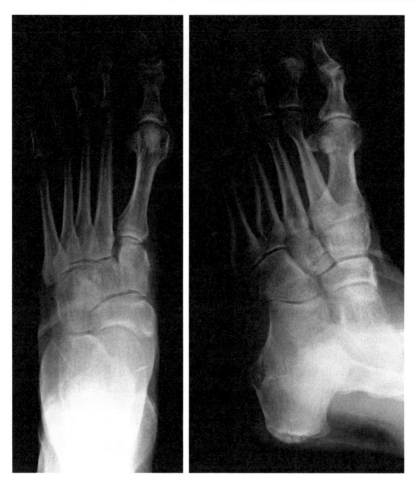

Fig. 78.1 The images show the anteroposterior and oblique view radiographs of a patient with metatarsalgia and hammertoe deformities affecting the second, third, and fourth toes. Note the relative shortness of the first metatarsal compared to the lesser metatarsals:

- ○ Results from an imbalance between intrinsic and extrinsic musculature
- ○ Associated with constricting shoe wear, hallux valgus, neuromuscular disorders, and inflammatory arthritis
- – Claw toe deformity—flexion of both PIP and DIP, hyperextension of MTP:
  - ○ Results from an imbalance between intrinsic and extrinsic musculature
  - ○ Associated with neuromuscular disorders
- – Crossover toe
- • Equinus deformity—persistent plantar-flexed foot generates increased stress on MT heads:
  - – Gastrocnemius-soleus complex tightness

- • Others: arthritis, tumor, infection, stress fracture of the metatarsal head/neck, and fracture malunion

Secondary: Indirectly Leads to Greater Loads on Forefoot

- • Trauma, metabolic disorders, gout, and rheumatoid arthritis (rheumatoid forefoot)
- • Morton's neuroma—irritation of the plantar interdigital nerves:
  - – May be associated with narrow space between MT heads, tight footwear, and trauma
  - – Most commonly affects the third interdigital nerve
- • Freiberg's infarction: avascular necrosis (AVN) of the metatarsal head

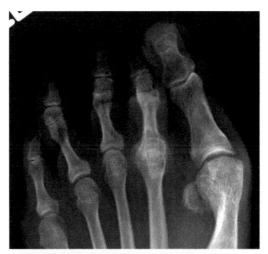

Fig. 78.2 The images show the anteroposterior and oblique view radiographs of a patient with iatrogenic second metatarsalgia and hammertoe deformity. The previous bunionectomy procedure resulted in shortening of the first metatarsal causing overload of the second metatarsal head, rupture of the plantar plate, and ultimately hammertoe deformity

Iatrogenic

- Nonunion or malunion after MT reconstructive surgery
- Excessive shortening of MT (Fig. 78.2)
- Partial MT head resection

Presentation

Symptoms

- Pain in forefoot region, exacerbated by walking, activity, or footwear

Signs [2, 3]

- Hyperkeratosis (thickened skin) on plantar aspect of foot
- Swelling or bruising
- Equinus contracture (common associated finding)

Evaluation

History

- Previous foot trauma or surgery
- Prior diagnosis of diabetes, peripheral neuropathy
- Equinus or cavus foot deformity and leg length discrepancy

Clinical Examination

- Inspect for hyperkeratosis on plantar aspect of foot:
  - May be diffuse or localized under affected MT heads

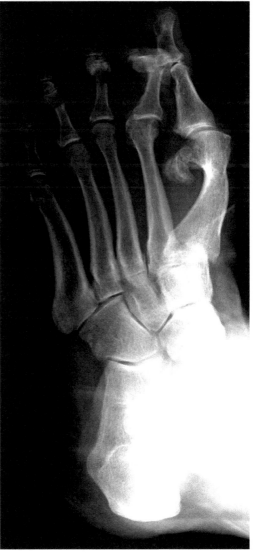

- Observe deformities including long second MT, hammertoes, and claw toes.
- Passive and active range of motion at MTP, PIP, and DIP joints.
- Palpation of MTP joints and intermetatarsal web spaces for tenderness.
- Range of motion of ankle: Silfverskiold's test to distinguish gastrocnemius versus Achilles tendon tightness.
- Check perfusion and sensitivity of distal toes.
- Weight-bearing foot posture:
  - Compare bilaterally.
  - Gait analysis, as necessary, to determine overload sites.

Radiology

- Obtain weight-bearing AP, lateral, and oblique views of the foot
- Evaluate:
  - Relative length of each MT.
  - MT cascade: second ray should be equal or shorter than the first.
  - Inclination of MT on lateral view.
  - Rule out subluxed or dislocated MTP joints and MT stress fractures.
  - Hallux deformities.

Treatment [1, 4]

Nonoperative

- Initial treatment for all patients.
- PT focused on stretching for heel cord tightness.
- Shoe modifications—for primary causes of metatarsalgia:
  - Wider toe box, appropriate length, softer sole, padding, lower heel, and metatarsal bars built into orthotics.
  - Rocker bottom sole reduces pressure at MT heads.
  - Nondisplaced ligamentous injury with or without avulsion fracture.

- Nondisplaced fractures through bases of first, second, or third MT.
- Corticosteroid injection (for Morton's neuroma, bursitis, and synovitis):
  - Frequency limited due to complications of subcutaneous fat atrophy and tendon rupture
- Alcohol injection (for Morton's neuroma) [5]:
  - Ultrasound guided, up to four injections
  - Pain relief with minimal side effects
- Shaving callus can reduce pain from chronic hyperkeratosis.

Operative

- Indicated after failure to respond to conservative management
- Distal oblique MT (Weil) osteotomy (for MTP joint instability and excessive MT length):
  - MT is shortened by intraarticular osteotomy; proximal translation of MT head relieves pressure during gait.
  - Three-step/triple Weil osteotomy (modified technique) limits relative plantarflexion of head (and shift in center of rotation) with coaxial shortening of shaft.
  - Contraindications: osteoporosis, hallux valgus causing second MT deformity.
- Midshaft segmental MT osteotomy: equalize lengths of lesser MT:
  - Shortening accomplished by segmental resection with plating
- Proximal MT osteotomy (correction of excessive MT declination/forefoot cavus):
  - Elevation of MT accomplished by dorsal wedge resection of proximal MT
- First TMT fusion: reduces instability of first TMT and associated overloading of 2–5 MT
- Tendon transfer for joint stabilization or lesser toe deformities:
  - EDB transfer or flexor-to-extensor transfer for treatment of crossover toes
- Achilles tendon lengthening or gastrocnemius recession for equinus contracture

Postoperative Rehabilitation

- After metatarsal shortening osteotomy, foot protected in neutral using stiff-soled shoe for 4–6 weeks, then progress range of motion

Complications [1, 3]

- Stiffness of MTP joint
- Dislocation at the MTP joint
- Floating toe deformity—toe fails to contact ground—associated with Weil osteotomy but minimized with three-step technique
- Nonunion or hardware failure
- Osteonecrosis of MT head
- Infection
- Neurovascular injury

References

1. Espinosa N, Brodsky JW, Maceira E. Metatarsalgia. J Am Acad Orthop Surg. 2010;18(8):474–85. doi:10.1111/j.1365-2036.2011.04609.x.
2. Maceira E, Monteagudo M. Transfer metatarsalgia post hallux valgus surgery. Foot Ankle Clin. 2014;19(2):286–307. doi:10.1016/j.fcl.2014.03.001.
3. Espinosa N, Maceira E, Mark M. Current concept review: metatarsalgia. Foot Ankle Int/Am Orthop Foot Ankle Soc [and] Swiss Foot Ankle Soc. 2008;29(8):871–9. doi:10.3113/FAI.2008.0000.
4. Myerson M. Reconstructive foot and ankle surgery: management of complications. 2nd ed. Philadelphia: Elsevier; 2010. doi:10.1016/B978-1-4377-0923-0.10012-8.
5. Pasquali C, Vulcano E, Novario R, Varotto D, Montoli C, Volpe A. Ultrasound-guided alcohol injection for Morton's Neuroma. Foot Ankle Int. 2014;36(1):55–9. doi:10.1177/1071100714551386.

Hallux Valgus

Satheesh K. Ramineni

Definitions

- Bunion: Any enlargement or deformity of the first MTP joint.
- Hallux valgus: Static subluxation of the first MTP joint characterized by lateral deviation of the great toe and medial deviation of the first metatarsal.
- Juvenile hallux valgus can originate due to lateral deviation of the articular surface of the first metatarsal head without subluxation of the first MTP joint.
- Hallux valgus can be associated with pes planus, contracted Achilles tendon, cerebral palsy, stroke, and rheumatoid arthritis.

Anatomy

- First MTP characterized by sesamoid mechanism, strong collateral ligaments, and sesamoid ligaments.
- Plantar plate – formed by condensation of the two tendons of flexor hallucis brevis, abductor and adductor hallucis, the plantar aponeurosis, and the joint capsule.

S.K. Ramineni
Orthopaedic Surgery, University of Toledo Medical Center, Toledo, OH, USA
e-mail: satheesh.ramineni@utoledo.edu

- Sesamoids – tibial (medial) and fibular (lateral) sesamoids located on the plantar aspect of the first metatarsal head separated by a bony ridge called crista.
- Sesamoids connected together by intersesamoidal ligament and to the base of the proximal phalanx by the plantar plate. They have no connections to the metatarsal head.
- The tendons and muscles that move the great toe are arranged around the MTP in four groups:
  - Dorsal group – long and short extensor tendons
  - Plantar group – long and short flexor tendons
  - Medial group – abductor hallucis
  - Lateral group – adductor hallucis
- The base of the metatarsal – mildly sinusoidal articular surface that articulates with the distal articular surface of the medial cuneiform.
- The first tarsometatarsal (TMT) joint has a slight medial plantar inclination. It permits motion in a dorsomedial to plantar-lateral plane.

Pathoanatomy

- Because no muscle inserts on the metatarsal head, it is vulnerable to extrinsic forces, in particular, and constricting footwear.
- Once the metatarsal head is destabilized and begins to sublux medially, the tendons around the metatarsal head drift laterally.

© Springer International Publishing AG 2017
A.E.M. Eltorai et al. (eds.), *Orthopedic Surgery Clerkship*, DOI 10.1007/978-3-319-52567-9_79

- The laterally drifted muscles becoming deforming forces as their pull is lateral to the longitudinal axis of the first ray.
- The soft tissues on the lateral aspect of the first MTP become contracted, and those on the medial side become attenuated.
- Deformity is associated with lateral displacement of the sesamoid sling and pronation of the hallux.
- Hallux valgus deformity is associated with transfer of more of the weight-bearing function to the lesser metatarsal heads which leads to the development of a transfer lesion beneath the second or third metatarsal head.

Demographics

- Age of onset – can develop before the age of 20 or during third to fifth decade of life. Early onset hallux valgus associated with increased distal metatarsal articular angle (DMMA).
- Gender – 90% patients are female.
- Majority of patients have bilateral hallux valgus deformities of differing magnitude.
- 2–4% incidence in the general population.

Etiology

- Extrinsic causes – constricting footwear and the type of occupation.
- Intrinsic causes – positive family history in up to 88% of patients, pes plans with pronation of hallux, hyper mobility of the metatarsocuneiform joint, ligamentous laxity, Achilles contracture, amputation of the second toe, and cystic degeneration of the medial capsule of the first MTP joint.

Angular Measurements

- Hallux valgus angle – angle between the long axis of the first metatarsal and the long axis of the proximal phalanx. Normal 15°, mild less than 20°, moderate 20–40°, and severe greater than 40°.

- 1–2 intermetatarsal (IM) angle – angle between the long axis of the first and second metatarsals. Normal is less than 9°, mild 11° or less, moderate 11–16°, and severe is greater than 16°.
- Hallux interphalangeus angle – angle between the long axis of the proximal phalanx and the long axis of the distal phalanx. Normal angle is less than 10°.
- Distal metatarsal articular angle (DMMA) – angle between the line perpendicular to the articular surface line of the distal metatarsal and the line along the longitudinal axis of the first metatarsal. Normal angle is 6° or less of lateral deviation.
- Proximal phalangeal articular angle (PPAA) – angle between the line perpendicular to the articular surface line of the proximal phalangeal articular surface and the line along the longitudinal axis of the proximal phalanx. Normal is 5° or less of valgus inclination.
- Metatarsophalangeal joint congruency – congruent or noncongruent hallux valgus deformity.
- Size of the medial eminence – distance from the line along the medial border of the diaphysis of the first metatarsal at the widest extent of the medial eminence.
- First metatarsocuneiform joint – straight MTC joint, curved MTC joint, or oblique MTC joint.

History and Physical

- Symptoms include pain over the medial eminence due to shoe wear and symptomatic metatarsalgia.
- Physical examination includes the severity of the deformity and any lesser toe deformities.
- Assess active and passive range of motion, tenderness over the MTP, mobility of the first MTC joint, vascular status of the foot, and a neurologic examination.

Conservative Treatment

- First line of treatment.
- Shoe modification with roomy footwear, a soft upper shoe with a wide toe box and a soft sole.

- The use of prefabricated custom orthotics is controversial. It has not been demonstrated that they prevent progression of the deformity.
- Orthotics may be useful to correct pes planus.

Surgical Treatment

- Type of surgical procedure based on the presence of congruent or incongruent joint, the presence of any degenerative joint disease in the first MTP or TMT joint, and the severity of the deformity.
- Mild to moderate hallux valgus with congruent joint with increased DMAA >11° – chevron procedure, double/triple first ray osteotomy, and akin procedure with exostectomy.

- Incongruent hallux valgus deformity:
  - Mild deformity with 1–2 IM angle <13° – Chevron osteotomy
  - Moderate deformity with 1–2 IM angle >13° – distal soft tissue procedure with or without proximal metatarsal osteotomy
  - Severe deformity – distal soft tissue procedure with or without proximal metatarsal osteotomy or MTP arthrodesis
- Hallux valgus deformity with degenerative joint disease of first MTP joint – first MTP arthrodesis.
- Hallux valgus deformity with hypermobile first TMT joint or degenerative joint disease of first TMT – Lapidus procedure (distal soft tissue procedure with arthrodesis of first TMT joint).

Heel Pain

80

Jordan Ernst and Brian Carpenter

Plantar Heel Pain

Etiology/Epidemiology

- Ten percent of people will experience during their lifetime, two million office visits per year [1]
- Mechanical
  - Most common
- Neurogenic
  - Often secondary to a mechanical derangement
  - Tarsal tunnel syndrome , Baxter's neuritis, S1 radiculopathy
- Traumatic
  - Calcaneal stress fracture, plantar fascia rupture
- Arthritic
  - Seronegative, rheumatoid, gouty
- Neoplastic, infectious
- Others – fat pad atrophy, chronic exertional compartment syndrome, flexor hallucis longus tendinitis, subcalcaneal bursitis, plantar fibromatosis

J. Ernst (✉)
Orthopedics, John Peter Smith, Fort Worth, TX, USA
e-mail: jernst@jpshealth.org

B. Carpenter, DPM, FACFAS
Department of Orthopaedic Surgery, John Peter
Smith Hospital, Fort Worth, TX, USA

Department of Orthopaedic Surgery, UNT Health
Science Center, Fort Worth, TX, USA

Anatomy

- Numerous structures in a confined area
  - Understanding the intricate relationships of these structures allows elucidation of heel pain etiology
- Dynamic changes from non-weight bearing to weight bearing
  - Structures simultaneously subjected to traction and compression during stance
    - ° Magnitude of these forces varies with body mass and activity level
- Calcaneus
  - Serves as an attachment for soft tissues of the heel
  - Calcaneal tuberosity – defined as the posterior limit of the plantar surface
    - ° Serves as the origin for:
      - Ligaments:
        - Long plantar – coursing from the calcaneus to the 2nd–4th metatarsal bases
        - Plantar fascia
          1. Three bands of longitudinally arranged collagen
          2. Central band divides distally into five digital bands inserting on the proximal phalanges
  - Muscles – first and second layer of plantar musculature
  - Neurovascular structures traversing across the plantar heel
    - ° Can also be a source of heel pain from compression

° First branch of the lateral plantar nerve
 – Site of compression thought to be between abductor hallucis fascia and medial process of calcaneal tuberosity
  • Nerve changes from vertical to horizontal orientation [1]

History and Physical

- Being thorough in this area will confer an accurate diagnosis in the vast majority of cases.
- Prior treatments and their level of success.
- Constitutional symptoms – if present may indicate a systemic cause.
- Pain unrelenting at rest or at night must raise suspicion for an infection or neoplasm.
- A history of lower back injuries may explain a radiculopathy-induced heel pain.
  – Often lacks localized tenderness to the plantar heel
- Pain after periods of rest (post-static dyskinesia).
  – Hallmark of plantar fascial pain
   ° Often the last component of pain to improve with conservative therapy
  – Purely neurogenic pain usually lacks this feature
  – Pain occurring after injury is more indicative of a plantar fascial rupture or calcaneal stress fracture
  – Rupture – tearing sensation, inability to perform a single-leg heel raise
  – Careful palpation will illicit the point of maximal tenderness (Fig. 80.1)
  – Plantar fascial pain is usually maximal at the medial process of the calcaneal tuberosity
  – Baxter's neuritis pain can often be provoked by palpation of the anterior medial calcaneal wall where the nerve courses deep to the abductor fascia
  – Squeezing the calcaneal wall (calcaneal squeeze test) posterior to the tuberosity will illicit the pain of a stress fracture or reaction
  – Pain to the central heel is often due to fat pad atrophy and the subsequent development of an adventitial bursa

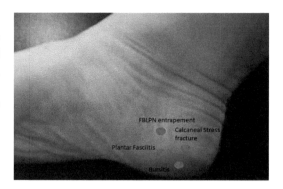

Fig. 80.1 Medial heel with superimposed sites of palpable tender areas in various heel pain conditions

Imaging/Other Diagnostics

- In most instances these are not needed for a diagnosis.
- May exclude less common causes of heel pain.
- Weight-bearing plain films may delineate why the plantar fascia is under excessive strain.
  – Calcaneal stress fracture/reaction can be seen 2–3 weeks after injury
   ° Should be ruled out when seeing a patient for the first time with chronic heel pain treated elsewhere
- Ultrasound – diagnosis of plantar fasciitis and quantification of fascial thickness.
- MRI – diagnosis of plantar fasciitis and visualization of space occupying lesions within the tarsal tunnel causing neuritic pain.
- Electrodiagnostics – a positive result may confirm neuritic source of heel pain, but negative results do not rule this out.
- HLA-B27 – although around 25% of plantar fasciitis is bilateral, consider this to rule out a seronegative spondyloarthropathy in patients with bilateral pain resistant to treatment.
- Other serology to consider – ESR, CRP, RF, ANA, CBC, uric acid.

Treatment

- Ninety percent of mechanically induced heel pain is treated successfully with conservative therapy [1]

- Neuritic heel pain tends to respond to the same treatment as plantar fasciitis
  - RICE, oral anti-inflammatory medication, stretching, orthoses
  - Physical therapy, night splints, corticosteroid injections
- Appropriate referral should be made for those with pain not found to be of a mechanical or neural origin
- Surgery may be indicated in cases of recalcitrant pain for appropriate patients

- Plantar fascial release
- Tarsal tunnel/Baxter's nerve release with or without lesion removal

Reference

1. DiGiovanni B, Dawson L, Baumhauer J. Plantar heel pain. In: Coughlin M, Saltzman C, editors. Mann's Surgery of the foot and ankle. Saunders, an imprint of Elsevier Inc: Philadelphia; 2014. p. 685–701.

Ankle Sprains and Fractures

81

Shane D. Rothermel and Paul Juliano

Anatomy [2, 3, 4]

Osseous Structure

- Complex hinge joint whereby a mortise joint is formed by the medial malleolus of the tibia, the plafond of the tibia, and the fibula with the talus.
- The talar dome is trapezoidal: 2.5 mm wider anteriorly than posteriorly. To accommodate for the talar geometry with dorsiflexion, the fibula externally rotates.

Lateral Ligamentous Complex

- Anterior talofibular (ATFL), calcaneofibular (CFL), posterior talofibular (PTFL)
- ATFL most commonly injured (i.e., the weakest lateral ligament) – prevents subluxation of the talus anteriorly, primarily in plantar flexion; anterior drawer laxity indicates injury.
- CFL second most commonly injured – positive talar tilt test indicates injury.
- CFL spans both tibiotalar and talocalcaneal joints.

- PTFL is the strongest lateral ligament: prevents posterior and rotatory subluxation of the talus.

Deltoid Ligament

- Superficial portion: arises from anterior colliculus; adds little to ankle stability
- Deep component: intra-articular origination from intercollicular groove and posterior colliculus. Fibers oriented transversely, primary medial stabilizer preventing lateral talar displacement

Distal Tibiofibular Syndesmosis

- Anterior inferior tibiofibular ligament (AITFL), posterior inferior tibiofibular ligament (PITFL), transverse tibiofibular ligament, interosseous ligament (IOL).
- PITFL is thicker and stronger than the AITFL.

Radiographic Imaging

Indications (Ottawa Ankle Rules) [8]

- Point tenderness near one or both malleoli plus one or more of the following:
  - Age >55
  - Inability to bear weight
  - Bone tenderness over the posterior edge or tip of either malleolus

S.D. Rothermel, MD (✉) • P. Juliano, MD
Department of Orthopaedics and Rehabilitation,
Penn State Health Milton S. Hershey Medical Center,
Hershey, PA, USA
e-mail: srothermel@hmc.psu.edu

© Springer International Publishing AG 2017
A.E.M. Eltorai et al. (eds.), *Orthopedic Surgery Clerkship*, DOI 10.1007/978-3-319-52567-9_81

Views [2, 4, 7]

AP (weight bearing if tolerated)

- >5 mm tibiofibular clear space is abnormal – syndesmotic injury
- <10 mm tibiofibular overlap is abnormal – syndesmotic injury
- Positive talar tilt test: varus stress shows >3° tilt compared to contralateral side or 10° overall tilt

Lateral (weight bearing if tolerated)

- Confirm talar dome is congruous with tibial plafond
- Can identify posterior tibial tuberosity fractures and direction of fibular displacement
- Positive anterior drawer test: stress radiograph shows >3 mm translation compared to opposite side, or an absolute value of 10 mm

Mortise (weight bearing if tolerated) – leg in approximately 15–20° internal rotation

- >4–5 mm medial clear space is abnormal – lateral talar shift
- <1 mm tibiofibular overlap is abnormal – syndesmotic injury
- Talocrural angle: angle between a line perpendicular to tibial plafond and a line intersecting the tips of the medial and lateral malleoli. Normal is 83 ± 4° or within 5° of the contralateral ankle or <2 mm difference from contralateral side
- Stress view: gentle external rotation of dorsiflexed foot with the leg stabilized or by allowing the ankle to rotate with the force of gravity (note: stress all isolated fibula fractures.)

Ankle Sprains

- High Ankle Sprains
  - Syndesmosis injury
- Low Ankle Sprains
  - Lateral ankle instability (ATFL and/or CFL injury)
  - ≈85% of all ankle sprains [9]

Classification of Acute Lateral Ankle Instability [7]

- Grade I: elastic deformation, no ligament disruption, minimal ecchymosis, swelling and tenderness, no weight-bearing pain
- Grade II: plastic deformation, ligament stretch without rupture, moderate ecchymosis, swelling and tenderness, mild weight-bearing pain
- Grade III: complete tear, severe ecchymosis, swelling and tenderness, severe weight-bearing pain

Treatment [7, 9]

Nonoperative

- Ninety percent of all acute ankle sprains resolve with RICE and early functional rehabilitation
- Full return to activity in 4–8 weeks

Operative Indications

- Continued pain and instability
- Bony avulsion
- The sprain that will not heal
  - Anterolateral impingement of thickened accessory AITFL (Bassett's ligament)
  - Osteochondral defect (OCD)
    - Medial – 50% due to trauma
    - Lateral – mostly due to trauma
  - Complex regional pain syndrome (CRPS)
  - Tarsal coalition
  - Lateral talar process fracture
  - Anterior calcaneal process fracture

Ankle Fractures

Classification Systems

Danis-Weber Classification: Basis of AO-OTA Classification

- Based on location of fibula fracture line in relation to level of syndesmosis

- Weber A: fracture distal to tibiofibular syndesmosis – infrasyndesmotic
- Weber B: most common, fracture at level of syndesmosis – transsyndesmotic
- Weber C: fracture proximal to syndesmosis – suprasyndesmotic

Anatomic Classification
- Isolated medial malleolar
- Isolated lateral malleolar
- Bimalleolar
- Trimalleolar
- Bosworth fracture-dislocation: posterior dislocation of fibula behind incisura fibularis

Lauge-Hansen Classification System (Fig. 81.1) [5]
- Based on a rotational mechanism of injury that utilizes radiographic patterns to describe the mechanism. (Note: This classification system was formulated from cadaveric studies.)
- First part of the classification identifies the position of the foot at time of injury (supination vs pronation).
- Second part of the classification relates to the force that is applied to the foot.
- Four injury patterns result from this classification schema: supination-adduction (SA), supination-external rotation (SER), pronation-abduction (PA), and pronation-external rotation (PER). Each injury pattern has a sequential order of injury.

Supination-Adduction
- Represents 20% of ankle fractures.
- Stage I: Disruption of the lateral collateral ligament or transverse avulsion-type fracture of the fibula.
- Stage II: Talus displaced toward medial malleolus. A vertical fracture develops from the medial axilla of the joint extending proximally through the metaphyseal cortex of the tibia. The medial malleolar fragment is typically a large shear fragment and only rarely comminuted. Often there will be an impaction injury of the medial tibial plafond.

- Vertical shear pattern of medial malleolus fracture is the essential component of SA injury

Supination-External Rotation
- Most prevalent ankle fracture pattern (40–75%)
- The fibula experiences a shearing force while the medial osteoligamentous complex experiences an avulsion-type force.
- Stage 1: Isolated anterior tibiofibular ligament (ATFL) injury
- Stage 2: Oblique fibula fracture with ATFL midsubstance rupture or avulsion fracture of ATFL tibial insertion with characteristic minimal displacement, fracture at the level of the syndesmosis but not affecting the syndesmosis, and fracture line orientation from distal anterior to proximal posterior.
- Stage 3: SER2 plus either a posterior tibiofibular ligament rupture or a posterior malleolus fracture
- Stage 4: SER2 plus progression to medial structures: medial malleolus osteoligamentous complex (MMOLC) injury. This may be an isolated deltoid ligament injury (SER4 "equivalent" lesion) or an isolated medial malleolus fracture or a combination of both an anterior colliculus fracture plus a deep deltoid ligament rupture.
- Indicators to distinguish SER4 equivalent injury from SER2 injury: evidence of anterior or posterior subluxation of the talus, more than 2 mm of fibular shortening, or mild lateral subluxation without any stress.

Pronation-Abduction
- Typically present as an avulsion-type medial malleolus fracture with a relatively transverse fibular fracture. The fibula fracture often has either a lateral butterfly fragment or comminution due to bending failure.
- The fibula fracture is usually 5–7 cm proximal to the joint.
- Anterolateral tibial plafond fracture may contribute to residual talar tilt or subluxation.

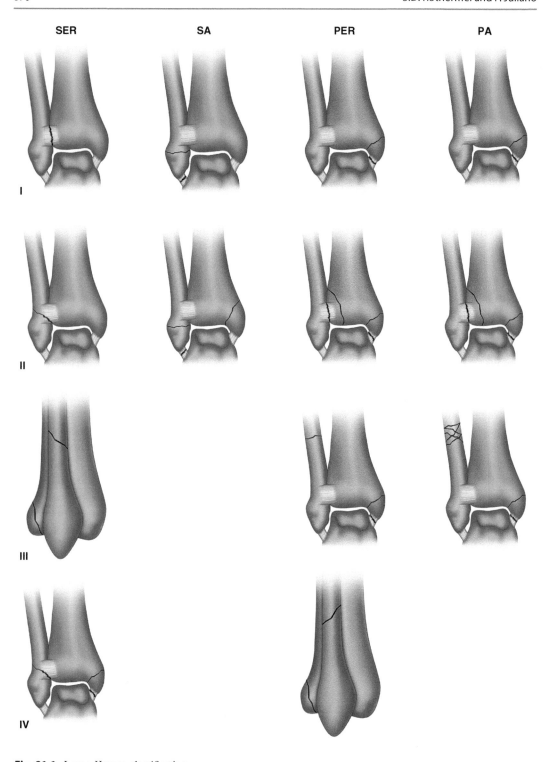

Fig. 81.1 Lauge-Hansen classification

- Stage I: Isolated deltoid ligament rupture or transverse medial malleolus fracture.
- Stage II: Chaput's tubercle fracture or anterior tibiofibular ligament sprain
- Stage III: Transverse or lateral comminuted fibula fracture.

Pronation External-Rotation

- *Stage I*: As in PA, isolated deltoid ligament rupture or transverse medial malleolus fracture.
- *Stage II*: Chaput's tubercle fracture or anterior inferior tibiofibular ligament disruption
- *Stage III*: Lateral short oblique or spiral fibular fracture, characteristically above the level of the syndesmosis oriented from distal posterior to proximal anterior.
- *Stage IV*: Posterior tibiofibular ligament rupture or posterior malleolus avulsion.
- Maisonneuve fracture: PER variant characterized by a proximal fibula shaft fracture. Suspect whenever an isolated medial malleolus fracture is seen and screen by palpation of the proximal fibula.
  - None of these classification systems addresses soft tissue aspects such as open fracture, blistering, or neurovascular compromise. In addition to fracture description, it is important to note and describe the soft tissue envelope in order to provide appropriate treatment.

Treatment

Nonoperative [3, 4, 6, 7]

- Indications
  - Nondisplaced, stable fractures with intact syndesmosis
  - Displaced fractures with stable anatomic reduction of the ankle mortise
  - Operative treatment contraindicated because of the condition of the patient or limb
- Stable fractures can be placed in short leg cast, removable boot, or functional brace for 4–6 weeks and allowed to weight bear as tolerated

- Unstable fractures treated with casting and nonweight bearing for a minimum of 4 weeks require frequent follow-up with radiographic confirmation that the talus remains reduced. Maintaining reduction in this fashion is difficult.

Operative [2, 3, 4, 6, 7]

- Indications
  - Failure to maintain reduction in a cast
  - Unstable fractures that may result in talar displacement or widened ankle mortise
  - Fractures that require abnormal foot position to maintain reduction
  - Open fractures
    - Goal is stable anatomic reduction of talus in ankle mortise (talar shift of 1 mm results in 40% decrease in tibiotalar contact area)
- ORIF postponed until general medical condition, ankle swelling, and soft tissue status allow. Swelling, blisters, and soft tissue typically stabilize 5–10 days after injury with RICE.
- Excellent results in 85–90% but may have prolonged recovery
- Factors associated with functional recovery: age, gender (better outcomes in males), diabetes mellitus, smoking, alcohol use
- Lateral malleolar fractures
  - Distal to syndesmosis: lag screw or Kirschner wires with tension banding
  - At or above syndesmosis, essential to restore fibular length and rotation typically done with lag screws and a plate
- Medial malleolar fractures
  - Can often be stabilized with cancellous screws or a figure-of-eight tension band.
  - Vertical shear fractures may require articular impaction reduction, bone void filling, and/or antiglide or buttress plate fixation.
- Posterior malleolar fracture
  - Indications for fixation: >25% of articular surface, >2 mm displacement, persistent posterior subluxation of talus (numbers are merely indicators, stability is the main factor)

- Fixation via indirect reduction and placement of anterior-to-posterior lag screw or directly utilizing a posterolateral approach and placement of a posterior-to-anterior lag screw or buttress plate. Posterolateral plate can sometimes lead to peroneal tendonitis.
- Syndesmosis
  - Following fixation of medial and lateral malleoli, syndesmosis should be stressed intraoperatively by lateral pull on the fibula with a bone hook or stress test.
  - One or two syndesmotic screws 1.5–2.0 cm proximal to plafond from fibula to tibia (syndesmotic hardware removal is controversial).
  - Screws can be tricortical or tetracortical (tetracortical screws are more likely to break).
  - Fixation of posterior malleolus may eliminate the need for syndesmotic fixation (as PITFL remains attached to fragment).

Postoperative Rehabilitation

- Baseline braking response time returns at 9 weeks after ankle surgery [9].

Complications [1, 3, 6, 7]

- Nonunion: rare.
- Malunion: lateral malleolus shortened and malrotated, widened medial clear space and large posterior malleolar fragment most predictive of poor outcome.
- Wound problems: skin edge necrosis (3%); decreased risk with minimal swelling, no tourniquet, and good soft tissue technique; fracture blisters or abrasions more than doubles complication rate.
- Infection: seen in <2% of closed fractures, up to 20% in diabetic patients.
- Immobilization time for the diabetic patient should be double that of the nondiabetic patient.
- Beware of the onset of Charcot arthropathy in the presence of neuropathy.

- Posttraumatic arthritis: rare with anatomic reduction, increased incidence with articular incongruity
- Complex regional pain syndrome (CRPS): rare
- Compartment syndrome of the foot or leg: rare
- Tibiofibular synostosis: associated with syndesmotic screw, typically asymptomatic
- Loss of reduction: 25% of unstable injuries treated nonoperatively
- Loss of ROM: the rule, not the exception

References

1. Chaudhary SB, Liporace FA, Gandhi A, Donley BG, Pinzur MS, Lin SS. Complications of ankle fracture in patients with diabetes. J Am Acad Orthop Surg. 2008;16(3):159–70.
2. Clanton TO, Waldrop NE. Athletic injuries to the soft tissue of the foot and ankle. In: Coughlin MJ, Saltzman CL, Anderson RB, editors. Mann's surgery of the foot and ankle. 9th ed. Philadelphia: Elsevier Saunders; 2014. p. 1531–687.
3. Davidovitch RI, Egol KA. Ankle fractures. In: Bucholz RW, et al., editors. Rockwood and Green's fractures in adults. 7th ed. Philadelphia: Lippincott Williams & Wilkins; 2010. p. 1975–2021.
4. Egol KA, Koval JK, Zuckerman JD. Injuries about the ankle. In: Hurley R, editor. Handbook of fractures. 4th ed. Philadelphia: Lippincott Williams & Wilkins; 2010. p. 476–506.
5. Lauge-Hansen N. Fractures of the ankle. II. Combined experimental-surgical and experimental-roentgenologic investigations. Arch Surg. 1950;60:957–85.
6. Sanders DW, Egol KA. Fractures of the ankle and tibial plafond. In: Boyer MI, editor. AAOS comprehensive orthopedic review. 2nd ed. Rosemont: American Academy of Orthopedic Surgeons; 2014. p. 443–60.
7. Spiguel A, Jo MJ, Gardner MJ. Ankle and pilon fractures. In: Chou LB, editor. Orthopedic knowledge update: foot and ankle. 5th ed. Rosemont: American Academy of Orthopedic Surgeons; 2014. p. 297–302.
8. Stiell IG, McKnight RD, Greenberg GH, et al. Implementation of the Ottawa ankle rules. JAMA. 1994;271(11):827–32.
9. Weiss DB, Milewski MD, Thompson SR, Stannard JP. Trauma. In: Miller MD, Thompson SR, Hart JA, editors. Review of orthopedics. 6th ed. Philadelphia: Elsevier Saunders; 2012. p. 697–813.

Talar Fracture

82

Kyle Duncan and Brian Carpenter

Anatomy

- The talus has no muscular or tendinous attachments; it should also be noted that approximately 70% of the talus is covered by cartilage [3].

Articulations

- Ankle joint – responsible for dorsiflexion and plantarflexion
- Subtalar joint – pronation and supination of the rearfoot
  - Posterior, middle, and anterior facets.
  - Posterior facet is located on the talar body while the middle and anterior facets are located on the talar head/neck.
- Talonavicular joint – primary pronation and supination of the midfoot

Blood Supply [3]

- Posterior tibial artery

K. Duncan (✉)
Department of Orthopaedic Surgery, John Peter Smith Hospital, Fort Worth, TX, USA
e-mail: kduncan01@jpshealth.org

B. Carpenter, DPM, FACFAS
Department of Orthopaedic Surgery, John Peter Smith Hospital, Fort Worth, TX, USA

Department of Orthopaedic Surgery, UNT Health Science Center, Fort Worth, TX, USA

  - Artery of the tarsal canal – main blood supply to the talar body
  - Calcaneal branches – posterior talus
- Anterior tibial artery
  - Supplies head and neck of the talus
- Perforating peroneal artery
  - Artery of the tarsal sinus – also supplies the head and neck of the talus
- Deltoid artery
  - Supplies talar body and can be the only remaining blood supply following talar neck fracture

Fracture Types and Classifications

Lateral Process Fracture

- Typically occurs when the foot is dorsiflexed and inverted with application of an axial force
- Snowboarding injury
- Classification [2]
  - Type 1 – no articular involvement
  - Type 2 – involve Subtalar and/or talofibular joints
  - Type 3 – comminuted fractures

Posterior Process Fracture

- Mechanism is one of forced plantarflexion where the posterior process is crushed between

© Springer International Publishing AG 2017
A.E.M. Eltorai et al. (eds.), *Orthopedic Surgery Clerkship*, DOI 10.1007/978-3-319-52567-9_82

the posterior malleolus of the tibia and the tuber of the calcaneus.
- May be indistinguishable from previously present os trigonum.
- Most reliable clinical sign of injury is pain with forced plantarflexion of the ankle, known as the nutcracker sign.

Talar Body Fracture

- High-energy injury, axial compression of the talus between the tibia and calcaneus
- Sneppen classification [4]
  - Type A – chondral or compression fracture
  - Type B – coronal shearing fracture
  - Type C – sagittal shearing fracture
  - Type D – fracture of the posterior process
  - Type E – fracture of the lateral process
  - Type F – crush fracture

Talar Neck Fracture (Fig. 82.1)

- High-energy injury, forced dorsiflexion where the anterior lip of the tibia strikes the talar neck
- Hawkins classification [1] (Table 82.1)

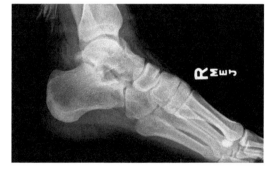

Fig. 82.1 Talar neck fracture

Table 82.1 Hawkins classification of talar neck fractures

Type	Findings	Incidence of AVN
I	Minimal displacement	7–15%
II	STJ subluxation	35–50%
III	Ankle dislocation	85%
IV	STJ/ankle/TNJ dislocation	100%

Treatment

- Closed reduction should be attempted at time of presentation

Nonoperative

- Non-displaced (<2 mm) fractures and Hawkins type I fractures
- Initially placed in posterior splint
- SLC application, NWB for 6–8 weeks

Operative

- Displaced (>2 mm) fractures or any fracture/dislocation where closed reduction failed
- Hawkins type II–IV

Surgical Approaches
- Anteromedial – medial to the tibialis anterior
- Anterolateral – between the tibia and fibula, in line with the fourth ray
- Combined approach – improved visualization of talar neck and body to better assess reduction

Fixation
- Dependent on fracture pattern.
- Typically with simple coronal fractures of the talar neck you can place two screws from anterior to posterior, across the fracture.
- Screws should be countersunk into the talar head, below the level of the articular surface.
- More comminuted fractures may require plate fixation, either medially or laterally (Fig. 82.2a, b).

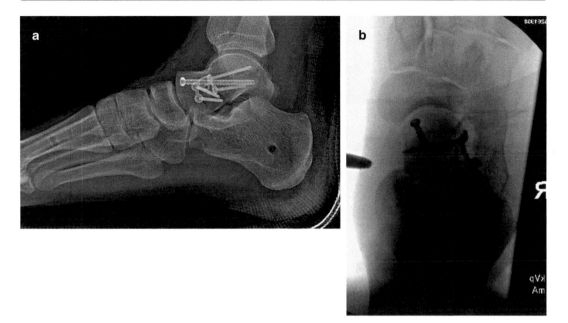

Fig. 82.2 Postoperative (**a**) lateral and intraoperative (**b**) AP view of the talus with interfragmentary screw and plate fixation due to associated comminuted fracture of the talar body

- Titanium implants may be beneficial as they create less artifact on MRI, which may be indicated during the postoperative course to assess for vascularity and viability of the talus.

Postoperative Course

- After ORIF, patient is typically NWB for 10–12 weeks
- Hawkins sign [3]
  - Lucency of the talar dome indicates vascularization of the talus. Best seen on ankle mortise X-ray.
  - Will not be seen until at least 6 weeks postop and may not appear until 12 weeks.
  - Lack of lucency, or sclerosis, can be indicative of AVN.
  - If after prolonged immobilization you do not see resorption of subchondral bone (Hawkins sign), MRI or technetium bone scan may be used to assess viability.

Complications

- Avascular necrosis
  - Primary concern is collapse of the talus
  - Prolonged NWB
  - May also consider patellar-tendon-bearing walking cast as prolonged immobilization, up to 8 months, may be impractical

References

1. Hawkins LGLG. Fractures of the neck of the talus. J Bone Joint Surg Am. 1970;52:991–1002.
2. Kirkpatrick DP, Hunter RE, Janes PC, et al. The snowboarder's foot and ankle. Am J Sports Med. 1998;26:271–7.
3. Schuberth J, et al. Talar fractures. In: Southerland JT, et al., editors. McGlamry's comprehensive textbook of foot and ankle surgery. 4th ed. Philadelphia: Lippincott Williams & Wilkins; 2013. p. 1707–38.Print.
4. Sneppen O, Christensen SB, Krogsoe O, et al. Fracture of the body of the talus. Acta Orthop Scand. 1977;48:317–24.

Calcaneus Fractures

83

Jyoti Sharma and Paul J. Juliano

Anatomy

- Calcaneus acts as a lever to increase the power of the gastrocnemius soleus complex.
- Insertion site of the Achilles tendon (posterior tuberosity).
- Articular facets:
  - Anterior facet – carries the facet of the calcaneocuboid joint.
  - Posterior facet – largest, major weight-bearing surface.
  - Flexor hallucis longus tendon runs just inferior to this facet and can be injured with screws/drills that are too long.
  - Anterior portion is perpendicular to the calcaneus long axis.
- Middle facet – anteromedial on sustentaculum tali
- Superior facet – contains three facets that articulate with the talus
- Sustentaculum tali
  - Projects medially and supports the talar neck, extension of the medial wall of the body
  - FHL passes beneath it
  - Contains the anteromedial facet, which remains constant in injury settings due to ligamentous attachments
- Sinus tarsi
  - Between the middle and posterior facets

Presentation

- Calcaneus is most commonly fractured tarsal bone
- Severe pain, may have deformity, open fracture

Mechanism

- Usually traumatic loading is primary mechanism
- May also have shear component which contributes to secondary fracture lines

Physical Exam

- Pain, diffuse tenderness to palpation of heel, accompanied by swelling
- May have a varus deformity of the heel, appear shortened and wide as compared to contralateral limb

J. Sharma, MD (✉) • P.J. Juliano, MD
Orthopaedic Surgery, Penn State Hershey
Medical Center, Hershey, PA, USA
e-mail: jsharma@hmc.psu.edu

Demographics

- More common in males
- Must rule out associated injuries like vertebral fractures (10%) and contralateral calcaneus fracture (10%)

Fracture Types

Intra-articular

- Up to 75% of fractures, result from axial loading
- Classification
  - Essex Lopresti: primary fracture line runs obliquely through the posterior facet creating two fracture fragments; the secondary fracture line runs either behind the posterior facet (joint depression fractures) or beneath the posterior facet exiting posteriorly (tongue-type fracture).
  - Sanders classification: coronal CT cut at the widest portion of the posterior facet used to classify fracture based on number of articular fragments seen (types i–iv).

Extra-articular

- Result from twisting forces on the hindfoot
- Posterior tuberosity avulsion fractures
  - Account for 1–3% of all calcaneus fractures.
  - Due to insertion of the Achilles tendon.
  - Fractures with significant displacement can threaten the skin posteriorly and require urgent reduction to prevent skin necrosis.
- Anterior process fractures
  - Avulsion secondary to bifurcate ligament

Imaging

Radiographs

- AP, lateral, oblique of foot

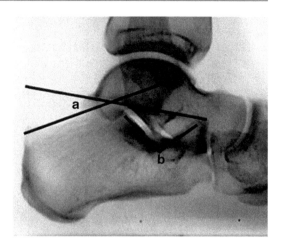

Fig. 83.1 Normal lateral radiograph of the foot showing (*a*) Bohler's angle and (*b*) crucial angle of Gissane (Image from *Core Knowledge in Orthopedics: Trauma*)

- Visualize decreased Bohler's angle (normal 20–40°), increased angle of Gissane (normal 130–145°), varus tuberosity, shortening of calcaneus (Fig. 83.1)
- AP ankle
  - Fibular impingement can be caused by lateral wall extrusion.
- Broden: posterior facet visualized
  - Ankle maintained in neutral dorsiflexion and X-ray beam moved to 10°, 20°, 30°, and 40° of internal rotation
- Harris: tuberosity visualized and assessed for shortening, widening, and varus position
  - Foot in maximal dorsiflexion with the X-ray beam at 45°

CT Scan

- Has become gold standard for imaging calcaneus fractures
- Sagittal view: shows tuberosity displacement
- Axial view: shows calcaneocuboid joint involvement
- Semicoronal view: shows posterior and middle facet displacement, used for Sander's classification (Fig. 83.2)

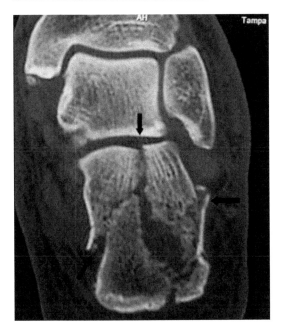

Fig. 83.2 Semicoronal view of the calcaneus on a CT scan used for the Sander's classification (Image from *Core Knowledge in Orthopedics: Trauma*)

- 3D reconstructions can aide in operative planning and understanding fracture patterns better.

MRI Scan

- Not routinely used unless diagnosis is unclear (stress fracture)

Treatment

Nonoperative

- Cast immobilization and non-weight bearing for at least 10–12 weeks
  - Indications: nondisplaced fractures, extra-articular fractures <1 cm with intact Achilles tendon, anterior process fractures <25% of calcaneocuboid joint, patients unable to undergo surgery due to medical comorbidities

Operative

- Closed reduction and percutaneous pinning
  - Indications: large extra-articular fractures, minimally displaced tongue-type fractures, mild shortening
- Open reduction internal fixation (ORIF)
  - Indications: displaced tongue-type fractures, large extra-articular fragments with detachment of the Achilles tendon. Anterior process fractures involving >25% of the joint, flattening of Bohler's angle, varus malalignment of tuberosity, posterior facet displacement >2 mm
  - Goals to restore calcaneal height, correct varus, and stabilize fracture
  - Wait up to 2 weeks for swelling to resolve prior to surgery (positive wrinkle sign)
  - Extensile lateral or medial approach most commonly utilized
    - Full-thickness skin flaps must be raised to maintain soft tissue integrity.
    - No-touch skin technique with the use of K-wires helps preserve the soft tissue envelope and prevent extra tissue damage from handling.
- Sinus tarsi approach
  - Best utilized in fracture patterns where anatomic reduction can be achieved through a small incision, such as Sanders type II fractures
  - Can be used in other types of calcaneus fractures, but achieving a congruent articular surface can be difficult through the small incision
- Primary subtalar arthrodesis
  - Combined with ORIF to restore height, Sanders type IV

Postoperative Rehabilitation

- Bulky U-splint initially after surgery
- Non-weight bearing for at least 10–12 weeks

- Can start subtalar range of motion exercises once incision healed after 2–3 weeks

Complications

- Wound complications (up to 25%)
  - Increased in smokers, diabetic patient, open fractures
- Posttraumatic subtalar arthritis
- Compartment syndrome (may result in claw toes)
- Lateral impingement with peroneal tendon irritation
- FHL damage
- Malunion

Outcomes

- Overall poor with 40% complication rate

Suggested Reading

1. Banerjee R, et al. Management of calcaneal tuberosity fractures. J Am Acad Orthop Surg. 2012;20:253–8.
2. Clare MP. Fractures of the calcaneus. Core Knowl Orthop: Trauma. 2008;23:386–402.
3. Heger L, Wulff K. Computed tomography of the calcaneus: normal anatomy. Am J Roentgenol. 1985;145:123–9.

Lisfranc Injuries

84

Tonya W. An, Alexander Kish, Matthew Varacallo, Amiethab A. Aiyer, and Ettore Vulcano

Anatomy and Function [1, 2]

Osseous

- Lisfranc joint complex consists of all midfoot articulations, including tarsometatarsal (TMT), intermetatarsal (IMT), and intertarsal (IT) joints.
- Base of second metatarsal (MT) is recessed into mortise between medial and middle cuneiform, providing frontal plane stability.
- Transverse arch of the foot is formed by trapezoidal shape of metatarsal bases, second MT base functions as the "keystone" for coronal plane stability.

T.W. An
Orthopedics Cedars-Sinai Medical Center, Los Angeles, CA, USA

A. Kish
Department of Orthopaedic Surgery, University of Mayland Medical Center, Baltimore, MD, USA

M. Varacallo
Department of Orthopaedic Surgery, Hahnemann University Hospital, Philadelphia, PA, USA

A.A. Aiyer (✉)
Department of Orthopaedic Surgery, University of Miami, Miami, FL, USA
e-mail: tabsaiyer@gmail.com

E. Vulcano
Department of Orthopedics, Mount Sinai Health System, New York, NY, USA

Ligamentous

- Lisfranc ligament originates from medial cuneiform, inserts on base of second MT
  - Strongest interosseous ligament of TMT joint complex
- Tightens with forefoot pronation and abduction, stabilizes midfoot arch

Vascular

- Dorsalis pedis artery lies between the first and second rays at the TMT articulation

Injury Classification [1]

- Quenu and Kuss: describes pattern of injury, but not prognosis (Fig. 84.1)
  - Homolateral: all 5 MT displaced in same direction
  - Isolated: 1–2 MT displaced from the others
  - Divergent: displacement of MT in both sagittal and coronal planes

© Springer International Publishing AG 2017
A.E.M. Eltorai et al. (eds.), *Orthopedic Surgery Clerkship*, DOI 10.1007/978-3-319-52567-9_84

Fig. 84.1 Quenu and Kuss classification of patterns of Lisfranc injury: homolateral, isolated, divergent (Reprinted with permission from *Netter's Sports Medicine*. 1st ed)

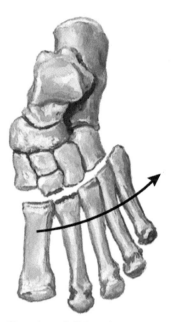 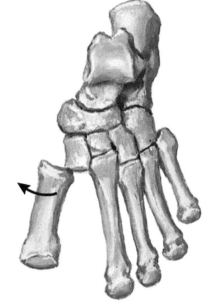

Homolateral dislocation.
All five metatarsals displaced
in same direction. Fracture
of base of 2nd metatarsal.

Isolated dislocation. One or two
metatarsals displaced; others in
normal position.

Pathophysiology

Definition

- Disruption of Lisfranc joint complex, can be ligamentous (sprain) or osseous (fracture, fracture dislocation) or both
- Associated with metatarsal or tarsal injuries

Cause of Injury [2]

- Direct trauma: motor vehicle accidents, crush injury
  - Frequently missed or delayed diagnosis in cases of multisystem trauma
- Indirect trauma: falls, athletic injury
  - Mechanism usually involves twisting – axial compression and abduction through plantar-flexed forefoot (Fig. 84.2)

- Historically observed in soldier falling from horse, with foot caught in stirrup

Presentation

Symptoms

- Severe midfoot pain
- Inability to bear weight

Signs

- Swelling, tenderness over TMT joint, plantar ecchymosis is considered pathognomonic [3]
- Pain reproducible by passive pronation and abduction of forefoot
- Instability: dorsal subluxation of TMT or separation of first and second metatarsals

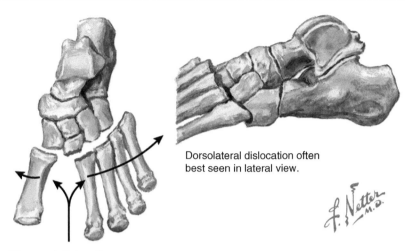

Dorsolateral dislocation often best seen in lateral view.

Divergent dislocation.
1st metatarsal displaced
medially, others superolaterally.

Fig. 84.2 (*Left*) classical mechanism of Lisfranc injury: axial load with abduction in a plantar-flexed foot causes disruption of Lisfranc ligament and dislocation of second metatarsal base (Reprinted with permission from *Netter's Sports Medicine*. 1st ed)

- Careful neurovascular exam to rule out dorsalis pedis injury

Radiology

- Obtain AP, lateral, and oblique view of the foot +/− CT scans
- Fluoroscopic stress views in the office or under sedation if in doubt: check for medial gapping at the first TMT joint in particular

Radiographic Signs of Injury [4]
- Loss of colinearity between medial border of second MT and medial border of middle cuneiform on AP view
- Widening of interval between first and second MT on AP view (Fig. 84.3)
- Loss of colinearity between medial border of fourth MT and medial border of cuboid, on oblique view
- MT base dorsal subluxation on lateral view
- Disruption of medial border congruity of navicular and medial cuneiform

Other Signs
- Fleck sign: bony fragment in first IMT space due to avulsion fracture of base of second MT on AP view (pathognomonic for Lisfranc injury)

Treatment [5]

Nonoperative

- Indicated for patients without instability.
  - Non-displaced ligamentous injury with or without avulsion fracture
  - Non-displaced fractures through bases of first, second, or third MT
- Other relative contraindications to surgery: nonambulatory, insensate foot, rheumatoid arthritis.
- Immobilize in short leg cast or boot for 6–8 weeks.
- Initially non-weight bearing, progress to weight bearing as tolerated.
- Repeat XR to detect osseous displacement around 2 weeks.

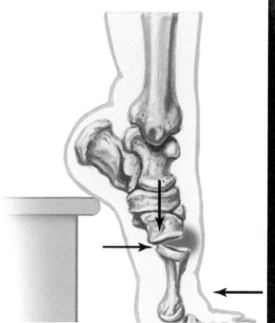 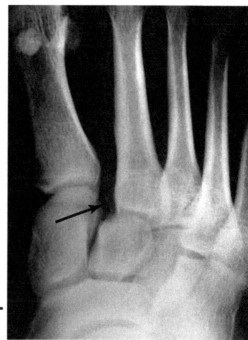

Lisfranc disruption x-ray.

Fig. 84.3 *Right* radiographic sign of widening between first and second metatarsal bases (Reprinted with permission from *Netter's Sports Medicine*. 1st ed)

- Physical therapy recommended for gait training and balance.
- Time to full recovery is approximately 4 months.

Operative [6]

- For any TMT displacement >2 mm
  - Best treated within 2 weeks of injury.
  - Surgery may be delayed further if severe foot swelling exists due to concerns over soft tissue healing.
- ORIF: focused on anatomic reduction of second MT base [6]
  - Rigid screw fixation preferred for 1–3 TMT joints, K-wire fixation acceptable for 4 and 5
    (a) K wires alone are at high risk of displacement
  - Comminuted fractures may be treated with dorsal bridge plating
  - Screw placed across second MT and medial cuneiform mimics Lisfranc ligament

- Closed reduction and percutaneous fixation: advocated in cases of minimal displacement
- Primary arthrodesis of first, second, and third TMT joints for primary ligamentous injury: shown to achieve good outcomes and reduced reoperation rate, compared to ORIF [7]
- Midfoot arthrodesis reserved for progressive arch collapse or failure of conservative management or missed injuries (~20%)

Postoperative Rehabilitation [5]

- Immobilize in cast or boot, non-weight bearing for 6–8 weeks
- Progressive weight bearing as tolerated to full weight bearing at 8 weeks post-op
- Can remove lateral column wire fixation at 8–12 weeks
- Keep screws for at least 4–6 months
- Physical therapy for gait training and balance

Complications [1]

- Posttraumatic arthritis
  - Dependent on initial injury and accuracy of reduction
  - Treated with orthotics, possible late medial column or midfoot arthrodesis
- Nonunion or hardware failure
- Compartment syndrome
  - Maintain high index of suspicious in early injury phases
- Infection
- Wound complications

References

1. Thompson MC, Mormino MA. Injury to the tarso-metatarsal joint complex. J Am Acad Orthop Surg. 2003;11(4):260–7.
2. Scolaro J, Ahn J, Mehta S. In brief: Lisfranc fracture dislocations. Clin Orthop Relat Res. 2011;469(7):2078–80. doi:10.1007/s11999-010-1586-z.
3. Glenn R, Cronin R, Hauzenblas J, Juliano P. Plantar ecchymosis sign: a clinical aid to diagnosis of occult Lisfranc tarsometatarsal injuries. J Orthop Trauma. 1996;10(2):119–22.
4. Siddiqui NA, Galizia MS, Almusa E, Omar IM. Evaluation of the tarsometatarsal joint using conventional radiography, CT, and MR imaging. Radiographics. 2014;34(2):514–31. doi:10.1148/rg.342125215.
5. Watson TS, Shurnas PS, Denker J. Treatment of Lisfranc joint injury: current concepts. J Am Acad Orthop Surg. 2010;18(12):718–28.
6. Kuo R, Tejwani N, DiGiovanni C, et al. Outcome after open reduction and internal fixation of Lisfranc joint injuries. J Bone Joint Surg Am. 2000;82(11):1609–18.
7. Ly TV, Coetzee JC. Treatment of primarily ligamentous Lisfranc joint injuries: primary arthrodesis compared with open reduction and internal fixation. Surgical technique. J Bone Joint Surg Am. 2007;89 Suppl 2:122–7. doi:10.2106/JBJS.F.01004.

Metatarsal Fractures

Megan R. Wolf and Lauren E. Geaney

Metatarsal Fracture

Background [1]

History

Etiology
- Direct crushing injuries (usually second to fourth metatarsals)
- Inversion-avulsion injuries (usually fifth metatarsal)
- Overuse injuries/stress fractures (second metatarsal most common)
- Head fractures usually result from shearing force or direct trauma

Physical Exam

- Swelling and ecchymosis especially on dorsal foot.
- Point tenderness over fracture site.
- Pain over midfoot with inability to bear weight.
- Must test for ligamentous stability as may present with Lisfranc joint fracture-dislocation.
- Neurovascular exam is mandatory as trauma may result in foot compartment syndrome.

Radiology

- AP, oblique, and lateral radiographs
  - Base fractures may be associated with Lisfranc joint fracture-dislocation.
  - Neck fractures often multiple and displaced.

Treatment

Nonoperative [10]
- Second through fourth metatarsal rarely need surgical treatment especially in isolation. (<10° of angulation and < 4 mm of translation)
  - Stiff-soled shoe or cast
  - Well-padded splint until swelling subsides
- Most metatarsal neck fractures can be treated with stiff-soled shoe and progressive weight bearing.

Operative [1]

Metatarsal Shaft Fractures
- Displaced first metatarsal shaft fractures
  - K-wire fixation after closed manipulation
  - ORIF if closed reduction unsuccessful
- Displaced second through fourth metatarsal fractures
  - Medial and lateral displacement and axial shortening may be treated like nondisplaced fractures.
  - Significant dorsal and plantar displacement should be fixed.

M.R. Wolf, MD • L.E. Geaney, MD (✉)
Department of Orthopaedic Surgery, UCONN Health, Farmington, CT, USA
e-mail: lageaney@uchc.edu

© Springer International Publishing AG 2017
A.E.M. Eltorai et al. (eds.), *Orthopedic Surgery Clerkship*, DOI 10.1007/978-3-319-52567-9_85

– Multiple consecutive metatarsal fractures are often unstable and should be
fixed.
  1. K-wire fixation after closed manipulation
  2. ORIF if closed reduction unsuccessful

Metatarsal Base Fractures [10]

- First metatarsal fractures should be treated
  with ORIF if comminuted and intra-articular.
- Rule out tarsometatarsal joint dislocation and
  instability.
- Treat second and third metatarsal base fractures with ORIF versus fusion if unstable and
  intra-articular.
- Rarely need to treat fourth and fifth metatarsal
  base fractures with ORIF.

Metatarsal Neck Fractures

- Closed reduction with K-wire fixation or
  ORIF if plantar displacement

Open Fractures

- Metatarsal fractures may be open due to
  crushing injuries and direct trauma.
- Irrigation and debridement, antibiotics, and
  delayed coverage.
- Stabilize early to allow for soft tissue healing
  with K-wire fixation or external fixation.

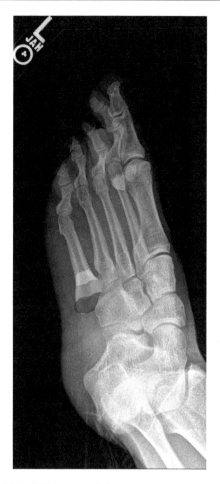

Fig. 85.1 Fifth metatarsal fracture zones

Table 85.1 Red shaded area - Zone I fracture; blue
shaded area - Zone 2 fracture; yellow shaded area - Zone
3 fracture

Zone I (pseudo-Jones)	Tuberosity avulsion which can extend into the TMT joint
Zone II (Jones)	Metaphyseal region at fourth/fifth metatarsal articulation (about 18 mm from base). No extension into intermetatarsal joint
Zone III (diaphyseal)	Proximal 1.5–3 cm, typically stress fracture

Fifth Metatarsal Fractures
(Fig. 85.1 and Table 85.1)

Background

Anatomy

- The fifth metatarsal is composed of the base,
  tuberosity, shaft, neck, and head.
- Muscle attachments:
  – Peroneus brevis attaches on the tuberosity
  – Abductor digiti minimi passes under the
    base with variable attachments
  – Origin of the flexor digit minimi on the base
  – Dorsal and plantar interossei originate on
    the shaft
- Plantar fascia attaches at the base.

Blood Supply

- The arterial supply to the tuberosity joins the
  supply to the proximal diaphysis in the area
  just distal to the tuberosity – this creates an
  area of low blood supply that may cause
  delayed healing or risk of stress fractures [8].

History

Mechanism of Injury [10]

Zone I (Fig. 85.2)
- Sudden inversion of hind foot with violent contracture of the lateral band of plantar aponeurosis

Zone II (Fig. 85.3)
- Large adduction force applied to forefoot while ankle is plantar flexed, such as a misstep onto the lateral border of the foot

Zone III
- Secondary to repetitive distraction force

Physical Exam

- Pain with passive inversion
- Pain with active eversion
- Tenderness at the base of the fifth metatarsal

Radiology [1]

Zones

Zone I (Pseudo-Jones Fracture)
- Tuberosity avulsion fracture which can extend into the tarsometatarsal joint

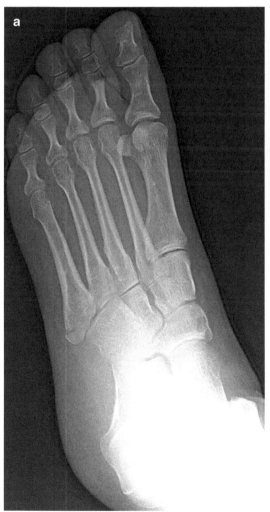
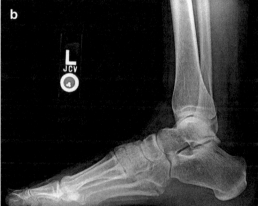

Fig. 85.2 Zone I fifth metatarsal fracture

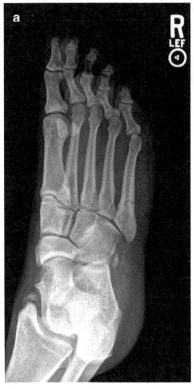
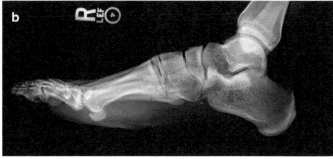

Fig. 85.3 Zone II fifth metatarsal fracture: Jones fracture

Zone II (Jones Fracture)
- At the metadiaphyseal region of the fifth metatarsal at the level of the fourth/fifth metatarsal articulation.
- True Jones fracture is a transverse fracture of the fifth metatarsal shaft about 18 mm from the base, with no extension into the intermetatarsal joint [2].
- Area between insertion of the peroneus brevis and tertius.

Zone III (Diaphyseal Stress Fracture)
- Pathologic fracture of proximal 1.5–3 cm of fifth metatarsal shaft
- Cortical hypertrophy, narrowing of medullary canal, and periosteal reaction

Treatment

Zone I

Nonoperative
- Nondisplaced fractures

- Hard-soled shoe, walking cast with protected weight bearing

Operative
- Rarely needed
- May be indicated in the setting of a symptomatic nonunion

Zone II

Nonoperative
- Nondisplaced fractures
- Non-weight-bearing immobilization for 6–8 weeks [6]
- Heals from medial to lateral direction, lagging behind clinical healing
- High risk of nonunion

Operative
- High-performance athletes or displaced fractures.
- Fractures that fail nonoperative treatment and remain symptomatic.

- Techniques include tension band wiring, cannulated screw fixation, or low-profile plates and screws.
- 6.5 m screws are torsionally stronger [3].
- Lag screws are stronger than intramedullary screws [4].

Zone III

Nonoperative
- Acute nondisplaced fractures require nonweight bearing and immobilization.

Operative
- Symptomatic nonunions
- Autograft can be considered for atrophic nonunion, intramedullary screw fixation

Outcomes

Zone II (Jones Fracture)
- One third of injuries went on to closed refracture [5]. Up to 50% treated nonoperatively result in nonunion [7].
- Patients treated nonweightbearing have a better rate of healing than those allowed to weightbear [6].

Zone III
- Healing in 93% of fifth metatarsal stress fractures with 7 weeks of non-weight-bearing immobilization [6]

Metatarsal Stress Fracture

Background
- Second metatarsal most often involved, then third [1]

History [9]

- "March fractures" – frequent occurrence in military personnel, especially new military recruits
- Runners near the end of the season
- Pain on a long march or increased running on hard pavement

- "Dancer's fracture" – stress fracture at the base of the second metatarsal

Physical Exam

- Tenderness, swelling, and ecchymosis over shaft of metatarsal

Radiographs [1]

- Radiographs lag behind clinical examination.
- Fine line in metatarsal shaft secondary to bone resorption.
- AP and oblique views most useful for detecting – usually show periosteal reaction by 2 weeks after onset.
  - First metatarsal stress fractures are usually proximal.
  - Second and third metatarsal stress fractures most commonly midshaft or neck.
  - Second metatarsal stress fracture may be at the base of the second metatarsal
  - Fourth metatarsal distal part of diaphysis
- Bone scan or MRI may be necessary for documentation in high-level athlete or for early diagnosis [9].

Treatment

Nonoperative
- Cessation of excess activity
- Stiff-soled shoe or short walking boot until fracture healed and no pain on exam
- Then training progressively advanced
- Pain usually subsides in 4–6 weeks

References

1. Coughlin M, Mann R, Saltzman C. Surgery of the foot and ankle. 8th ed. Philadelphia: Elsevier; 2007.
2. Steward IM. Jones's fracture: fracture of base of fifth metatarsal. Clin Orthop. 1960;16:190–8.
3. Horst F, Gilbert BJ, Glisson RR, Nunley JA. Torque resistance after fixation of Jones fractures with intramedullary screws. Foot Ankle Int. 2004;25(12): 914–9.

4. Moshirfar A, Campbell JT, Molloy S, Jasper LE, Belkoff SM. Fifth metatarsal tuberosity fracture fixation: a biomechanical study. Foot Ankle Int. 2003;24(8):630–3.

5. Quill GE. Fractures of the proximal fifth metatarsal. Orthop Clin North Am. 1995;26(2):353–61.

6. Torg JS, Balduini FC, Zelko RR, Pavlov H, Peff TC, Das M. Fractures of the base of the fifth metatarsal distal to the tuberosity. Classification and guidelines for non-surgical and surgical management. J Bone Joint Surg Am. 1984;66(2):209–14.

7. Kavanaugh JH, Brower RD, Mann RV. The Jones fracture revisted. J Bone Joint Surg Am. 1978;66(6):776–82.

8. Shereff MJ, Yan QM, Kummer FJ, Frey CC, Grennidge N. Vascular anatomy of the fifth metatarsal. Foot Ankle 1991;11:350–3.

9. Schenck RC, Heckman JD. Fractures and Dislocations of the Forefoot: operative and nonoperative treatment. J Am Acad Orthop Surg. 1995;3(2): 70–8.

10. Bucholz RW, Heckman JD, Court-Brown C. Rockwood and Green's Fracturs in Adults. 6th ed. Philadelphia, PA: Lippincott Williams & Wilkins; 2006.

Pilon Fractures

86

John Tidwell and Paul Juliano

Introduction

Pilon or tibial plafond fractures are characterized by high-energy mechanisms of injury that typically involve a distal tibial intra-articular fracture with associated comminuted metaphyseal fractures. The soft tissue envelope can be more significant than the bony injury itself and usually guides management.

Anatomy

Tibiotalar (Ankle) Joint

- A hinge joint providing ankle dorsiflexion and plantar flexion (-10 to $35°$) that allows small amounts of axial rotation
- Medial stability provided by medial malleoli (distal tibia) and deltoid ligament

- Lateral stability provided by lateral malleoli (fibula), both anterior and posterior talofibular ligaments, and calcaneofibular ligament
- Fibula positioned posterior to distal tibia in incisura

Ankle Syndesmosis

- Consists of the interosseous membrane (IOM), interosseous ligament (IOL), transverse tibiotalar ligament, anterior inferior tibiofibular ligament (AITFL), and posterior inferior tibiofibular ligament (PITFL)
- Functions to provide stability in a relative motion environment for the distal tibiofibular junction

Vascular

- Anterior tibial artery: runs in anterior compartment just anterior to IOM with deep peroneal nerve terminating in the foot as the dorsalis pedis artery (palpated at dorsal most prominence of navicular)
- Posterior tibial artery: runs in deep posterior compartment with tibial nerve terminating in the foot medially as plantar arteries (palpated posterior to medial malleoli)

J. Tidwell
Department of Orthopaedics,
UCSF Fresno, Fresno, CA, USA

P. Juliano (✉)
Department of Orthopaedics, Penn State,
Hershey, PA, USA
e-mail: pjuliano@hmc.psu.edu

© Springer International Publishing AG 2017
A.E.M. Eltorai et al. (eds.), *Orthopedic Surgery Clerkship*, DOI 10.1007/978-3-319-52567-9_86

- Peroneal artery: runs also in deep posterior compartment between tibialis posterior and flexor hallucis longus terminating in the foot as calcaneal branches (difficult to palpate)
- Vascular injury relatively uncommon given fracture limb shortening

Neurological

- Deep peroneal nerve (DPN): runs in anterior compartment with anterior tibial artery providing motor innervation to that compartment and supplying sensation to the first web space
- Superficial peroneal nerve (SPN): runs in lateral compartment providing motor innervation to that compartment and supplying sensation to the dorsum of the foot
- Tibial nerve: runs in deep posterior compartment with posterior tibial artery providing innervation to both superficial and deep posterior compartment's musculature and supplying sensation to the plantar aspect of the foot via the plantar nerves

Imaging

Radiographs

- Injury radiographs consisting of three views of the ankle (AP, lateral, and mortise) are most important imaging modality as they best represent fracture energy and initial displacement: AP/lateral views shown (Fig. 86.1a, b).
- Imaging of joint above and below fracture is necessary in trauma patients to rule out concomitant injury (knee, tibia, and foot films in addition to ankle).

CT Scan

- Dedicated ankle thin cut (1 mm) with coronal and sagittal reconstructions to be obtained prior to definitive fixation but after any planned staged treatment (external fixation) procedure

- Preoperative planning for fixation and approach based on this modality
- 3D reconstructions (if available) with talar subtraction may provide additional details especially for surface characteristics and comminution of fracture
- Axial CT cut showing named standard fracture components (Fig. 86.2)

Classification

AO/OTA Fracture Classification (4-tibia,3-distal)

- 43-A (extra-articular), 43-B (partial-articular), 43-C (intra-articular)
- Classified by amount of joint involvement and level of comminution (Fig. 86.3)
- Fibula fracture: present in ~75% of cases

Gustilo and Anderson Classification for Soft Tissue Injury in Open Fractures

- Grade I: wound up to 1 cm length, low energy, low level contamination, wound closeable with local tissue only, minimal fracture comminution
- Grade II: wound 1–10 cm length, moderate energy, moderate contamination, wound closeable with local tissue only, moderate fracture comminution
- Grade III: wound >10 cm, high energy, severe contamination, severe fracture contamination
  - Grade IIIA: wound does not require flap coverage (or skin graft only).
  - Grade IIIB: wound requires free flap coverage.
  - Grade IIIC: extremity requires revascularization procedure.

Tscherne Classification for Soft Tissue Injury in Closed Fractures

- Grade 0: minimal soft tissue damage from low-energy mechanism with simple fracture pattern

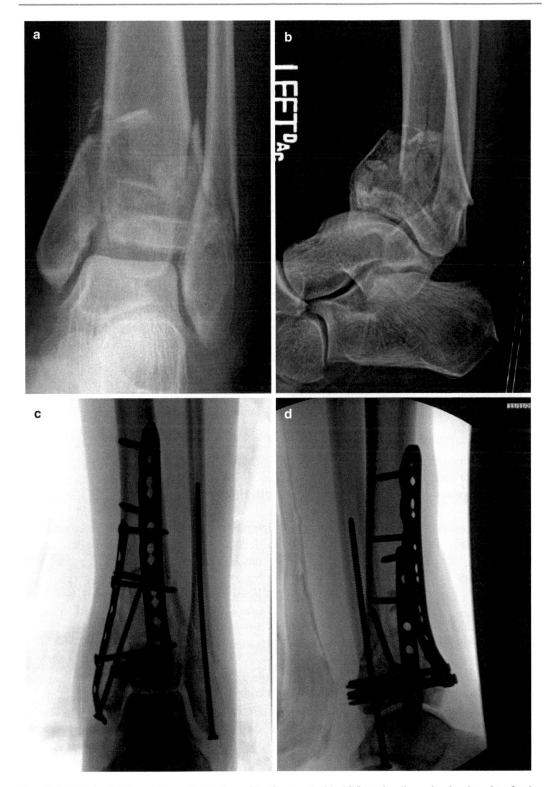

Fig. 86.1 AP/lateral injury radiograph of valgus pilon fracture (**a**, **b**). AP/lateral radiographs showing plate fixation (**c**, **d**) [5]

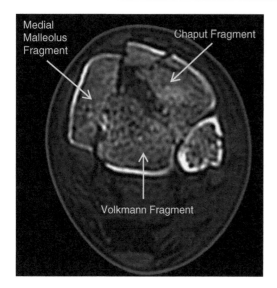

Medial Malleolus Fragment

Chaput Fragment

Volkmann Fragment

Fig. 86.2 Pilon fracture axial CT scan

- Grade 1: soft tissue skin contusion from low-energy mechanism with moderate fracture pattern
- Grade 2: soft tissue muscle contusion from direct high-energy mechanism with severe fracture pattern
- Grade 3: severe soft tissue damage from high-energy mechanism and/or crush injury that may result in compartment syndrome or subcutaneous avulsion

Presentation

Epidemiology

- Incidence:
  - 3–10% of all fractures of the tibia.
  - <1% of all fractures of the lower extremity.
  - 30–50% of patients have associated injuries (polytrauma).
  - 10–30% of patients have open fractures.
- Demographics: there is a significant male dominance with age range 25–40 typical.
- Mechanism of action: often high-energy motor vehicle crashes or falls from heights greater than 8 ft.
- Concurrent injuries: axial load injuries causing lumbar spine fractures, tibial plateau

fractures, calcaneal fractures, and talus and other forefoot fractures.

History and Physical Exam

- Determine medical and traumatic comorbidities for overall picture of patient.
- Specific history of smoking, vascular disease, and diabetes for patient risk stratification and prognosis.
- ATLS (Advanced Trauma Life Support) protocol and general orthopedic secondary examination for concomitant injury evaluation.
- Evaluate for bony deformities and/or dislocations.
- Palpate for Doppler dorsalis pedis and posterior tibialis arterial pulses.
- Examine sensation and motor function level for sural, saphenous, DPN, SPN, and tibial nerve.
- Always consider signs and symptom of compartment syndrome.
- Inspect soft tissues for skin tenting from fractures, blisters, and open wounds.

Treatment

Initial Treatment

Open Fracture Management
- Tetanus and antibiotic prophylaxis in accordance with open fracture grade.
- Secure picture of wound for documentation of initial wound and further orthopedic team evaluation of wound without taking down dressing.
- Irrigate/remove loose debris and place sterile gauze dressing over wound.

Subluxated or Dislocated Joint Management
- Urgently reduce joint to minimize damage to cartilage and protect skin and soft tissue from further injury.
- Stabilize fracture and soft tissue with splint.
- Determine need for ankle-spanning external fixator based on length stability of fracture at time of injury.

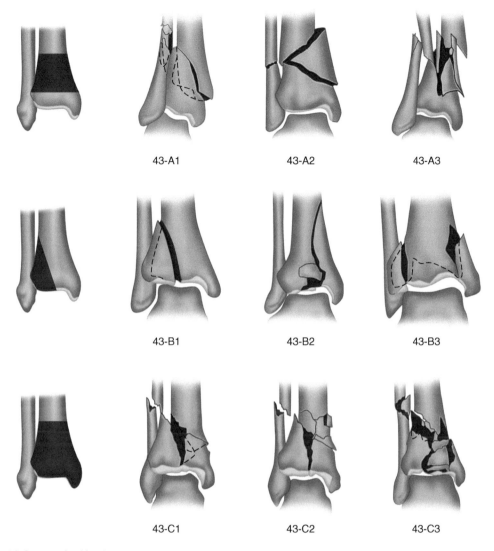

Fig. 86.3 AO fracture classification

Nonsurgical Treatment

- Close reduce fracture to best of ability and treat with long leg cast.
- Option for patients that are not good surgical candidates.
- Articular step-off likely cannot be reduced anatomically.
- Wound complications can still exist with need for casting which doesn't allow monitoring of soft tissue easily.

Surgical Treatment

- Primarily consists of temporary ankle-spanning external fixation followed by delayed surgical open reduction and internal fixation (ORIF) by experienced orthopedic trauma and/or orthopedic foot and ankle surgeon

Ankle-Spanning External Fixation

- Temporizing solution to maintain fracture length for ease of delayed reduction and fixation and to stabilize the fracture to calm soft tissue inflammation (usually left in place 10–14 days).

- Usually performed by connecting carbon fiber rods between a transcalcaneal pin and two tibial Schanz pins to form an A-frame (Fig. 86.4).
- Strict postoperative elevation is necessary to decrease extremity swelling.

Delayed ORIF
Common approaches

- Approach decisions.
  - Initial fracture displacement
    1. *Varus* fractures more likely to need *medial* buttress
    2. *Valgus* fractures more likely to need *lateral* buttress
  - Location of major fracture displacement (approach on this side)
  - Soft tissue injury (avoid areas of significant damage)
  - Location and/or presence of fibula fracture (must coordinate approach with same or extra incision to address fibula fracture)

- Anterolateral (Böhler).
  - Interval between peroneal brevis (SPN) and peroneus tertius (DPN).
  - Access to tibiotalar joint, distal tibia (except medial aspect of joint and malleolus), and fibula.
  - SPN must be identified superficially as it generally crosses the incision from lateral to medial.
  - DPN and anterior tibial artery must be protected under extensor tendons throughout case with gentle retraction.
  - Lower risk of soft tissue complications but difficult access to medial fracture lines.
- Anteromedial (extensile).
  - Interval between tibialis anterior laterally and medial malleolus medially.
  - Access to tibiotalar joint and medial malleolus.
  - Avoid the tendon sheath of tibialis anterior tendon.
  - Must protect DPN and anterior tibial artery with gentle retraction under extensor tendons while minimizing dissection.
  - Improved overall access to entire tibiotalar joint but higher incidence of soft tissue complications.

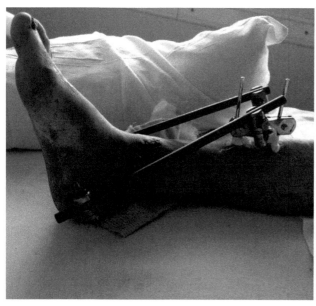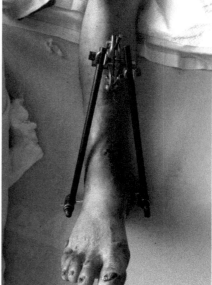

Fig. 86.4 Picture of an ankle spanning external fixator

- Separate approach to fibula fracture may be necessary.
- Posteromedial and posterolateral are utilized although less commonly for posterior fracture involvement.

Surgical goals

- Anatomic reduction of distal tibial articular surface
- Regain length of distal tibia and/or fibula
- Reconstruct distal tibial metaphyseal segment
- Reattach articular block to metaphyseal segment
- Avoid infection and soft tissue complications
- AP/lateral radiographs showing ORIF (Fig. 86.1c, d)

Circular Ring Fixation

- In the experienced hands, can be alternative treatment for patients with:
  - Significant bone loss
  - Need for surgical flap coverage
  - Continued soft tissue injury making ORIF risky for infection
  - Otherwise at risk of infection from ORIF or with previous failure of ORIF due to infection

Prognosis

- Generally poor outcomes that improve with improved articular reduction
- Poor prognostic indicators
  - Low socioeconomic status
  - Diabetes/smoker
  - Married
  - Two or greater comorbidities
  - Infection

Complications

- Overall common with high-energy pilon fractures
- Postoperative wound dehiscence/superficial infection (up to 20%)
- Infection/chronic osteomyelitis
  - Decreased rates with careful attention to soft tissue envelope prior to definitive fixation
  - Increased rates with increased Gustilo-Anderson open fracture grade
- Malunion/nonunion (up to 33%)
- Post-traumatic tibiotalar arthritis
  - Up to 50%
  - Increases with C-type fractures
- Tibiotalar joint stiffness (most patients experience decreased range of motion)

References

1. Barei D. Pilon fractures. In: Bucholz RW, Heckman JD, Court-Brown CM, Tornetta P, editors. Rockwood and Green's fractures in adults. 7th ed. Philadelphia: Lippincott Williams & Wilkins; 2010. p. 1929–73.
2. Ketz JP, Sanders RW. Pilon fractures. In: Coughlin MJ, Saltzman CL, Anderson RB, editors. Mann's surgery of the foot and ankle. 9th ed. Philadelphia: Elsevier Saunders; 2014. p. 1973–2002.
3. Bartlett III CS, Putnam RM, Endres NK. Fractures of the tibial pilon. In: Browner BD, Jupiter JB, Levine AM, Trafton PG, Krettek C, editors. Skeletal trauma: basic science, management, and reconstruction. 4th ed. Philadelphia: Elsevier Inc; 2009. p. 2453–514.
4. Crist BD, Khazzam M, Murtha YM, Della Rocca GJ. Pilon fractures: advances in surgical management. J Am Acad Orthop Surg. 2011;19:612–22.
5. Allen D. Tibial plafond fractures. In: Orthobullets. org[Internet]. Cambridge: Lineage Medical, LLC [updated 18 Aug 15]. Available from: http://www.orthobullets.com/trauma/1046/tibial-plafond-fractures.

87 Achilles Tendon Pathology

Ryan J. McNeilan and Grant L. Jones

Anatomy

- The achilles tendon is a confluence of distal gastrocnemius and soleus muscles, 10–15 cm in length, surrounded by a prominent paratenon
- Inserts on posterior superior calcaneus
- Largest and strongest tendon in the human body

Spectrum of Disorders

- Retrocalcaneal bursitis/insertional achilles tendinopathy
- Achilles tendinosis/tendonitis
- Achilles tendon rupture

Presentation

Retrocalcaneal Bursitis/Insertional Achilles Tendinopathy

- Insidious-onset heel pain at distal aspect of achilles tendon
- Enlarged posterosuperior calcaneal tuberosity may be palpable and/or visible
- Lateral imaging of ankle or foot film may show prominent posterosuperior calcaneal tuberosity (aka Haglund's deformity) (Fig. 87.1) and soft tissue swelling
- MRI not necessary for diagnosis but will show enhancement surrounding Haglund's deformity and achilles insertion

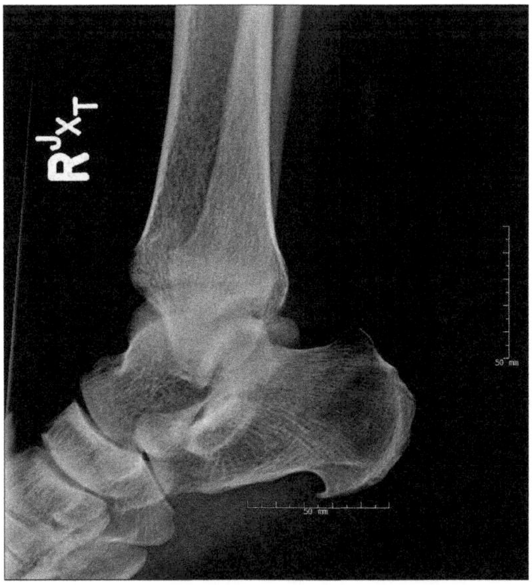

Fig. 87.1 Posterior superior calcaneal prominence aka Haglund's deformity

R.J. McNeilan (✉) • G.L. Jones
Department of Orthopaedics, The Ohio State University Wexner Medical Center, Columbus, OH, USA
e-mail: ryan.mcneilan@osumc.edu

A.E.M. Eltorai et al. (eds.), *Orthopedic Surgery Clerkship*, DOI 10.1007/978-3-319-52567-9_87

Achilles Tendinosis/Tendonitis (Non-insertional)

- Acute (more common in tendonitis) or chronic (more common in tendinosis) pain in the midsubstance of the achilles, worse with activity
- Pain exacerbated by passive ankle dorsiflexion, resisted ankle plantarflexion
- Radiographs typically normal but may demonstrate soft tissue swelling
- MRI not necessary for diagnosis but will demonstrate thickening of the tendon (tendinosis/tendinopathy) with or without intrasubstance enhancement

Achilles Tendon Rupture

- Acute onset of posterior ankle pain, commonly associated with feeling of being kicked or hit in the posterior ankle during an explosive sporting activity
- Tenderness at site of rupture commonly with a palpable gap
- Thompson test (Fig. 87.2) – with patient in prone position, squeeze the calf, and inspect motion of the foot; lack of plantarflexion is consistent with rupture of the tendon

- Radiographs demonstrate soft tissue swelling, asymmetry of achilles soft tissue shadow – bony avulsion or calcifications may be present though less common
- Ultrasound/MRI – both are effective methods for diagnosis and will demonstrate discontinuity of the tendon but neither are necessary for diagnosis

Treatment

Retrocalcaneal Bursitis/Insertional Achilles Tendinopathy

Nonoperative: First-Line Management Strategy
- Anti-inflammatory medications, activity modifications, eccentric stretching, shoe pads/bracing for comfort
- Corticosteroid injections controversial secondary to concerns of increased rupture rate

Operative: Indicated After Failed Nonoperative Management
- Open or endoscopic medial, lateral, or midline approach to the posterosuperior calcaneal tuberosity with excision of the bony prominence and debridement of the retrocalcaneal bursa with or without achilles elevation and repair

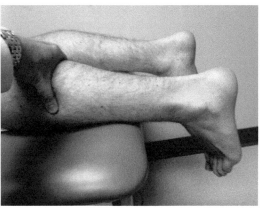 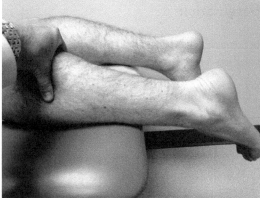

Fig. 87.2 Thompson test. Passive ankle plantarflexion with manual squeeze of the gastrocnemius-soleus muscle complex suggests an intact achilles tendon, as depicted below. Lack of ankle plantarflexion with squeeze of gastrocnemius-soleus complex is indicative of achilles tendon rupture

Achilles Tendinosis/Tendonitis (Non-insertional)

Nonoperative: First-Line Management Strategy
- Eccentric training
- Anti-inflammatory medications, activity modifications, shoe pads/bracing for comfort, immobilization in severe disease

Operative: Refractory Tendinosis or Tendinitis
- Percutaneous or endoscopic tenotomies
- Open paratenon release, debridement and tubularization of tendon
- Open debridement with tendon transfer, most commonly FHL, but use of FDL and plantaris has been reported

Achilles Tendon Rupture

Nonoperative
- Casting or bracing in equinus with graduated decrease in plantarflexion until reaching neutral
- Functional rehabilitation with early weight bearing and protected range of motion

Operative
- Acute
  - Open end-to-end repair with nonabsorbable suture is gold standard technique
  - New percutaneous techniques reported; however, risk of iatrogenic sural nerve damage remains a concern
- Chronic – FHL transfer

Outcomes Retrocalcaneal Bursitis/Insertional Achilles Tendinopathy

Nonoperative
- Success rates of 70–95% have been reported, though less likely with increasing size of the posterosuperior bony prominence.

Operative
- High success rates with no definitive superiority of aforementioned surgical treatment options

Achilles Tendinosis/Tendonitis (Non-insertional)

Nonoperative
- Success rates approach 90%.
- Eccentric training results in decreased tendon volume, decreased intratendinous signal, and improved clinical outcome [1].
- 82% of patients satisfied and returned to prior level of sport with eccentric stretching/strengthening program [2].

Operative
- Good/excellent success rates range from 60 to 90% across techniques.

Achilles Tendon Rupture

Nonoperative
- Functional rehabilitation with early weight bearing and protected range of motion has demonstrated re-rupture rates and functional outcomes similar to operative repair [3]

Operative
- Overall excellent results with most returning to prior activity level without strength deficits
- Re-rupture rates 2–5% [4–7]
- Higher complication rates than nonoperative secondary to soft-tissue-related problems

References

1. Shalabi A, Kristoffersen-Wilberg M, Svensson L, Aspelin P, Movin T. Eccentric training of the gastrocnemius-soleus complex in chronic Achilles tendinopathy results in decreased tendon volume and intratendinous signal as evaluated by MRI. Am J Sports Med. 2004;32(5):1286–96.

2. Mafi N, Lorentzon R, Alfredson H. Superior short-term results with eccentric calf muscle training compared to concentric training in a randomized prospective multicenter study on patients with chronic Achilles tendinosis. Knee Surg Sports Traumatol Arthrosc. 2001;9(1):42–7.
3. Soroceanu A, Sidhwa F, Aarabi S, Kaufman A, Glazebrook M. Surgical versus nonsurgical treatment of acute Achilles tendon rupture: a meta-analysis of randomized trials. J Bone Joint Surg Am. 2012;94(23):2136–43.
4. Nilsson-Helander K, Silbernagel KG, Thomeé R, Faxén E, Olsson N, Eriksson BI, Karlsson J. Acute Achilles tendon rupture: a randomized, controlled study comparing surgical and nonsurgical treatments using validated outcome measures. Am J Sports Med. 2010;38(11):2186–93.
5. Willits K, Amendola A, Bryant D, Mohtadi NG, Giffin JR, Fowler P, Kean CO, Kirkley A. Operative versus nonoperative treatment of acute Achilles tendon ruptures: a multicenter randomized trial using accelerated functional rehabilitation. J Bone Joint Surg Am. 2010;92(17):2767–75.
6. Cetti R, Christensen SE, Ejsted R, Jensen NM, Jorgensen U. Operative versus nonoperative treatment of Achilles tendon rupture. A prospective randomized study and review of the literature. Am J Sports Med. 1993;21(6):791–9.
7. Möller M, Movin T, Granhed H, Lind K, Faxén E, Karlsson J. Acute rupture of tendon Achillis. A prospective randomised study of comparison between surgical and non-surgical treatment. J Bone Joint Surg Br. 2001;83(6):843–8.

Other Foot Fractures

88

Brady W. Rhodes

Cuboid (Fig. 88.1)

Anatomy

- Most lateral bone of the five tarsal bones
- Superior surface faces superior lateral
- Inferior faces inferomedial
- Peroneus longus runs along the plantar ridge referred to as the peroneal ridge [1]

Fractures

- Fractures of the cuneiforms and cuboid constitute 8.4% of all tarsal fractures and 0.24% of all fractures [2]
- Often occur in conjunction with fifth metatarsal or calcaneal fractures
- Rare for there to be displacement of the cuboid
- Either classified as avulsion of body fractures
- Avulsion from the pull of the inferior calcaneocuboid ligament, occurs with adduction of the cuboid on the calcaneus [3]

B.W. Rhodes, DPM
Department of Orthopedics, John Peter Smith Hospital, Fort Worth, TX, USA
e-mail: brhodes@jpshealth.org

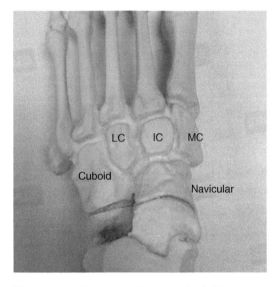

Fig. 88.1 Navicular, cuneiforms, and cuboid comprise the five most distal tarsal bones of the foot

Mechanism

- Foot hits the ground in a plantar-flexed position with axial forces directed up the lateral column
- "Nutcracker"
  - Described by Hermel and Gershon-Cohen
  - Caught like a nut in a nutcracker between the base of the fourth and fifth metatarsal and the calcaneus [4]

© Springer International Publishing AG 2017
A.E.M. Eltorai et al. (eds.), *Orthopedic Surgery Clerkship*, DOI 10.1007/978-3-319-52567-9_88

Treatment

Avulsion and Non-displaced Fractures
- 6–8 weeks in SLC and NWB

ORIF for Depressed Fractures

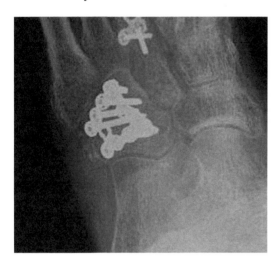

- Spanning ex-fix for compressed cuboid fractures

Complications

- CC arthritis
- Peroneal tendon subluxation/tendonitis

Navicular

Anatomy

- Previously called the scaphoid.
- Dorsal surface is convex.
- Plantar surface is continuous medially with the tuberosity.
- Groove for the PT tendon separates the plantar surface with the tuberosity.
- Plantar calcaneonavicular (spring) attaches to the plantar surface.
- PT tendon inserts on the tuberosity.
- Tuberosity can form secondary ossification center, "os tibiale externum" [1].

Fractures

- Body fractures represent 29% of all navicular fractures [2]
  - Classified as:
    ○ Non-displaced vertical/horizontal
    ○ Crush, stress, or displaced
    ○ Non-displaced vertical/horizontal most common [5]

Mechanism
- Fall with foot striking in plantar flexion [6]
- Plantar flexion and abduction at the MTJ [7]

Treatment

- Non-displaced fractures, 6–8 weeks SLC
- Displaced body fractures, closed reduction is difficult and ORIF recommended [8]

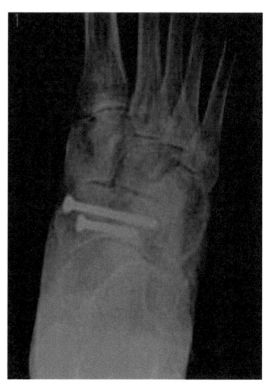

- Ex-fix for navicular crush injury

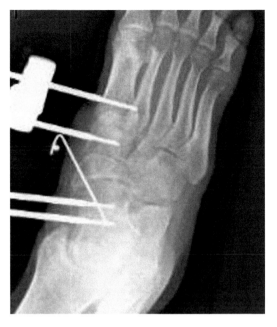

- Avulsion medially due to TA tendon
- Body fractures due to direct trauma or axial forces
- Isolated are difficult to see secondary to stable ligamentous complex about cuneiforms
- With dislocation, typically will be dislocated dorsally due to weaker dorsal ligaments [1]

Treatment

- Generally heal with SLC 6–8 weeks
- CT scan if difficult diagnosing
- Percutaneous pinning if dislocated
- ORIF rarely indicated due to stable nature of anatomy

Complications

- NC arthritis
- Nonunion

Complications

- TN arthritis
- Nonunion
- Central third of navicular relatively avascular [9]

Cuneiforms

Anatomy

- Apex of the medial cuneiform directed dorsally
- Other two cuneiforms apex directed plantarly
- Articulate with the navicular and met bases 1–3 [1]

Fractures

- Represent 4.2% of tarsal fractures
- 1.7% are isolated injuries and 2.5% associated with other F&A trauma [6]

References

1. Khan MA. Lower limb anatomy. 5th ed. Des Moines University; 2010, p. 7.
2. Eichenholtz SN, Levibe DB. Fractures of the tarsal navicular bone. Clin Orthop. 1964;34:142–57.
3. Day AJ. The treatment of injuries to the tarsal navicular. J Bone Joint Surg. 1947;26:359–66.
4. Hermel MB, Gershon-Cohen J. the nutcracker fracture of the cuboid by indirect violence. Radiology. 1953;60:850–4.
5. Goldman F. Fractures of the midfoot. Clin Podiatry. 1985;2:259–85.
6. Wilson PD. Fractures and dislocation of the tarsal bones. South Med J. 1933;26:833–45.
7. Eftekhar NM, Lyddon DW, Stevens J. An unusual fracture dislocation of the tarsal navicular. J Bone Joint Surg Am. 1969;51:577–781.
8. Ashurst PAC, Crossan ET. Fractures of the tarsal scaphoid and the os calcis. Surg Clin North Am. 1930;10:1477–87.
9. Torg JS, Pavlov H, Cooley LH, et al. Stress fracture of the tarsal navicular: a retrospective review of twenty one cases. J Bone Joint Surg Am. 1982;64:700–12.

The Diabetic Foot

Brad Wills and Michael D. Johnson

Abbreviations

ABI   Ankle-brachial index
TAL   Tendoachilles lengthening

Diabetes

Systemic disease marked by high blood glucose affecting the nervous, vascular, immune, integumentary, and musculoskeletal systems.

Types

- Type 1: Autoimmune destruction of B cells in the pancreas leading to insulin deficiency
- Type 2: Normal insulin production with developed insulin resistance

B. Wills, MD • M.D. Johnson, MD (✉)
Surgery – Orthopaedics, University of Alabama at Birmingham, Birmingham, AL, USA
e-mail: bradleywills@uabmc.edu;
michaeljohnson@uabmc.edu

Epidemiology

- 22.3 million Americans with diabetes in 2012, incurring an estimated $306 billion in direct medical costs [1]
- Estimated 15% lifetime risk of developing a foot ulcer

Pathophysiology

Nervous System

- Affects motor, sensory, and autonomic divisions via microvascular changes leading to focal nerve fiber loss
  - Typically presents with symmetric peripheral polyneuropathy
    - Inability to respond to mechanical stress due to neuropathy is often responsible for initial skin breakdown.
  - Autonomic nervous system helps regulate perspiration, skin temperature, and arteriovenous shunting [2].
    - Loss of autonomic regulation leads to thick skin that dries and cracks from loss of perspiration generating an avenue for infection.
    - Motor neuropathy is less common, but caused by demyelination [2].

Vascular System

- Microvascular disease contributes to the development of neuropathy, nephropathy, and retinopathy.
- Macrovascular disease can lead to peripheral artery disease, lower extremity infection, and amputation.

Immune System

- Alters polymorphonuclear leukocyte function creating an environment favorable for bacteria and impairing wound healing [3]

The Diabetic Foot

Evaluation

- Inspect the foot for bony prominences that may lead to pressure ulcers and for any ulcers that may have already developed. Record sizes and depth of ulcers.
- Neurologic evaluation:
  - Semmes-Weinstein test: Test foot sensation using a 5.07 monofilament. It is thought that if a patient has sensation to the 5.07 monofilament, then their protective sensation is intact [4].

Vascular Evaluation

- Ankle-brachial index (ABIs): Measurement of macrovascular involvement
  - Ratios greater than 1.0 are concerning for vessel calcification.
  - Ratios less than 0.9 are concerning for vascular disease, less than 0.45 is severe disease.
- Toe pressures: More accurate for assessing healing potential than ABIs
  - Greater than 45 mm Hg is need to heal an ulcer [4].
- Transcutaneous oxygen diffusion: Most accurate means of evaluating local perfusion
  - Greater than 30 mm Hg is associated with wound healing [4].

Radiographs

- Plain radiographs: Good for evaluating fractures and may provide evidence of osteomyelitis.
- MRI: Good for the diagnosis of osteomyelitis, although difficult to differentiate osteomyelitis from Charcot Foot on MRI. May characterize soft tissues and help evaluate for abscess formation.
- Technetium-99 bone scan is sensitive for detecting early osteomyelitis and may help differentiate from Charcot arthropathy.

Ulceration

Classifications

Brodsky Depth-Ischemia Classification [5]
- Class O: Intact skin, but foot at risk
- Class I: Superficial ulceration, not infected
- Class II: Deep ulceration with exposed tendon or joints, with or without infection
- Class III: Deep ulceration with exposed bone, deep infection, or abscess

Wagner Classification [5]
- Grade 0: Skin intact, but at risk
- Grade 1: Superficial ulcer
- Grade 2: Deeper, full-thickness extension to tendon or capsule
- Grade 3: Deep abscess formation or osteomyelitis, extends to bone
- Grade 4: Partial gangrene of forefoot
- Grade 5: Extensive gangrene

Treatment

- Brodsky Class 0 and I/Wagner Grade 0 and 1: Conservative
- Brodsky Class II and III/Wagener Grade 2: Wound care, surgical debridement, total contact casting, and antibiotics if infected
- Brodsky Class III/Wagener Grade 3: Surgical debridement, antibiotics, total contact casting
- Wagner Grade 4 and 5: Amputation

Conservative Treatment

- Footwear modification, patient education, total contact casts, local wound care

Surgical Management

- Osteotomy with or without tendoachilles lengthening (TAL) to help resolve areas under pressure at risk of ulceration.
- Evaluate need for gastrocnemius recession or TAL in patients with forefoot ulcers.
- With partial or complete gangrene patient may require amputation.

Associated Conditions

- Infection/osteomyelitis: diagnose with deep, surgical cultures and treat with the appropriate antibiotic.

Infection

Microbiology
- Commonly polymicrobial with aerobic and anaerobic bacteria

Treatment

- Initial treatment is broad-spectrum antibiotics.
- Antibiotics tailored to the bacteria grown from cultures:

- Gold standard for diagnosis of osteomyelitis is bone biopsy.
- Vascular supply must be adequate enough to perfuse the affected area with antibiotics; if not, then the patient may need surgical debridement or amputation.
- Fractures: Takes longer for diabetics to heal fractures, typically need to double the non-weight-bearing time.
- Neuropathic changes: Discussed in the chapter on Charcot foot.
- Amputation:
  - Performed in patient unable to heal ulcers secondary to impaired vascularity.
  - Common amputations include digital, ray, transmetatarsal, and below the knee amputations.
  - Tissue must be resected to healthy, bleeding tissue in order to maximize chances of healing.

References

1. American Diabetes Association. Economic costs of diabetes in the U.S. in 2012. Diabetes Care. 2013;36(4):1033–46.
2. Laughlin RT, et al. The diabetic foot. J Am Acad Orthop Surg. 1995;3:218–25.
3. Uhl RL, et al. Diabetes mellitus: musculoskeletal manifestations and perioperative considerations for the Orthopedic surgeon. J Am Acad Orthop Surg. 2014;22(3):183–92.
4. Coughlin ML, et al. Mann's surgery of the foot and ankle. Philadelphia: Saunders/Elsevier; 2014.
5. Lavery LA, et al. Classification of diabetic foot wounds. J Foot Ankle Surg. 1996;35(6):528–31.

Charcot Neuroarthropathy

90

Megan N. Severson and Michael D. Johnson

Background

- Definition: A destructive, non-infective process of bones and joints that occurs due to the loss of protective sensation that occurs with peripheral neuropathy
- Associations:
  - In the USA, most commonly associated with longstanding diabetes mellitus
  - Other associations include leprosy, tabes dorsalis, Charcot-Marie-Tooth, and alcohol abuse
- Patient burden: Commonly painless but associated with progressive deformity of the foot and joint instability leading to altered gait mechanics and load bearing
  - Increased risk for pressure ulcers, infections, and ultimately amputations
  - Increased patient morbidity and decreased quality of life

Pathophysiology

It is not clearly understood but there are currently two theories which both hinge on the idea that the patient's continued weight bearing in the face of injury leads to progressive destruction of the involved bones and joints [2–4].

Neurotraumatic Destruction

- Joint destruction, fractures, and foot collapse occur due to cumulative mechanical trauma.
- Can be major, minor, or microtrauma that the patient does not recognize due to lack of protective sensation in the foot.
- Continued activity and weight bearing propagate the destruction and inhibit the healing process.

Neurovascular Destruction

- Trauma or another trigger causes a state of hyperemia due to vasomotor autoneuropathy.
- Dysregulation of blood flow leads to cytokine mediated bone resorption and ligamentous weakening.
- Leads to bone breakdown and joint dislocation with progressive deformity due to continued high levels of pro-inflammatory cytokines.

M.N. Severson, MD
Division of Orthopedic Surgery, Department of Surgery, University of Alabama – Birmingham Hospital, Birmingham, AL, USA

M.D. Johnson, MD (✉)
Department of Orthopaedics, University of Alabama – Birmingham, Birmingham, AL, USA
e-mail: michaeljohnson@uabmc.edu

© Springer International Publishing AG 2017
A.E.M. Eltorai et al. (eds.), *Orthopedic Surgery Clerkship*, DOI 10.1007/978-3-319-52567-9_90

Presentation and Evaluation

Most present with a red, warm, swollen foot with a history of diabetes and no recollection of injury.

- Patients often present initially with a red, hot, swollen foot that is commonly misdiagnosed as cellulitis or osteomyelitis.
- Key finding in differentiating Charcot is that the erythema and swelling resolves with elevation of the limb. Osteomyelitis, cellulitis, or other infection will remain erythematous despite elevation.
- Will have evidence of peripheral neuropathy with decreased sensation with monofilament testing.
- May have concomitant vascular disease and workup with ankle-brachial indices (ABI's) and toe pressures may be warranted.
- Radiographs may show erosive changes and even new bone formation but lack the surrounding osteopenia associated with osteomyelitis. Joint subluxations and dislocations are commonly seen in advanced cases.
- Bone biopsy may be useful in differentiating between Charcot changes and osteomyelitis.

Staging/Classification

Modified Eichenholtz stages of Charcot arthropathy [5]

- Clinical/prefragmentation stage:
  - Red, hot, swollen foot with significant inflammation
  - Often confused with cellulitis and infection
  - Minimal changes on x-rays
- Dissolution/fragmentation stage:
  - Significant edema, warmth, erythema persists
  - Radiographs will show joint dislocation, bone fragmentation, and regional demineralization
- Coalescence:
  - Erythema, edema, and inflammation decreased
  - Bone debris absorbed, new periosteal bone formation, and early healing seen on x-rays

- Resolution:
  - Complete resolution of erythema, edema, and warmth
  - X-rays will show consolidation of healing with smooth bone edges and bony or fibrous ankyloses
  - Will likely have continued progression of deformity over time

Brodsky Anatomic Classification [1]

- Type 1 – involves the midfoot
  - Most common, about 60% of Charcot joints
  - Usually requires shorter treatment duration for healing
  - Progresses to classic "rocker bottom" foot deformity
  - High risk of development of pressure ulcers and associated infection
- Type 2 – involves the hindfoot joints: subtalar, talonavicular, calcaneocuboid
  - Significant instability but pressure sores and infection are less common
- Type 3 – tibiotalar joint involvement
  - Least common
  - Significant deformity, instability, and disability
  - Usually require significant bracing and/or surgical treatment

Treatment

- Goals are to preserve stability and alignment while the Charcot process evolves.
  - Initial treatment is total contact casting and protected weight bearing
  - Duration of casting depends on deformity and patient's ability to comply with non-weight bearing
  - Transition to AFO, Arizona brace, or CROW boot once initial warmth and swelling resolves
  - Shoe modification to unload pressure from bony prominences
  - If non-operative treatment fails, surgical treatment is considered. Options include

tendon Achilles lengthening, exostectomy, and fusion of affected joints

References

1. Ergen FB, Sanverdi SE, Oznur A. Charcot foot in diabetes and an update on imaging. Diabet Foot Ankle. 2013. doi: 10.3402/dfa.v4i0.21884. PubMed central PMCID: PMC3837304.
2. Johnson JE, Klein SE, Brodsky JW. Chapter 27: Diabetes. In: Coughlin MJ, Saltzman CL, Anderson RB, editors. Mann's surgery of the foot and ankle – expert consult, vol. 2. 9th ed. Philadelphia: Elsevier; 2014. p. 1385–480.
3. Kadakia AR, Irwin TA. Chapter 6: disorders of the foot and ankle. In: Miller MD, Thompson SR, Hart JE, editors. Review of Orthopedics. 6th ed. Philadelphia: Elsevier; 2012. p. 488–90.
4. Milne TE, Rogers JR, Kinnear EM, Martin HV, Lazzarini PA, Quinton TR, Boyle FM. Developing an evidence-based clinical pathway for the assessment, diagnosis and management of acute Charcot Neuro-Arthropathy: a systematic review. J Foot Ankle Res. 2013;6:30. PubMed CMID PMCID: PMC3737070.
5. Rosenbaum AJ, DiPreta JA. Classifications in brief: eichenholz classification of charcot arthropathy. J Clin Ortho Relat Res. 2015;473(3):1168–71.

Tarsal Tunnel Syndrome

Henry C. Hilario

Overview

- Tarsal tunnel syndrome (TTS) is a painful entrapment neuropathy caused by impingement of the tibial nerve as it passes through the tarsal tunnel.
- The tarsal tunnel is a fibro-osseous canal located posterior to the medial malleolus

Intrinsic Causes of TTS

- Space-occupying lesions such as a ganglion cyst, lipoma, tumor, osteophytes, or neurilemmoma
- Varicose veins
- Hypertrophy of tendons in the canal caused by trauma or overuse
- Accessory muscle that passes through the tunnel

Extrinsic Causes of TTS

- Trauma
- Foot Structure – flatfoot, subtalar joint coalition
- Postsurgical changes
- Shoe gear

H.C. Hilario, DPM
Department of Orthopedics, John Peter Smith Hospital, Fort Worth, TX, USA
e-mail: hhilario@jpshealth.org

Anatomy of the Tarsal Tunnel

Borders of the Tunnel

- Medially: flexor retinaculum that covers the contents of the tunnel
- Laterally: the calcaneus and talus
- Inferiorly: abductor hallucis muscle belly

Contents of the Tunnel Include Anterior to Posterior- (Pneumonic: *Tom Dick & A Very Nervous Harry*) (Fig. 91.1)

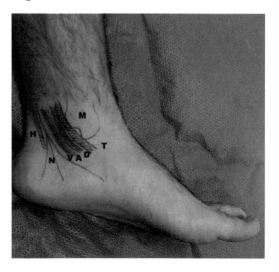

Fig. 91.1 *M* medial malleolus of ankle, *T* tibialis posterior tendon, *D* flexor digitorum longus tendon, *A* posterior tibial artery, *V* posterior tibial vein, *N* tibial nerve, *H* flexor hallucis longus tendon

A.E.M. Eltorai et al. (eds.), *Orthopedic Surgery Clerkship*, DOI 10.1007/978-3-319-52567-9_91

- Tibialis posterior tendon
- Flexor digitorum longus tendon
- Posterior tibial artery and vein
- Tibial nerve
- Flexor hallucis longus tendon

Tibial Nerve

- Branch of sciatic nerve, responsible for sensory innervation of plantar foot, motor innervation of intrinsic foot musculature
- Enters the canal as one nerve, branching into medial plantar nerve, lateral plantar nerve, and medial calcaneal nerve

Clinical Signs

History

- Commonly a diffuse pain at medial ankle, plantar foot that is poorly localized.
- Medial heel pain, burning, and paresthesias.
- Pain is worse with activity and long periods of standing.
- Relief with rest.

Physical Exam

- Tinel's sign – percussion of tibial nerve at medial ankle can illicit pain that radiates distally to plantar foot; feeling of "pins and needles"
- Neuritis that can radiate proximally as well (Valleix phenomenon)
- Compression with manipulation – plantarflexion and inversion of the ankle

Diagnostic Tests

- Clinical diagnosis is key for tarsal tunnel syndrome.

- Weight-bearing X-rays – to evaluate for any osseous coalition or trauma.
- Ultrasound can be technician dependent and can diagnose ganglia and varicose veins.
- MRI – Good for evaluating any space-occupying lesions.
- EMG, NCV – can help confirm diagnosis, can have some false negatives:
  - Medial plantar nerve to abductor hallucis muscle should be <6.2 ms.
  - Lateral plantar nerve to abductor digiti minimi muscle should be <7.0 msec.
  - If difference is greater than 1 ms, it can indicate tarsal tunnel syndrome.
  - EMG is considered more sensitive.
- Other differential diagnoses:
  - Radiculopathy – this will have a + straight leg test, calf muscle atrophy, low back radiating pain
  - Sensory polyneuropathy – bilateral presentation, absent Tinel's
  - Important to test for diabetes, thyroid disease, alcoholism in cases of neuropathy
- Of the three following findings – neuritic symptoms, positive NCV, + Tinel's sign:
  - If you have none of these, it can eliminate tarsal tunnel syndrome as differential.
  - If one finding present, can keep as differential. If two, high chance of tarsal tunnel

Treatment

Nonoperative

- Dependent on etiology of the pain
- Not indicated if there is a mass present causing symptoms
- Nonsteroidal anti-inflammatories, oral vitamin B_6
- Selective serotonin reuptake inhibitors or anti-seizure medications (gabapentin)
- Compression stockings – in cases of venous congestion
- Bracing, orthotics – for those with rearfoot instability

Operative

- Release of the entire flexor retinaculum
- Also recommended to release the deep fascia of abductor muscle belly which is another area of nerve compression along the tunnel

Outcomes

- Those with removal of space-occupying lesions that are etiology of the tunnel syndrome tend to do better.
- Approximately 75% of those treated surgically have some pain relief compared to pre-op.

Complications

- Recurrence – repeat surgery not often recommended
- Scar tissue – avoid excessive dissection
- CRPS type 2 – edema, allodynia, hyperalgesia, skin color, temperature change

Suggested Reading

1. Coughlin MJ, Saltzman CL, Anderson RB. Mann's surgery of the foot and ankle. Tarsal tunnel syndrome. Mosby; 2013. Print..
2. Kelikian AS, Sarrafian SK, Sarrafian SK. Sarrafian's anatomy of the foot and ankle. Philadelphia: Wolters Kluwer Health/Lippincott Williams & Wilkins; 2011. Print
3. McGlamry ED, Southerland JT. Mcglamry's comprehensive textbook of foot and ankle surgery. Philadelphia: Wolters Kluwer Health/Lippincott Williams & Wilkins; 2013. Print
4. Pinzur MS. Orthopedic knowledge update: foot and ankle. Rosemont: American Academy of Orthopedic Surgeons; 2009. Print.

Peroneal Tendon Pathology

92

Christopher Arena and Paul Juliano

Anatomy

Peroneus Longus (PL)

- Insertion: first metatarsal, medial cuneiform
- Action: plantar flexion of first ray and ankle
- At level of lateral malleolus: posterior to PB
- Os peroneum: <20% population, sesamoid within PL substance plantar to cuboid or lateral to calcaneus [5]

Peroneus Brevis (PB)

- Insertion: fifth metatarsal (MT) base
- Action: primary evertor of the foot
- At level of lateral malleolus: anterior/medial to PL
- "Brevis = bone" – closer to the fibula at level of the lateral malleolus (Fig. 92.1)

C. Arena, MD (✉)
Department of Orthopaedics and Rehabilitation, Penn State Milton S. Hershey Medical Center,
Hershey, PA, USA
e-mail: carena@hmc.psu.edu

P. Juliano, MD
Orthopaedics, Penn State, Hershey, PA, USA

Force Couples: Opposing Pulling Forces

- Tibialis anterior vs. peroneus longus.
- Tibialis posterior vs. peroneus brevis.
- Tendons travel superficial to calcaneofibular ligament (CFL).
- Innervation: superficial peroneal nerve (lateral compartment of the leg).

Tendon Stability

- Superior peroneal retinaculum (SPR) – primary restraint in peroneal tendon stability. Attaches from posterior ridge of fibula to lateral wall of calcaneus
- Inferior peroneal retinaculum
- Fibula sulcus – distal to fibula, concave

Anomalies

- Low-lying PB muscle belly (normally tendinous 2–3 cm proximal to tip of fibula), peroneus quartus muscle, and hypertrophied peroneal tubercle [1]
- Leads to laxity of SPR and peroneal tendon pathology

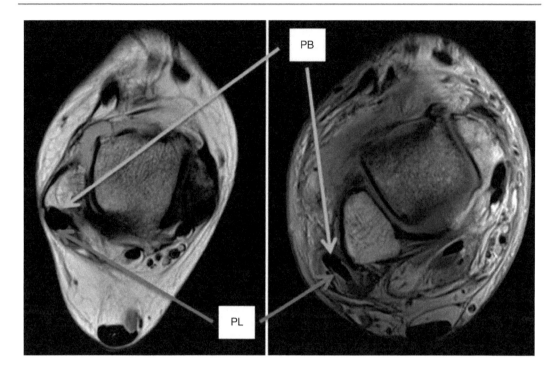

Fig. 92.1 Comparison of normal anatomy vs. peroneus longus subluxation. The figure on the left demonstrates normal peroneal tendon anatomy with the peroneus brevis ("brevis = bone") anterior and medial to the peroneus longus and closer to the fibula in the retromalleolar groove. The figure on the right demonstrates subluxation of the peroneal tendons with disruption of the superior peroneal retinaculum (Courtesy of S.A. Bernard, MD., Penn State Hershey Medical Center, Department of Radiology)

Tendon Subluxation

- Injury sustained during forceful contraction of peroneal tendons with foot plantar flexion and inversion. Patients with hindfoot varus more prone to injury [1]
- Shallow retromalleolar groove: more prone to anterior subluxation of tendon
- Skiing
- Differentiate from ankle sprains
    - Sprain: pain over anterior talofibular ligament
    - Peroneal tendon: retromalleolar pain
- Exam: lateral ankle pain, posterior fibular pain, pain with resisted eversion, passive inversion, resisted plantar flexion of first MT. Popping/crepitus of the distal fibula during forceful eversion and dorsiflexion of the ankle

Imaging

- Weight bearing XR – fleck avulsion of distal fibula – SPR injury.
- Ultrasound.
- CT – osseous anatomy – peroneal tubercle hypertrophy, calcaneal fractures, and convexity of distal fibula (risk factor for tendon subluxation).
- MRI: T2-weighted signal may indicate tenosynovitis, tendinosis, and tear. Tendons may lay lateral or anterior to fibula (Fig. 92.1). Fluid collection within the common peroneal tendon sheath [4].
- Magic angle artifact: increased signal on MRI with short echo time (T1) in linear tissues at an angle approximately 55° to magnetic field may be mistaken for fluid signal (i.e., tendonitis) (Fig. 92.2) [4].

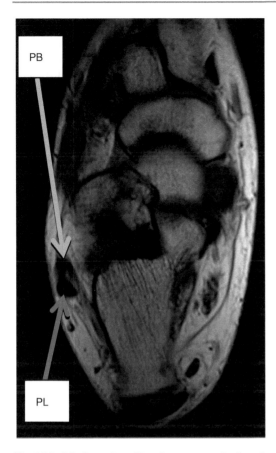

Fig. 92.2 Magic angle artifact demonstrates the "magic angle artifact" affecting the peroneus brevis (anterior) but not the peroneus longus in this axial MRI. Increased peroneus brevis (*PB*) signal artifact may be mistaken for pathologic fluid signal compared to normal-appearing low-signal peroneus longus (*PL*) in this image (Courtesy of S.A. Bernard, MD., Penn State Hershey Medical Center, Department of Radiology)

Treatment

- Conservative treatment: compressive dressing reinforced with a splint fabricated with keyhole pad over lateral malleolus providing support to SPR and peroneal tendon. Transition to plantar flexed/inverted cast for 6 weeks followed by ankle proprioception and strengthening rehabilitation [1]
- Surgical: stabilize peroneal tendons [2]
  - Bony procedures: peroneal groove deepening, bone block

- Soft tissue procedures: SPR repair – plication, advancement, and reattachment to malleolar ridge. Achilles tendon sling used to reinforce SPR. Re-route tendons beneath calcaneal fibular ligament
- Correct hindfoot varus if present – lateralizing calcaneal osteotomy

Peroneus Brevis Tears

- Occurs during anterior subluxation of tendon out of the groove and is tensioned over posterior ridge of fibula [1]
- Retromalleolar pain, history of chronic ankle sprains/instability
- Imaging: MRI – split PB appears as a "C-shaped" lesion at or below level of lateral malleolus [4]
- Treatment
  - Conservative: usually unsuccessful (NSAID, activity modification)
  - Surgical: assess SPR competence, incise SPR (tension and repair during closure), and evaluate location of tear [2, 3]
    ◦ Anterior one third tear: excise
    ◦ Middle tear: primary suture repair
    ◦ >50% tendon involvement/fraying: excision and tenodesis to peroneus longus tendon

Peroneus Longus Tears

- Uncommon
- Risk factors: diabetes, hyperparathyroidism, rheumatoid arthritis, psoriasis, ankle instability, hindfoot varus, and hypertrophied peroneal tubercle [1]
- Causes: direct trauma and long-standing tenosynovitis
- Exam: pain with plantar flexion of first MT
- Imaging: MRI may see fracture of os perineum [4]
- Treatment
  - Conservative: NSAID and activity modification

– Surgical: debridement, tubularization, end-to-end repair, and tenodesis to PB if distal tear with side-to-side suture repair [2]

Painful Os Peroneum Syndrome

- Sesamoid found in the peroneus longus tendon adjacent to cuboid
- History: lateral ankle trauma or supination-inversion injuries
- Exam
  – Tender over peroneus longus distal to fibula
  – Exacerbated by resisted plantar flexion of first ray, heel rise phase of gait cycle
  – Weak/painful foot eversion
- Imaging: MRI, XR – migration of os perineum, multipartite os, and enlarged peroneal tubercle compared to contralateral foot
- Treatment
  – Conservative: cast immobilization (4–6 weeks), corticosteroid injections

– Surgical
  ◦ Excision of os peroneum with primary peroneus longus tendon repair [2, 3]
  ◦ Excision of os peroneum with PB tenodesis [2, 3]

References

1. Padanilam T. Disorders of the anterior tibial, peroneal, and achilles tendons. In: Chou LB, editor. Orthopedic knowledge update: foot and ankle 5: American Academy Orthopedic Surgeons; 2014. p. 357–61.
2. Philbin TM, et al. Peroneal tendon injuries. J Am Acad Orthop Surg. 2009;17:306–17.
3. Jones CJ. Tendon disorders of the foot and ankle. J Am Acad Orthop Surg. 1993;1:87–94.
4. Recht MP, et al. Magnetic resonance imaging of the foot and ankle. J Am Acad Orthop Surg. 2001;9:187–99.
5. Sobel M, Pavlov H, Geppert MJ, Thompson FM, DiCarlo EF, Davis WH: Painful os peroneum syndrome: A spectrum of conditions responsible for plantar lateral foot pain. Foot Ankle Int 1994;15:112–24.

Adult-Acquired Flat Foot Deformity

93

Satheesh K. Ramineni

Definition

- Also called as posterior tibial tendon dysfunction.
- It results from insufficiency of posterior tibial tendon.

Anatomy and Function

- Origin: from the interosseous membrane and adjacent surfaces of the proximal one-third of the tibia and fibula.
- Course: behind the medial malleolus in a groove and held in place by the flexor retinaculum.
- Insertion: has eleven insertions which include the navicular; the sustentaculum tali; the medial, middle, and lateral cuneiforms; the cuboid; and the bases of the second, third, and fourth metatarsals.
- Function: Inversion of the subtalar joint, adduction and supination of the forefoot, and an accessory plantar flexion of the ankle.
- The tendon sheath runs approximately 45 mm proximal to the apex of the medial malleolus

and continues approximately 26 mm distal to the tip of medial malleolus.
- The excursion of the tendon is only 2 cm.
- The tendon receives blood supply from the posterior tibial artery at the level of the musculotendinous junction and the periosteal vessels at the tendon-bone interface at the insertion which are the branches of the medial plantar branch of the posterior tibial artery and by the medial tarsal artery, a branch of the dorsalis pedis artery.
- It stabilizes the hindfoot against valgus forces or eversion.
- It is a stance phase muscle, firing from heel strike to shortly after heel lift-off.
- It decelerates the subtalar joint pronation following heel strike through eccentric contraction.
- It stabilizes the midtarsal joints at midstance.
- During the propulsive phase, it adducts the transverse tarsal joint initiating inversion of the subtalar joint.

Pathophysiology

- Due to its limited excursion, any insult that lengthens the tendon has an adverse effect on its function.
- The valgus deformity of the hindfoot results from dysfunction of the posterior tibial tendon

S.K. Ramineni
Orthopaedic Surgery, University of Toledo Medical Center, Toledo, OH, USA
e-mail: satheesh.ramineni@utoledo.edu

© Springer International Publishing AG 2017
A.E.M. Eltorai et al. (eds.), *Orthopedic Surgery Clerkship*, DOI 10.1007/978-3-319-52567-9_93

which alters the mechanical pull of the Achilles tendon.

- The Achilles tendon is placed lateral to the axis of the subtalar joint allowing it to become an everter of the hindfoot accelerating the valgus deformity.
- Inability of the posterior tibial tendon to lock the transverse tarsal joint results in loss of rigid lever arm of the foot at push off which accelerates attrition of the spring ligament with each gait cycle.

Etiology

- Trauma and inflammation were proposed as the most common possible etiological factors.
- Vascular cause was suggested by other authors.
- Zone of hypovascularity (14 mm long) presents approximately 40 mm proximal to the insertion of the posterior tibial tendon.
- Two anatomic theories exist as to posterior tibial tendon attrition.
  - The first potential agent is the overlying constricting flexor retinaculum which can cause compression and constriction of the tendon.
  - The second possible factor is the sharp turn or angle behind the medial malleolus that creates excessive friction with physical activity.
- Congenital pes planus is strongly associated with later development of PTT dysfunction.
- The presence of accessory navicular has a high correlation with the development of PTT dysfunction.
- The cause is most likely multifactorial and patient specific.

Physical Exam

- Evaluate in standing and sitting.
- Hindfoot valgus from the front and behind.
- Collapse of the medial arch.
- Swelling or fullness about the medial malleolus in early stages.

- Abduction of the forefoot (too many toes sign).
- Forefoot develops compensatory varus from hindfoot valgus.
- Tenderness along the PTT, sinus tarsi, and subfibular region.
- Loss of inversion strength of the PTT.
- Positive single heel rise test.

Clinical Staging

- Stage 1: Tenosynovitis of the PTT. No flatfoot deformity. Pain and tenderness along the medial ankle. Preserved length of the tendon. Patient will be able to perform single heel rise, but repetitive heel rise may reproduce pain.
- Stage 2: Flexible flatfoot deformity. Pain along the medial ankle. Elongation and degeneration of the tendon. Patient is unable to perform single heel rise. Divided into stages 2A and 2B:
  - Stage 2A: No abduction of forefoot with >50% coverage of the talar head by navicular
  - Stage 2B: Abduction of the forefoot with <50% coverage of the talar head by navicular
- Stage 3: Rigid flatfoot deformity. Tight gastrocnemius-soleus complex with fixed forefoot varus of atleast 10–15°. Often, pain along the medial ankle is absent, and complains of pain along the lateral ankle and hindfoot. Unable to perform single heel rise. Degenerative joint disease of the subtalar, talonavicular, and calcaneocuboid joints.
- Stage 4: Rigid flatfoot deformity with valgus deformity of the ankle joint due to attenuation of the deltoid ligament.

Imaging

- Standard views include standing AP, mortise, and lateral views of the ankle and standing AP, oblique, and lateral views of the foot.
- AP view:
  - The talocalcaneal angle, the talometatarsal angle, and the articular congruity angle

- Talocalcaneal angle: Angle between the longitudinal axis of the talus and the calcaneus
- Talometatarsal angle: Angle between the longitudinal axis of the talus and the first metatarsal
- Articular congruity angle: Angle between the perpendicular lines to the articular surface of the talus and navicular
- Lateral view: The lateral talometatarsal angle – The angle between the longitudinal axis of the talus and the first metatarsal.

MRI

- MRI is an excellent modality for detecting sheath inflammation, soft tissue resolution, and anatomic detail of the tendon.
- Stage 1: Fluid filled synovial sheath, increased diameter of the tendon, split tears of the tendon on T1 images.
- Stage 2: Elongation of the tendon with increase in diameter of the tendon.
- Stage 3: Complete rupture is often visualized on T1 images, sinus tarsi syndrome with decreased T1 signal in sinus tarsi and subfibular impingement.

Conservative Treatment

- Resting or relieving the tension on the tendon with the use of a lace-up ankle brace and a CAM walker or a cast in patients with severe pain for 4–6 weeks.

- Anti-inflammatory medication for a complete 2-week course.
- Oral and injectable corticosteroids are not recommended.
- Physical therapy modalities with dexamethasone iontophoresis and cryotherapy. Ultrasound not recommended.
- PTT strengthening once the acute pain has subsided.
- Medial arch support for stage 2 dysfunction.
- Bracing with custom molded Arizona or University of California at Berkeley Laboratories (UCBL) for patients with stage 3 and stage 4 dysfunction.
- Conservative treatment attempted for 3–6 months unless a severe structural deformity is present for stage 2 or 3 dysfunction and 6-week trial for stage 1 dysfunction.

Surgical Treatment

- Stage 1: Tenosynovectomy
- Stage 2A: Flexor digitorum longus tendon transfer with medial displacement calcaneal osteotomy
- Stage 2B
  - Flexor digitorum longus tendon transfer with medial displacement calcaneal osteotomy, lateral column lengthening
  - Fixed forefoot varus more than 10°: Plantar flexion osteotomy of the medial cuneiform
- Stage 3: Triple arthrodesis (arthrodesis of subtalar talonavicular, and calcaneocuboid joints)
- Stage 4: Triple arthrodesis with ankle arthrodesis

Plantar Fasciitis

Andrew E. Hanselman and Robert D. Santrock

Introduction

Epidemiology and Etiology [1–3]

- Two-million patients in the United States treated for heel pain annually, representing 1% of all visits to orthopedic surgeons.
- Plantar fasciitis accounts for 80% of patients with heel pain symptoms.
- Peak incidence between ages 40 and 60 years old. Affects men and women equally.
- Risk factors include body mass index (BMI) > 30 kg/m², prolonged standing, equinus contracture, and runners.

Pathophysiology [1–3]

- Likely a degenerative process of the plantar fascia, as opposed to an inflammatory process, that involves fascial microtears, myxoid degeneration, angiofibroblastic hyperplasia, and collagen necrosis.
- Chronic overuse and repetitive trauma.

A.E. Hanselman, MD (✉) • R.D. Santrock, MD
Department of Orthopedics, Health Sciences South,
PO Box 9196, Morgantown, WV 26506, USA
e-mail: ahansel1@hsc.wvu.edu;
rdsantrock@hsc.wvu.edu

- Although "heel spurs" may be seen in patients with plantar fasciitis, there is no direct correlation.

Anatomy

Plantar Fascia
- Thick, fibrous aponeurosis that originates on the anteromedial aspect of the calcaneal tuberosity and inserts onto the bases of the proximal phalanges
- Helps to support the arch of the foot and functions as a key component to the "windlass mechanism" of the foot

Heel Fat Pad
- Subcutaneous fat surrounding the heel that acts as a hindfoot cushion
- Begins to deteriorate after age 40, but rarely of clinical significance

Clinical Evaluation

History

- Most commonly a diagnosis based on the patient's history and physical exam findings
- Gradual onset of medial heel pain

© Springer International Publishing AG 2017
A.E.M. Eltorai et al. (eds.), *Orthopedic Surgery Clerkship*, DOI 10.1007/978-3-319-52567-9_94

- Worse in the morning or after prolonged sitting/standing ("start-up pain")
- Improves with ambulation, however, worse at the end of the day

Physical Exam

- Pain concentrated at the plantar medial heel (medial tubercle of the calcaneus) that is exacerbated with passive dorsiflexion of ankle and toes.
- Achilles stiffness (equinus contracture) resulting in limited ankle dorsiflexion.
- Pes planus or cavus deformities may be present.

Imaging

- Limited role and often not required to make diagnosis.
- Radiographs, magnetic resonance imaging (MRI), bone scans, and ultrasound may be used to rule out other causes of heel pain.

Differential Diagnoses

- Numerous other causes of heel pain, such as tarsal tunnel syndrome, peripheral neuropathy, calcaneal stress fracture, systemic arthroses, fat pad atrophy, Achilles tendinitis, subtalar arthritis, and posterior tibial tendinitis

Treatment [1–3]

Nonsurgical

Overview
- Most patients respond to nonoperative treatment.
  - Studies have shown 90% success in patients treated conservatively for 6–10 months.
- American Orthopaedic Foot and Ankle Society (AOFAS) recommends minimum 6–12 months of nonoperative treatment before surgical intervention.

Stretching
- Achilles stretching to treat the equinus contracture is shown to be the best solution for long-term resolution.
- Addition of a plantar fascia-specific stretch protocol (PFSS) shown to have increased effectiveness and to be the most satisfactory to patients.

Splinting
- Night splinting keeps ankle dorsiflexed and prevents plantar fascia from contracting during periods of inactivity.
- Patient compliance may be an issue.

Casting
- May be beneficial in certain patient populations unresponsive to other nonoperative therapies, however, not common first-line treatment

Foot Orthoses
- Better patient compliance compared to night splinting.
- Custom-made orthotics has not been shown to be more beneficial than lower-cost prefabricated orthotics.

NSAIDs
- Some studies have shown a trend toward symptom improvement, however, not fully supported in literature.

Injections
- Corticosteroid injection
  - Often combined with a local anesthetic
  - Common intervention, although efficacy not supported in the literature
  - Risk of plantar fascia rupture and fat pad atrophy
- Botulinum toxin type A (Botox) injection
  - Although limited, benefits are shown in several smaller studies.
- Several new treatments still under investigation
  - Hyaluronic acid
  - Amniotic membrane
  - Platelet rich plasma

Extracorporeal Shock Wave Therapy (ESWT)

- Based on lithotripsy technology with shock waves targeted at the plantar fascia
- Theorized to induce injury which results in localized inflammation, neovascularization, and repair of tissue
- Low energy: more frequent treatments and does not require sedation but shown to have lower efficacy
- High energy: less frequent treatment and requires sedation or regional anesthesia but shown to have higher efficacy
- Good results supported in literature

Surgical

Plantar Fascia Release

- Partial vs full release
- Open vs endoscopic
- May include releases of the proximal and distal tarsal tunnel

Gastrocnemius Recession

- May be performed in isolation or in combination with plantar fascia release

References

1. Aiyer A. Plantar fasciitis. www.orthobullets.com.
2. DiGiovanni BF, Dawson LK, Baumhauer JF. Plantar heel pain. In: Coughlin MJ, Saltzman CL, Anderson RB, editors. Mann's surgery of the foot and ankle. 9th ed. Philadelphia: Elsevier; 2014. p. 685–705.
3. Neufeld SK, Cerrato R. Plantar fasciitis: evaluation and treatment. J Am Acad Orthop Surg. 2008;16(6):338–46.

Morton's Neuroma

David Arsanious and Kafai Lai

Introduction

- Interdigital (Morton's) neuroma is a benign enlargement of, most commonly, the third common digital branch of the medial plantar nerve. The majority of the literature reports that the neuroma usually involves the third webspace, but neuromas in the second webspace have been noted. An interdigital neuroma of the first or fourth webspace probably does not exist as a clinical entity [1].
- Demographics: Women are up to ten times more likely than men to be affected; age at presentation is typically 40–60 years [3].

Anatomy

- The third common plantar digital nerve, which passes between the third and fourth metatarsal heads in the third webspace, is a branch of the medial plantar nerve. The common plantar

digital nerves pass deep to the deep transverse metatarsal ligament [6] (Fig. 95.1).
- In approximately one in four individuals, there is also a communicating branch that connects the medial and lateral plantar nerves. The increased thickness of the third common plantar digital nerve due to the communicating branch from the lateral plantar nerve suggests that it may be predisposed to entrapment, explaining why

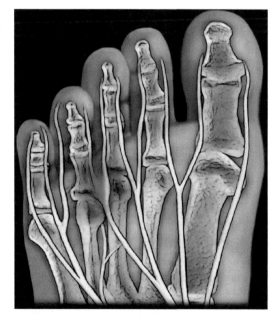

Fig. 95.1 Course of the medial and lateral plantar nerve. A communicating branch occurs in about 27% of patients

D. Arsanious (✉)
University of Vermont College of Medicine,
Burlington, VT, USA
e-mail: david.arsanious@med.uvm.edu

K. Lai
Orthopaedics, The University of Toledo Medical
Center, Toledo, OH, USA
e-mail: Kafai.Lai@utoledo.edu

the third webspace is the most frequently encountered location [3, 6] (Fig. 95.1).

Pathogenesis

- Four main differing opinions on the underlying pathological process [3, 5, 6] – true pathology likely multifactorial:
  - Trauma theory – repetitive trauma occurs to the forefoot, particularly aggravated during walking
  - Ischemic theory – supported by degenerative arterial changes, thrombosis, and incomplete recanalization seen in resected lesions
  - Intermetatarsal bursitis theory – an inflamed bursa in the third webspace will lie close to the common digital neurovascular bundle and cause fibrosis of the nerve
  - Entrapment theory – the common digital nerve becomes trapped by the deep transverse metatarsal ligament during ambulation

Histopathology

- Perineural fibrosis, increased number of intravascular arterioles with thickened walls, demyelinization and degeneration of nerve fibers, endoneural edema, and bursal tissue frequently accompanies specimen [6].
- The term neuroma is actually a misnomer in this condition. Axonal proliferation seen in traumatic neuromas is not seen. The pathological process is degenerative and not proliferative [6].

Clinical Presentation

History and Physical Findings [1, 2, 5]

- Burning, aching, or cramping plantar pain in the third webspace.
- Neuroma may be palpable.
- Duration varies from few weeks to many years.
- Pain is aggravated by walking in shoes with a narrow toe box or high heels.

- Pain is relieved by rest, removing the shoe, or massaging the forefoot.
- About half of patients report pain radiating to the toes or that be associated with paresthesia in some cases.
- Plantar tenderness in the webspace is the most common physical exam finding.
- Usually unilateral.

Provocative Tests

- Mulder's sign – the first and fifth metatarsal heads are manually squeezed together with one hand, and the thumb and index finger of the other is used to compress the site of the suspected neuroma. A click may be audible when the neuroma slides past the deep transverse metatarsal ligament [2, 3] (Fig. 95.2).
- Digital nerve stretch test – toes on either side of the affected webspace are passively extended and the ankle dorsiflexed, with both feet on the examiner's knees. Pain or discomfort in the webspace indicates a positive test [2, 3].

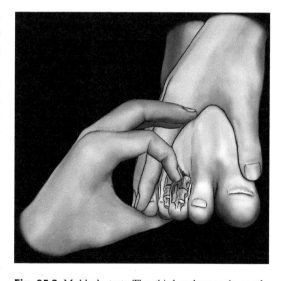

Fig. 95.2 Mulder's test: The third webspace is gently compressed between the examiner's index finger (plantar) and thumb (dorsal). With the opposite hand, the examiner compresses the forefoot mediolaterally with the other hand. A click with reproduction of the patient's pain is sometimes appreciated

- MTP joint plantarflexion – causes little pain in the setting of Morton's neuroma, but suggests MTP joint synovitis [2, 3].

Imaging

- Diagnosis is most often clinical, on the basis of the history and physical exam. Radiological investigations should be reserved for unconvincing presentations or suspected multiple lesions or to rule out another pathology [2].

Differential Diagnosis

- Metatarsophalangeal joint synovitis
- Freiberg osteochondrosis
- Stress fracture of the metatarsal neck
- Metatarsalgia
- Tarsal tunnel syndrome
- Peripheral neuropathy
- Lumbar radiculopathy
- Unrelated soft tissue tumor (ganglioma, lipoma, etc.)

Nonoperative Treatment

- Modifications to footwear: avoidance of high heels, shoe with wide toe box, metatarsal pads placed just proximal to the metatarsal heads, orthotics [1, 3, 7].
- Oral anti-inflammatory medications: steroids or NSAIDs [1, 3, 7].
- (Ultrasound guided) Corticosteroid and local anesthetic injections – 40 mg Depo-Medrol and 1 cc 0.25% Marcaine [5] (Fig. 95.3)
  - This may be both therapeutic and diagnostic. For it to be of diagnostic value, caution must be exercised so as not to flood the area with anesthetic, rather carefully directing a small quantity into the common digital nerve. Steroids should be used with caution as they can cause fat pad atrophy, skin discoloration, and/or MTP joint capsule laxity [5].

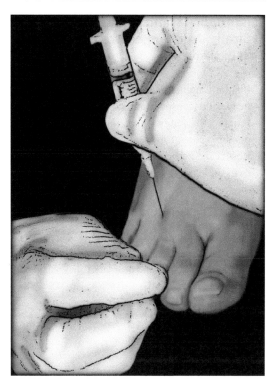

Fig. 95.3 Injection of local anesthetic + steroid through a dorsal approach into the common plantar digital nerve of the affected webspace. The needle must be plantar to the deep transverse metatarsal ligament

- (Ultrasound guided) Alcohol sclerosing solution injection – 70% Carbocaine-adrenaline and 30% ethyl alcohol [5].
- Radiofrequency ablation [5].

Operative Treatment

Dorsal Approach is Most Common [4, 5]

- Dorsal longitudinal incision 3–4 cm proximal to the webspace.
- Lamina spreader is used to spread the third and fourth metatarsal necks to visualize the deep transverse metatarsal ligament, which is then released.
- The neuroma becomes visible immediately after release of the ligament.
- The nerve is followed proximally to the level of the metatarsal head to ensure that there is no tethering of the nerve to the fat pad; this is the most common reason for recurrence.

Longitudinal Plantar Incision: Typically Used for Recurrent/Failed First Excision [4, 5]

- Plantar longitudinal incision 3–4 cm just proximal to the webspace and continue proximally.
- Expand the longitudinal incision through the plantar aponeurosis.
- Resect the nerve 2–3 cm proximal to the deep transverse intermetatarsal ligament and release the ligament.

References

1. Adams 2nd WR. Morton's neuroma. Clin Podiatr Med Surg. 2010;27(4):535–45.

2. Ebraheim NA. Morton's neuroma – everything you need to know – Dr. Nabil Ebraheim. YouTube. YouTube, 27 July 2011. Web. 9 July 2015.

3. Jain S, Mannan K. The diagnosis and management of Morton's neuroma: a literature review. Foot Ankle Spec. 2013;6(4):307–17.

4. Richardson D. Morton's neuroma and revision Morton's neuroma excision. In: Easley M, editor. Operative techniques in foot and ankle surgery. Philadelphia: Lippincott Williams & Wilkins; 2011. p. 263–70.

5. Richardson EG. Interdigital neuroma (Morton Toe). In: Canale ST, Beaty JH, editors. Campbell's operative orthopedics, vol. 4. 11th ed. Philadelphia: Mosby Elsevier; 2008.

6. Schon LM, Mann RA. Interdigital plantar neuroma. In: Coughlin MM, Mann RA, Saltzman CL, editors. Surgery of the foot and ankle. Philadelphia: Mosby Elsevier; 2007. p. 614–36.

7. Thomson CE, Gibson JN, Martin D. Interventions for the treatment of Morton's neuroma. Cochrane Database Syst Rev. 2004;(3):CD003118.

Foot and Ankle Arthritis

96

Megan R. Wolf and Lauren E. Geaney

Ankle

Background [2–4]

- Ankle arthritis is usually the result of a traumatic event (about 70% of the time).
- Incidence of ankle arthritis is nine times lower than hip or knee.
- Ankle cartilage differs from knee and hip cartilage [5].
- Thinner, smaller area of contact with higher peak contact stresses
  - Ankle cartilage deteriorates less rapidly with age due to the tensile strength of ankle cartilage.

History

- History of fractures, recurrent sprains
- Other etiologies: hemophilia, gout, talar avascular necrosis, septic arthritis, Charcot neuroarthropathy, inflammatory arthritis
- Loss of ankle motion
  - Pain with walking uphill due to loss of dorsiflexion
  - Difficulty going downstairs due to loss of plantar flexion

M.R. Wolf, MD • L.E. Geaney, MD (✉)
Department of Orthopaedic Surgery, UConn Health,
Farmington, CT, USA
e-mail: mwolf@uchc.edu; lageaney@uchc.edu

Physical Exam [1]

- Points of maximal tenderness along anterior ankle joint line.
- Decreased ankle dorsiflexion and plantar flexion.
- Varus or valgus alignment on standing exam.
- Sitting exam should include vascular, neurologic, skin, and nail assessments for etiology and surgical planning.
- Injection into the ankle joint may be useful to assess etiology of pain if more than one focal source of pain.

Radiology (Fig. 96.1)

- Standing AP, lateral, and mortise views
  - Tibiotalar joint space narrowing, sclerosis, subchondral cysts ± osteophytes
  - AP and mortise views will show varus or valgus alignment-Hindfoot alignment views can be helpful to show deformity

Treatment

Nonoperative
- NSAIDS
- Corticosteroid injections
- Mechanical unloading devices:
  - Cane or walker
  - Custom braces: AFO, Arizona brace
- Shoe modifications: rocker bottom shoe

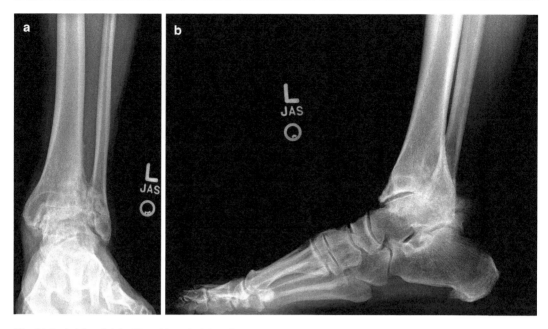

Fig. 96.1 Ankle arthritis. AP and lateral of the left ankle in a patient with advanced ankle arthritis. (**a**) AP of a left ankle shows joint space narrowing (**b**) Lateral ankle x-ray shows joint space narrowing, anterior and posterior osteophytes and subchondral sclerosis

Operative

- Indication: failed nonoperative treatment, with functional limitations
  - Arthrodesis
  - Position of fusion:
    - Neutral dorsiflexion/plantar flexion
    - 5° varus/valgus
    - Equal or slightly more externally rotated than contralateral side
  - Fusion rate is 60–100%
- Total ankle arthroplasty
  - Indicated in older, low demand individual with minimal deformity
  - Complications: osteolysis, wound infection due to minimal tissue envelope, wound healing problems due to poor vascular supply to anterior wound, aseptic loosening, infection

Hindfoot [1, 6]

Background

- Hindfoot includes talonavicular, subtalar, and calcaneocuboid joints.
- The hindfoot provides inversion and eversion motion and adduction and abduction.

History

- Pain on uneven surfaces due to subtalar joint arthritis
- Previous trauma, such as calcaneus fractures
- Other etiologies: Charcot-Marie-Tooth disease, inflammatory disease, tarsal coalition

Physical Exam

- Valgus or varus deformity of the hindfoot
- Tenderness at the sinus tarsi may indicate subtalar arthritis or impingement
- Loss of inversion/eversion
- Painful active and/or passive inversion/eversion

Radiographs

- Weight-bearing AP, lateral, and hindfoot alignment films, calcaneus films if history of calcaneal fractures
- Varus or valgus alignment on hindfoot alignment films
- Joint space narrowing, sclerosis, subchondral cysts +/− osteophytes of involved joint

Treatment

Nonoperative

- NSAIDs, corticosteroid injections
- Bracing: AFO, over-the-counter ankle stabilizing braces

Operative

- Arthrodesis of the hindfoot
  - Reliable improvement in pain
  - Isolated talonavicular fusion has highest nonunion rate

Midfoot [1, 7]

Background

- May be the result of trauma, such as Lisfranc joint fracture or dislocation
- May be spontaneous, as in osteoarthritis or inflammatory arthritis
- May represent Charcot arthropathy if no history of trauma in setting of peripheral neuropathy
- Most commonly involved joints included second and third tarsometatarsal joints

History

- Pain in the longitudinal arch with weight bearing
- Worsened pain with tightly laced shoes
- May have nerve-type symptoms in the distribution of the superficial peroneal nerve (i.e., numbness, burning, paresthesias) due to nerve impingement on osteophytes

Physical Exam

- Tender dorsal osteophytes
- Passive abduction and pronation stress of forefoot elicits maximal pain
- Piano key test: dorsal stress at each tarsometatarsal joint articulation elicits pain

Radiology (Fig. 96.2)

- Weight-bearing AP, lateral, and internal rotation oblique radiographic views

- Findings:
  - Sagging of the medial column
  - Midfoot abduction in severe cases
  - Joint space narrowing
  - Dorsal osteophytes

Treatment

Nonoperative

- Soft or rigid custom-made orthoses to provide support to longitudinal arch
- Shoe modifications: stiff insole, rocker-bottom sole
- Ankle-foot orthosis
- Cast immobilization or short leg brace-cortisone injections (may require fluoroscopic or ultrasound guidance for most accurate injections)

Operative

- Arthrodesis of first, second or third TMT joints
  - Reestablish normal alignment of midfoot
- Interposition arthroplasty for lateral column arthritis due to increased motion through the fourth and fifth tarsometatarsal joints

---

Hallux Rigidus

Background

- Restricted motion (dorsiflexion) and dorsal osteophytes at the first metatarsal phalangeal joint.
- Classic location for cartilage loss is on the dorsal 1/2 to 2/3 of the metatarsal head [8, 9].
- 1 in 40 people over 50 years old develop hallux rigidus [10].
- Most common etiology is trauma.
- Other etiologies include flattened or chevron-shaped joint, hallux valgus interphalangeus, metatarsus adductus, positive family history, female gender [11, 12]

History

- Stiffness with ambulation
- Pain with dorsiflexion
- Pain localized to first metatarsal phalangeal joint that is aggravated by walking and standing and relieved by rest

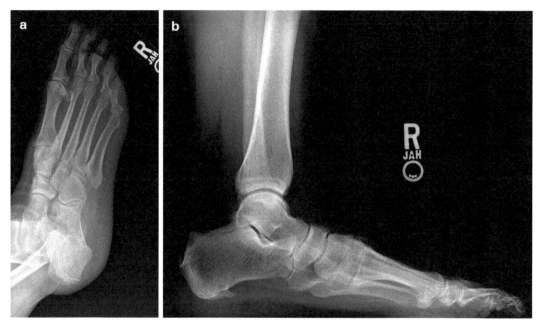

Fig. 96.2 Midfoot arthritis. Oblique and lateral views of a right foot with midfoot arthritis. Joint space narrowing is seen on oblique views, and dorsal osteophytes are visualized on the lateral view

Physical Exam

- Classic finding is restricted dorsiflexion with normal or adequate plantar flexion.
- Bony osteophytes on dorsal and dorsolateral aspect of first metatarsal head with skin irritation.
- Proximal phalanx can become positioned in plantar flexion.
- May have tingling and hyperesthesia over dorsal digital nerve in first web space from compression from osteophyte.
- Differentiate pain at midrange of motion from pain at end range of motion alone for surgical planning.

Radiographs (Fig. 96.3)

- Standing AP, lateral, and sesamoid radiographs.
- AP radiograph shows nonuniform joint space narrowing, flattening of first metatarsal head, subchondral sclerosis and cysts.
- Oblique radiograph can demonstrate adequate joint space.

- Lateral radiograph shows dorsal metatarsal osteophyte and/or dorsal proximal phalanx.
  - May use dorsiflexion stress view to demonstrate dorsal impingement
- Hypertrophy of sesamoids.

Treatment

Nonoperative
- NSAIDs, intra-articular corticosteroid
- Taping to decrease dorsiflexion excursion
- Stiff insole and Morton's extension (extended steel or fiberglass shank) to decrease excursion of first metatarsal phalangeal joint
- Shoe with low heel and roomy upper to reduce pressure against osteophyte

Operative
- Consider surgical intervention when symptoms restrict activity
- Synovial thickening without radiographic arthritis

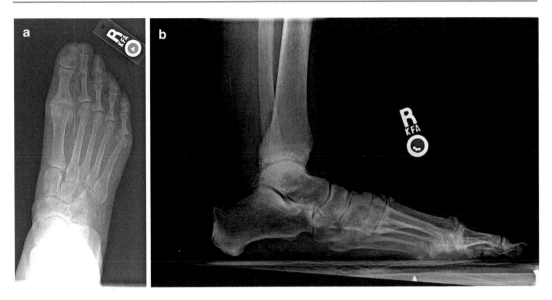

Fig. 96.3 Hallux rigidus. Lateral and oblique views of the right foot demonstrating dorsal and lateral osteophyte formation. Also noted is decreased joint space in the first metatarsal phalangeal joint

– Synovectomy
• Osteochondral defect
    – Removal of loose fragments, microfracture
    – OATs procedure in younger patient
    – Dorsal closing wedge osteotomy in juvenile
• Dorsal osteophyte with maintained joint space
    – Cheilectomy is mainstay of treatment.
    – May have continued pain due to cartilage destruction.
    – May have inadequate bone resection – recommend removing dorsal 1/3 of metatarsal head.
• Severe osteoarthritis
    – Arthrodesis
    – Arthroplasty – excisional, interpositional, prosthetic replacement
        ○ Prosthetic replacement not recommended due to poor clinical outcomes

References

1. Coughlin M, Mann R, Saltzman C. Surgery of the foot and ankle. 8th ed. Philidelphia: Elsevier; 2007.
2. Cushnaghan J, Dieppe P. Study of 500 patients with limb joint osteoarthritis. I. Analysis by age, sex, and distribution of symptomatic joint sites. Ann Rheum Dis. 1991;50(1):8–13.
3. Huch K, Kuettner KE, Dieppe P. Osteoarthritis in ankle and knee joints. Semin Arthritis Rheum. 1997;26(4):667–74.
4. Wilson MG, Michet CJ, Ilstrup DM, Melton LJ. Idiopathic symptomatic osteoarthritis of the hip and knee: a population-based incidence study. Mayo Clin Proc. 1990;65(9):1214–21.
5. Kempson GE. Age-related changes in the tensile properties of human articular cartilage: a comparative study between the femoral head of the hip joint and the talus of the ankle joint. Biochim Biophys Acta. 1991;1075(3):223–30.
6. Greisberg J, Sangeorzan B. Hindfoot arthrodesis. J Am Acad Orthop Surg. 2007;15(1):65–71.
7. Patel A, Rao S, Nawoczenski D, Flemister AS, DiGiovanni B, Baumhauer JF. Midfoot arthritis. J Am Acad Orthop Surg. 2010;18(7):417–25.
8. Hattrup SJ, Johnson KA. Subjective results of hallux rigidus following treatment with cheilectomy. Clin Orthop Relat Res. 1988;226:182–91.
9. Moberg E. A simple operation for hallux rigidus. Clin Orthop Relat Res. 1979;(142):55–6.
10. Gould N, Schneider W, Ashikaga T. Epidemiological survey of foot problems in the continental United States: 1978–1979. Foot Ankle. 1980;1(1):8–10.
11. Coughlin MJ, Shurnas PS. Hallux rigidus. Grading and long-term results of operative treatment. J Bone Joint Surg Am. 2003;85-A(11):2072–88.
12. Coughlin MJ, Shurnas PS. Hallux rigidus: demographics, etiology, and radiographic assessment. Foot Ankle Int. 2003;24(10):731–43.

Vertebral Disc Disease

97

Jeffery Pearson, Thomas E. Niemeier, and Steven M. Theiss

Intervertebral Disc

Composition of the Disc

Annulus Fibrosus
- Cartilage ring surrounding central nucleus pulposus
- Concentric ring of fibers (lamellae)
- Fibroblastic-like cells (produce both type I and II collagen)
- Only outer layers have blood supply [5]

Nucleus Pulposus
- Central part of disc
- Gelatinous composition (high water content)
- Embryonic remnant of notochord
- Chondrocyte-like cells
  - Produce only type II collagen [5]
- Function of vertebral disc and biomechanical properties
  - Function as shock absorber for the spine
  - Annulus has high tensile strength
  - Nucleus has high compressibility
- Figure 97.1 (Anatomy of Vertebral Disc)

Intervertebral Disc Degeneration

- Degenerative disc disease often indistinguishable from aging.
- Clefts and tears develop in the annulus.
- Blood supply of outer annulus recedes.
- Annulus and nucleus become indistinguishable [5].
- The aging disc leads to decreased water content, decreased proteoglycans, and decreased height [2, 3].

Disc Herniation and Neural Compression

- Types of disc herniation
  - Protrusion: when outer annular lamellae remain intact
  - Extrusion: outer annular lamellae are disrupted
  - Sequestration: the herniation is completely detached from body of disc [3]
- Nerve root anatomy
  - Nerve roots of cervical spine exit above vertebral body of that number
    - C4 nerve root exits above the body of C4.
    - This "fixes" itself after C8 exits above the body of T1.
    - As a result of cervical anatomy, paracentral disc herniation at C4 C5 affects transversely exiting C5 nerve, which exits above C5.

J. Pearson • S.M. Theiss (✉)
Orthopedic Surgery, UAB, Birmingham, AL, USA
e-mail: Jpearson@uabmc.edu; stheiss@uabmc.edu

T.E. Niemeier
University of Alabama at Birmingham,
Birmingham, AL, USA

© Springer International Publishing AG 2017
A.E.M. Eltorai et al. (eds.), *Orthopedic Surgery Clerkship*, DOI 10.1007/978-3-319-52567-9_97

Fig. 97.1 Anatomy of an intervertebral disc

NORMAL DISC

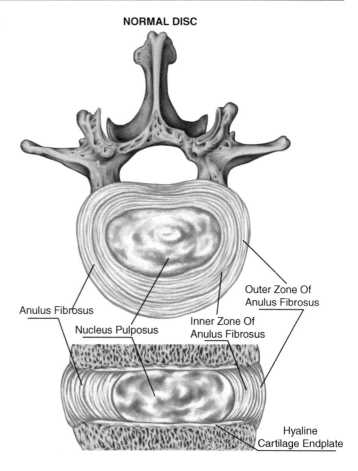

Anulus Fibrosus

Nucleus Pulposus

Inner Zone Of
Anulus Fibrosus

Outer Zone Of
Anulus Fibrosus

Hyaline
Cartilage Endplate

- Nerve roots of lumbar spine exit below vertebral body of that number.
  ○ L5 nerve root exits below body of L5 [1].
  ○ As a result of lumbar anatomy, L4 L5 disc herniation affects crossing L5 nerve root which exits below L5.

Radiculopathy (Nerve Root Compromise)

- Clinical syndrome resulting from compression of nerve root
- Characterized by pain in distribution of affected nerve root
  - Numbness, tingling, decreased strength, decreased reflexes
  - Pain increased with provocative signs
    ○ Spurling sign in cervical spine

- Extend and rotate neck to involved side.
- Reproduction of arm pain is positive.
- Straight leg raise in lumbar spine
  - Flex hip and extend knee of the involved leg.
  - Reproduction of leg pain is positive.

Myelopathy (Spinal Cord Compression)

- Clinical syndrome resulting from compression to the spinal cord
  - Can apply to any cervical and thoracic spine herniation (above the cauda equina)
- Characterized by gait instability, decreased hand dexterity if involving the cervical spine (classically problems buttoning shirt), motor weakness

– Stepwise deterioration
– Compression on spinal cord will have UMN signs
  ◦ Hoffmann's sign
    – Flicking distal phalanx long finger leads to spontaneous contraction of index and thumb
  ◦ Hyperreflexia [4]
– Figure 97.2 *(Herniated disc impinging on spinal canal)*

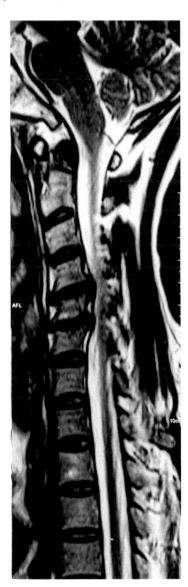

Fig. 97.2 MRI of a cervical spine (T2) demonstrating multiple level degenerative disc disease resulting in compression of the spinal cord

References

1. Chhabra A, Katolik L, Pavlovich R, Cole B. Sports medicine. In: Miller M, editor. Review of orthopedics. 4th ed; Philadelphia: Elsevier Saunders publishing; 2003.
2. Biyani A, Andersson GB. Low back pain: pathophysiology and management. J Am Acad Orthop Surg. 2004;12(2):106–15.
3. Boos N, Weissbach S, Rohrbach H, Weiler C, Spratt KF, Nerlich AG. Classification of age-related changes in lumbar intervertebral discs: 2002 Volvo Award in basic science. Spine (Phila Pa 1976). 2002;27(23):2631–44.
4. Lebl D, Bono C. Update on the diagnosis and management of cervical spondylotic myelopathy. J Am Acad Orthop Surg. 2015;23(11):648–60.
5. Roberts S, Evans H, Trivedi J, Menage J. Histology and pathology of human intervertebral disc. J Bone Joint Surg Am. 2006;88(Suppl 2):10–4.

Spondylolysis and Spondylolisthesis

98

Hossein Elgafy and Mark Oliver

Applied Anatomy

The Vertebral Arch (Fig. 98.1a)

- The portion of the vertebra dorsal to the vertebral body that surrounds and protects the spinal canal.
- The arch is attached to the superior aspect of the posterior wall of the vertebral body by the pedicle.
- The transverse processes extend laterally from this level, and the superior articular processes extend superiorly.
- Dorsally, the arch comes together to form the lamina and spinous process.
- Superior and inferior articular processes extend from the upper and the lower border of the lamina, respectively. The articular processes contain the articular facets, which contact and articulate with the adjacent vertebrae.

Pars Interarticularis (Fig. 98.1b)

- The region of the arch connecting the lamina with the pedicle, which lies between the superior and inferior articular processes, is known as the pars interarticularis.

H. Elgafy, MD, FRCSEd, FRCSC (✉)
M. Oliver, MD
Department of Orthopedic Surgery, University of
Toledo Medical Center, Toledo, OH, USA

- This relatively thin section of bone is stressed during extension of the spine by forces through the adjacent facet joints. These forces may cause fractures (spondylolysis) to occur at this point.

Spinal Cord and Nerve Roots

- The spinal cord terminates at conus medullaris at the level of the L1 vertebra.
- Below this point, the individual nerves continue distally in the spinal canal as the cauda equine. Each nerve exits caudal to the pedicle of its respective vertebra.
- L5 nerve root will exit inferior to the L5 pedicle. The space through which it exits is the intervertebral foramen. The pars interarticularis forms the dorsal aspect of the foramen, which means that an L5 pars fracture is adjacent to the exiting L5 nerve root.

Definition [1]

Spondylolysis (also Known as a Pars Fracture)

- The term spondylolysis comes from the Greek "spondylos," meaning "vertebra," and "lysis," which is "decomposition, dissolving, or disintegration."

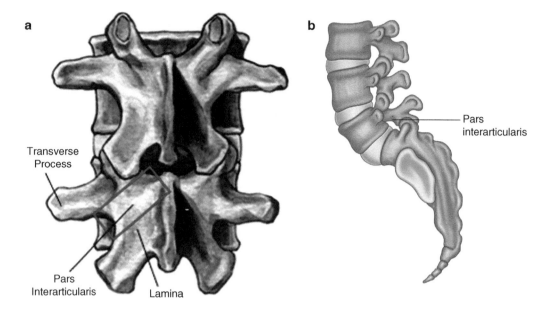

Fig. 98.1 (**a**) Posterior view of the spine showing the posterior arch. (**b**) Side view of the spine showing the Pars interarticularis

- Spondylolysis, then, is a defect in the vertebra. Spondylolysis may be unilateral or bilateral and occurs across the region of the vertebra known as the pars interarticularis.
- Spondylolysis most commonly affects the L5 vertebra and generally develops in children or adolescents.

Table 98.1 Meyerding grade

Meyerding grade	Slip percentage
1	0–25%
2	25–50%
3	50–75%
4	75–100%
5	>100%

Spondylolisthesis (Forward Slip of One Vertebra Relative to Another)

- "Oliothesis" means "dislocation or slipping." Accordingly, spondylolisthesis is the forward slip of one vertebra relative to another.
- This may occur in the presence or absence of spondylolysis.
- The lower lumbar vertebrae and lumbosacral junction are most commonly affected.
- The extent of the forward slip may be measured in millimeters or assigned a grade based on the percentage of the vertebral body that is no longer positioned above the adjacent vertebra, called the Meyerding grade (Table 98.1 and Fig. 98.2).
- Furthermore, spondylolisthesis can be classified based on the mechanism of the slip according to the Wiltse-Newman classification

(Table 98.2). The isthmic and degenerative types are the most common.

Clinical Presentation

- In general, the most common presentation is low back pain that increases with activity and improves with rest. Some patients present with radicular pain down one or both lower extremities, usually in the distribution of L5 nerve root dermatome, which is lateral side of the leg and the top of the foot to the big toe. In rare cases, patient may present with a weakness in the lower extremity usually foot drop or cauda equina syndrome that involves loss of the knee, ankle reflexes, as well as loss of bowel and bladder control.

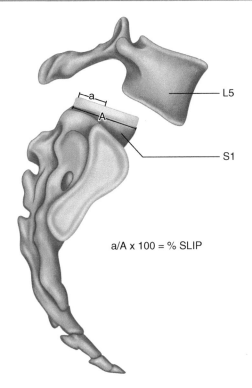

a/A x 100 = % SLIP

Fig. 98.2 Meyerding grade of slip percentage

Table 98.2 Wiltse-Newman classification of spondylolisthesis types

Type I	Dysplastic (congenital)
Type IIA	Isthmic – pars stress fracture
Type IIB	Isthmic – pars elongation
Type IIC	Isthmic – acute pars fracture
Type III	Degenerative (usually seen in older patient)
Type IV	Traumatic (from fall or car accident)
Type V	Pathologic (from tumor or infection)
Type VI	Iatrogenic (occurred after spine surgery)

- The classification of spondylolisthesis is important because the clinical presentation of each type is different.

Type I Dysplastic Spondylolisthesis

- It is a congenital anomalous development of the facet joint results in loss of the normal spine stability and usually occurs between L5 and S1.
- There is anterior displacement of a vertebra without interruption of the pars, which means there is spondylolisthesis without spondylolysis.

- The unstable anatomy means that the condition has a high rate of continued progression compared to other forms of spondylolisthesis (32% vs. 4% for isthmic) and as a result is also more likely to require surgical stabilization.
- As the vertebra slips forward, pulling the intact vertebral arch with it, spinal stenosis develops. This lumbar stenosis compresses the L5 and sacral nerve roots, which can lead to L5 radiculopathy and cauda equina syndrome.

Type II Isthmic Spondylolisthesis

- The three subtypes of isthmic spondylolisthesis have in common a defect in the normal anatomy of the pars. In these cases, the spondylolisthesis results from spondylolysis.
- Type IIA involves a fatigue failure of the pars (stress fracture).
- Type IIB is a sequela of repeated microtrauma; healing processes lead to elongation of the pars in the absence of fracture. The abnormal length of the pars allows for vertebral slippage to occur.
- Type IIC is the result of an acute fracture of the pars.
- These pars abnormalities are frequently the results of repetitive hyperextension activities, as seen in divers, gymnasts, and football linemen. The hyperextension places significant stress on the thin pars. Stress reactions from these activities may heal with rest and immobilization but may progress to well-defined defects when left untreated. As a result of ongoing hyperextension stress, elite-level divers and gymnasts have been found to have an incidence of spondylolysis of 47%.
- They are more common in boys, while girls are more likely to experience slip progression. There is also genetic variation, with rates as low as 1.1% among African-American females and as high as 50% in Eskimos; 4–6% of the population at large will develop spondylolysis.
- Patients tend to be younger and experience back and/or leg pain often worse with activity and improve when lying down. As the body responds to the injury and instability of the pars, cartilage and fibrous tissue accumulate

in an attempt to heal and stabilize the spine. This narrows the spinal foramina through which the exiting nerve root passes. The leg pain in a patient with spondylolysis and isthmic spondylolisthesis is more likely to occur in a dermatomal distribution of the nerve root exiting at the level of the spondylolisthesis.

- They may have midline tenderness with or without palpable step off, decreased flexion, and hamstring muscle spasm.

Type III Degenerative Spondylolisthesis

- More common in older people and will occur without spondylolysis. Men are four to five times more likely to be affected than women. L4–5 is the level most commonly affected by degenerative spondylolisthesis.
- Instability results from age-related disc degeneration, which allows the vertebra to slip forward. Like with dysplastic spondylolisthesis, the vertebral arch remains intact, which results in stenosis of the spinal canal.
- The exiting nerve root will have left the spine cranial to the level of the slip, so the stenosis differs from isthmic spondylolisthesis in that it affects the traversing nerve root at the level of the slip. That is to say that a degenerative L4–5 spondylolisthesis will more likely impinge on the L5 nerve root. Neurological symptoms may present in the form of radiculopathy or neural claudication; this distinction is important to keep in mind while developing a differential

diagnosis, as patients of this age group may also suffer from vascular claudication (Table 98.3). Similarly, the radicular symptoms of spinal stenosis/spondylolisthesis may mimic the symptoms of hip osteoarthritis. 11–17% of patients with degenerative spondylolisthesis may have concurrent hip osteoarthritis. Intra-articular injection of the hip is a useful diagnostic test; relief of symptoms following injection suggests the patient's leg pain is more likely to originate at the hip than in the spine.

- Type IV traumatic spondylolisthesis will be associated with acute injury and rapid onset of symptoms.
- Type V pathologic varieties will occur secondarily, such as in the presence of tumor or infections that affect the stability of the spine.
- Type VI iatrogenic spondylolisthesis is a potential sequela of spinal surgery. Frequently, these patients will have undergone prior laminectomies. If insufficient osseous structure is preserved during the procedure, the pars will be weakened and more likely to fracture. Patients with iatrogenic spondylolisthesis present with persistent back pain and radicular leg pain after lumbar spine surgery.

Risks Factors Associated with Slip Progression

- Type 1 dysplastic spondylolisthesis.
- Diabetes (weakened collagen cross-linking).
- Oophorectomy (estrogen deficiency.)

Table 98.3 Differentiation between neurogenic and vascular claudication

Claudication	Neurogenic (from spinal stenosis)	Vascular (from circulation insufficiency)
Provocative factors	Walking, standing	Walking
Walking uphill	Less painful than downhill	More painful
Relieving factors	Sitting, forward flexion	Standing, rest
Shopping cart sign	Present	Absent
Bicycling	Does not provoke symptoms	Painful
Pulses	Normal	Absent/diminished
Skin	Normal	Hair loss, shiny
Weakness	Occasional	Rare
Back pain	Common	Occasional

- Orientation of the facet joints has been implicated in instability and progression. More sagittally oriented (lying side by side) lumbar facet joints are less able to withstand stress from the anterior movement of the vertebra than coronally oriented (lying front to back) facet joints.
- Certain radiographic measurements may also be predictive of progression of spondylolisthesis such as the slip angle:
    - It measures the degree of lumbosacral kyphosis.
    - It is associated with progression when it exceeds 50°.
    - This angle is measured at the intersection of a line drawn along the superior endplate of L5 and a line drawn perpendicular to the posterior cortex of the sacrum (Fig. 98.3).

Diagnosis [2–5]

Plain Radiographs

- Diagnosis of spondylolisthesis is easily performed with standing radiographs in most cases.
    - Studies should include standing AP and lateral films in addition to flexion/extension

lateral radiographs. These films demonstrate the presence and severity of the slip as well as its stability (Fig. 98.4). Spondylolisthesis is considered unstable when 2 mm slip progression is seen in flexion compared to extension lumbar spine plain radiographs.

- Often, spondylolistheses may reduce in the supine position, as in supine radiographs or MRI/CT studies, leading to failure to recognize the condition if standing films are not obtained. For this reason, measuring or grading of a slip (Meyerding grade) should be performed using the standing lateral view.
- An oblique view provides better visualization of the pars and can be used to identify spondylolysis. It is in this view that the "scotty dog sign" may be visualized; spondylolysis appears as a "collar" around the dog's neck (Fig. 98.5).

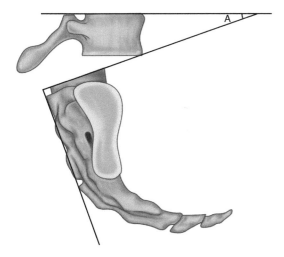

Fig. 98.3 The slip angle (*A*) as measured between the intersection of a line drawn along the superior endplate of L5 and a line drawn perpendicular to the posterior cortex of the sacrum

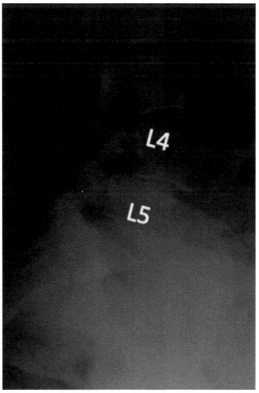

Fig. 98.4 Plain radiograph lateral view showing L4–5 grade I degenerative spondylolisthesis

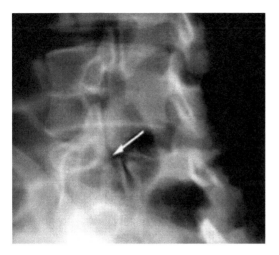

Fig. 98.5 Plain radiograph oblique plain view showing scotty dog sign "collar around the dog's neck" (*arrow*), which represent the pars interarticularis defect in spondylolysis

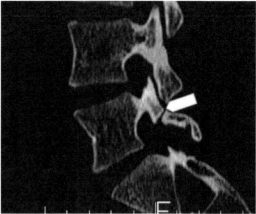

Fig. 98.6 CT scan sagittal reformate showing the pars interarticularis defect at L5 (*arrow*) in spondylolysis

CT and MRI Scans

- If there is strong clinical suspicion for spondylolysis but inconclusive radiographic evidence, a single-photon emission CT (SPECT) scan is recommended. This is the most effective method for detecting spondylolysis, and it can also provide information regarding the acuity of an identified pars defect. A positive SPECT scan suggests an acute rather than chronic spondylolysis. This has implication on the treatment methods as an acute pars defect responds well and has a higher chance of healing with bracing compared to a chronic pars defect.
- A CT scan may also be used to confirm the diagnosis of spondylolysis (Fig. 98.6).
- MRI should be performed in the presence of neurological symptoms to evaluate for spinal canal and foramina stenosis.

Management [6–9]

Non-operative Management

- Though the treatment of choice varies depending on the type of spondylolisthesis, the majority of cases should be managed initially with conservative treatment.
- In the case of a child or adolescent with a stress fracture of the pars (spondylolysis), the patient

should be placed in a lumbosacral orthosis (LSO) brace for 6–12 weeks. The brace may be discontinued when there is pain-free lumbar extension or repeat CT scan demonstrates boney healing. The absence of pain without evidence of bony union on CT scan is usually the result of fibrous union, which often leads to good outcomes and is sufficient to allow the patient to return to sport activities. Evidence supports early bracing achieved improved outcomes compared to activity restriction without bracing.
- In older patients with degenerative spondylolisthesis, modifications of activities, physical therapy, NSAIDs, and sometime epidural steroid injections should be tried before considering surgical management.

Operative Management

- Indications
  - Spondylolysis
    - Persistent pain despite 6–12 weeks of bracing with nonhealing pars stress fracture in children and adolescents
  - Spondylolisthesis
    - High-grade slip in isthmic spondylolisthesis
    - Progressive dysplastic spondylolisthesis
    - Degenerative spondylolisthesis that failed non-operative management
    - Traumatic spondylolisthesis after injury as the spine is unstable

- ◦ Iatrogenic spondylolisthesis that presents with persistent back pain after spine surgery
- • Surgical Options
  - – Spondylolysis
    - ◦ Pars repair using iliac crest bone graft and different instrumentation options such as wires, screws or hooks
  - – Spondylolisthesis
    - ◦ Posterolateral fusion in situ with hyperextension casting in children
    - ◦ Decompression, instrumentation, and fusion with iliac crest bone graft or allograft in adults
- • Regardless of the cause of the spondylolysis or spondylolisthesis, the goals of surgical management remain the same. These goals include pain relief, resolution of neurological deficits, restoration of spinal stability, and development of a solid arthrodesis at the level of the fusion.

References

1. Beutler WJ, et al. The natural history of spondylolysis and spondylolisthesis: 45-year follow-up evaluation. Spine. 2003;28:1027–35.

2. Anderson K, et al. Quantitative assessment with SPECT imaging of stress injuries of the pars interarticularis and response to bracing. J Pediatr Orthop. 2000;20:28–33.

3. Blanda J, et al. Defects of pars interarticularis in athletes: a protocol for nonoperative treatment. J Spinal Disord. 1993;6:406–11.

4. Roca J, et al. Direct repair of spondylolysis using a new pedicle screw hook fixation: clinical and CT-assessed study: an analysis of 19 patients. J Spinal Disord Tech. 2005;18:S82–9.

5. Ivanic GM, et al. Direct stabilization of lumbar spondylolysis with a hook screw: mean 11-year follow-up period for 113 patients. Spine. 2003;28:255–9.

6. Herkowitz HN, et al. Degenerative lumbar spondylolisthesis with spinal stenosis. A prospective study comparing decompression with decompression and intertransverse process arthrodesis. J Bone Joint Surg Am. 1992;74:729.

7. Fischgrund JS, et al. 1997 Volvo Award winner in clinical studies. Degenerative lumbar spondylolisthesis with spinal stenosis: a prospective, randomized study comparing decompressive laminectomy and arthrodesis with and without spinal instrumentation. Spine (Phila Pa 1976). 1997;22:2807–12.

8. La Rosa G, et al. Pedicle screw fixation for isthmic spondylolisthesis: does posterior lumbar interbody fusion improve out-come over posterolateral fusion? J Neurosurg. 2003;99(2 Suppl):143–50.

9. Harris IE, et al. Long-term follow-up of patients with grade-III and IV spondylolisthesis: treatment with and without posterior fusion. J Bone Joint Surg Am. 1987;69:960–9.

Spinal Stenosis

99

J. Mason DePasse and Alan H. Daniels

Cervical Spinal Stenosis

Definition

- Central canal diameter <13 mm (normal is 17 mm)

Causes

- Congenital
- Traumatic arthritis
- Degenerative arthritis

Evaluation

History
- Often asymptomatic.
- Advanced stenosis may cause cervical myelopathy, ask about clumsiness with buttons and other hand dexterity tasks.
- May also cause radiculopathy.

J. Mason DePasse, MD (✉)
Department of Orthopedic Surgery, Division of
Pediatric Surgery, Warren Alpert Medical School
of Brown University, Providence, RI, USA
e-mail: jmdepasse@gmail.com

A.H. Daniels, MD
Department of Orthopaedic Surgery,
Division of Spine Surgery, Rhode Island Hospital,
Providence, RI, USA

Physical Exam
- Neurologic exam, with special attention to myelopathy
- Check for Hoffman's sign
- Check all reflexes
- Observe for steady gait

Imaging
- AP, lateral, flexion, extension plain radiographs of the cervical spine may show canal narrowing.
  - Measure Torg-Pavlov ratio, which is the ratio of the width of the canal to the width of the vertebral body (<0.8 is abnormal).
- MRI.

Treatment
- If asymptomatic, may observe.
- If myelopathy, perform decompression +/− fusion.
- If radiculopathy, consider injection vs. decompression +/− fusion.
- Athletes – may not participate in sports if history of neurologic symptoms, even if transient
  - Interpretation of Torg ratio is controversial.

© Springer International Publishing AG 2017
A.E.M. Eltorai et al. (eds.), *Orthopedic Surgery Clerkship*, DOI 10.1007/978-3-319-52567-9_99

Lumbar Spinal Stenosis

Types

- Central stenosis <100 mm² on CT scan
- Lateral recess stenosis, narrowing lateral to the dura, and medial to the pedicle
  - Usually compresses the traversing root, which is the lower nerve root, e.g., L5 at the L4–L5 level.
- Foraminal stenosis
  - Usually compresses the exiting root, which is upper root in the lumbar spine, e.g., L4 at the L4–L5 level.

Causes

- All types may be caused by bulging or herniated discs, depending on where the disc presses on the neurologic structures.
- Central stenosis may be caused by ligamentum flavum hypertrophy or degenerative spondylolisthesis.
- Lateral recess and foraminal stenosis may be caused by degenerative spondylolisthesis or arthritic facets, which can hypertrophy or form synovial cysts.

Evaluation

History
- Patients complain of "pressure" and pain in their buttocks and lower extremities.

- Neurogenic claudication – pain and weakness in the lower extremities that is worst in lumbar extension and relieved by lumbar flexion, which opens the central canal.
- May have bladder dysfunction.

Physical Examination
- Neurologic exam.
- Phalen test – extend back for 1 min, then flex forward. Exacerbation and relief of symptoms is a positive test.
- Kemp sign – radicular pain worsened by extension.

Imaging

- AP, lateral, flexion, extension plain radiographs may show degenerative disease or spondylolisthesis.
  - May see instability in flexion/extension
- MRI, though may note stenosis in asymptomatic patients.

Treatment

- Anti-inflammatories, physical therapy, and cortisone injections may improve symptoms.
- Decompression alone should be performed for persistent symptoms if conservative therapy fails or for neurologic deficits.
- Decompression and fusion should be performed if there is evidence of instability, such as in some cases of degenerative dynamic spondylolisthesis.

Spinal Cord Injury

Hossein Elgafy and Nathaniel Lempert

Epidemiology

- Estimated annual incidence of spinal cord injury (SCI) in the USA is 12,000 new cases each year.
- Approximately 50% of new injuries involved patient's age 16–30 with majority (81%) male.

Age Distribution: Bimodal

- First peak young adults and adolescents.
- Second peak adults older than 60.
- Percentage of SCI's occurring older adults has nearly doubled due to the aging US population.

Location

- 50% cervical spine
- 35% thoracic/thoracolumbar
- 11% lumbar/lumbosacral

Pathophysiology [1]

- Two-step process: Primary and secondary

Primary Injury

- Immediate neuronal cell damage
- Mechanisms: acute compression, laceration, shear, distraction, and impaction

Secondary Injury

- Begins immediately but may extend for weeks to months.
- This is the body's response to primary injury and is the cellular cascade, which results in additional damage.

Glial Scarring

- The body's attempt to contain the injury via a tough, cellular barrier.
- Detrimental because it prevents axonal growth and regeneration in the affected area.

Acute Management

- Prehospital treatment
  - Immediate stabilization and transport

H. Elgafy, MD, FRCSEd, FRCSC (✉) • N. Lempert, MD
Department of Orthopedic Surgery,
University of Toledo Medical Center,
Toledo, OH, USA
e-mail: hossein.elgafy@utoledo.edu

- Physical exam
  - ATLS protocol first and foremost.
  - The spinal column should be inspected from occiput to sacrum, looking for ecchymosis, posterior midline tenderness to palpation, and step-offs or interspinous widening.
- Neurogenic shock
  - Hypotension, bradycardia, and decreased cardiac output due to decreased sympathetic output
  - Treatment: IV fluids, vasopressors (i.e., dopamine, dobutamine)
- Spinal shock
  - Refers to the period of time immediately following injury (usually 24–48 h) where there is complete loss of motor, sensory, reflexes below the level of the injury.
  - The end of spinal shock is defined by the return of the bulbocavernosus reflex.
  - Long-term neurologic deficit cannot be determined until this phase is over.

Classification [2]

- Complete versus incomplete
  - (i) Complete
    - No motor or sensory function below the affected level
      - ◦ No voluntary anal contraction and no perianal sensation.
      - ◦ Bulbocavernosus reflex is present (patient not in spinal shock).
  - (ii) Incomplete
    - Palpable or visible muscle contraction and sensation present below injury level
    - Voluntary anal contraction present
    - Perianal sensation present
- American Spinal injury Association (ASIA) classification for grading the injury

ASIA classification	Function
A (complete)	No sensory or motor function is preserved below the level of injury including the sacral segments S4–S5
B (incomplete)	Sensory function is spared, but there is no motor function below the level of injury except for the preservation of sacral segments S4–S5

ASIA classification	Function
C (incomplete)	Motor function is preserved below the neurologic level, and more than half of the key muscles below the neurologic level have muscle strength less than grade 3
D (incomplete)	Motor function is preserved below the neurologic level, and at least half of the muscles below the neurologic level have muscle strength of at least grade 3
E (normal)	Normal function

- ASIA score was developed by the American Spinal Injury Association for neurological assessment of patients with a spinal cord injury. This is based on scores as assessed by the examiner. These minimal elements are strength assessment of ten muscles on each side of the body and pin-prick discrimination assessment at 28 specific sensory locations on each side. The level of the SCI can be determined by indentifying the sensory level as well as the most distal functioning muscle. Figure 100.1 is a sheet used to calculate the ASIA score.

Common Syndromes (Incomplete Injuries)

Central Cord Syndrome

- Most common of incomplete syndromes
- Motor deficit which preferentially effects upper >lower extremities due to injury to the centrally located descending corticospinal tracks

Brown-Sequard Syndrome

- Traumatic hemisection of the spinal cord
  - Ipsilateral loss of motor and most sensory function (light touch, vibration, and proprioception)
  - Contralateral loss of pain and temperature
  - Best prognosis

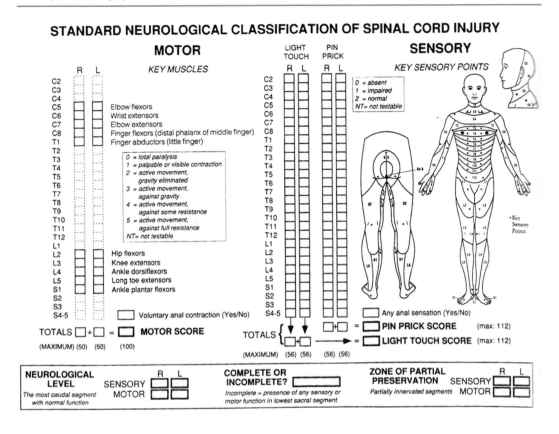

Fig. 100.1 A sheet used to calculate the ASIA score

Anterior Cord Syndrome

– Bilateral loss of motor function distally (lateral corticospinal tracks)
– Bilateral loss of pain in temperature sensation distally (lateral spinothalamic tracts)
– Worst prognosis

Posterior Cord Syndrome

– Bilateral loss of proprioception and vibration
– Rarest

Conus Medullaris Syndrome

• Injury typically occurs after fractures of the T12–L1 level causing damage to the tip of the spinal cord:
  – Mild to moderate back pain

– Unilateral radicular symptoms more common
– Bowel and bladder dysfunction
– Sexual dysfunction common
– Often mixed upper motor neuron and lower motor neuron signs

Cauda Equina Syndrome

• Injury to the cauda equina collection of L1–S5 nerve roots.
• Constellation of symptoms:
  – Severe lower back pain
  – Often *bilateral* lower extremities radicular pain
  – Saddle anesthesia (decrease perianal sensation)
  – No or weak voluntary anal contraction
  – Areflexia (absent deep tendon reflexes in the lower extremities)

- Neurogenic bladder dysfunction (i.e., urinary retention followed by overflow incontinence)
- Treatment is urgent surgical decompression within 48 h.

Imaging [3]

- Extremely important to obtain imaging of the entire spinal column in the setting of trauma due to the high rate of noncontiguous concomitant injury

CT Scan

- Advantage of being quick and readily available.
- Disadvantage is the increased exposure to radiation.
- Best imaging modality for assessing bony structures and fractures.
- Sensitivity for correctly identifying spine fractures is >95%.

MRI

- Warranted in patients with new neurologic deficit
- Best imaging modality for soft tissue (e.g., intervertebral disks, ligamentous structures, and neural structures)

Treatment/Therapies [4, 5]

- Surgical decompression and stabilization
  - Indications:
    ◦ Neurological deficit
    ◦ Unstable spine fracture
- Non-operative (i.e., bracing/observation)
  - Indications: Stable fracture in a neurologically intact patient
- Neuroprotective medications
  - Methylprednisolone:

    ◦ Potential to inhibit inflammatory damage to the spinal cord and exert a cell-stabilizing effect by impeding lipid peroxidation, decreasing the neurotoxicity of excitatory amino acids, increasing blood perfusion in the spinal tissue, and slowing the traumatic shift of ions.
    ◦ According to NASCIS III, must be given within 8 h of non-penetrating spine cord injury.
    ◦ Still highly controversial as there is increased risk of sepsis and death in those receiving high dose steroids.
    ◦ Steroids are an option, not the standard of care
  - Tirilazad mesylate:
    ◦ Shown to decreased lipid peroxidation in rat models
  - GM1 ganglioside:
    ◦ Shown to reduce neuronal edema by promoting activation of sodium, potassium, and magnesium pumps
    ◦ Also shown to increase the presence of endogenous neurotrophic factors with may stimulate neuritic "sprouting"
  - Riluzole:
    ◦ Blocks voltage gated sodium channels.
    ◦ This mechanism may reduce secondary injury due to excitotoxicity.
    ◦ This therapy remains unproven and is an area of active research.

Complications

- Urinary tract infection
- Respiratory tract infections
- Venous thromboembolic disease
- Neuropathic pain
- Osteoporosis
- Pressure ulcers
- Autonomic dysreflexia:
  - Occurred in SCI at or above T6 due to uncontrolled sympathetic activity of splanchnic nerves as a result of loss of sympathetic inhibitory impulse that originates above T6

Presentation

- Elevated blood pressure, pounding headache, sweating, flushing, and piloerection in response of noxious stimuli such as tight clothing, ingrown toenail, fecal impaction, full bladder, sexual activity, or menstrual cramp

Treatment

- Locate and remove stimuli
- Head elevation
- Consider antihypertensive (nitroprusside, clonidine, hydralazine. Do not use beta blockers.)

Rehabilitation

- Spasticity
  - Non-pharmacologic
    - Proper posture and stretching activities
  - Pharmacologic
    - Baclofen, diazepam, tizanidine, dantrolene
- Anticipated outcomes by neurologic level of injury in patients with complete SCI

Level	Patient function
C1–C3	Ventilator dependent Electric wheelchair with blink or head control Dependent in daily activities
C4	Initially ventilator dependent but can become independent Electric wheelchair with chin control Dependent in daily activities
C5	Ventilator independent Biceps, deltoid intact and can flex elbow but lacks wrist extension Arm-controlled wheelchair Dependent in daily activities

Level	Patient function
C6	Wrist extensors intact that results into better function: Able to bring hand to mouth to feed oneself Able to independently transfer with sliding board Independent living Manual wheelchair with sliding board transfer Can drive a car with manual control
C7	Improved triceps strength but limited hand dexterity Independent living
C8–T1	Improved hand and finger strength and dexterity Fully independent transfers
T2–T12	Normal upper extremity function Improved trunk control Wheelchair dependent
L1–L2	Ambulating with long leg braces in household
L3–L5	Community ambulating with long leg possible short leg braces
S1–S5	Walking with minimal or no assistance Some return of bowel/bladder control and sexual function

References

1. Mayle RE, Eismont FJ. Spinal cord injury: pathophysiology, classification, treatment, and complications. Orthop Knowl Online J. 2012;10. http://www.aaos.org/OKOJ/vol10/issue1/SPI046/.
2. Tay BK, Eismont FJ. Spinal cord injury. Orthop Knowl Online J. 2004;2.
3. Inaba K, Munera F, McKenney M, Schulman C, de Moya M, Rivas L, Pearce A, Cohn S. Visceral torso computed tomography for clearance of the thoracolumbar spine in trauma: a review of the literature. J Trauma. 2006;60(4):915–20.
4. Fehlings MG, Wilson JR, Frankowski RF, Toups EG, Aarabi B, Harrop JS, Shaffrey CI, Harkema SJ, Guest JD, Tator CH, Burau KD, Johnson MW, Grossman RG. Riluzole for the treatment of acute traumatic spinal cord injury: rationale for and design of the NACTN Phase I clinical trial. J Neurosurg Spine. 2012;17(1 Suppl):151–6.
5. Koc RK, Akdemir H, Karakücük EI, Oktem IS, Menkü A. Effect of methylprednisolone, tirilazad mesylate and vitamin E on lipid peroxidation after experimental spinal cord injury. Spinal Cord. 1999;37(1):29–32.

Cervical Fracture and Dislocation

101

J. Mason DePasse and Alan H. Daniels

Cervical Spine Trauma

- High-energy trauma patients or other patients suspected of cervical spine injuries placed in a collar in the field.
- Primary and secondary surveys performed by general surgery trauma team include cervical spine assessment.
- Trauma team may clear the cervical spine by physical exam if the patient is fully awake, denies neck pain, and has no distracting injuries.
  - Radiologic clearance, usually with CT scan, required otherwise.
- Important to have high suspicion in patients with a fused cervical spine, either from previous surgery, ankylosing spondylitis, or diffuse idiopathic skeletal hyperostosis (DISH).
  - Missed injuries in these circumstances can rapidly lead to paralysis or death.

J. Mason DePasse, MD (✉)
Department of Orthopedic Surgery, Division of Pediatric Surgery, Warren Alpert Medical School of Brown University, Providence, RI, USA
e-mail: jmdepasse@gmail.com

A.H. Daniels, MD
Department of Orthopaedic Surgery, Division of Spine Surgery, Rhode Island Hospital, Providence, RI, USA

Occipito-Cervical Junction Injuries

- High mortality
- Occipital condyle fractures
  - Three types
    - Type 1 – comminuted impaction fracture
    - Type 2 – condyle fracture with associated basilar skull fracture
    - Type 3 – alar ligament avulsions
  - Most treated with cervical orthosis
    - Halo vest for type 1 with collapse
    - Occipito-cervical fusion for type 3 with instability
- Occipito-cervical dissociation or atlanto-occipital dissociation
  - Majority die in the field.
  - Measurements used to make the diagnosis:
    - Powers ratio – ratio of distance from basion to posterior arch to distance from opisthion to anterior arch, 1 is normal.
      - Powers ratio > 1 concerning for anterior dislocation
      - Powers ratio < 1 concerning for posterior dislocation
    - Harris rule of 12 – if vertical distance from basion to dens or horizontal distance from basion to posterior axial line is greater than 12 mm, concerning for occipito-cervical dissociation
  - Treated with fusion.

Atlas or C1 Ring Injuries

- Low risk of neurologic injury because C1 injuries expand the canal
- Types:
  - Anterior or posterior arch fracture
  - Burst or "Jefferson" fracture and bilateral anterior and posterior arch fractures from axial load
  - Lateral mass fracture
- Stability determined by the transverse atlantal ligament (TAL)
  - May evaluate TAL on open-mouth odontoid view or CT scan.
  - Rule of Spence: if lateral masses displaced more than 6.9 mm (8 mm with radiographic magnification), then TAL is disrupted, and fractures unstable.
  - May also evaluate ligaments on lateral view with atlanto-dens interval (ADI):
    ○ ADI 3–5 mm concerning for injury to TAL
    ○ ADI >5 mm concerning for injury to TAL, as well as supporting alar ligaments
  - Treated with a cervical orthosis if stable or fusion if unstable.

Axis or C2 Fractures

- Odontoid or dens fracture is the most common.
  - Bimodal: high energy in the young, simple falls in the elderly
  - Types: classified by Anderson and D'Alonzo
    ○ Type 1 – oblique fracture through the odontoid tip
    ○ Type 2 – fracture through the base of the dens
      - poor healing due to the watershed area
    ○ Type 3 – fracture involving the C2 vertebral body

- Treatment depends on the age and type
  ○ Type 1 – treated with a cervical orthosis
  ○ Type 2 – treated with a cervical orthosis in elderly patients who are not surgical candidates, treated with fusion in elderly patients, treated with halo-vest immobilization or surgery in young patients
  ○ Type 3 – treated with cervical orthosis
- Traumatic spondylolisthesis, also called "hangman's fracture"
  - Bilateral pars fracture caused by hyperextension
  - Types
    ○ Type 1 – <3 mm displacement, indicating C2–C3 disc intact
    ○ Type 2 – >3 mm displacement, ruptured C2–C3 disc and PLL, notable angulation
    ○ Type 2A – horizontal fracture line, angulation with no displacement
    ○ Type 3 – same as Type 1 with associated C2–C3 facet dislocation
  - Treatment depends on the type
    ○ Type 1 – treated with a cervical orthosis
    ○ Type 2 – reduction with halo traction or surgery
    ○ Type 2A – no traction, reduction with hyperextension in halo
    ○ Type 3 – surgical reduction and fusion

Subaxial Spine Injuries

Facet Dislocations

- Bilateral or unilateral.
  - Unilateral facet dislocations missed frequently on plain radiographs
- May cause radiculopathy (more common with unilateral) or significant spinal cord injury (more common with bilateral).
- CT may demonstrate "hamburger sign" on axial views, which is the superior facet now lying posterior to the inferior facet.

- Prereduction MRI often performed, though timing of MRI is controversial and dependent on the institution and surgeon.
- Reduction with Gardner-Wells tongs and hanging weights.
  - Can be a large amount of weight to reduce unilateral dislocations, though they are more stable after reduction.
- Surgical fixation after reduction.
  - MRI always performed before surgery to ensure that an ACDF is not required for a herniated disc. ⟶ *Anterior cervical discectomy and Fusion*
    Anterior corpectomy, discectomy and Fusion.

Fractures

- Compression fractures are failure of the anterior column or anterior vertebral body.
  - May include disruption of posterior ligamentous complex
- Burst fractures include failure of the anterior and middle columns, often with retropulsion of fracture into the spinal canal.
- Flexion teardrop fractures result from failure of the inferior anterior column in compression and the posterior column in tension.

- Extension teardrop fractures are avulsions of the anterior longitudinal ligament.
- Stable compression fractures and extension teardrop fractures treated with a cervical orthosis.
- Unstable compression fractures, burst fractures, and flexion teardrop fractures treated with decompression and fusion, sometimes including corpectomy and grafting.

Central Cord Syndrome

- May be caused by trauma in the context of cervical stenosis
- Characterized by more pronounced motor weakness in the upper extremities than the lower extremities
- Treated with a cervical orthosis or operative intervention, depending on the degree of injury and surgeon
- May cause permanent difficulties with manual dexterity

Instability Based on Three column Concept of Spinal stability and
White + Panjabi classification
  ⟶ > 3.5 mm of Translation
  ⟶ > 11° Kyphosis angulation.

Thoracolumbar Fractures

102

Scott D. Daffner

Anatomy

"Three-Column" Model

- Anterior column – anterior longitudinal ligament, anterior 2/3 of vertebral body and disk
- Middle column – posterior 1/3 of vertebral body and disk, posterior longitudinal ligament
- Posterior column – pedicles, lamina, spinous process, facets (and capsules), ligamentum flavum, intraspinous and supraspinous ligaments
- "Instability" (in this model) defined as disruption of at least two columns

Posterior Ligamentous Complex (PLC)

- Structures: facet capsules, ligamentum flavum, intraspinous ligament, supraspinous ligament
- Functions as posterior tension band to resist flexion, rotation, translation, and distraction
- Disruption usually necessitates surgical fusion as ligaments do not heal well

Imaging Studies

Plain Radiographs

- Anteroposterior (AP) views may show widening of interpedicular distance (burst fracture) or superior-inferior splaying of spinous processes (flexion-distraction injury).
- Lateral views may show retropulsion of the bone, kyphosis, or bony flexion-distraction injuries.
- Obtain images with the patient upright (e.g., standing) if possible.

Computed Tomography (CT)

- Better delineation of bony injuries noted on plain radiography
- May note subtle bony injury
- Frequently obtained first as part of trauma evaluation (e.g., CT of chest/abdomen/pelvis)
- Axial imaging useful to demonstrate splits through vertebral body or degree of spinal canal impingement

Magnetic Resonance Imaging (MRI)

- Should obtain in all patients with neurological deficit to assess neurologic structures
- Evaluate degree of neural compression, edema in the cord, presence of hematoma, etc.
- Can help assess degree of disruption of PLC

S.D. Daffner, MD
Department of Orthopaedics, West Virginia University, Morgantown, WV, USA
e-mail: sdaffner@hsc.wvu.edu

© Springer International Publishing AG 2017
A.E.M. Eltorai et al. (eds.), *Orthopedic Surgery Clerkship*, DOI 10.1007/978-3-319-52567-9_102

475

Classification Systems

Denis Three-Column Classification (1983)

- Describes fracture morphology and mechanism of injury
- Four "major" injury types described
  - Compression fractures (mechanism: flexion)
  - Burst fractures (mechanism: axial load)
  - "Seat-belt type" injuries (mechanism: flexion-distraction) – *Chance Fx*
  - Fracture dislocations (mechanism: flexion-rotation, flexion-distraction, shear)

Thoracolumbar Injury Classification and Severity Score (TLICS; 2005)

- Scoring system developed to help direct operative vs. nonoperative treatment
- Includes fracture morphology, neurologic status, and injury to the PLC
- Points assigned for each category and summed score directs treatment (Table 102.1)

- Score ≤ 3 – nonoperative treatment
- Score = 4 – operative or nonoperative treatment (at surgeon's discretion)
- Score ≥ 5 – operative treatment

AOSpine Thoracolumbar Spine Injury Classification System (2013)

- Includes fracture morphology, neurological status, and relevant patient-specific modifiers
- Morphological classification (three basic types) (Figs. 102.1, 102.2, and 102.3)
  - Type A – compression injuries
  - Type B – tension band disruption
  - Type C – displacement or translational injuries
- Neurological deficit grading
  - N0 – neurologically intact
  - N1 – transient neurological deficit (which has resolved)
  - N2 – signs or symptoms of radiculopathy
  - N3 – incomplete spinal cord injury or cauda equina injury
  - N4 – complete spinal cord injury (ASIA A)
  - NX – unable to assess neurological function due to concomitant injuries or conditions

Table 102.1 Point allocation for the thoracolumbar injury classification and severity score (TLICS)

Injury morphology		
Type	Qualifiers	Points
Compression		1
	Burst	1
Translational/rotational		3
Distraction		4
Integrity of posterior ligamentous complex		
PLC disruption		Points
Intact		0
Suspected/indeterminate		2
Injured		3
Neurologic status		
Involvement	Qualifiers	Points
Intact		0
Nerve root		2
Cord, conus medullaris	Complete	2
	Incomplete	3
Cauda equine		3

Adapted from Vaccaro et al. [6]

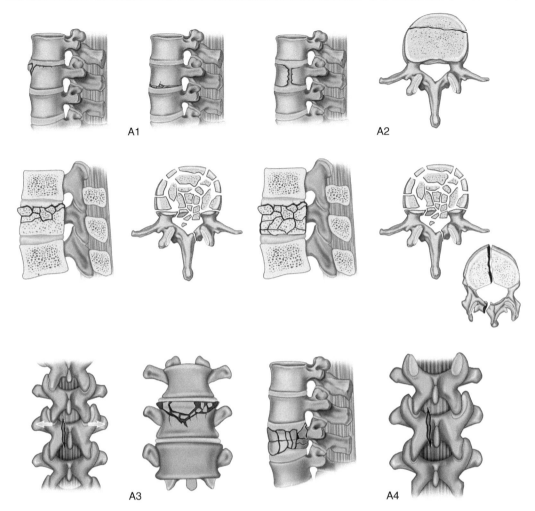

A1

A2

A3

A4

Fig. 102.1 AOSpine is a clinical division of the AO Foundation—an independent medically guided nonprofit organization. The AOSpine Knowledge Forums are pathology focused working groups acting on behalf of AOSpine in their domain of scientific expertise. Each forum consists of a steering committee of up to 10 international spine experts who meet on a regular basis to discuss research, assess the best evidence for current practices, and formulate clinical trials to advance spine care worldwide. Study support is provided directly through AOSpine's Research department and AO's Clinical Investigation and Documentation unit. (© Copyright AO Foundation, Switzerland)

- Case-specific modifiers (applied when relevant)
  - M1 – indeterminate injury to PLC
  - M2 – patient-specific comorbidity which might impact surgical decision-making (e.g., ankylosing spondylitis, osteoporosis, burns overlying the area of injury, etc.)
- The morphology, neurology, and modifiers are then combined to describe the injury

  - For example, a "B2N0" injury at T12-L1 would describe a patient with bony and/or ligamentous disruption of the posterior tension band who is neurologically intact.
  - In cases where another type of fracture coexists (e.g., a type B fracture with an incomplete burst fracture of the same vertebral body), the fracture types may be combined before adding the neurologic description ("B2A3N3").

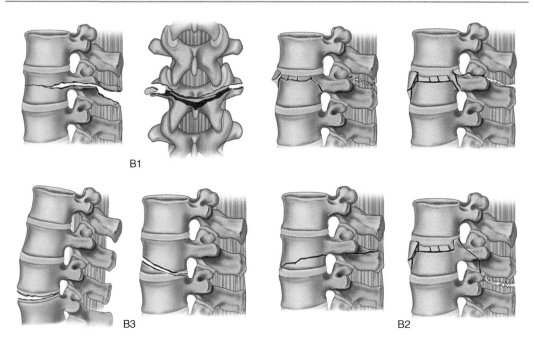

Fig. 102.2 AOSpine thoracolumbar injury classification system type B injuries. Type B1 denotes a monosegmental bony injury to the posterior tension band (i.e., the classic bony Chance fracture). Type B2 denotes a disruption of the posterior tension band with or without bony involvement. Type B3 denotes a hyperextension injury with disruption of the anterior tension band (anterior longitudinal ligament). (© Copyright AO Foundation, Switzerland) https://aospine.aofoundation.org/Structure/research/KnowledgeForum/Documents/AOSpine%20Thoracolumbar%20Classification%20System_poster.pdf

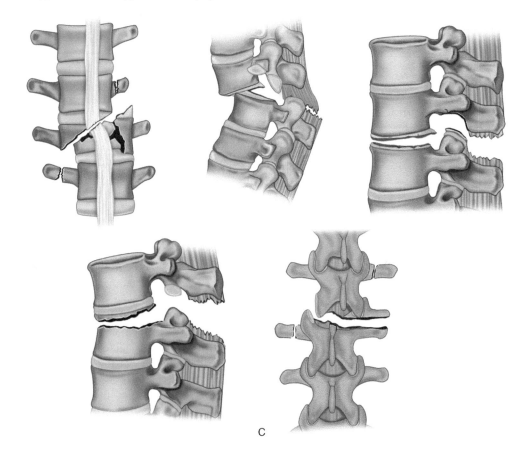

Treatment

Goals of Treatment

- Prevent neurologic deterioration, enhance neurologic recovery
- Facilitate early motion and rehabilitation
- Prevent late pain and deformity

Nonoperative Treatment

- Types of injury
  - Compression fractures
  - Stable burst fractures (no PLC disruption)
  - Pure bony flexion-distraction (Chance) fractures (no ligamentous involvement)
  - Referral for osteoporosis treatment if low-energy injury
- Bracing for 8–12 weeks
  - Thoracolumbosacral orthosis (TLSO) or Jewett brace
  - For bony flexion-distraction (Chance) fractures, brace in hyperextension
  - Increasing evidence that bracing may not be required for AO type A fractures
- Close clinical follow-up
- Long-term data show better clinical outcomes for nonoperative treatment compared to surgery for stable burst fractures

Surgical Treatment

- Indications
  - Kyphosis >30° (or any kyphosis at thoracolumbar junction)
  - Neurologic injury
  - Instability as defined by disruption of PLC
  - Failure of nonoperative treatment (e.g., progressive kyphosis or development of neurologic symptoms)
  - Degree of canal compromise and vertebral body height loss are no longer considered reliable indicators

Approaches

- Anterior
  - Allows direct decompression of canal via corpectomy
  - Reconstruct with strut graft or cage and possibly plate
  - May combine with posterior procedure
- Posterior
  - Decompress neurologic elements, if needed
    - Ligamentotaxis
    - Laminectomy
    - Tamp fragments beck into vertebral body
  - Addresses disruption of PLC, allows reconstruction of posterior tension band
  - Posterior fusion with instrumentation
- Percutaneous pedicle screw fixation (without fusion)
  - Increasing evidence to support in certain fracture patterns
  - Functions as "internal brace" allowing fracture healing
  - Typically remove hardware 6–12 months post fixation, once fracture healed
    - Allows restoration of motion at affected levels
    - Frequently see mild progression of kyphosis after hardware removal

Fig. 102.3 AOSpine thoracolumbar injury classification system type C injuries represent translational or shear injuries with displacement of the cranial and caudal parts of the spine beyond the physiologic range. (© Copyright AO Foundation, Switzerland)

References

1. Bailey CS, Urquhart JC, Dvorak MF, Nadeau M, Boyd MC, Thomas KC, Kwon BK, Gurr KR, Bailey SI, Fisher CG. Orthosis versus no orthosis for the treatment of thoracolumbar burst fractures without neurologic injury: a multicenter prospective randomized equivalence trial. Spine J. 2014;14:2557–64.
2. Barbagallo GM, Yoder E, Dettori JR, Albanese V. Percutaneous minimally invasive versus open spine surgery in the treatment of fractures of the thoracolumbar junction: a comparative effectiveness review. Evid Based Spine Care J. 2012;3:43–9.
3. Denis F. The three column spine and its significance in the classification of acute thoracolumbar spinal injuries. Spine. 1983;8:817–31.
4. Kim YM, Kim DS, Choi ES, Shon HC, Park KJ, Cho BK, Jeong JJ, Cha YC, Park JK. Nonfusion method in thoracolumbar and lumbar spinal fractures. Spine. 2011;36:170–6.
5. Ge CM, Wang YR, Jiang SD, Jiang LS. Thoracolumbar burst fractures with a neurological deficit treated with posterior decompression and interlaminar fusion. Eur Spine J. 2011;20:2195–201.
6. Vaccaro AR, Lehman RA, Hurlbert J, Anderson PA, Harris M, Hedlund R, Harrop J, Dvorak M, Wood K, Fehlings MG, Fisher C, Zeiller SC, Anderson DG, Bono CM, Stock GH, Brown AK, Kuklo T, Oner FC. A new classification of thoracolumbar injuries: the importance of injury morphology, the integrity of the posterior ligamentous complex, and neurologic status. Spine. 2005;30:2325–33.
7. Vaccaro AR, Oner C, Kepler CK, Dvorak M, Schnake K, Bellabarba C, Reinhold M, Aarabi B, Kandziora F, Chapman J, Shanmuganathan R, Fehlings M, Vialle L, AOSpine Spinal Cord Injury & Trauma Knowledge Forum. AOSpine thoracolumbar spine injury classification system: fracture description, neurological status, and key modifiers. Spine (Phila Pa 1976). 2013;38:2028–37.
8. Vanek P, Bradac O, Konopkova R, DeLacy P, Lacman J, Benes V. Treatment of thoracolumbar trauma by short-segment percutaneous transpedicular screw instrumentation: prospective comparative study with a minimum 2-year follow-up. J Neurosurg Spine. 2014;20:150–6.
9. Wood KB, Butterman GR, Phukan R, Harrod CC, Mehbod A, Shannon B, Bono CM, Harris MB. Operative compared with nonoperative treatment of a thoracolumbar burst fracture without neurological deficit: a prospective randomized study with follow-up at sixteen to twenty-two years. J Bone Joint Surg Am. 2015;97:3–9.

Lumbar Strain and Lumbar Disk Herniation

Ryan Scully and Raj Rao

Lumbar Strain

Definition

Lumbar strain is a stretching injury to the paraspinal musculature and tendons.

Epidemiology and Natural History [5]

- Affects all age groups and socioeconomic classes.
- 70–80% of people get affected over their lifetime (developed countries).
- Most people recover without lasting difficulty or loss of function.
- 60–70% will have severe enough symptoms to require work absence.
- 80–90% return to work by 12 weeks.

Clinical Presentation

- Onset may be acute following injury or trauma or gradual and progressive from repetitive activity (physical labor, sports).
- Pain described as localized back spasm or nonspecific ache.
- Physical exam may reveal paraspinal or midline tenderness.
- Red flags:
  - Atypical complaints such as night pain, nonmechanical pain, or radicular symptoms warn of an alternative diagnosis
  - History of significant trauma
    ∘ Look for endplate fracture or compression fracture
  - Infection (osteomyelitis, epidural abscess)
    ∘ Systemic complaints (fever, chills, malaise, anorexia)

    ∘ Risk factors (IVDU, immunosuppressed, diabetes, recent infection)
  - Tumor
    ∘ Night pain
    ∘ Established diagnosis of malignancy
    ∘ Unexplained weight loss
  - Cauda equina syndrome
    ∘ Saddle paresthesias
    ∘ Urinary and/or fecal incontinence
    ∘ Poor rectal tone
    ∘ Decreased perianal sensation
    ∘ Diffuse lower extremity weakness and/or numbness
    ∘ Hyporeflexia

R. Scully, MD (✉) • R. Rao, MD
Department of Orthopaedic Surgery,
George Washington University Medical Center,
Washington, DC, USA
e-mail: rdscully6@gmail.com; rrao@mfa.gwu.edu

© Springer International Publishing AG 2017
A.E.M. Eltorai et al. (eds.), *Orthopedic Surgery Clerkship*, DOI 10.1007/978-3-319-52567-9_103

Investigations

- Back strain is a clinical diagnosis and one of exclusion
- In the absence of red flag signs or symptoms, imaging is not initially indicated
- If pain persists despite appropriate treatment and beyond the expected course, plain radiographs can be obtained

Treatment

Overlying Principles
- Resuming function early as possible will minimize complications and prevent chronicity
- Rule out red flag conditions
- Surgery never indicated in pure lumbar strain

Pharmacotherapy
- NSAIDs (both over the counter and prescription) are frequently used
  - Prolonged use can lead to gastric ulcer, bleeding, tinnitus
  - Avoid in patients with renal disease
  - Recent FDA warning on potential cardiac side effects
- Acetaminophen
  - Effective and appropriate for acute pain management
  - Avoid long-term use and in patients with a history of alcohol abuse or liver disease
- Muscle relaxants can provide relief for severe, acute pain
- Opioid analgesics
  - Reserve for recalcitrant pain after ruling out other diagnoses
  - Avoid dependency and abuse by limiting use to brief periods

Activity Modification
- Transient modifications in strenuous activities that precipitate symptoms

Physical Therapy and Exercise
- Avoids deconditioning
- Strengthening abdominal provides increased lumbar support
- Strengthening and stretching paraspinal musculature

Other
- Massage therapy, acupuncture, and transcutaneous electrical nerve stimulation (TENS) are alternative therapies with little clinical data supporting their use.
- Low-risk modalities can be considered in chronic cases as second-line therapy.

Pearls and Perils

- Most common cause of low back pain
- Diagnosis of exclusion
- Surgery is not indicated – treat conservatively
- Rule out other pathology using red flag symptoms and exam findings

Lumbar Disk Herniation

Definitions

Containment
- Contained herniation – displaced contents remain covered by outer annulus or PLL
- Uncontained herniation – disk material passes beyond boundary of annulus or PLL

Geographic Location [4]
- Central
  - Disk herniation in central zone of posterior annulus
- Paracentral
  - Disk herniation lateral to both thecal sac and nerve root

- Axillary ("shoulder")
  - Disk herniation between thecal sac and nerve root origin from thecal sac
- Far lateral (extra-foraminal)
  - Disk herniation beyond lateral-most aspect of pedicle
- Degree of displacement of disk contents (annulus, nucleus pulposus) beyond normal anatomic peripheral boundary of disk
- Disk bulge: >25% diffuse protuberance of annulus fibrosus with loss of disk height
  - Disk material remains contained
- Disk protrusion: disk material displaces through partial thickness of annulus
  - Base of protrusion is wider than the apex
- Disk extrusion: disk material displaces through complete disruption in annulus, with some residual continuity with disk space
  - Base of extrusion is narrower than the apex
- Sequestered disk: herniated contents are no longer continuous with the disk space

Epidemiology and Natural History

- Most common between ages 40 and 50
- Herniations are not always symptomatic
  - Approximately 24% of individuals may have an asymptomatic disk herniation [2]
  - Males more likely to have symptomatic herniation
- Nearly 90% of patients will have significant improvement within 3 months of initial onset and ultimately avoid surgery
  - Disk fragments can resorb

Anatomy

Intervertebral Disk Anatomy

- Intervertebral disk is a collagen-based shock absorber composed of outer annulus fibrosis (type I collagen) and gelatinous central nucleus pulposus (type II collagen)

- Nutrition of the disk occurs via diffusion through porous cartilaginous (hyaline) end plates
- Outermost region of annulus fibrosus is innervated, remainder of disk lacks innervation

Lumbar Spine Anatomy

- Nerve roots in lumbar spine exit below same named pedicle
  - For example, at the L3–4 interspace – L4 nerve root traverses vertically across the disk near the midline before exiting laterally under L4 pedicle into neural foramen
- Neurologic presentation will be determined by the anatomic level and location of disk herniation
  - Posterolateral disk herniation affects traversing nerve root
  - Far lateral disk herniation affects nerve root that has exited at level above
  - Central disk herniation
    - Can compress both traversing nerve roots or thecal sac leading to cauda equina
    - May cause back pain without radiculopathy

Pathophysiology

- Unclear but likely multifactorial

Degenerative Changes

- With aging, the desiccated disk loses the elastic properties necessary for tolerating forces dissipated through spine
- Annulus can become fissured and torn – this causes pain when the outermost innervated aspect of the annulus is affected

Mechanical Stress

- Heavy lifting
- Altered loading of vertebral endplates secondary to disk desiccation

Chemical Cascade

- Disk contents within the epidural space incite inflammatory response
- Multiple cytokines, enzymes, and other signaling molecules have been implicated in nociception
  - IL-1, IL-6, TNF-alpha, prostaglandin E2, nitric oxide, matrix metalloproteinases

Clinical Presentation

Both Back and/or Leg Pain Are Common

- Leg pain is generally indicative of nerve root inflammation
- Back pain is generally indicative of annular pathology or central herniations that can irritate the posterior longitudinal ligament
- Both indolent and acute onset symptoms are possible
  - Acute cases may be precipitated by heavy lifting or a less forceful event such as a sneeze

Radiculopathy

- Varying amount of pain, paresthesias, weakness corresponding to dermatome, and myotome affected by nerve root compression
- Ankle jerk may be diminished or lost with S1 radiculopathy; knee jerk may be diminished or lost with L3 radiculopathy
- Positive straight leg raise
- Contralateral straight leg raise for more specific nerve tension sign

Cauda Equina

- Large central herniations can cause marked thecal sac compression and cauda equina syndrome
- Congenital stenosis of the spinal canal may increase the likelihood
- Neurologic findings can be patchy and include:
  - Numbness or paresthesias in the perianal region
  - Motor and sensory deficits in the lower extremities

- Decreased rectal tone, urinary and fecal incontinence
- Urgent surgical decompression helps with neurologic recovery

Treatment

- Initial trial of nonsurgical management warranted in most cases
  - 50% will have adequate symptom relief to return to work and activities within 6 weeks

Multimodal Approach

- Activity modification and brief period of rest may be helpful
  - Supine position decreases pressure on disk

Physical Therapy

- Avoids deconditioning and improves ergonomics
- Muscle stretching and strengthening

Pharmacotherapy

- NSAIDs (both over the counter and prescription)
  - Beneficial and considered a mainstay of treatment
  - Beware of gastric ulcerations, bleeding, tinnitus, and renal and cardiac side effects that can occur
- Muscle relaxants
  - Helpful adjunct acutely
- Oral steroids
  - Useful over a short course in patients with severe radicular pain
  - Potential risks and benefits must be discussed with patient
- Manipulation and lumbar traction
  - Poor evidence to support these modalities

Epidural Steroid Injections

- Target inflamed nerve roots via transforaminal or interlaminar fluoroscopic-guided approach
- Some data suggests effective symptomatic relief and potential decreased need for surgery

Operative

- Surgery indicated for intractable pain, progressive or profound neurologic findings, or when at least 6 weeks of conservative management has failed
- Microdiskectomy
  - Magnification and illumination used in conjunction with dilators or specialized retractors
  - Lumbar laminotomy performed to facilitate disk visualization
  - Herniated fragments removed to decompress nerve
- Wiltse approach
  - Far lateral disk herniations cannot be accessed through standard direct midline approach
  - Wiltse approach can be used for these herniations by developing the interval between the longissimus and multifidus paraspinal muscles

Outcomes

Nonoperative

- Saal et al. [6]: 64 patients with symptomatic lumbar disk herniation – aggressive strengthening program
  - 90% good to excellent results, 92% returned to work
  - 4/6 patients requiring surgery were found to have stenosis

Operative

- Yorimitsu et al. [9]: long-term follow-up (10 years) after diskectomy
  - Favorable results but residual low back pain in 75%
  - Decreased disk height on follow-up radiographs associated with worse outcome but less likely to have recurrent herniation

Comparative

- SPORT trial [8] – prospective randomized cohort study
  - Surgical group achieved greater improvement at 4-year follow-up with regard to pain and satisfaction but not work status
- Atlas et al. [1] – prospective cohort study with analysis of symptoms, functional status, work status, satisfaction at 8–10 years
  - Surgical patients – worse baseline symptoms and functional status but greater satisfaction, symptom relief
  - No significant difference in disability or work status
- Weber [7] – patients randomized to surgery or conservative management
  - Better outcomes at 1 year in surgical group but no statistically significant difference at 4 years and 10 years

Complications of Surgery

- Failed back surgery syndrome (persistent or recurrent pain)
  - Recurrent herniation – as high as 20% in some studies
  - Inadequate lateral recess decompression
- Wrong-level surgery
  - Watch for transitional segments in lumbar sacral anatomy
  - Utilize intraoperative radiography or fluoroscopy to confirm level
- Nerve root injury – lacerations or contusion from excessive retraction
- Dural tear – 8–16% [3]
  - Higher in revision surgery
- Infection
  - Surgical site, wound
  - Diskitis
    - Elevated ESR, CRP

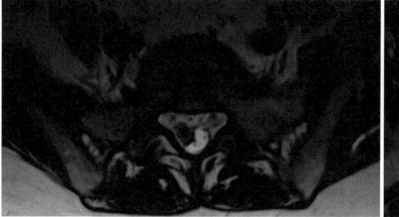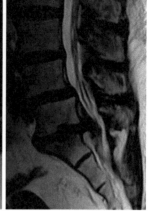

Fig. 103.1 Lumbar disk extrusion. Axial and sagittal T2 MRI images demonstrating a disk extrusion at L5–S1, causing stenosis of the right lateral recess and central canal at this level. The patient presented with acute pain in the S1 distribution on the right side, superimposed on low-grade chronic intermittent low back pain, likely from the degenerative spondylolisthesis at the L4–L5 level

○ Endplate erosion on radiographs, increased signal on T2 MRI sequence
○ Generally responds to targeted antibiotic therapy after percutaneous biopsy and culture

Pearls and Pitfalls

• Not all herniations noted on imaging studies are symptomatic.
• Many patients will respond well to cautious observation and nonoperative care.
• Rule out cauda equina syndrome.
• 10–20-year outcomes may be similar with operative or nonoperative care (Fig. 103.1).

References

1. Atlas SJ, Keller RB, Wu YA, et al. Long-term outcomes of surgical and nonsurgical management of sciatica secondary to a lumbar disc herniation: 10 year results from the maine lumbar spine study. Spine. 2005;30(8):927–35.
2. Boden SD, Davis DO, Dina TS, et al. Abnormal magnetic-resonance scans of the lumbar spine in asymptomatic subjects. A prospective investigation. J Bone Joint Surg Am. 1990;72(3):403–8.
3. Espiritu MT, Rhyne A, Darden BV. Dural tears in spine surgery. J Am Acad Orthop Surg. 2010;18(9):537–45.
4. Fardon DF, Milette PC. Nomenclature and classification of lumbar disc pathology: recommendations of the combined task forces of the North American Spine Society, American Society of Spine Radiology, and American Society of Neuroradiology. Spine. 2001;26(5):93–113.
5. Rao RD, editor. Orthopedic knowledge update: spine 4. Rosemont: American Academy of Orthopedic Surgeons; 2012.
6. Saal JA, Saal JS. Nonoperative treatment of herniated lumbar intervertebral disc with radiculopathy: an outcome study. Spine. 1989;14(4):431–7.
7. Weber H. Lumbar disc herniation: a controlled, prospective study with 10 years of observation. Spine. 1983;8:131–40.
8. Weinstein JN, Lurie JD, Tosteson TD, et al. Surgical versus non-operative treatment for lumbar disk herniation: four-year results for the Spine Patient Outcomes Research Trial (SPORT). Spine. 2008;33(25):2789.
9. Yorimitsu E, Chiba K, Toyama Y, et al. Long-term outcomes of standard discectomy for lumbar disc herniation: a follow-up study of more than 10 years. Spine. 2001;26(6):652–7.

Adult Spine Deformity

104

John France

Introduction

Normal Spine Anatomy

- Coronal – normal alignment is neutral through the entire spine.
- Sagittal – ranges of normal alignment are regional: cervical, lordotic; thoracic, kyphotic; lumbar, lordotic; and sacral, kyphotic.

Adult Deformity

- Coronal plane deformity – scoliosis
  - Scoliosis also includes components of sagittal and rotational deformity.
- Sagittal plane deformity – abnormal kyphosis, lordosis, or sagittal imbalance

Adult Deformity Etiology

Scoliosis
- Childhood deformity extending into adult life
- De novo degenerative – asymmetric disk and facet wear
- Iatrogenic as a result of surgical intervention

- Decompression instability
- Fixed from fusion in poor alignment
- Adjacent to fusion

Sagittal Imbalance: Commonly Loss of Lumbar Lordosis or Exaggerated Thoracic Kyphosis
- Degenerative
- Iatrogenic
  - Fusion altering the sagittal alignment, "flat back" deformity
  - Decompression instability
- Post-traumatic
- Ankylosing spondylitis
- Persistent from childhood (e.g., Scheuermann's disease, neurofibromatosis, or congenital)

Describing and Measuring Deformity

Scoliosis

- Curve description as either "left" or "right" depending on apex of convexity (i.e., curve with the convex apex to the patient's left described as a left curve).

J. France
Department of Orthopaedic Surgery,
West Virginia University, Stewart Hall,
Morgantown, WV 26506, USA
e-mail: jfrance@hsc.wvu.edu

© Springer International Publishing AG 2017
A.E.M. Eltorai et al. (eds.), *Orthopedic Surgery Clerkship:* DOI 10.1007/978-3-319-52567-9_104

- Location of the vertebral body at the curve's apex determines whether it is a thoracic (T2-10), thoracolumbar (T11-L1), or lumbar curve (L2-5).
- Measured using Cobb angle (Fig. 104.1) – lines drawn at the endplates of the most tilted vertebrae superior and inferior to the apex are used to measure the curve.

Sagittal Imbalance

- Predictive of outcome, greater imbalance results in worse outcome in operative and non-operative patients (Glassman 2005) [2]

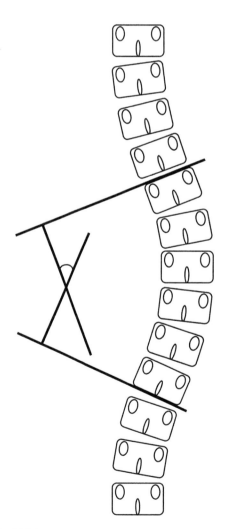

Fig. 104.1

- Components of sagittal balance
  - Thoracic kyphosis (10–40o)
  - Lumbar lordosis (40–60o)
  - Pelvic parameters
- Sagittal vertical axis (SVA) (Fig. 104.2) – measured by drawing plumb line from the C7 vertebral body
  - Neutral occurs when line intersects the S1 posterior-superior corner.
  - Positive imbalance: plumb line falls anterior to neutral.
  - Negative imbalance: plumb line falls posterior to neutral.
- Pelvic parameters (Fig. 104.3)
  - Positionally variable – changes with pelvic version
    - Sacral slope (SS)
    - Pelvic tilt (PT)
  - Positionally static – fixed and unique to that patient
    - Pelvic incidence (PI)

Presentation

History

- Patients may describe back and/or leg pain that progressively worsens throughout the day, difficulty maintaining an upright posture, and difficulty ambulating.
- Cone of economy (Fig. 104.4) – narrow range within which the body remains balanced without external support and with minimal effort (1 – Dubousset); imbalance places patient's torso outside of "the cone," which increases effort to maintain an upright posture.

Physical Exam

Neurological Exam
- Motor strength: hip flexion, quadriceps extension, tibialis anterior, extensor hallucis longus, gastroc-soleous complex function
- Sensation: L2 to S1 dermatomes
- Reflexes: abdominal, patellar, Achilles, Babinski's, clonus, Hoffman's

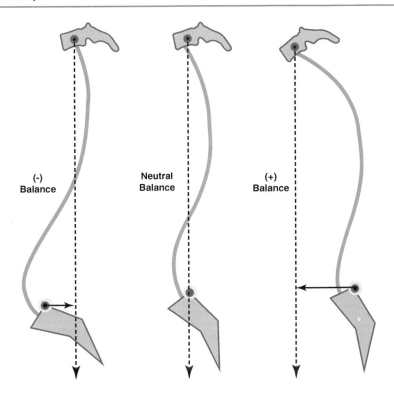

Fig. 104.2

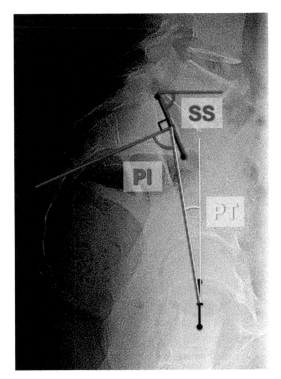

Fig. 104.3

Scoliosis
- Coronal imbalance: can be appreciated from examining upright patient from behind

Sagittal Imbalance
- Sagittal imbalance: ability to stand with head over pelvis; patients will use compensatory mechanisms (retroverting pelvis, flexing or extending hips, standing with knees in flexed position)
  - Have patient stand with knees in locked in extension – evaluate head position over pelvis, if forward or negative. If imbalanced, patient will often be unable to maintain this position for long.
  - Assess for hip flexion contractures.

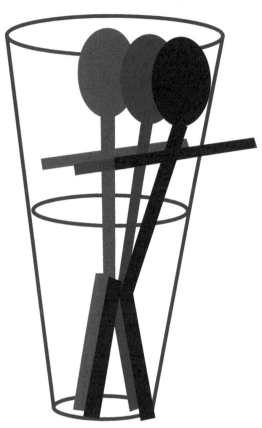

Fig. 104.4

Treatment: Adult Kyphoscoliosis

Nonoperative

- Successful in 27% of patients (Schwab & Farcy 1997) [3] – all successful patients had two intact caudal disks and sagittal malalignment <4 cm.

Indications
- No progressive neurologic decline, new patients without prior treatment
- Medically ill patients – high risk cardiac/pulmonary/renal history with high risk of complications and mortality

Symptomatic Relief
- Treat imbalance and the muscle strain trying to fight imbalance (therapy)
- NSAIDs, tramadol

Physical Therapy
- Aerobic conditioning
- Core and hip extensor strengthening
- Improve flexibility/posture (i.e., for hip/knee contractures)
- Low-impact/low-gravity exercises

Bracing
- Ineffective in preventing progression. Can be effective for symptomatic relief – use with caution as it can weaken core if abused.

Injections
- Can be useful if neurologic/root symptoms secondary to convexity of curvature or secondary degenerative changes
  - Pain consistent with distribution – necessary
  - Diagnostic test and symptomatic relief
  - Nerve root blocks, epidural steroid injections, facet joint injections, trigger point injections

Operative (Fig. 104.5)

Indications
- Curve progression
- Failed 6 months conservative treatment
- Severe deformity/debility
- Healthy enough for high-risk surgery
- Relative contraindications: psychiatric disorder, diabetic/osteoporotic, substantial cardiopulmonary disease, poor family/social support (high-risk surgery with significant pre- and postoperative rehabilitation required)

Goals
- Clinical: restore balance, improve pain, improve activity tolerance, improve quality of life
- Radiographic: SVA <5 cm, PT <20°, PI-LL <10° (Glassman 2005) (Shwab 2010)

Preop Work-Up
- Complete imaging (standing scoliosis PA/lat XR, full spine CT scan to eval for mobility of

Fig. 104.5

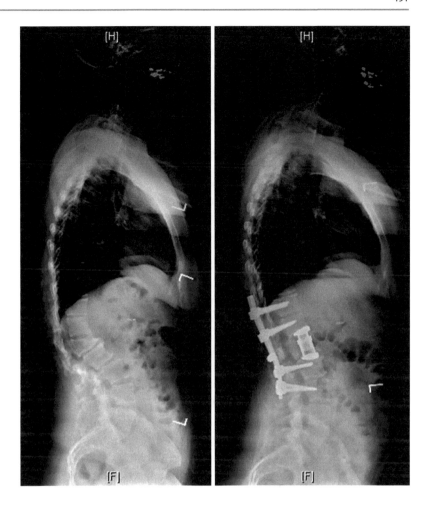

segments and sites of autofusions, MRI or CT myelogram to evaluate sites of compression).
- Medically optimize (generally deconditioned and sick patients). May require pulmonary function tests for baseline diseases such as ankylosing spondylitis or severe scoliosis with secondary restrictive pulmonary disease. Cardiac work-up/fine tuning.
- Quit smoking.
- Optimize nutrition and improve glycemic control (if DM).

Surgical Options
- Multiple. Must be tailored to each patient/deformity and individual combinations of local, regional, and global expression [5]

– Totally flexible spine
  ○ Correct balance through patient positioning
  ○ IPSF ± anterior interbody fusions to "fix in place"
– Partially flexible – stiff section with compensation (flexibility) in remainder segments resulting in overall better global balance
  ○ Manipulate mobile segments to compensate for stiff segments through anterior interbody fusions and posterior Ponte/Smith-Petersen osteotomies.
  ○ Posterior segmental instrumentation and fusion to fuse "in place" after the above osteotomies provide the corrections.

- Totally inflexible spine – does not correct meaningfully through remaining mobile segments (if any). No correction in recumbent position
  ○ One- or more three-column osteotomies with posterior instrumented spinal fusion
  ○ High risk of neurologic injury, root or cord level
- Regardless of type – neuromonitoring for high risk of neurologic complications (increases with more osteotomies and higher with vertebrectomies than pedicle subtraction osteotomies), type and cross units for high volume blood loss surgery, postoperative ICU warranted
- High complication rate of approximately 40%

Postoperative Rehabilitation

- Aggressively mobilize post-op day 1 – improves conditioning and pulmonary rehabilitation and decreases thromboembolic event.
- Remove Foley promptly (drives patient to mobilize and reduces infection risk).
- Be conscientious: high-risk ileus, high-risk wound/instrument/perioperative complications if baseline debility severe.
- Avoid early aggressive anticoagulation if mobilizing well and if no baseline hypercoagulable disorder or medical issue requiring anticoagulation (prosthetic valve, stents, chronic DVT history).
- Optimize nutrition in hospital – dietary consult – double protein diet, protein supplements with every meal. For those with extended ileus, limited use of total parenteral nutrition may be required (infection risk).

Long Term

- Adult deformity alters lifestyles and activity levels.
- Adult deformity surgery cannot "erase time"
- *Controversial*: permanent restriction in lifting
- *Controversial*: permanent restriction to strenuous activities (twisting/bending activities)
- High risk of nonunions and breakdown – long-term follow-up required
- Adjacent segment breakdown and proximal junctional kyphosis – 5–10% per year for every remaining year of life
- Postoperative outcomes depend not only on surgical skill and techniques but on realistic preoperative expectations. Must be set early and set concretely.

References

1. Dubousset J. Three-dimensional analysis of the scoliotic deformity. In: Weinstein SL, editor. The pediatric spine: principles and practice. New York: Raven Press; 1994. p. 479–96.
2. Glassman SD, Bridwell K, Dimar JR, et al. The impact of positive sagittal balance in adult spinal deformity. Spine. 2005;30:2024–9.
3. Farcy JP, Schwab F. Management of flatback and related kyphotic decompensation syndromes. Spine. 1997;22:2452–7.
4. Schwab F, Lafage V, Patel A, et al. Sagittal plane considerations and the pelvis in the adult patient. Spine. 2009;34:1828–33.
5. Schwab F, Patel A, Ungar B, et al. Adult spinal deformity postoperative standing imbalance: how much can you tolerate? An overview of key parameters in assessing alignment and planning corrective surgery. Spine. 2010;35:2224–31.

Tumors of the Spine

105

Sean Kraekel and Raj Rao

Clinical Presentation

Patient Age [1, 4]

- Two-thirds spinal column tumors in patients <18 years old are benign.
- Three-fourths spinal column tumors in patients >18 years old are malignant.
- In patients >50 years old, suspect metastatic disease, multiple myeloma, or lymphoma.

Location [1, 4]

- Seventy percent of lesions confined to the posterior elements (spinous process, lamina, pedicle, etc.) are benign.
- Seventy-five percent of lesions confined to the anterior elements (vertebral body) are malignant.
- The thoracic spine has higher rate of metastases due to blood supply (Batson venous plexus).

S. Kraekel, MD (✉) • R. Rao, MD
Department of Orthopedic Surgery,
The George Washington University,
2300 M Street, NW 5th Floor/5-507,
Washington, DC 20037, USA
e-mail: skraekel@gmail.com

Symptoms/Signs [4]

- Eighty-five percent of patients present with pain for more than 3 months (especially at night and with recumbence).
- Neurological deficits – 55% of malignant lesions and 35% of benign lesions.
- Palpable mass/deformity (less common).

Imaging [5] (XR, CT, MRI, bone scan, PET)

- Orthogonal radiographs
  - Limited utility early in disease course; 30–50% vertebral trabecular resorption is required to detect on radiographs.
  - Loss of normal curvature (particularly in children), generally due to muscle spasm but occasionally from bone collapse.
- Computed tomography – detects bony destruction
- Magnetic resonance imaging – detects soft tissue and nerve involvement
- Bone scan/PET – useful as a screening tool for metastatic/distant skeletal lesions

Labs [1] CBC, BMP, Ca + 2, PSA, alkaline phosphatase, CEA, TSH, SPEP, and UPEP

Biopsy [1] Core needle or excisional biopsy should be carried out within future resection planes to avoid contamination of normal tissue, best coordinated by musculoskeletal oncologic surgeon.

A.E.M. Eltorai et al. (eds.), *Orthopedic Surgery Clerkship*, DOI 10.1007/978-3-319-52567-9_105

Staging [1, 4] Histologic grade, size, local extent of the primary mass, and presence of metastasis

- Enneking surgical staging system of benign and malignant tumors [1]
  - For reproducible prognostic decision-making for bone tumors of mesenchymal origin
    ○ Less useful for myeloma, lymphoma, Ewing sarcoma, metastatic carcinomas, etc.
  - Limited for spine tumors given the continuous epidural compartment and functional limitations associated with resecting spinal cord and nerve
- The Weinstein-Boriani-Biagini classification [4]
  - Complex division of spine into 12 zones and five layers to aid planning for en bloc resection
- The Tomita surgical classification system [4]
  - Intracompartmental (confined to vertebral body), extracompartmental (extends beyond the vertebral body), and contiguous vertebral segment involvement

Classification of Tumors of the Spinal Column [1, 4, 5]

- Primary tumors – Arise within the spinal column.
- Secondary tumors – Arise outside but spread to the spinal column.
- Tumors of the spinal column are considered extradural tumors.
- Intradural *tumors* (both extramedullary and intramedullary) are a separate topic excluded from this text.

Secondary Tumors

Metastatic Tumors [1, 4]

- Presentation: The spinal column is the third most common site for metastasis after the lung and liver; 70% of metastatic carcinoma to the

bone involves the axial skeleton; fifth decade and older; pain; unplanned weight loss; and symptoms associated with primary tumor
- Location: Thoracic >> lumbar > cervical; can involve multiple levels; anterior elements >> posterior elements
- Most common types of metastases and radiographic appearance of lesion: The lung (lytic), breast (mixed), prostate (blastic), thyroid (lytic), and kidney (lytic) [BLT Kosher Pickle]
- Imaging: XR (include flexion/extension), CT, and MRI/CT myelogram full spine [5]
- Treatment: The goal is pain control, preservation of neurological status, and stabilization of spine
- Tokuhashi and Tomita scoring systems – predict prognosis [5]
- If life expectancy >3–6 months → Decompressive surgery and postoperative radiotherapy

Lymphoma [4]

- Presentation: Usually a secondary process; primary lymphoma (rare) has better prognosis; >50% non-Hodgkin lymphoma involves spine; fifth/sixth decade; "B symptoms" fever, night sweats, or weight loss; and progressive neurological deficits
- Location: Lumbar > cervical, thoracic, and sacral; anterior elements > posterior elements; and multiple lesions
- Laboratory tests: Lymphocytosis; anemia; thrombocytopenia; B- and T-cell-specific markers (i.e., CD19, CD5, and CD23 would indicate B cells); and elevated LDH
- Imaging: X-ray shows lytic, sclerotic, or mixed lesions; MRI shows mass that is hypointense to cord on T1 and hyperintense on T2; evaluate for distant sites with bone scan and CT of the chest, abdomen, and pelvis [5]
- Histology: Monoclonal B or T cells (both types affect spine), typically non-Hodgkin lymphoma [2]
- Treatment: Medical oncologist will typically treat with radiation and chemotherapy regimen cytoxan, adriamycin, oncovin, and prednisone (CHOP); surgical decompression if needed

Primary Tumors: Malignant

Multiple Myeloma/Plasmacytoma [1, 3, 4]

- Presentation: The most common primary bone malignancy; persistent bone pain; 2:1 M:F; and >50 years old
- Location: Thoracic > lumbosacral and cervical; posterior element > anterior elements
- Laboratory tests: Hypercalcemia; Bence Jones protein in urine; SPEP (M-Spike); and anemia
- Imaging: Skeletal survey shows multiple "punched out" bone lesions; bone scans often negative; and PET scan positive [5]
- Histology: Bone marrow infiltrated by malignant monoclonal plasma cells [2]
- Treatment: Combination chemotherapy (bortezomib, thalidomide, lenalidomide, dexamethasone) with radiation; may be followed by autologous stem-cell transplantation; bisphosphonates to inhibit bone resorption; cement augmentation via kyphoplasty or vertebroplasty used for pathologic vertebral body fractures; and surgical decompression and reconstruction may be necessary in cases of cord compression from fractures [3]

Ewing Sarcoma [1, 4]

- Presentation: The most common pediatric spinal malignancy; number one nonmyeloproliferative vertebral column tumor; M > F; second decade; pain; and neurologic deficits frequent
- Location: Sacrum > thoracolumbar > cervical; posterior elements > anterior elements
- Laboratory tests: Anemia; leukocytosis; ↑ESR; and ↑LDH
- Imaging: X-ray shows eroded "moth-eaten" vertebra and large paraspinal soft-tissue mass; FDG-PET/CT scans positive [5]
- Histology: Sheets of small round blue cells; genetics t(11;22); and EWS-FLI1 [2]
- Treatment: Multidrug chemotherapy regimen sometimes curative, however it is often followed by radiation or surgery

Chondrosarcoma [1, 4]

- Presentation: Number two nonmyeloproliferative vertebral column tumor; M:F 2–4:1, fifth/sixth decade
- Location: Thoracic and lumbar, 15% anterior elements, 40% posterior elements, and 45% both
- Imaging: X-ray shows expansive, lytic, and chondrogenic "ring and arc" calcification; MRI shows hypointense T1 and hyperintense T2, usually not midline (unlike chordoma) [5]
- Histology: Well-differentiated hyaline cartilage and mitotic figures [2]
- Treatment: Wide resection alone (chemotherapy and radiation generally ineffective)

Osteosarcoma [1, 4]

- Presentation: Number three nonmyeloproliferative vertebral column tumor; M:F 1.6:1; primary osteosarcoma, first to third decades; secondary osteosarcoma, elderly (following Paget's disease or prior radiation treatments); mass often palpable; and neurologic deficit frequent
- Location: Thoracic and lumbar > cervical and sacral; 80% posterior elements with some anterior involvement; and can involve multiple levels
- Laboratory tests: ↑Alk phos and ↑LDH
- Imaging: PET/CT used for staging and variable appearance based on matrix [5]
- Histology: Osteoid producing; destructive; large tissue mass; hemorrhage; and vascular invasion [2]
- Treatment: Neoadjuvant and postsurgical chemotherapy and wide resection

Chordoma [1, 4]

- Presentation: The most common tumor of the sacrum; locally aggressive; M > F; fifth/sixth decade; indolent growth; sensation of rectal fullness; and sacral nerve root deficits
- Location: 50% sacrococcygeal and 33% base of skull

- Imaging: X-ray shows midline lobulated expansive lytic lesion with calcifications; MRI shows hypointense lesion on T1 and hyperintense on T2 [5]
- Histology: Soap bubble cells (vacuolated cytoplasm) and hemosiderin [2]
- Treatment: Wide resection and proton beam; high recurrence rate

Primary Tumors: Benign

Hemangioma [1, 4]

- Presentation: The most common benign primary tumor; M = F; all ages; typically an incidental finding on imaging studies; symptomatic lesions (i.e., lesions expanding the cortex or causing spinal cord compression); and higher incidence in pregnancy
- Location: Predominantly found in anterior elements; 30% of people have multiple lesions
- Imaging: X-rays show coarse vertical striations "corduroy cloth"; MRI shows lesions hyperintense on T1- and T2-weighted sequences [5]
- Histology: Benign and vascular [2]
- Treatment: Generally no intervention; if symptomatic, treat with radiation, arterial embolization, or surgical decompression

Osteoid Osteoma (<2 cm)/ Osteoblastoma (>2 cm) [1, 4]

- Presentation: 3:1 M:F; 5–25 years old; painful (worse at night); pain typically relieved by NSAIDs; and scoliosis (apex of curve away from lesion)
- Location: Posterior element involvement; 60% lumbar, 30% cervical, and 10% thoracic
- Imaging: X-rays and CT scans show radiolucent "nidus" <2 cm (osteoblastoma >2 cm) with central density and surrounding sclerosis; PET scans show intense uptake locally [5]
- Histology: Vascular spindle cell stroma, abundant irregular osteoid, and mineralized bone [2]
- Treatment: Osteoid osteoma, NSAIDs, percutaneous radiofrequency ablation; Osteoblastoma, resection

Aneurysmal Bone Cyst (ABC) [1, 4]

- Presentation: 15% of primary spine tumors; F > M; <30 years old or associated with other bone lesions (GCTs, hemangioma, osteoblastoma, chondroblastoma); pain; and neurological deficit
- Posterior elements > anterior elements; lumbar > thoracic and cervical
- Imaging: Multilobulated lytic "soap bubble" with cortical shell and fluid-fluid levels (MRI/CT) [5]
- Histology: Benign and blood vessels [2]
- Treatment: Embolization (reduce bleeding) and curettage; 10% 10-year recurrence

Giant Cell Tumor [1, 4]

- Presentation: Locally aggressive, F > M, 10–40-year-olds
- Location: Sacrum (the second most common sacral tumor) > thoracic > cervical > lumbar; anterior elements > posterior elements
- Imaging: X-rays show expansive lytic cavity [5]
- Histology: Mononuclear stromal cells, mononuclear monocytes, and multinucleated giant cells [2]
- Treatment: Curettage with adjuvant (cryotherapy, chemicals, heat) and denosumab

Eosinophilic Granuloma/Langerhans Cell Histiocytosis [1]

- Presentation: Rare; M > F; first decade; pain (worse at night), and neurologic symptoms more common with cervical lesions
- Cervical > thoracic > lumbar; anterior elements > posterior elements
- Imaging: X-rays show a flattened "coin on end" or "pancake vertebra" known as vertebra plana; MRI shows lesion that is isointense on T1, hyperintense on T2, and enhances strongly with gadolinium; and adjacent disks are preserved [5]
- Histology: Histiocytes with coffee bean-shaped nuclei and eosinophils [2]
- Treatment: NSAIDs; may spontaneously resolve

References

1. David KS, et al. Primary and metastatic spine tumors. In: Rao RD, editor. Orthopedic knowledge update spine. 4th ed. Rosemont: American Academy of Orthopedic Surgeons; 2012. p. 491–507. Print.
2. Kumar V, Abbas A, Aster J, Robbins S. Robbins basic pathology. Philadelphia: Elsevier/Saunders; 2013. Electronic.
3. Palumbo A, Rajkumar SV. Multiple myeloma: chemotherapy or transplantation in the era of new drugs. Eur J Haematol. 2010;84(5):379–90.
4. Panchal RR, et al. Primary malignant and benign tumors of the spine. In: Kim DH, editor. Surgical anatomy & techniques to the spine. 2nd ed. Philadelphia: Elsevier Saunders; 2013. p. 622–32. Electronic.
5. Van den Hauwe L, et al. Spinal tumours. In: Herkowitz HN, editor. Rothman simeone the spine expert consult. 6th ed. London: Elsevier Health Sciences; 2011. p. 1316–44. Electronic.

Infections of the Spine

Scott D. Daffner

Pyogenic Discitis and Osteomyelitis

Epidemiology

- Incidence: 0.4–1 per 100,000 (general population)
- Risk Factors – often patients have no identifiable risk factors:
  - IV drug use
  - Chronic renal insufficiency (especially on dialysis)
  - Diabetes
  - Immunocompromise
  - Chronic steroid use
  - Rheumatoid arthritis
- Bimodal age distribution (peaks at age 7 and age 50)
- Distribution within the spine
  - Lumbar (45–50%)
  - Thoracic (35%)
  - Cervical (20%)

Anatomy

- Vascular anatomy of the disc-endplate interface contributes to risk.
  - Blood vessels end in blind loop at endplate (within the vertebral body)
  - Creates sluggish blood flow, allowing transfer of bacteria
- Batson's plexus (valveless venous plexus of the spine).
  - Sluggish, large-volume flow
  - Predisposes to transfer of bacteria through retrograde flow
- Disc itself is avascular.
  - Creates difficulty in treating infection

Microbiology

- Usually caused by hematogenous spread of bacteria
- *Staphylococcus aureus* is most common organism overall
  - MRSA increasingly common
- Other common organisms
  - *Streptococcus* species
  - *Escherichia coli*
  - *Enterococcus*
  - *Proteus*

S.D. Daffner, MD
Department of Orthopaedics, West Virginia
University, Morgantown, WV, USA
e-mail: sdaffner@hsc.wvu.edu

© Springer International Publishing AG 2017
A.E.M. Eltorai et al. (eds.), *Orthopedic Surgery Clerkship*, DOI 10.1007/978-3-319-52567-9_106

- Some conditions/patients frequently associated with specific organisms
  - Urinary tract infection – *Escherichia coli*, *Proteus*
  - IV drug users – *Pseudomonas aeruginosa*, *Klebsiella*, fungal species
    - *Staphylococcus aureus* is still the most common in this population.
  - Immunocompromised – mycobacterial species, fungal species

Clinical Presentation

- Initially, symptoms are nonspecific and insidious in onset.
  - Often leads to delay in diagnosis
- Back or neck pain, ± tenderness to palpation, ± paraspinal muscle spasm.
- Symptoms exacerbated by movement.
- Constitutional symptoms (e.g., fever, chills, weight loss) less common.
- Radicular pain may be present in up to 1/3 of patients.
- Focal neurologic deficit (motor or sensory) rare.
  - More likely in cervical or thoracic involvement

Diagnostic Studies

Laboratory Studies
- Complete blood count (CBC) with differential
  - WBC may be normal in up to 50% of patients.
- Erythrocyte sedimentation rate (ESR)
- C-reactive protein (CRP)
  - Elevated in over 90% or patients with spinal infections
  - Normalizes more quickly than ESR, so can be used to assess a patient's
  - response to treatment

- Blood cultures
  - May be negative in up to 75% of patients
  - If positive, may be used to direct antimicrobial treatment
- Other labs to assess potential cause of infection or factors that impact treatment
  - Urinalysis (and culture)
  - Nutrition labs
  - Renal function

Imaging Studies (Table 106.1)
- Plain radiographs (Fig. 106.1)
  - May appear normal early in the course of the disease.
  - Radiographic changes lag behind clinical symptoms (2–8 weeks).
  - Bony destruction may take 8–12 weeks to become evident.
  - Initially, disc space narrowing.
  - Endplate irregularities and sclerosis.
  - Findings of coronal or sagittal malalignment or instability.
  - Frank bony destruction.
  - Upright (weight-bearing) radiographs preferred as they demonstrate
  - instability better.
- Computed tomography (CT) (Fig. 106.2)
  - Provides better assessment of bony integrity.
  - May allow assessment of associated soft tissue abscess.
- Magnetic resonance imaging (MRI) (Fig. 106.3)
  - High sensitivity, specificity, and diagnostic accuracy (94%)

Table 106.1 Sensitivity, specificity, and diagnostic accuracy (percentage) of imaging studies for diagnosis of discitis/osteomyelitis (Adapted from Modic et al.)

Modality	Sensitivity	Specificity	Accuracy
Plain radiography	82	57	73
Bone scan	90	78	86
Bone scan + gallium scan	90	100	94
MRI	96	92	94

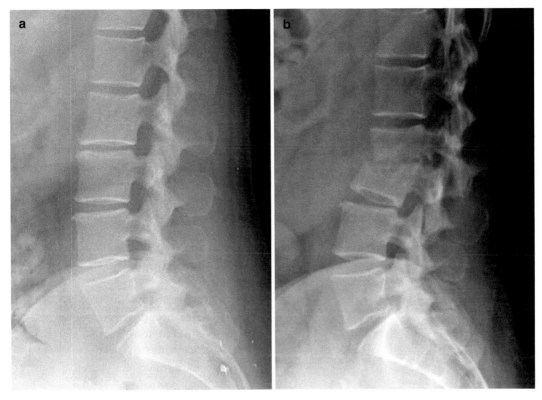

Fig. 106.1 It may take weeks for radiographic changes to appear in the setting of discitis. (**a**) Lateral radiograph of a 40-year-old woman obtained after complaining of back pain for 6 weeks. There is subtle narrowing of the L2–L3 disc space, easily mistaken for mild degenerative change. (**b**) After an additional 3 months of persistent, worsening symptoms, repeat imaging shows significant bony destruction of the L2 and L3 endplates with associated kyphotic deformity

- Preferably performed with gadolinium contrast, if able
- Decreased T1 signal, increased T2 signal
- May help differentiate pyogenic infection from granulomatous infection or neoplastic process
- May be unremarkable early in disease process
- Serial MRI not useful to monitor treatment or follow resolution of infection
- Radionuclide studies
  - Useful in patients who cannot undergo MRI.
  - Three-phase technetium (Tc-99) bone scan: sensitive, but not specific.
  - Addition of gallium (Ga-67) citrate scan improves sensitivity, specificity, and diagnostic accuracy to that of MRI.

Medical Management

- Initial treatment is almost always nonoperative, except for:
  - Severe or progressive neurologic deficit
  - Structural instability
  - Systemic sepsis
- Obtain tissue biopsy prior to treatment – positive in 70% of cases.

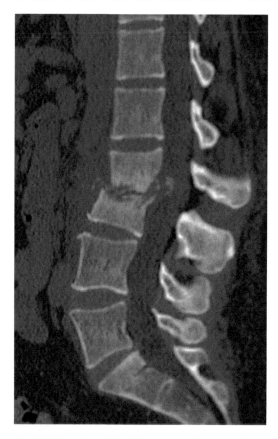

Fig. 106.2 Sagittal CT of the same patient gives better detail of the degree of bony destruction

- – Interventional radiology-guided biopsy
- – Send for microbiology
  - ○ Aerobic and anaerobic cultures
  - ○ Fungal
  - ○ Acid-fast bacilli (AFB)
- – Send for pathology to rule out neoplastic process
- Involve infectious disease specialist.
- Broad-spectrum intravenous antibiotics initially.
- Taper antibiotics to fit results of culture and sensitivity studies when results available.
- Typically 6–12 weeks duration of antibiotics.
- Optimize host factors (e.g., nutrition, glucose control).

- Immobilization of the spine in a rigid orthosis may promote healing:
  - – Decreases pain, facilitates ambulation
  - – Allows affected levels to autofuse in anatomic alignment
- Efficacy of treatment is based on:
  - – Improvement and resolution of clinical symptoms.
  - – Normalization of ESR and CRP.
  - – Repeat MRI is not useful in determining resolution of infection.
- Nonoperative treatment is successful in 75–85% of patients.

Surgical Management

Surgical Indications
- The presence or progression of neurologic deficit due to compressive lesion
- Loss (or impending loss) of structural stability (e.g., significant bony destruction, sagittal or coronal imbalance)
- Need to drain an abscess causing systemic sepsis
- Failure of appropriate nonoperative treatment
- Recurrent infection
- Need to obtain tissue diagnosis
- Intractable pain

Goals of Surgery
- Debridement of all infected or necrotic tissue
- Decompression of neural elements (when involved)
- Correction of deformity
- Reestablish structural stability

Surgical Approach Options
- Anterior
- Posterolateral extracavitary (e.g., costotransversectomy)
- Combined anterior-posterior approach
  - – Significant kyphotic deformity
  - – Multilevel infections
  - – Poor bone quality (e.g., osteoporosis)

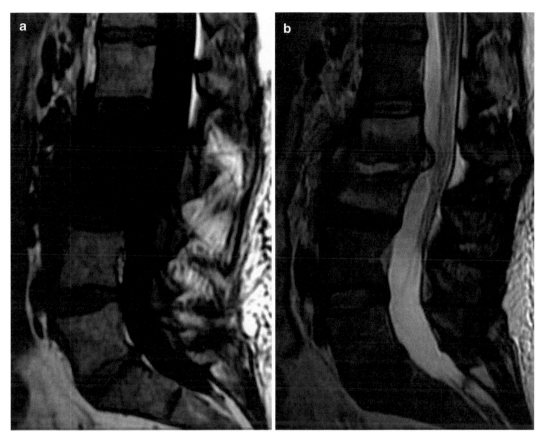

Fig. 106.3 (**a**) Sagittal T1 MRI of the same patient shows decreased signal intensity within the involved disc space and bone. (**b**) On T2 imaging, there is increased signal intensity. Also note a small ventral epidural abscess

Reconstruction Options
- Interbody space
  - Structural autograft.
  - Structural allograft.
  - Titanium mesh cage.
  - All have been shown to be safe and effective.
- Structural support
  - Anterior (lateral) plate
  - Posterior pedicle screws
- Surgical approach and reconstruction options will vary based on location and degree of pathology as well as patient-specific factors (Fig. 106.4):
  - Continue culture-specific antibiotics 6–12 weeks postoperatively

Pyogenic Spinal Abscess

Epidural Abscess

- Most frequent is extension of infection from disc space or bone
- Occasionally may result from direct seeding of bacteria into the epidural space

Clinical Presentation
- Often appear more systemically ill than discitis-osteomyelitis patients
- Localized ± radicular pain pattern
- May progress to neurologic deficit including paresis

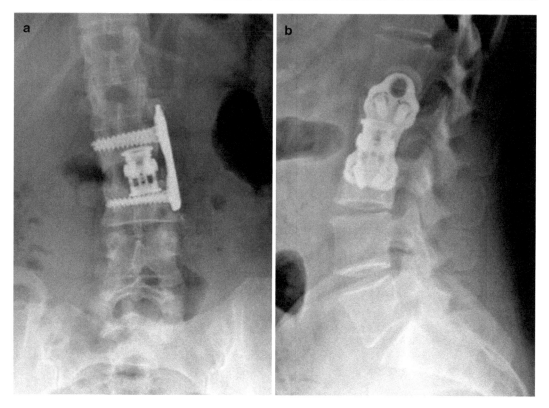

Fig. 106.4 Anteroposterior (**a**) and lateral (**b**) imaging of the same patient 9 months postoperatively. She was treated by stand-alone anterior debridement and fusion. Imaging shows restoration of spinal alignment

Radiographic Findings

- Best seen on MRI.
- Abscess lies dorsal to the thecal sac 75% of the time.

Treatment

- Medical management alone (rare) if:
  - No neurologic deficit
  - Poor surgical candidate
  - Complete neurologic deficit for >72 h
- Surgical management:
  - Goal is decompression of neural elements and evacuation of abscess.
  - Surgical approach depends on location of the abscess:
    - Posterior laminectomy (if no associated vertebral osteomyelitis/discitis)
    - Anterior only or combined anterior-posterior (if lesion lies in anterior

epidural space or is due to vertebral osteomyelitis/discitis)
  - Surgical treatment followed by IV antibiotics, usually for 6 weeks
- Intradural or intramedullary abscess can occur but are rare.

Granulomatous Spinal Infection

- Most commonly seen in immunocompromised patients or developing countries
- Causes:
  - Mycobacteria (e.g., tuberculosis), fungi, *Spirochetes*
  - Usually due to hematogenous spread from established foci of disease
- Radiographic findings
  - Disc space often preserved

○ Anterior abscess from one vertebra to the adjacent level

○ Underneath the anterior longitudinal ligament

– Can result in significant spinal deformity and/or bony destruction

• Treatment
  – Prolonged antimicrobial therapy
  – Surgery to address spinal deformity, instability, and/or neurologic compromise

Postoperative Wound Infection

• Incidence: around 2% (range 0–15%)

Risk Factors

• Diabetes
• Suboptimal timing of perioperative antibiotics
• Elevated blood glucose perioperatively
• Obesity (BMI > 30.0 kg/m^2)
• Smoking

Treatment

Prevention

• Optimize medical comorbidities perioperatively
• Administration of perioperative antibiotics

Surgical Debridement

• Evacuate any abscess, obtain cultures
• Debride necrotic tissue, including unincorporated bone graft material
• Usually retain spinal instrumentation
• Culture-specific antibiotics (usually at least 6 weeks)

References

1. Butler JS, Shelly MJ, Timlin M, Powderly WG, O'Byrne JM. Nontuberculous pyogenic spinal infection in adults: a 12-year experience from a tertiary referral center. Spine. 2006;31:2695–700.
2. Cheung WY, Luk KD. Pyogenic spondylitis. Int Orthop. 2012;36:397–404.
3. Karikari IO, Powers CJ, Reynolds RM, Mehta AI, Isaacs RE. Management of a spontaneous spinal epidural abscess: a single-center 10-year experience. Neurosurgery. 2009;65:919–23.
4. Modic MT, Feiglin DH, Piraino DW, Boumphrey F, Weinstein MA, Duchesneau PM, Rehm S. Vertebral osteomyelitis: assessment using MR. Radiology. 1985;157:157–66.
5. Murray MR, Schroeder GD, Hsu WK. Granulomatous vertebral osteomyelitis: an update. J Am Acad Orthop Surg. 2015;23:529–38.
6. Olsen MA, Nepple JJ, Riew KD, Lenke LG, Bridwell KH, Mayfield J, Fraser VJ. Risk factors for surgical site infection following orthopedic spinal operations. J Bone Joint Surg Am. 2008;90:62–9.
7. Tay BK, Deckey J, Hu SS. Spinal infections. J Am Acad Orthop Surg. 2002;10:188–97.

Pelvic Ring Fractures

107

James Reagan, Jeffery Kim, and James Day

Introduction

Epidemiology

- Incidence is 37 per 100,000 persons per year.
- If >35 years old, more common in females; if <35 years old, more common in males.
- Mortality for closed fractures is 15–25% in higher energy patterns, but for open fractures can be as high as 50%.
- Most common cause of mortality overall is hemorrhage.
- Most common mechanism is lateral compression.

Mechanism

- High energy: motor vehicle accidents (MVA), motorcycle accidents, crush injuries, falls

J. Reagan
Department of Orthopaedic Surgery, Cabell
Huntington Hospital/Marshall University School of
Medicine, Huntington, WV, USA

J. Kim
Department of Orthopaedics Surgery, Cabell
Huntington Hospital/Marshall University School of
Medicine, Huntington, WV, USA

J. Day (✉)
Director of Orthopaedic Trauma, Department of
Orthopaedic Surgery, Joan C. Edwards School
of Medicine, Marshall University,
Huntington, WV, USA
e-mail: day62@marshall.ed

from height, auto versus pedestrian injuries, and sports
  - Blunt force trauma
  - Young and old victims
  - Higher likelihood of concomitant injuries and instability patterns
- Low energy
  - Falls from standing height
    ○ Predominantly elderly patients
    ○ Lower incidence of instability
  - Avulsions
    ○ Athletics
    ○ Muscular attachments in pelvis

Anatomy

Osteology

Sacrum
- Caudad extent of spinal column
- Keystone of pelvic ring and mechanical nucleus of axial skeleton

Innominate Bones
- Formed by fusion of three ossification centers through triradiate cartilage
  - Ilium
  - Ischium
  - Pubis
- Connect anteriorly at the pubic symphysis
- Connect to sacrum posteriorly at paired sacro-iliac (SI) joints

Ligaments

- Large contribution to stability of pelvic ring.
- In general, transversely oriented ligaments help to provide rotational stability and vertically oriented ligaments help to provide vertical stability.
- Sacroiliac ligamentous complex:
  - Attaches sacrum to ilium.
  - Divided into posterior and anterior ligaments.
  - Posterior SI ligaments are the strongest and most important for pelvic stability.
- Sacrotuberous ligament:
  - Connects posterolateral sacrum and dorsal ilium to ischial tuberosity
  - Oriented more vertically and therefore important to vertical pelvic stability
- Sacrospinous ligament:
  - Connects lateral sacrum and coccyx to ischial spine
  - Oriented more transversely and therefore important to rotational pelvic stability
- Symphyseal ligaments.
- Iliolumbar and lumbosacral ligaments:
  - Iliolumbar: connects L4 and L5 transverse processes to posterior iliac crest.
  - Lumbosacral: connects transverse process of L5 to sacral ala.
  - It is not uncommon to see concomitant L4 or L5 transverse process fractures in high-energy vertically unstable pelvic ring injuries due to these ligamentous attachments.

Evaluation

Clinical Evaluation

- ATLS primary assessment (ABCs).
  - The pelvis represents a large potential space that can accommodate potentially life-threatening volumes of internal hemorrhage.
- Gently rock the pelvis to test stability.
  - Low sensitivity.
  - Only perform once because the first clot is the best clot.
- Carefully inspect perineum and skin.
- Asymmetry of lower extremities.
  - Neurological exam of lower extremities.
  - Rectal exam: sphincter tone and rule out occult open fractures.
  - Urogenital exam: gross hematuria, blood at meatus, and high riding prostate.
  - Vaginal exam: evaluate for occult open fractures (mucosal tears).

Associated Injuries

Vascular Injury

- Typically due to disruption of venous plexus in posterior pelvis
- Can be arterial
  - Superior gluteal artery
  - Pudendal artery

Bowel Injury

- Occult open fracture
- High diverting colostomy indicated if fecal stream contacts fracture site or open injury

Urologic Injury

- Up to 20% incidence
- Retrograde urethrogram indicated with high suspicion
- Bladder rupture
  - Intraperitoneal: repair
  - Extraperitoneal: observe
- Urethral injuries repaired on delayed basis

Neurologic Injury

- Lumbosacral plexus injuries.
- Injuries of nerve roots L2–S4 are possible.
- L5 and S1 are the most commonly injured.
- Higher incidence of neurologic injury with more medial sacral fractures.
- Decompression of sacral foramina may be indicated if progressive deficits manifest with imaging that correlates.

Other Associated Injuries

- *Head injury*: most common cause of mortality in a lateral compression-type pelvis fracture

- *Chest injury*
- *Abdominal injury*
- *Acetabulum fractures*
- *Long bone fractures*
- *Morel-Lavallée lesion*: fasciocutaneous degloving injury (see also Fractures of the Acetabulum)

Imaging

Radiographs

- Anteroposterior (AP) pelvis (Fig. 107.1):
  - Part of the standard initial trauma radiographs
  - Good for anterior ring injury and as a screen for pelvic injury

- Inlet pelvis (Fig. 107.2a):
  - Particularly useful to detect anterior-posterior displacement

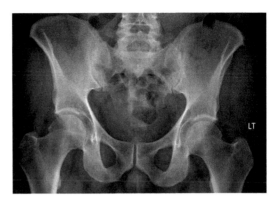

Fig. 107.1 Anteroposterior (AP) radiograph of normal pelvis

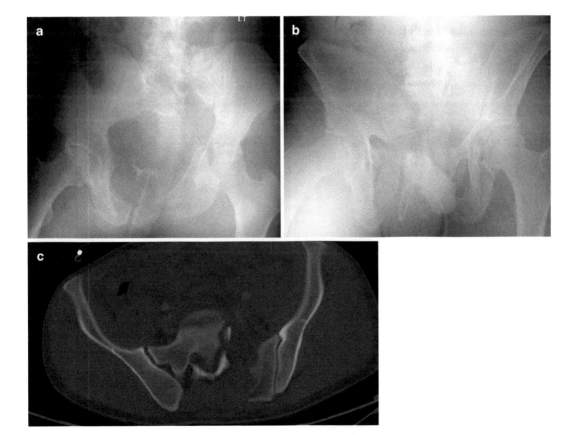

Fig. 107.2 Thirty-three-year-old male involved in a high-speed MVA demonstrating posterior displacement and a vertical shear pattern of instability of the left hemipelvis with noted bilateral superior and inferior pubic rami fractures, a comminuted left vertical sacral fracture, as well as a left acetabulum fracture shown on the inlet pelvis radiograph (**a**). Outlet radiograph demonstrating superior displacement of the left hemipelvis, consistent with a VS injury pattern (**b**). Axial CT image of pelvis demonstrating complete disruption through posterior pelvic arch (Denis zone 2 sacral fracture) with resultant posterior displacement (**c**)

- Also good for detecting rotational deformities and sacral impaction injuries
- Adequate image when S1 vertebral body overlies S2 vertebral body
• Outlet pelvis (Fig. 107.2b):
  - Useful in detecting vertical displacement
  - Also provides AP of the sacrum and allows assessment of sacral fractures and foramina
  - Adequate image when pubic symphysis overlies S2 body
• Stress radiographs with manipulation under anesthesia may aid in identifying instability and directing treatment.

Computed Tomography (CT)
(Fig. 107.2c)

• Better detail in terms of bony involvement, displacement, and fracture definition
• Particularly useful in evaluation of posterior portions of pelvic ring

Classification

Young and Burgess Classification: Based on Mechanism and Injury Pattern

• Lateral Compression (LC) – internal rotation injury patterns
  - Anterior injury = pubic rami fractures (can be ipsilateral or contralateral to side of impact)
  - LC 1 (Fig. 107.3a)
    ◦ Anterior pubic rami fractures
    ◦ Posterior sacral compression fracture on ipsilateral side of impact
    ◦ Most common pelvic ring injury pattern
  - LC 2 (Fig. 107.3b)
    ◦ Anterior pubic rami fractures
    ◦ "Crescent" fracture (posterior iliac wing) on ipsilateral side of impact
  - LC 3 (Fig. 107.3c)
    ◦ "Windswept" pelvis

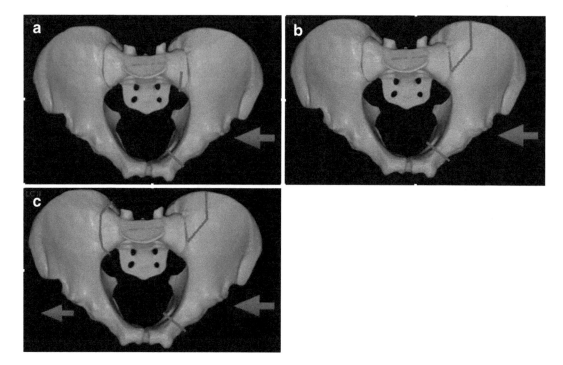

Fig. 107.3 Schematic depicting lateral compression (LC) pelvic ring fractures: LC 1 (**a**), LC 2 (**b**), LC 3 (**c**)

- Ipsilateral LC 1 or LC 2 injury with contralateral external rotation "open book" pelvis injury
- Unstable injury pattern with high rate of neurovascular injury due to traction at the SI joint on the external rotation side of the injury
- Anteroposterior compression (APC) – external rotation injury patterns
  - Anterior injury = pubic symphyseal diastasis or longitudinal pubic rami fractures
  - APC 1 (Fig. 107.4a)
    - Pubic symphyseal diastasis <2.5 cm.
    - Anterior SI ligaments may be stretched.
    - Intact posterior ligaments.
  - APC 2 (Fig. 107.4b)
    - Pubic symphyseal diastasis >2.5 cm
    - Widening of anterior SI joint
    - Rupture of sacrotuberous, sacrospinous, and anterior SI ligaments
    - "Open book" pelvis with posterior SI ligaments intact
  - APC 3 (Fig. 107.4c)
    - Complete symphyseal diastasis
    - Complete disruption of ligamentous structures, including posterior SI ligaments
    - Extreme rotational instability and lateral hemipelvis displacement
    - Highest rate of associated vascular injuries and blood loss
- Vertical shear (VS) (Figs. 107.2a–c and 107.5)
  - Vertically applied forces that commonly result in extreme instability of the involved hemipelvis in a posterior superior direction.

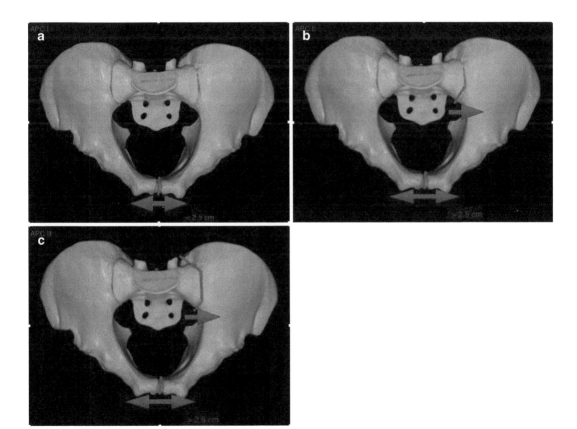

Fig. 107.4 Schematic depicting anterior-posterior compression (APC) pelvic ring fractures: APC 1(**a**), APC 2 (**b**), APC 3 (**c**)

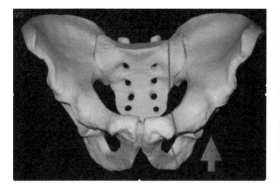

Fig. 107.5 Schematic depicting a vertical shear variant

- – Anteriorly: symphyseal diastasis or rami fractures
- – Posteriorly: iliac wing fractures, sacral fractures, or SI dislocation
- – High incidence of associated neurovascular injuries
- • Combined – Most commonly combined vertical shear and lateral compression

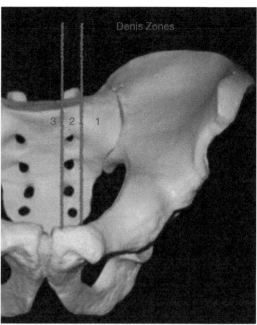

Fig. 107.6 Schematic depicting Denis classification of sacral fractures

Tile Classification

- • Addresses stability of pelvis
- • Type A – stable pelvic ring; posterior arch intact
- • Type B – rotationally unstable, but vertically stable; incomplete disruption of posterior arch
- • Type C – rotationally and vertically unstable; complete disruption of posterior arch

Denis Classification of Sacral Fractures (Figs. 107.2c and 107.6)

- • Zone 1 – Fracture is lateral to foramen with a 6% incidence of neurological injury.
- • Zone 2 – Fracture is through foramen with a 30% incidence of neurological injury.
- • Zone 3 – Fracture is medial to foramen into spinal canal with a 60% incidence of neurological injury.

Treatment

Initial Emergency Room Management

- • ATLS protocol (ABCs)
- • Hemorrhage
  - – Volume resuscitation.
  - – Massive transfusion protocol is 1:1:1 (platelets/PRBC/FFP).
  - – Rule out other sources of volume loss.
  - – Close pelvic volume down provisionally with binder or sheet at level of greater trochanters for APC injuries with pelvic widening (open book).
  - – May require angiography and embolization with interventional radiology.
  - – Emergent anterior external fixation with subsequent laparotomy and open packing of retroperitoneum.
- • Skeletal traction for vertically unstable injury patterns

- Appropriate tetanus prophylaxis and antibiotics for open fractures

Nonoperative Treatment

- Most LC1 and APC1 injuries are regarded as stable patterns and may be treated nonoperatively.
- Weight bearing as tolerated versus protected weight bearing with serial post mobilization radiographs.
- If there is secondary displacement of the posterior ring >1 cm, then weight bearing is halted and operative intervention is considered.

Operative Indications

- Emergent absolute indications
  - Open fractures
  - Continued hemodynamic instability with associated unstable pelvic ring fractures
- Relative indications
  - Symphyseal diastasis >2.5 cm
  - Anterior and posterior SI ligament disruption
  - Vertical instability of posterior hemipelvis
  - Sacral fractures with >1 cm displacement
  - Continued intractable pain with conservative treatment
  - Spinopelvic dissociation

Operative Options

- In general, if posterior instability exists, both anterior and posterior disruptions require stabilization
- Anterior stabilization
  - Plate open reduction internal fixation (ORIF)
  - Anterior external fixation

- Posterior stabilization
  - Percutaneous iliosacral screws:
    ∘ Pelvic outlet view ensures that screws stay out of sacral foramina.
    ∘ Inlet view for proper placement in the S1 sacral body.
    ∘ Lateral sacral view helps to minimize risk to L5 nerve root as it travels over anterior sacral ala.
  - Anterior SI plate ORIF.
  - Posterior transiliac bars or tension band plate ORIF.
  - Lumbopelvic fixation can be an option in vertically unstable injuries or spinopelvic dissociation injury patterns.

Postoperative Management

- Early mobilization
- Aggressive pulmonary toilet
- Venous thromboembolic disease (VTE) prophylaxis
- Protected versus non-weight bearing on effected lower extremity for at least 8–12 weeks
- Full weight bearing at 12 weeks

Complications

- Hemorrhage
- Urological injury
- Sexual dysfunction
- Neurological deficit
- Malunion
- Nonunion
- Heterotopic ossification (HO)
- Functional impairment
- Deep vein thrombosis (DVT) and/or pulmonary embolism (PE)
- Infection – especially with open fractures or a Morel lesion that is opened
- Mortality
  - Open fractures
  - Hemodynamic instability

- – LC: head injury is most common cause of death
- – APC: pelvic and visceral injury major causes of death

References

1. Tile M, Helfet D, Kellman J. Fractures of the pelvis and acetabulum. Philadelphia: Lippincott Williams & Wilkins; 2003.

2. Egol KA, Koval KJ, Zuckerman JD. Handbook of fractures. Philadelphia: Lippincott Williams & Wilkins; 2010.

3. Weiss DB, et al. Trauma. In: Miller MD, et al., editors. Review of orthopedics. 6th ed. Philadelphia: Elsevier; 2012. p. 735–8.

4. Rockwood CA, Green DP, Heckman JD, Bucholz RW. Rockwood and green's fractures in adults. Philadelphia: Lippincott Williams & Wilkins; 2001.

5. Guyton JL. Fractures of acetabulum and pelvis. In: Canale ST, et al., editors. Campbell's operative orthopedics. 12th ed. Philadelphia: Elsevier; 2013. p. 2799–828.

Charles Bishop, Jeffery Kim, and James Day

Anatomy

- Junction of three bones
  - Ilium
  - Ischium
  - Pubis
- Cup-shaped structure acting as a socket for the femoral head
  - Superiorly there is the dome or sourcil
  - Anterior wall
  - Posterior wall
  - Inferiorly transverse acetabular ligament
  - Central fovea where the ligament to the head of the femur originates
  - Anteverted approximately 20°
- Two-column theory (Fig. 108.1)
  - Anterior column
    ◦ Extends from the iliac crest down to the symphysis pubis
    ◦ Includes anterior wall

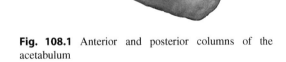

Fig. 108.1 Anterior and posterior columns of the acetabulum

  - Posterior column
    ◦ Extends from the greater sciatic notch to the ischial tuberosity
    ◦ Includes posterior wall

C. Bishop, MD
Department of Orthopaedics, Marshall University School of Medicine, Huntington, WV, USA

J. Kim, MD
Department of Orthopaedics Surgery, Cabell Huntington Hospital/Marshall University School of Medicine, Huntington, WV, USA

J. Day, MD, PhD (✉)
Director of Orthopaedic Trauma, Department of Orthopaedic Surgery, Joan C. Edwards School of Medicine, Marshall University, Huntington, WV, USA
e-mail: day62@marshall.edu

© Springer International Publishing AG 2017
A.E.M. Eltorai et al. (eds.), *Orthopedic Surgery Clerkship*, DOI 10.1007/978-3-319-52567-9_108

Etiology

- High-energy injuries in young patients
  - High-speed motor vehicle collision (MVC)
  - Fall from height
  - Skiing, horseback riding contact sports, etc.
- Low-energy injuries possible in older patients with poor bone quality
  - Fall from standing height
  - Direct blow

Evaluation

Physical Exam

- Remember the ABCs of trauma
- Check the lower extremity, e.g., knee-dashboard injury
- Obtain a good neurovascular exam
- Check for Morel-Lavallée lesion
  - Subcutaneous degloving injury
  - High incidence of infection

Associated Injuries Common

- Vascular
  - Superior gluteal artery or vein in posterior fractures
  - Retroperitoneal hematoma
- Neurologic
  - Sciatic nerve
    ◦ Up to 30% of cases
    ◦ Usually partial involving the peroneal division
  - Superior gluteal nerve
  - Traumatic brain injury
- Visceral organ
  - Liver
  - Lung
  - Kidney
  - Bladder
  - Spleen

- Musculoskeletal
  - Patella fracture
  - Femoral shaft fracture
  - Ligamentous injury
  - Pelvic ring injury
  - Spinal fractures

Radiographs

- X-rays
  - Anteroposterior (AP) pelvis
  - Judet views
    ◦ Taken 45° oblique to AP pelvis
    ◦ Obturator oblique
      i. Anterior column
      ii. Posterior wall
    ◦ Iliac oblique
      i. Posterior column
      ii. Anterior wall
  - Lines
    ◦ Ilioischial line – posterior column
    ◦ Iliopectineal line – anterior column
    ◦ Anterior and posterior rim
- Computed tomography (CT) scan for details of fracture

Classification

- Letournel
  - Simple patterns
    ◦ Anterior wall (Fig. 108.2)
    ◦ Anterior column (Fig. 108.3)
    ◦ Posterior wall (Fig. 108.4)
    ◦ Posterior column (Fig. 108.5)
    ◦ Transverse (Fig. 108.6)
  - Complex
    ◦ Transverse + posterior wall (Fig. 108.7)
    ◦ Anterior column posterior hemitransverse (Fig. 108.8)
    ◦ T-shaped (Fig. 108.9)
    ◦ Both columns (Fig. 108.10)
    ◦ Posterior column + posterior wall (Fig. 108.11)

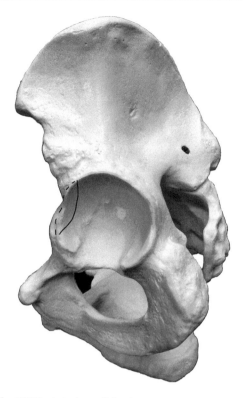

Fig. 108.2 Anterior wall fracture

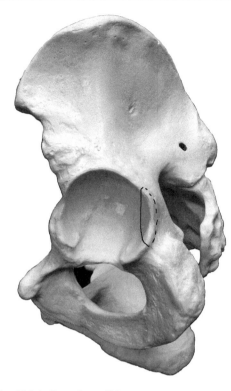

Fig. 108.4 Posterior wall fracture

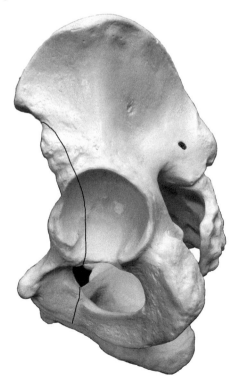

Fig. 108.3 Anterior column fracture

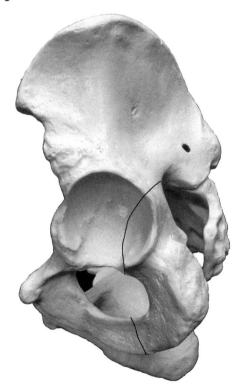

Fig. 108.5 Posterior column fracture

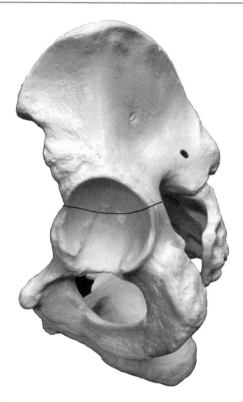

Fig. 108.6 Transverse fracture

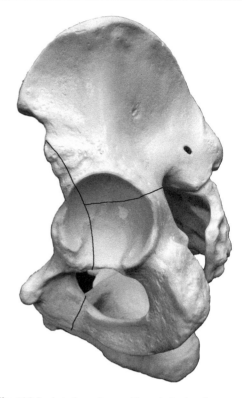

Fig. 108.8 Anterior column with posterior hemitransverse fracture

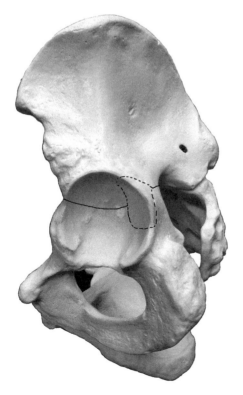

Fig. 108.7 Transverse with posterior wall fracture

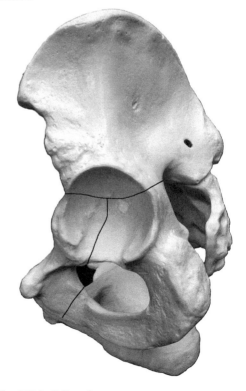

Fig. 108.9 T-Type fracture

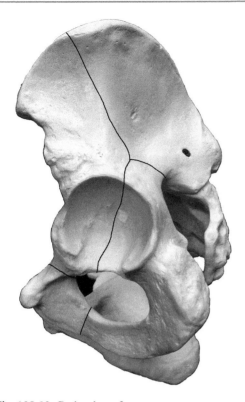

Fig. 108.10 Both column fracture

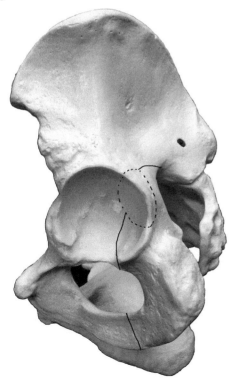

Fig. 108.11 Posterior column with posterior wall

Treatment

Non-operative

Indications
- No femoral head subluxation
- Less than 40% width involvement of the posterior wall
- Roof arc measurements on Judet views >45° (traditional method)
- No fracture of weight-bearing dome
- <2 mm displacement articular surface

Management
- Traction
  - Take pressure off of the articular cartilage
  - May help realign bony fragments and maintain limb length
  - Maintain femoral head reduction
  - May be definitive in poor surgical candidates
- Non-weight bearing

Operative

Emergent Situations
- Irreducible hip dislocations
- Progressive neurologic deficit
- Open fracture
- Vascular compromise

Indications
- Displacement >2 mm
- Intra-articular fragments
- Lack of secondary congruence
- >25% width of posterior wall
- Otherwise non-emergent but should be done as soon as possible
  - Easier to reduce
  - Better results
- Open reduction internal fixation
  - Anatomic reduction of articular surface
  - Predictive of outcome
- Closed reduction percutaneous fixation
  - Considered for elderly
  - Fractures with minimal displacement

Complications
- Nonunion
- Infection
- Avascular necrosis (AVN) of the femoral head
- Post-traumatic arthritis
- Heterotopic ossification (HO)
- Thromboembolism
  - Deep vein thrombosis (DVT)
  - Pulmonary embolus (PE)

Approaches
- Kocher-Langenbeck
  - Posterior wall fractures
  - Posterior column fractures
  - Transverse fractures
  - T-shaped fractures (may be in combination to other approach)
- Ilioinguinal
  - Anterior wall
  - Anterior column
  - Anterior column posterior hemitransverse
  - Associated both columns
- Extended iliofemoral
  - Considered if delayed fixation of associated fractures
  - Both columns, transverse or t-shaped under certain circumstances
- Combined
  - Transtectal transverse fractures
  - Anterior + posterior hemitransverse

- T-shaped
- Associated both columns

Postoperative Care
- DVT prophylaxis – can consider pelvic DVT screening
  - Chemoprophylaxis
  - Caval filter
- Toe touch or non-weight bearing 8–12 weeks
- Heterotopic ossification prophylaxis
  - Indomethacin
  - Low-dose radiation (XRT): 600–700 centigray in single or two doses
- Postoperative antibiotic prophylaxis

References

1. Rockwood CA, Green DP, Heckman JD, Bucholz RW. Rockwood and green's fractures in adults. Philadelphia: Lippincott Williams & Wilkins; 2001.
2. Porter SE, Schroeder AC, Dzugan SS, Graves ML, Zhang L, Russel GV. Acetabular fracture patterns and their associated injuries. J Orthop Trauma. 2008;22:165–70.
3. Egol KA, Koval KJ, Zuckerman JD. Handbook of fractures. Philadelphia: Lippincott Williams & Wilkins; 2010.
4. Letrounel E, Judet R. Fractures of the acetabulum. Heidelsberg: Springer-Verlag; 1993.
5. Tile M, Helfet D, Kellman J. Fractures of the pelvis and acetabulum. Philadelphia: Lippincott Williams & Wilkins; 2003.

Dominic J. Gargiulo

Genu Valgum (Knock Knee)

- There is a normal progression of coronal plane alignment in children's legs from varus to valgus (Fig. 109.1).
- Must differentiate between pathologic and physiologic process.

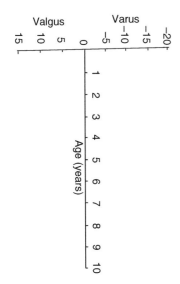

Fig. 109.1

D.J. Gargiulo, DO
Pediatric Orthopedics, Children's Hospital
New Orleans, New Orleans, LS, USA
e-mail: dgargi@lsuhsc.edu

- Genu varum can arise from either the distal femur or proximal tibia.
- Beware of lower limb rotation causing the appearance of lower extremity angular deformity; external rotation and knee flexion may resemble bowing.

Pathologic Etiology

Bilateral Genu Valgum
- Rickets
- Renal Osteodystrophy
- Skeletal dysplasias
  - Morquio's syndrome
  - Spondyloepiphyseal dysplasia

Unilateral Genu Valgum
- Damage to growth plate from trauma, vascular injury, or infection
  - Proximal tibial metaphyseal (Cozen's) fracture (Fig. 109.2) can cause late presentation of genu valgum (up to 18 months after injury; almost always remodels without intervention).
  - Rickets can occasionally be unilateral.
- Tumors
  - Fibrous dysplasia
  - Ollier's disease
  - Osteochondroma

© Springer International Publishing AG 2017
A.E.M. Eltorai et al. (eds.), *Orthopedic Surgery Clerkship*, DOI 10.1007/978-3-319-52567-9_109

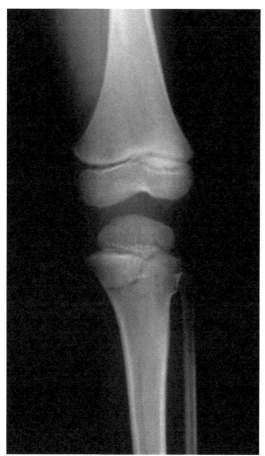

Fig. 109.2

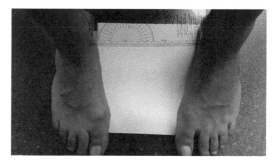

Fig. 109.3

Normal Physiologic Process of Genu Valgum

- Between 3 and 4 years of age children have up to 20° of genu valgum.
  - Genu valgum rarely worsens after age 7.
  - After age 7 valgus should not be worse than 12°.
  - After age 7 the intermalleolar distance should be <8 cm (Fig. 109.3).

Treatment

- Observation
  - Physiologic genu valgum
  - <15° in patients <6 years old
- Bracing
  - Rarely used

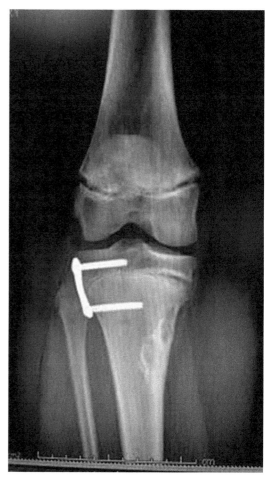

Fig. 109.4

- Operative
  - Hemiepiphysiodesis, medial physeal tethering/stapling in skeletally immature patient (Fig. 109.4)

- ○ Indication: >15–20° valgus in child <10 years
- ○ If mechanical axis falls in lateral quadrant of the tibia in child >10 years (Fig. 109.5)
- – Distal femoral varus osteotomy
  - ○ Skeletally mature patient or insufficient growth remaining to correct deformity

Genu Varum (Bow Legged)

- Physiologic varus deformity (bow legged) (Fig. 109.6)
  - – Normal until age 18 months

- Pathologic tibia vara (Blount's disease)
  - – Progressive varus deformity of the tibia
    - ○ Infantile
    - ○ Adolescent (>age 10)
- Infantile Blount's disease
  - – Pathologic tibia vara in children age 0–3 years
  - – More common than adolescent Blount's disease
  - – Usually bilateral
- Adolescent Blount's disease
  - – Pathologic tibia vara age > 10 years
  - – Usually less severe
  - – May be unilateral

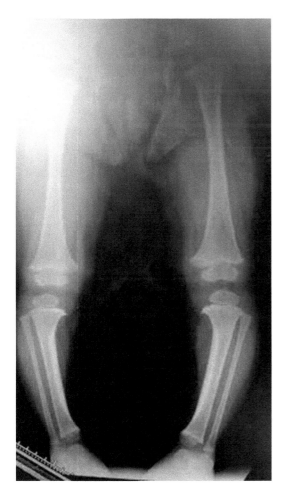

Fig. 109.5

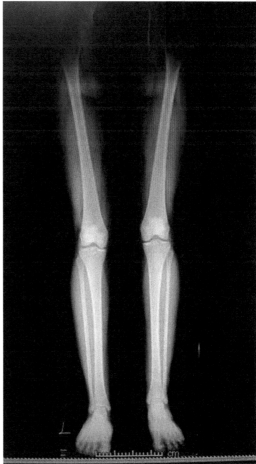

Fig. 109.6

Etiology

- Overloading of medial tibial growth plate in genetically susceptible individuals
- Risk factors: overweight, African American/Latino children, who begin walking early (<1 year)

Infantile Blount's Disease

Physiologic Varus

- Normal for children <2 years to be bow legged
- Alignment near neutral at 18–24 months
- Peak valgus alignment approx. age 3 years (Fig. 109.1)

Pathologic Process

- Can be difficult to determine pathologic versus physiologic in young children
- Usually bilateral disease in infants
- Differential Dx
  - Rickets
  - Osteogenesis imperfecta
  - Trauma
  - Skeletal dysplasia
- Findings suggestive of Blount's disease
  - Severe deformity
  - Asymmetric deformity
  - Progressive deformity
  - Varus knee thrust while ambulating

Radiographs

- Standing or lying AP hips to ankle films to measure mechanical axis
  - Patella must be facing forward (Fig. 109.7)
- Metaphyseal-diaphyseal angle/Drennan's angle (Fig. 109.8)

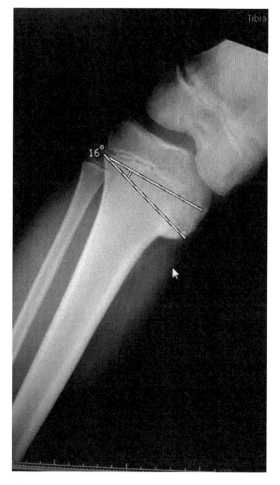

Fig. 109.7

  - Angle between metaphyseal beaks and the longitudinal axis of the tibia
    ∘ >16° is associated with pathologic progression
    ∘ <10° is physiologic

Langenskiold Classification
(Fig. 109.9)

- There is a normal progression of coronal plane alignment in children's legs from varus to valgus (Fig. 109.1)

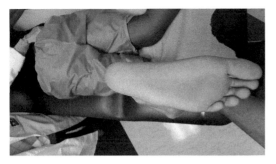

Fig. 109.8

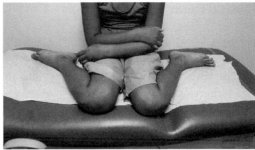

Fig. 109.10

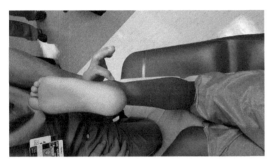

Fig. 109.9

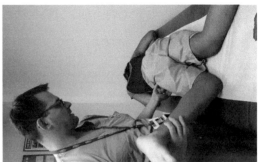

Fig. 109.11

Treatment

- Bracing with knee-ankle-foot orthosis (KAFO) (Fig. 109.10)
  - Indicated in stage I–II in children <3 years
  - Worn for approx. 2 years

Operative

- Indications
  - Stage I–II in age > 3 years
  - Stage III–VI in age < 3 years
  - Failure of brace treatment
  - Should be done prior to age 4 to prevent recurrence
- Proximal tibial osteotomy
  - Overcorrect 10–15° due to medial physeal pathology.
  - Resect bony bars as needed.

- Elevate medial plateau in severe disease.
- Consider prophylactic anterior compartment fasciotomy.
- Proximal tibial lateral hemiepiphysiodesis (Fig. 109.11)
  - Hueter-Volkman principle – compression across a growth plate slows longitudinal growth. Reversible phenomenon

Adolescent Blount's Disease

Pathologic Varus (Children >10 years)

- More likely unilateral limb involvement
- Less severe deformity
- Less common than infantile Blount's disease
- May have femoral and tibial components contributing to varus deformity

Physical Exam

- Obese
- May have lateral collateral ligament laxity
- May have limb length discrepancy due to deformity

Radiographs

- Standing hip to ankle radiograph measure mechanical axis
  - Patella must face forward
  - Metaphyseal-diaphyseal angle/Drennan's angle (Fig. 109.8)
    - >16° suggests pathology

Treatment

- Observation
  - Genu varum may progress
    - Leads to early degenerative changes to medial knee compartment

- Operative intervention
  - Proximal tibial lateral hemiepiphysiodesis/epiphysiodesis (permanent or temporary with growth guidance plate)
    - Include femur if involved
    - Skeletally immature patients
  - Proximal tibia/fibular osteotomy
    - More severe cases.
    - Skeletally mature patients.
    - Often have associated leg length deficiency. Treatment with a frame (i.e., Ilizarov, Taylor Spatial Frame, etc.) can correct length and angulation simultaneously.

Suggested Readings

1. Staheli L. Practice of pediatric orthopedics. 2nd ed. Philadelphia: Lipincott Williams & Wilkins; 2006. p. 77–103.
2. Tolo S. Master techniques in orthopedic surgery; pediatrics. Philadelphia: Lipincott Williams & Wilkins; 2008. p. 297–302, 313–24.

Principles of Pediatric Fracture Treatment

110

LeeAnne Torres, Dana Lycans, and Viorel Raducan

Structure and Biomechanics [2]

- Bones have two epiphyses (proximal and distal) and two metaphyses (proximal and distal) with a diaphysis in between. The physis lies between the epiphysis and metaphysis on each end of the bone.
- Organic component – matrix proteins, type I collagen, and proteoglycans
- Inorganic component – hydroxyapatite (compressive strength)
- Periosteum – thick peripheral osteogenic fibrous membrane. Very thick in children and helps to minimize fracture displacement as well as provide additional stability
  - Haversian channels – larger in children with secondary increase in porosity and corresponding change in biomechanical properties. This allows for more frequent failure in compression.

Physis [2]

- Area of specialized cartilage interposed between the epiphysis and the metaphysis
- Function: appositional growth (lengthwise)

Anatomy [2]

- Resting zone – distal-most zone. Supplies chondrocytes to the proliferative zone
- Proliferative zone – highest metabolic activity: matrix synthesis and cell turnover
- Hypertrophic zone – enlarged cells participating in mineralization
- Perichondrial ring of LaCroix – at the bone/cartilage junction. Responsible for 80% of distraction strength
- Groove of Ranvier – contains proliferative cells for circumferential growth

Biomechanics [1]

- Maximum resistance to distraction
- Least resistance to torsion
- Weak link in the mechanical characteristics of the pediatric bone. Periarticular injuries in children will result in physeal fracture, while the same injury in adults will result in ligamentous injury.
- The fracture plane is through the plane between the calcified and uncalcified cartilage layers

L. Torres, MD • D. Lycans, MD
Department of Orthopaedic Surgery,
Marshall University/Cabell Huntington Hospital,
Huntington, WV, USA

V. Raducan, MD (✉)
Department of Orthopaedic Surgery,
Marsashall University School of Medicine,
Huntington, WV, USA
e-mail: raducan@marshall.edu

© Springer International Publishing AG 2017
A.E.M. Eltorai et al. (eds.), *Orthopedic Surgery Clerkship*, DOI 10.1007/978-3-319-52567-9_110

529

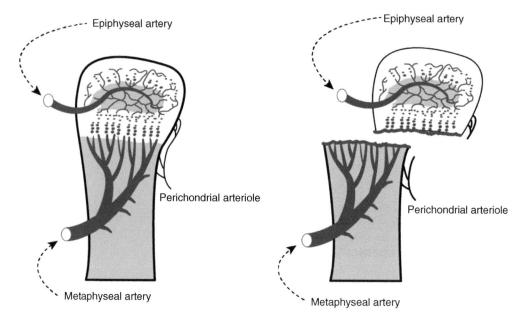

Fig. 110.1 Physeal Blood Supply

Blood Supply (Fig. 110.1) [3]

- Epiphyseal artery – for the resting and proliferative zones. Its injury has high risk of growth
  arrest.
- Metaphyseal artery – for the remained of the
  physis. Its injury has less propensity for
  growth arrest.
- Intra-articular epiphyses have a more tenuous blood supply – high risk of avascular
  necrosis (proximal femoral physis has highest risk).
- Epiphyses with soft tissue attachments have
  as a consequence a more robust blood supply
  and less propensity for avascular necrosis.
- Perichondrial arteries – at the level of the ring
  of LaCroix and groove of Ranvier.

Embryology [2]

- Upper limb evident at 26 days after fertiliza-
  tion as an elevation on the ventrolateral body
  wall at the level of pericardial swelling.

- Interaction between the apical ectodermal
  ridge and progress zone is critical for limb
  development.
- Three axes of limbs.
  - Anteroposterior
  - Dorsoventral
  - Proximal-distal
- Order of appearance
  - Early seventh week: cartilage anlage of
    entire upper limb skeletal elements, except
    the distal phalanges, is present; process in
    foot occurs 1 week later.
  - Ossification centers.
    ◦ First bones to ossify are the clavicle,
      mandible, and maxilla at weeks 6–7.
    ◦ Just prior to birth, ossific centers appear
      in the calcaneus, talus, cuboid, distal
      femoral epiphysis, and proximal tibial
      epiphysis.
    ◦ Elbow: capitellum (1 year), radial head
      (3–4 years), medial epicondyle
      (5–6 years), trochlea (8–9 years),
      olecranon (10–11 years), lateral epicon-
      dyle (12–13 years).

Limb Growth [1]

- Lower extremity grows 23 mm/year, with most growth at the knee (15 mm/year).
  - Proximal femur: 3 mm/year
  - Distal femur: 9 mm/year
  - Proximal tibia: 6 mm/year
  - Distal tibia: 5 mm/year
- Upper extremity growth.
  - Proximal humerus contributes about 80% of humerus growth.
  - Distal radius contributes 80% of radius growth (5 mm/year) and 40% of upper extremity growth.

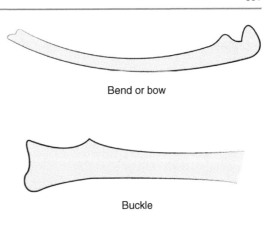

Bend or bow

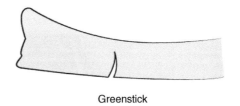

Buckle

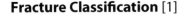

Fracture Classification [1]

Extra-physeal

- Incomplete fractures (Fig. 110.2)
  - Buckle/torus fractures – compression failure near the metaphysis (highest porosity)
  - Greenstick fractures – occur when the bone is angulated beyond its limits to bend. Failure of tension side, with bending at the compression side
  - Traumatic bowing of bone – plastic deformation: bending without acute angular deformity and ability to straighten back
- Complete fractures
  - Described by location (diaphyseal, metaphyseal) and pattern (oblique, spiral, transverse, butterfly) (Fig. 110.3)

Greenstick

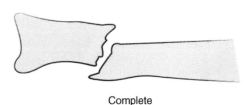

Complete

Fig. 110.2 Extra-physeal Fractures

Physeal Fractures [3]

- Constitute 1/3 of pediatric skeletal trauma
- Risks of limb shortening and angulation due to damage to physis and risk of subsequent growth arrest
- Salter-Harris classification (Fig. 110.4)
  - Type 1: fracture lines follow the growth plate; physeal separation (Fig. 110.5).

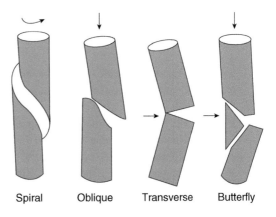

Spiral   Oblique   Transverse   Butterfly

Fig. 110.3 Fracture Patterns

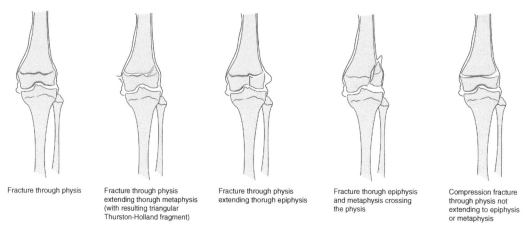

Fracture through physis | Fracture through physis extending thorugh metaphysis (with resulting triangular Thurston-Holland fragment) | Fracture through physis extending thorugh epiphysis | Fracture thorugh epiphysis and metaphysis crossing the physis | Compression fracture through physis not extending to epiphysis or metaphysis

Fig. 110.4 Salter-Harris Classification

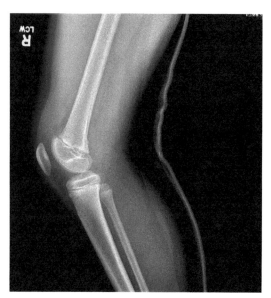

Fig. 110.5 Salter-Harris 1

- Type 2: fracture crosses the physis and exits the metaphysis (most common) (Fig. 110.6).
  ◦ Thurston Holland fragment: small portion of metaphyseal bone can be carried with epiphysis.
- Type 3: fracture crosses the physis and exits through epiphysis (Fig. 110.7).
- Type 4: fracture traverses the epiphysis, physis, and metaphysis.
- Type 5: severe compression of physis due to axial loading.

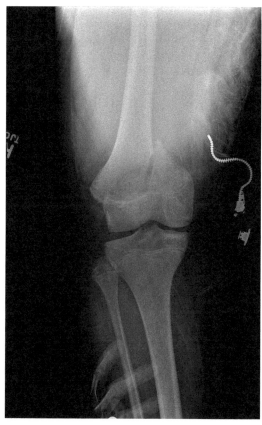

Fig. 110.6 Salter-Harris 2

Open Fractures [1]

- Direct communication with the fracture site
- Increased risk of infection
- Higher energy mechanism

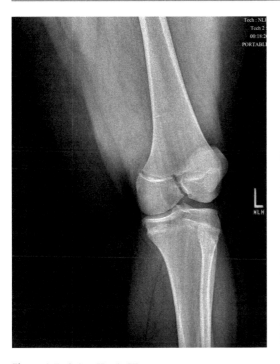

Fig. 110.7 Salter-Harris III

- Longer time to union
- Closed fractures: skin intact

Evaluation [1, 2]

- Check neurovascular status.
  - Before and after manipulation
- Skin examination for integrity. Any laceration indicates open fracture.
- Imaging.
  - Orthogonal X-rays – AP/lateral views

Treatment [2]

Nonoperative

- Cast immobilization and closed reduction (if necessary)
  - Respect to physeal integrity is critical, and additional physeal injury should be avoided.
    ○ Do not manipulate growth plate fracture >7–10 days after injury.

- Periosteal flap may get entrapped in fracture site, or sharp fracture fragment may buttonhole through the periosteum which may prevent reduction.
- Cast should span one joint above and below the fracture.

Operative

- Indications: open fractures, soft tissue compromise, neurovascular injury, compartment syndrome, inability to maintain adequate reduction, Salter-Harris III and IV fractures with displacement (intra-articular).
- Fixation across physis is temporary with smooth implants that are removed at 3–6 weeks.

Remodeling [2]

- Open physes allow for significant remodeling in cases of severe deformity (average 1°/month up to 10°/year).
- Remodeling potential depends on growth remaining (which depends on age of patient), proximity to physis, and growth potential of physis.
  - The proximal humerus and distal radius will remodel more than fractures around the elbow, ankle, and knee.
  - Fractures around knee have higher risk of growth arrest.
  - Remodeling is maximized in the plane of maximal range of motion.
  - Malrotation does not remodel.

Complications [1, 2]

- Early
  - Soft tissue compromise
  - Neurovascular injury
  - Compartment syndrome
  - Lost reduction
- Late
  - Nonunion (rare)
  - Malunion (common)
  - Growth arrest

References

1. Egol KA, Koval KJ, Zuckerman JD, Koval KJ. Pediatric orthopedic surgery: general principles. In: Handbook of fractures. Philadelphia: Wolters Kluwer/Lippincott Williams & Wilkins Health; 2010.

2. Morrissy RT, Weinstein SL, editors. Lovell and Winter's pediatric orthopedics. 6th ed. Philadelphia: Lippincott Williams & Wilkins; 2006.

3. Rang M, Wenger DR, Pring ME. The physis and skeletal injury. In: Rang's children's fractures. 3rd ed. Philadelphia: Lippincott Williams & Wilkins; 2005.

Radial Head Dislocation

111

Amit Momaya and Reed Estes

Radial Head Dislocation

Congenital Dislocation

- Rare entity (0.06–0.16% incidence).
- Often bilateral.
- Associated with other congenital anomalies.
- Most patients are asymptomatic until adolescence when elbow pain or lack of motion becomes an issue.
- Most commonly posterior dislocation.
- Symptoms.
  - Pain or limited range of motion when symptomatic
- Physical examination.
  - Radial head prominence
  - Limited elbow range of motion
- Radiographs.
  - Bilateral comparison view
  - Convex radial head and hypoplastic capitellum
- Treatment.
  - Nonoperative – often successful
  - Radial head resection
    ◦ May provide substantial pain relief, but only modest improvement in forearm

rotation and no improvement in flexion/extension

Monteggia Fracture

- Radial head dislocation with associated ulna fracture/plastic deformation.
- Isolated radial head dislocations are extremely rare, and one must maintain a high suspicion for a Monteggia fracture.
- Classification.
  - Bado classification is most commonly used (Table 111.1).
    ◦ Bado type I is the most common type of pediatric Monteggia fracture
- Imaging.
  - Radiographs will show a radial head that is no longer in line with the capitellum (Fig. 111.1)
  - The ulna may show a fracture or subtle plastic deformation
- Treatment.
  - Nonsurgical

Table 111.1 Bado classification of Monteggia fractures

Bado type	Ulnar fracture apex	Radial head dislocation
I	Anterior	Anterior dislocation
II	Posterior	Posterior dislocation
III	Lateral	Lateral dislocation
IV	Any direction	Proximal dislocation with fracture

A. Momaya, MD • R. Estes, MD (✉)
Department of Surgery, Division of Orthopedic Surgery, University of Alabama at Birmingham, Birmingham, AL, USA
e-mail: reede44@uab.edu; reed.estes@gmail.com

© Springer International Publishing AG 2017
A.E.M. Eltorai et al. (eds.), *Orthopedic Surgery Clerkship*, DOI 10.1007/978-3-319-52567-9_111

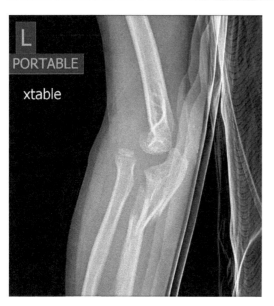

Fig. 111.1 The lateral elbow X-ray shows an anterior radial head dislocation with an ulna fracture

- elastic titanium intramedullary nail fixation.
  - • Comminuted ulna fractures are treated with plate and screws.
  - ∘ Chronic fractures.
    - • Generally those fractures that are greater than 2–3 weeks from injury
    - • Should undergo fixation
      - i. Numerous techniques have been described including a combination of ulnar osteotomy with fixation, open reduction of radial head, and repair of the annular ligament
- • Complications.
  - – Posterior interosseous nerve palsy can occur (10% of acute injuries), but most will resolve spontaneously.
  - – Missed Monteggia fractures in adolescents can result in debilitating deformities.

  - ∘ Often successful in children.
  - ∘ Establishing ulnar length is key to maintaining radial head reduction.
  - ∘ Bado type I and III fractures are usually casted with the forearm in supination.
  - – Surgical
    - ∘ Acute fractures that are open or unstable require operative fixation.
      - • Transverse or short oblique fractures of the ulna are often treated with an

References

1. Bengard MJ, Calfee RP, Steffen JA, Goldfarb CA. Intermediate-term to long-term outcome of surgically and nonsurgically treated congenital, isolated radial head dislocation. J Hand Surg Am. 2012;37(12):2495–501.
2. Beutel BG. Monteggia fractures in pediatric and adult populations. Orthopedics. 2012;35(2):138–44.

Viorel Raducan

Epidemiology [1]

- Age – peripubertal (10–14)
- Risser I/open triradiate cartilages
- Usually in obese children – BMI >35
- Racial preponderance:
  - Highest in Polynesians, Hispanics, and African Americans

Etiology *Unknown*; *idiopathic* in the majority of cases.

Endocrine 5–8%

- Hypothyroidism
- Panhypopituitarism
- Growth hormone deficiency/treatment
- Hyperparathyroidism
- Hypogonadism
- Down syndrome (associated hypothyroidism)

Renal Osteodystrophy

- Secondary hyperparathyroidism.
- The pathology involves the metaphysis.
- Control of the hyperparathyroidism will prevent progression.

Radiation Therapy

- 10% will develop SCFE.

Mechanical factors *Increased/abnormal stress on the physis*

- Coxa vara
- Femoral retroversion
- Coxa profunda (deep sockets)
- Obesity [4]

Pathological Anatomy

Macro

- The epiphysis is fixed in the acetabulum.
- The neck and shaft displace anteriorly and in external rotation.
- Consequences: the leg is externally rotated/the metaphysis impinges on the rim of the acetabulum.

V. Raducan, MD, FRCS(C)
Department of Orthopaedic Surgery,
Marsashall University School of Medicine,
Huntington, WV, USA
e-mail: raducan@marshall.edu

Micro

- The proximal femoral physis is disorganized – thick hypertrophic zone; the proliferative zone is hypocellular.
- The displacement occurs through the abnormal zones – hypertrophic/proliferative.

Diagnosis

Clinical Presentation

- Lower extremity pain: usually around the hip and *sometimes isolated to the knee*. The onset is acute or insidious, without or with minimal trauma.
- Antalgic limp.
- Decreased internal rotation of the hip.
- Obligatory hip external rotation during hip flexion.
- High BMI [4].
- Peripubertal age.
- Critical – ability to bear weight.
- Affected limb in external rotation.

Imaging Studies

- X-rays – AP/frog
  - Frog view more sensitive
  - Kline's line
  - Southwick angle
- MRI scan – minimal indications:
  - Evaluate the contralateral side.
  - If high index of suspicion (will identify the abnormal physis if X-rays are negative).

Classification

Radiological: *Southwick Angle*

- Mild – <30°
- Moderate –30°–50°
- Severe – >50°

Clinical

- Onset/duration:
  - Acute – sudden onset
  - Chronic – slow onset/long duration of symptoms
  - Acute on chronic – acute exacerbation of symptoms of long duration

Stable/Unstable

- Stable – ability to bear weight
- Unstable – unable to bear weight even with walking aides
- Utmost prognostic significance
- Critical to document

Natural History

Short Term

- 80% unilateral at presentation, of which half will progress to the other side, usually within 18 months
- 20% bilateral at presentation
- Risk factors of progression to the other side: known etiology and younger age (open triradiate cartilages) [3]

Long Term: Early OA, Poor Hip Function

- All untreated SCFE's will progress.

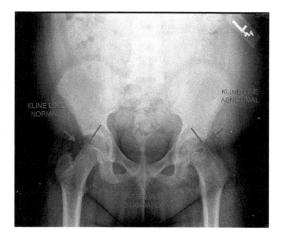

Fig. 112.1

- Poor prognostic factors:
  - Severity
  - Delay of treatment
  - Unstable slip
  - Complications

Treatment

Rationale

- Prevent progression.
- Prevent/minimize long term complications – OA.
- Admit to hospital as soon as diagnosis made.
- Non-weight-bearing affected lower extremity.
- Treat within 24 h (? emergently for unstable SCFE).
- Goals:
  - Proximal femoral epiphysiodesis (which will prevent further displacement).
  - Minimize deformity.

The Treatment Is Surgical

- Percutaneous in situ cannulated screw fixation [5]
  - One or two screws
  - Direction – perpendicular to the plane of the base of the epiphysis (will maximize epiphyseal screw purchase and minimize the risk of intraarticular penetration)
  - Will not correct the deformity
- Open hip dislocation with open reduction and internal fixation [6].
  - Will correct the deformity (minimize the risk of early OA)?
  - High risk of avascular necrosis (up to 32%).
  - Its usage is increasing.

Complications

Avascular Necrosis [2]

- Causes
  - Direct injury to the vessels

- Increased intracapsular pressure (intraarticular hematoma) [7]
- Risk factors
  - Unstable slip
  - Delay of treatment
  - Open treatment
  - Young age
  - Female sex
  - Severe slip
- Percutaneous cannulated screw fixation – 0–5%
- Open treatment – up to 32%

Chondrolysis

- Cartilage lysis – femoral head and acetabulum.
- Unknown mechanism.
- Diagnosis – persistent pain and stiffness 2 weeks after treatment.
- Triad of pain/stiffness/decreased joint space.
- Predisposing factors – *iatrogenic*.
  - Any treatment
  - Most – hip spica (historical interest only)
  - Open procedure
  - Least – PCCSF (percutaneous cannulated screw fixation)
- Prognosis – highly variable, from full recovery to joint destruction. No factors are identified to predispose either outcome.

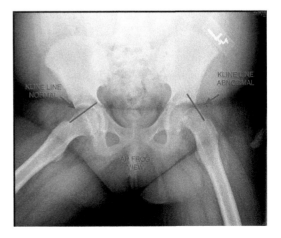

Fig. 112.2 Percutaneous cannulated screw fixation with contralateral slip

- Treatment – NSAIDS/physical therapy for range of motion.
- End stage – fusion/arthroplasty.

Osteoarthritis

- End stage
- Pathogeny – joint incongruity
- Severity related to:
  - Degree of residual deformity
  - Complications

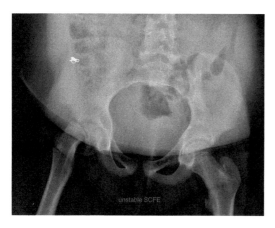

Fig. 112.3 Kline line - essential for the radiological diagnosis of SCFE

SCFE Essentials

- *10–16 YO/high BMI.*
- *Lower extremity pain.*
- *Inability to bear weight.*
- *Pelvis X-rays – AP and frog/Kline's line.*
- *Admit as soon as diagnosis is made.*

References

1. Castro Jr FP, Bennett James T, Kevin D. Epidemiological perspective on prophylactic pinning in patients with unilateral slipped capital femoral epiphysis. J Pediatr Orthop. 2000;20(6):745–8.
2. Kennedy JG, Hresko TM, Kasser JR. Osteonecrosis of the femoral head associated with slipped capital femoral epiphysis. J Paediatr Orthop. 2001;21(2):189–93.
3. Popejoy D, Emara K, Birch J. Prediction of contralateral slipped capital femoral epiphysis using the modified Oxford bone age score. J Paediatr Orthop. 2012;32(3):290–4.
4. Body mass index in patients with slipped capital femoral epiphysis. J Pediatr Orthop. 2006;26(2):197–9.
5. Loder RT, Dietz FR. What is the best evidence for the treatment of slipped capital femoral epiphysis? J Paediatr Orthop. 32(Suppl 2):S158–65.
6. Tibor LM, Sink EL. Risks and benefits of the modified Dunn approach for the treatment of moderate to severe slipped capital femoral epiphysis. J Paediatr Orthop. 2013;33(Suppl 1):S99–S102.
7. Crepeau A, Birbaum M, Have V, et al. Intracapsular pressures after stable slipped capital femoral epiphysis. J Paediatr Orthop. 2015;35(8):e90–2.

Viorel Raducan

Definition

It is an abnormal in utero development of the hip joint – the spectrum includes instability, dysplasia, subluxation, and frank dislocation.

Embryology

- Origin – mesenchymal cells.
- Cleft at 7 weeks
- Complete development at 11 weeks.
- The acetabulum develops from the triradiate cartilage.
- The proximal femoral ossification center appears between the fourth and seventh weeks.
- The key factor in normal hip development is *acetabular growth around a spherical, centrally located femoral head.*

Etiology

- Genetics – familial preponderance
- Intrauterine position – packaging
  - Breech
  - Oligohydramnios

- Neuromuscular
  - Myelomeningocele
- Postnatal factors – swaddling

> N.B. *Ligamentous laxity* – not a causal relationship. Children have documented ligamentous laxity without hip instability. DDH is not a hallmark of systemic hyper laxity syndromes – Marfan, Down, Ehlers-Danlos.

Epidemiology/Risk Factors

- Incidence: 1–2/1000 live births. Variable with ethnicity/geographical location
- Ethnicity
  - Highest – Laplanders
  - Lowest – African Americans
- Female sex
- First born
- Breech
- Positive family history
- Oligohydramnios
- Metatarsus adductus
- Torticollis

V. Raducan, MD, FRCS(C)
Department of Orthopaedic Surgery,
Marshall University School of Medicine,
Huntington, WV, USA
e-mail: raducan@marshall.edu

© Springer International Publishing AG 2017
A.E.M. Eltorai et al. (eds.), *Orthopedic Surgery Clerkship*, DOI 10.1007/978-3-319-52567-9_113

Pathology

- *Shallow acetabulum with insufficient anterior and lateral coverage*
- Coxa valga
- Redundant capsule
- Inverted labrum
- Elongated ligament teres
- Tight iliopsoas tendon
- Redundant fibrous tissue in the joint – pulvinar

> The normal development of the hip joint is dependent on the uninterrupted contact of the acetabulum with a spherical and centrally located femoral head. The consequences of dysplasia and the response to treatment are directly related to the time allowed for the abnormal relationship to persist. This means that the clinical presentation, the investigation, the treatment, and the outcome will depend on the time of diagnosis and stage of child development at the time of diagnosis.

Clinical Presentation (See Above)

- Newborn to 6 months
  - Barlow maneuver – the located hip is dislocated.
  - Ortolani – the dislocated hip is relocated.
  - They are usually performed concomitantly, are interchangeable, and have equal diagnostic value.
  - They become ineluctable after 3 months.

An irreducible hip in the nursery with limited abduction is the hallmark of teratological DDH, usually present in systemic conditions – 2% of all nursery diagnosed DDH.

The "hip click" has no diagnostic significance.

- Six months to walking age
  - Limited hip abduction – hallmark

- Galeazzi sign – apparent femoral shortening
- Asymmetrical gluteal folds
- Limb length inequality

Bilateral DDH – more difficult to diagnose especially after 3–6 months (Barlow/Ortolani are absent); the findings are symmetrical.

- After walking age
  - Limited abduction
  - Limp – due to abductor weakness (relative shortening, Trendelenburg)
  - Waddling gait – bilateral DDH, bilateral Trendelenburg gait
  - Lumbar hyperlordosis

Imaging Studies

- Ultrasound
  - Noninvasive and operator dependent
  - Evaluates
    - Hip anatomy – see (Fig. 113.1)
    - Location of the femoral head.
    - Degree of femoral head coverage.
    - Above in static and dynamic modes.
  - High false positive rate (over diagnosis)/low false negative rate
  - Critical information
    - Alpha and beta angles (alpha angle >60° is normal)
    - Percentage of femoral head coverage (>50% is normal)
  - Indications in the United States
    - Screening for high-risk newborns
    - Follow-up while treatment in brace
    - After age 3 weeks
- *X-rays – pelvis (AP and frog lateral)*
  - Timing – after 3 months of age/when the proximal epiphyses are present
  - Landmarks – see (Fig. 113.1)
  - Normal hip parameters
    - The proximal femur/epiphysis projects in the inferomedial quadrant.
    - Acetabular index <30°.
    - Continuous Shenton line.

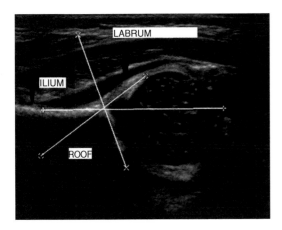

Fig. 113.1 Bilateral hip dysplasia: the femoral epiphyses are outside the inferior medial quadrant, the Shenton lines are broken

- ◦ Symmetrically developed proximal epiphyses.
- ◦ Symmetrical hip abduction with the femoral epiphyses projecting centrally in relationship with the triradiate cartilage on the frog view.
- – Arthrogram – used to assess the adequacy of closed reduction in the operating room
- – CT scan – same indications as the arthrogram
- – MRI scan – limited indications, need for general anesthesia
- • Natural history – degenerative joint disease
- – Dysplasia without subluxation – the progression and severity of DJD is not related to the radiograph's findings.
- – Dysplasia with subluxation – severity related to the degree of subluxation.

Treatment – Age Dependent

- • Zero to 6 months – Pavlik harness
- – Prevents hip adduction and extension
- – Allows abduction and flexion/promotes reduction/stabilization
- – Duration: until hip stabilizes. If Ortolani positive: 6–12 weeks
- – 95% successful
- – Contraindications

- ◦ Neuromuscular etiology
- ◦ Syndromic generalized ligamentous laxity – Ehlers-Danlos
- ◦ Teratological DDH, i.e., arthrogryposis
- ◦ Age >6 months – child too active, 50% failure
- – Complications – secondary to
- ◦ Persistent use despite failure – persistent dislocation/subluxation
- ◦ Inappropriate application
- ◦ Consequences – femoral head and acetabular damage, femoral nerve palsy.
- • 6 months to 2 years
- – Closed reduction and spica application
- ◦ Under general anesthesia
- ◦ Well-molded spica
- ◦ Arthrogram documentation of reduction before spica application
- ◦ CT scan documentation of reduction after spica application and follow-up
- ◦ Duration – 6–12 weeks
- ◦ Postcasting – hip abduction orthosis until age 18–24 months
- – Open reduction and spica application
- ◦ Indications: failed/lost reduction/irreducible dislocation
- ◦ Spica for 12 weeks
- ◦ Hip abduction orthosis postcasting
- – Additional procedures
- ◦ Femoral shortening – if reduction not possible intraoperatively
- ◦ Periacetabular osteotomy – to increase anterior coverage/deepen the acetabulum
- ◦ Varus/derotation femoral osteotomy – in conjunction with the above (will allow centralization of the femoral head – the essential condition of normal hip development).

Complications: Proximal Femoral Growth Disturbance

- • Usually iatrogenic
- • Avascular necrosis of the femoral head
- – Injury to the medial circumflex femoral artery

- Indirect – excessive abduction during closed/open reduction
- Direct injury during open reduction.
- Possibly prevented by femoral shortening during open reduction
• Persistent malreduction – abnormal pressure on the femoral head

Conclusions
• DDH is a complex entity.
• Natural history is uniformly bad with lifelong disability.

• Early diagnosis is imperative – mandatory screening.
• Screening in the United States is by clinical evaluation with ultrasound recommended for high-risk/ambiguous cases.
• The outcome depends on early diagnosis and treatment.
• Successful treatment means a hip that at maturity has:
  - Full coverage of the femoral head
  - Shenton lines in continuity
  - Normal tear drop

Congenital Coxa Vara

114

Evan Sheppard and Reed Estes

Background

- Description
  - Abnormal decrease in the femoral neck-shaft angle
    - Normal at 1 year of age is ~148°
    - Adult is 120°
  - Shortening of the femoral neck
  - Relative overgrowth of the greater trochanter
- 1 in 25,000 live births
- Males and females affected equally
- Most commonly unilateral
  - Bilateral cases more likely seen with generalized skeletal dysplasia
- Usually associated with a short femur

Anatomy

- Common proximal femoral physis between the greater trochanter and the capital femoral epiphysis.
- As growth continues, the physis divides in a balanced way that favors the capital femoral epiphysis and leads to a normal neck-shaft angle.

E. Sheppard, MD • R. Estes, MD (✉)
Department of Surgery, Division of Orthopedic
Surgery, University of Alabama at Birmingham,
Birmingham, AL, USA
e-mail: reede44@uab.edu; reed.estes@gmail.com

- Femoral deformity is present in the subtrochanteric region:
  - Bone is bent.
  - Thickened cortices.
- The femur is often retroverted.

Pathogenesis

- Primarily a cartilaginous defect in the femoral neck:
  - Defect in endochondral ossification of the medial portion of the femoral neck
  - Unequal growth in the common femoral physis before differentiating into the greater trochanteric apophysis and the capital physis
- As the neck-shaft angle changes from horizontal to vertical, the shearing force increases across the physis:
  - Results in less growth of the femoral neck medially compared to the lateral side
- Histology shows disorganized islands of cartilage cells in reduced numbers.

Physical Exam

- Most present at walking age.
- May have skin dimpling in the groin region.
- External rotation of the femur with valgus deformity of the knee may be noted.
- Waddling caused by abductor weakness from abnormal tension.

- Leg length discrepancy.
- Limited abduction and internal rotation.
- Look for other dysplasias.

Imaging

- AP and frog lateral.
- Decreased neck-shaft angle.
- Widening of the capital epiphysis.
- Measure the amount of deformity on the AP pelvis radiograph:
  - Neck-shaft angle → not useful in prognosis
  - Head-shaft angle → more accurately reflects severity and likelihood of progression
    ○ Angle between the axis of the shaft and a line perpendicular to the base of the femoral epiphysis
  - Hilgenreiner's epiphyseal angle → good prognostic value
    ○ Angle between Hilgenreiner's line and a line parallel to the proximal femoral physis on an AP X-ray with the hips in neutral.
    ○ Normal is 0–25°.
    ○ Greater than 60° = progression and merits surgical correction.
    ○ Less than 45° = stable or improve.
    ○ Between 45 and 60 = monitor with serial X-rays.

Treatment

- Goals of treatment
  - Stimulate ossification and healing of the defective femoral neck.
  - Restore head-shaft angle.
  - Restore normal mechanical muscle function.
- H-E angle greater than 60°
  - Valgus osteotomy
- H-E angle 45–59°
  - Monitor those without symptoms with serial radiographs.
  - Valgus osteotomy for those with symptoms.
- H-E angle less than 45°
  - Assess for limb length inequality.
  - Follow radiographically.
- Timing of correction
  - Balance between limited fixation in young patients and the severity of acetabular dysplasia with increasing age
    ○ Correct when there is sufficient deformity and there is adequate bony development.

Suggested Reading

1. Tachdjian MO, et al. Congenital coxa vara. In: Tachdjian's pediatric orthopedics. 4th ed. Philadelphia: Saunders/Elsevier; 2008. p. 897–901. Print.

David Cealrey

Osteochondritis Dissecans

Overview

Etiology

- Remains unclear. Despite the nomenclature, inflammation is not likely.
- Repetitive microtrauma:
  - History of injury reported in up to 40% of cases [1].
  - Fairbanks [2] described repetitive impingement from tibial spine.
  - Stanitsky and Aichroth reported association with discoid lateral meniscus [3, 4].
- Vascular Insufficiency:
  - Similar histology and pathophysiology to osteonecrosis
  - May be due to poor blood supply to the area of the medial femoral condyle near the insertion of the PCL [5]
- Hereditary:
  - Association of OCD with dwarfisms and Legg-Calve-Perthes and Stickler syndrome
  - May be explained by patterns of abnormal ossification of the distal femoral condyles

Incidence <1% [6]

- Male/female = 2:1 [1]
- Most patients between 10 and 15 years of age

Anatomic Considerations

- Classically located on the lateral aspect of the medial femoral condyle.
- Other locations can include the patella and the lateral femoral condyle.
- As the subchondral bone undergoes structural changes, the overlying articular cartilage is subject to damage from the lack of support.

Classifications

Guhl's Arthroscopy [7]

- Type I: Softening of the articular cartilage
- Type II: Stable but breached cartilage
- Type III: Partially detached fragment (flap)
- Type IV: Full-thickness cartilage defect with intraarticular loose body

Dipaola: MRI [8]

- Stable vs. unstable based on fluid signal between cartilage and subchondral bone

Clinical Presentation

- Presents most commonly as pain in the knee often accompanied by swelling and usually associated with activity.

D. Cealrey, MD
Associate Professor of Orthopedics,
Augusta University, Augusta, GA, USA
e-mail: dcearley@gru.edu

© Springer International Publishing AG 2017
A.E.M. Eltorai et al. (eds.), *Orthopedic Surgery Clerkship*, DOI 10.1007/978-3-319-52567-9_115

- More advanced stages may present with mechanical symptoms such as locking, popping, or "giving way." If these symptoms are severe, it may indicate the presence of a loose body.
- Physical exam should include testing for meniscal and ligamentous pathology as well as for any malalignment:
  - "Wilson's Test" [9]
    ◦ Reproduction of pain with internal rotation and extension of the knee from 90 to 30°.
    ◦ This is thought to cause impingement of the tibial spine on the OCD.

Imaging

- Plain radiographs
  - Usually diagnostic for the presence of the lesion.
  - Determine the status of the physes (i.e., open or closed).
  - Not reliable for staging or determining stability of lesion.

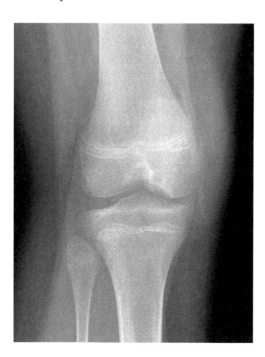

- MRI
  - Useful for accurately measuring size of the lesion
  - Stability assessed by presence of fluid signal behind the cartilage and whether a breach of the articular surface is seen.

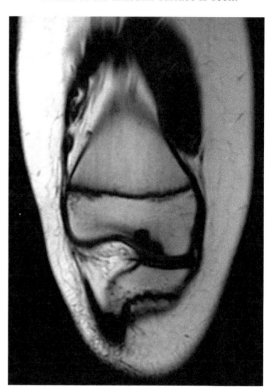

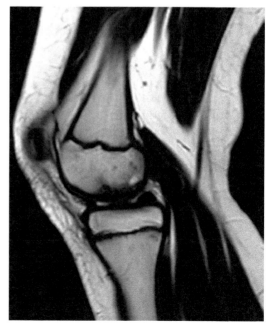

Prognosis

- Small, stable lesions (<4 mm) in younger patients with open growth plates often heal without surgery.
- Older patients with signs of instability or articular disruption on MRI tend to fail conservative treatment [10].
- If left untreated, patients are at risk of developing osteoarthritis if lesions are located on weight bearing surface of joint.

Treatment

Nonsurgical
- Activity modifications with elimination of sports and high-impact activities
- Crutches, braces for pain relief, and cast immobilization in extreme cases or when compliance is questionable
- NSAIDs/acetaminophen

Surgical
- Arthroscopy
  - Classify lesion based on Guhl's criteria.
  - Antegrade drilling to stimulate vascular ingrowth and healing of subchondral bone recommended for stable lesion with intact cartilage.
  - Internal fixation recommended for unstable lesions or full-thickness lesions in the acute setting.
- Treatment of late-stage or very large lesions
  - Microfracture – retrograde drilling of exposed subchondral bone to create a clot that will produce a fibrocartilage "scar" to fill the defect
  - Autologous chondrocyte implantation
  - Osteochondral allograft

Osgood-Schlatter Disease

Overview

- Osteochondrosis affecting the tibial tubercle in skeletally immature patients first described by Osgood and Schlatter in 1903

- Etiology likely related to repeated and/or forceful contracture of the quadriceps on the developing bone of the tibial tubercle apophysis [11]

Anatomy

- The patellar tendon, which is the continuation of the quadriceps muscle, inserts on the tibial tubercle.
- In children this area consists of physeal cartilage. Sites of tendon insertions into cartilaginous growth plates are known as apophyses.
- During periods of growth, with puberty in particular, the tissue undergoes ossification.
- It is believed that repetitive or forceful traction from the patellar tendon at these times results in inflammation either in the tendon itself or through small avulsion fractures of incompletely developed bone of the tubercle [1].

Clinical Presentation

- Usually presents in girls 8–12 or boys 10–15 due to the earlier onset of puberty in females.
- Male/Female = 3:1.
- Patients frequently are involved in running or jumping sports and activities.
- Physical exam [12]:
  - Pain and tenderness directly over the tibial tubercle
  - Pain with resisted knee extension
  - Often present with localized swelling
  - Important to verify active knee extension to rule out acute tubercle avulsion fracture

Imaging
- Plain radiography is usually all that is necessary [12]:
  - Often negative in early stages or in very young patients prior to ossification.
  - Soft tissue swelling may be seen.
    - May show pattern of abnormal ossification of tubercle in older patients and even ossicles or bony fragments located within the tendon.

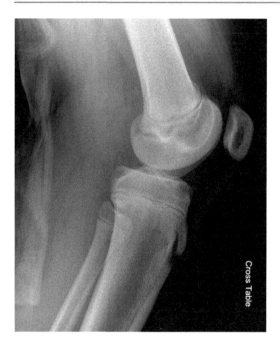

Cross Table

Natural History

- Vast majority of cases show complete resolution of symptoms by skeletal maturity with a low incidence of associated patellar instability [13].
- Many patients do continue to complain of a tender bony prominence into adulthood that often prevents comfortable kneeling [13].

Treatment

Nonoperative
- Mainstay of treatment.
- Rest, ice, and NSAIDs.
- Limitation of sports and other activities as indicated by severity of symptoms.
- Use of braces may be beneficial and even brief periods of cast immobilization can be employed for relief of pain in more severe cases, although prolonged immobilization should be avoided to prevent knee stiffness.

Operative
- Almost never indicated in skeletally immature patients.

- Rarely, patients will continue to report painful symptoms into adulthood.
- Surgery usually not necessary, as early reports showed little benefit with significant rate of postoperative complications [12].
- More recently, good results have been reported in cases of unresolved Osgood-Schlatter disease with resection of ossicles within the tendon combined with a tubercleplasty to relieve the bony prominence [14].

Complications

- Early closure of the tibial tubercle with resultant genu recurvatum has been reported in severe cases [15].
- Surgical complications include persistent or worsened bony prominence, wound dehiscence, and recurvatum if the patient is skeletally immature at time of surgery [12].

References

1. Crawford D. Osteochondritis dissecans of the knee. J Am Acad Orthop Surg. 2006;14:90–100.
2. Fairbank HAT. Osteochondritis dissecans. J Bone Joint Surg Br. 1933;21:67–73.
3. Stanitski C. Juvenile osteochondritis dissecans of the lateral femoral condyle after lateral discoid meniscus surgery. Am J Sports Med. 2004;32:797–801.
4. Aicroth P. Congenital discoid lateral meniscus in children: a follow up study and evolution of management. J Bone Joint Surg Br. 1991;73:932–6.
5. Reddy A. Evaluation of the interosseous blood supply to the distal femoral condyles. Am J Sports Med. 1998;26:415–9.
6. Linden B. The incidence of osteochondritis dissecans in the condyles of the femur. Acta Orthop Scand. 1976;47:664–7.
7. Guhl J. Arthroscopic treatment of osteochondritis dissecans. Clin Orthop. 1982;167:65–74.
8. Dipaola J. Characterizing osteochondritis dissecans lesion by magnetic resonance imaging. Arthroscopy. 1991;7:101–4.
9. Wilson J. A diagnostic sign in osteochondritis dissecans of the knee. J Bone Joint Surg Am. 1967;49:477–80.
10. Pill S. Role of magnetic resonance imaging and clinical criteriain predicting successful non-operative treatment of osteochondritis dissecans in children. J Pediatr Orthop. 2003;23:102–8.

11. Lazarte G. Quad contracture produces avulsion fracture of incompletely developed bone. Am J Path. 1958;34(4):803–15.

12. Herring JA. Tachdjian's pediatr orthop. 3rd ed. WB Saunders. Philadelphia: PA; 2002. p. 812–4.

13. Krause B. A natural history of osgood-sclatter disease. J Pediatr Orthop. 1990;10(1):65–8.

14. Weiss J. Surgical treatment of unresolved osgood-schlatter disease: ossicle resection with tibial tubercleplasty. J Pediatr Orthop. 2007;27(7): 844–7.

15. Lynch M. Tibia recurvatum as a complication of osgood-schlatter disease: a report of two cases. J Pediatr Orthop. 1991;11:543.

Osteogenesis Imperfecta

116

Evan Sheppard and Reed Estes

Background

- Genetic defect in Type I collagen
- Variety of phenotypes
- Linked to 150 mutations of the COL1A1 and COL1A2 genes
  - Encode Type I procollagen.
- Incidence of Type I osteogenesis imperfecta→3–5/100,000

Classification

Type	Inheritance	Long bone deformity	Bone fragility	Teeth	Lethal	Sclerae
I	AD	Moderate	Less severe	Normal or involved	No	Blue
II	AR	Severe	Extreme	Unknown	Yes	Blue
III	AR	Progressive bowing	Severe	Involved	No	Blue as an infant, becomes white
IV	AD	Moderate	Moderate	Normal or involved	No	Normal

E. Sheppard, MD • R. Estes, MD (✉)
Department of Surgery, Division of Orthopedic
Surgery, University of Alabama at Birmingham,
Birmingham, AL, USA
e-mail: reede44@uab.edu; reed.estes@gmail.com

© Springer International Publishing AG 2017
A.E.M. Eltorai et al. (eds.), *Orthopedic Surgery Clerkship*, DOI 10.1007/978-3-319-52567-9_116

- Type I
  - 50% of the normal amount of Type I collagen due to ineffective mRNA for pro-α1 collagen
  - Generalized osteoporosis
  - Blue sclera
- Type II
  - Extreme fragility leads to perinatal death
- Type III
  - Moderate fragility makes this the most severe type that children can survive with.
  - Due to stress on the abnormal bone, kids develop progressive and marked deformity and have severe growth retardation.
- Type IV
  - Osteoporosis, bone fragility, and long bone deformities are variable.
  - New forms that do not have Type I collagen defects but have similar phenotypes.
- Type V→ AD
  - Hypertrophic callus formation after fracture
  - Calcification of the interosseous membrane in the forearm
  - Hyperdense metaphyseal bands
  - Normal sclerae
- Type VI
  - Frequent fracture
  - Vertebral compression
  - Long bone deformity
  - Normal sclerae
  - No tooth involvement
  - Elevated Alk Phos
- Type VII→ AR
  - Rhizomelic limb shortening
  - Coxa vara

Pathophysiology

- Type I collagen is comprised of two α-1 chains and one α-2 chain that form a triple helix:
  - Triple helix forms because every third amino acid is a glycine.
- Mutations in COL1A1 and COL1A2 substitute glycine with another amino acid, interfering with normal formation.

- Formation of both endochondral and intramembranous bone is disturbed.
- Increased quantity of woven bone.
- Bone trabeculae are thin without organization.
- Physis is broad and irregular.
- Proliferative and hypertrophic zones are disorganized.
- Microfracture over time causes progressive deformity.

Physical Exam

- Varies based on subtype.
- Patient may present with multiple fractures after minimal trauma:
  - Rule out non-accidental trauma.
- The femur is more often fractured than the tibia.
- Fractures heal at a normal rate:
  - Callus is wispy.
- Short stature:
  - Can be secondary to multiple epiphyseal microfractures
- Bowing long bones:
  - Results from multiple transverse fractures with muscle contraction across the weakened diaphysis.
  - Anterolateral bow or proximal varus deformities of the femur develop.
  - Saber shins.
- Blue sclera.
- Poor dentition.
- Deafness.
- Olecranon apophyseal avulsion fracture.
- Basilar invagination.

Imaging

- Bone is osteopenic
- Wormian bones in the cranium
  - Detached portions of the primary ossification centers of the adjacent membrane bones

Treatment

Conservative Treatment

- Bisphosphonates
  - Inhibit osteoclastic resorption of the bone (which is increased in OI).
  - Alendronate reduces frequency of fracture and improves ambulatory status.
  - Braces and wheelchairs.

Surgical Treatment

- Management of long bone fractures
  - Age dependent (splinting/casting in younger kids)
  - Intramedullary devices
  - ORIF
- Management of deformity
  - Realignment osteotomy with rod fixation
  - Telescoping devices
- Scoliosis
  - Spinal fusion for curves greater than 45°
  - Supplemental fixation/decreased correction secondary to decreased bone quality
- Basilar Invagination
  - May require decompression and posterior fusion

References

1. Burnei G, Vlad C, Georgescu I, Gavriliu TS, Dan D. Osteogenesis imperfecta: diagnosis and treatment. J Am Acad Orthop Surg. 2008;16(6):356–66.
2. Tachdjian MO, et al. Metabolic and endocrine bone diseases. In: Tachdjian's pediatric orthopedics. 4th ed. Philadelphia: Saunders/Elsevier; 2008. p. 1944–68. Print

Child Abuse

Susan A. Scherl

Introduction

- Child abuse is a real, common problem.
- The diagnosis is clinical and can be difficult to make.
- There are adverse sequelae to both under- and overdiagnosis.
- A multidisciplinary approach to diagnosis and reporting can be helpful.

Background

- 1962: "Battered Child Syndrome" described by Kempe, et al., in *JAMA*.
  - Estimated that 25% of fxs in children <1, and 10–15% in children <3, are the result of abuse [4].
- 1967: All 50 states instituted mandatory reporting laws.
- 1968: Green and Haggerty estimated that an abused child returned to an unsafe home environment is at 50% risk for additional injury and 10% risk of death [2].

Statistics

- Collected every year from all 50 states by the US Department of Health and Human Services, Department of Children and Families.
- Published every December in a yearly report entitled "Child Maltreatment."
  - As of this writing the latest available statistics are for 2013 [7].
- There are about 3.5 million reports per year, involving about 6.4 million children.
- About 60% of reports are investigated and about 20% of reports are substantiated, for a total of 680,000 unique victims.
- The estimated incidence of abuse is ~9.1/1000 children in the USA.
- There were 1520 fatalities in 2013, for an incidence of 2.0/100,000.
- 74% of fatalities are children less than 3 years old.
- 27% of victims are less than 3 years old.
- An additional 20% are 3–5 years old.
- 10–70% of abused children sustain skeletal injury.
- 30–50% of abused children are referred to the care of an orthopedist.

Types of Abuse

- Emotional
  - Difficult to define and quantify
- Medical neglect

S.A. Scherl, MD
The University of Nebraska, Department of
Orthopaedic Surgery, Omaha, NE, USA
e-mail: sscherl@unmc.edu

(i) Very common
  ◦ Often manifests as failure to thrive
- Sexual
  - True incidence is unknown.
  - Estimated to occur in 13% of reported cases of physical abuse.
- Physical abuse
  - Soft tissue injuries
  - Burns
  - Abusive Head trauma—"shaken baby syndrome"
  - Internal injuries
  - Fractures

Soft Tissue Injuries: Types

- Bruises
- Welts
- Lacerations
- Rope burns
- Bites

Soft Tissue Injuries: Characteristics

- Clustered
- Shaped
- In various stages of healing
- In unusual locations:
  - Back
  - Buttocks/thighs
  - Mucosal surfaces

Burns

- Immersions/scalds:
  - Well-demarcated borders corresponding to the level of immersion.
  - Scaldings are considered an endpoint of progressive, severe abuse because of degree of planning and premeditation involved.
- Cigarette:
  - Often to palms and soles.
  - Cigarette burns to the eyes and face are often accidental and occur when a child runs into an adult holding a cigarette in their hand with their arm at their side.
- Brandings:
  - Patterned or shaped

Abusive Head Trauma

- Subdural hematoma
- Subarachnoid hemorrhage
- Retinal hemorrhage

Internal Injuries

- Abdominal wall injuries
- Solid and hollow viscus rupture:
  - Spleen
  - Liver
  - Kidney
  - Intestines
  - Bladder

Fractures

- 50% of fractures secondary to abuse occur in children less than 1 year old.
- The incidence of non-accidental fractures decreases with increasing age.
- No particular fracture pattern, location, or morphology is pathognomonic of abuse.
  - However, some fracture findings are more specific to abuse than others.
- Long bone spiral fractures are *not* pathognomonic of child abuse!
  - In fact, a single, transverse fracture is the most common long bone fracture pattern seen in cases of child abuse [1, 5].
  - The most frequently fractured long bone varies in large series (humerus, tibia, femur).

High-Specificity Fracture Findings

- Multiple fractures in various stages of healing
- Posterior rib fractures

- Bilateral acute fractures
- Metaphyseal corner fractures, also known as classic metaphyseal lesions or CMLs
  - Caused by a characteristic mechanism of combined torsion and traction
- Complex skull fractures
- Long bone fractures in nonambulatory children
- Sternal and scapular fractures
  - Usually caused by very-high-energy mechanisms (motor vehicle accidents or falls from heights)
- Transphyseal distal humerus fractures

Low-Specificity Fracture Findings

- Isolated long bone shaft fractures in ambulatory children
- Simple skull fractures
- Clavicle fractures
- Supracondylar humerus fractures

Elements of the History

- Caretaker's account of injury
  - Consistency
  - Plausibility
- Caretaker's attitude toward child and medical personnel
- Child's demeanor
- Social factors:
  - Blended families
  - Unemployment
  - Addiction
  - Chronic illness

Physical Exam

- Systemic exam of the skin and entire skeleton.
- Neurovascular exam.
- Eye exam.
- Consider a genitourinary exam, performed by appropriate personnel, if sexual abuse is suspected.

Radiologic Exam

- Biplanar (A/P and lateral) X-rays, with obliques as needed, for areas suspected of fracture
- Skeletal survey
- U/S
- Bone scan
- MRI/PET scan

Skeletal Survey

- Consists of 20–30 separate images (Fig. 117.1)
  - A/P and lateral of each segment of all extremities, including hands and feet.
  - A/P and lateral of entire spine, including a separate rib series.
  - Skull series.
  - A "babygram" is not an acceptable skeletal survey!
- Indications
  - All children less than 1, with evidence of any medical neglect.
  - All children less than 2, with evidence of any physical abuse.
  - Consider in children less than 5 with a suspicious acute fracture.
  - Consider a follow-up skeletal survey 2–4 weeks after initial evaluation.
    ◦ 21% of follow-up skeletal surveys reveal new findings [3].
- Consider getting a skeletal survey on siblings of the index child [6].
  - Skeletal survey is positive in 12% of siblings less than 24 months of age.
  - Twins are particularly at risk.

Ultrasound

- *May be useful in demonstrating*:
  - Acute subperiosteal hemorrhage
  - Occult long bone fractures
  - Costochondral injuries

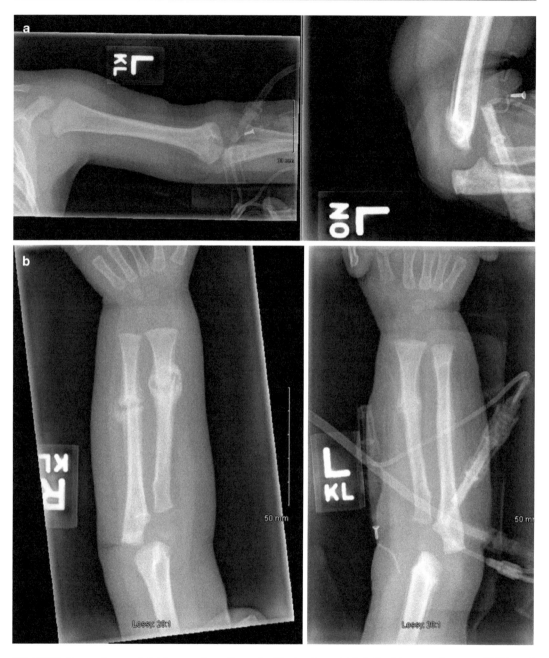

Fig. 117.1 Images from a skeletal survey in an 8-month-old, showing a (**a**) left distal humerus fracture, (**b**) bilateral distal radius and ulna fractures, (**c**) bilateral proximal and distal tibia and fibula fractures, and (**d**) skull fracture

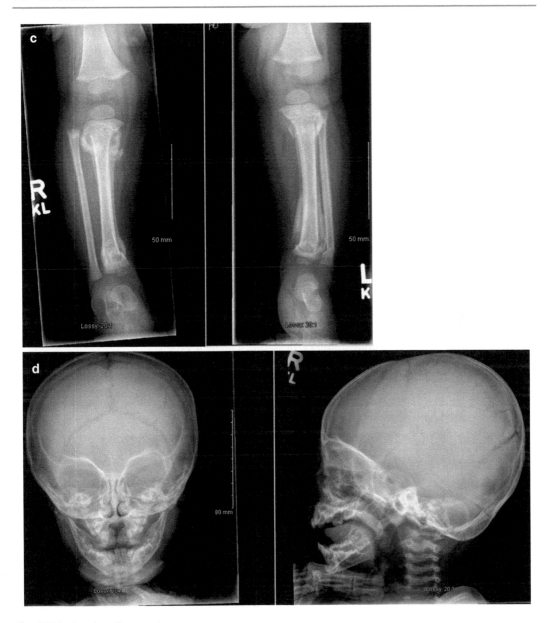

Fig. 117.1 (continued)

Bone Scan

- Indicated when clinical suspicion for fracture is high, but standard X-rays are negative.
- Difficult to interpret in cases of:
  - Bilateral fracture
  - Fractures near growth plates

MRI/PET Scan

- Indications and protocols still being determined
- Sensitive and specific for fracture and can also be used to diagnose visceral injury

- No radiation involved, but most children require sedation or general anesthesia to perform the studies

Estimating Fracture Age

- Periosteal reaction peaks at about 14 days.
- Callus is visible at 3–6 weeks.
- Remodeling occurs between 3 months and 1 year.

Differential Diagnosis

- Birth trauma:
  - Usually the clavicle or humerus.
  - Typically there is a history of high birth weight and/or traumatic delivery.
  - Callus should appear within 2 weeks of life.
- Caffey's disease (infantile cortical hyperostosis):
  - Painful, self-limited condition in children less than 1 year old.
  - Mandibular involvement is characteristic.
    (a) Metabolic bone disease variants:
  - Osteogenesis imperfecta.
  - Rickets.
  - Osteopenia of chronic illness:
    ◦ Renal disease
    ◦ Steroids/seizure medications
    ◦ Nonambulators (i.e., patients with cerebral palsy)
  - Fracture patterns in pathologic bone can mimic those highly specific for abuse.
  - A workup to rule out metabolic bone disease will:
    ◦ Potentially decrease the incidence of erroneous reports.
    ◦ Enable children to obtain treatment if necessary.
    ◦ Help with addressing the issue of possible metabolic bone disease if it arises in court.
  - *Metabolic bone disease workup*:
    ◦ Labs: BUN, Cr, Alp, Ca++, and PO4
    ◦ DEXA scan

- *Rickets*:
    ◦ Some child abuse experts maintain that children with OI and other chronic illnesses are more likely to be abused than others, but the literature does not support or refute this claim.
    ◦ A family of conditions in which mineralization of osteoid is abnormal.
    ◦ The diagnosis can usually be made based on history, physical exam, labs, and X-rays.
    ◦ There is a characteristic X-ray appearance of physes in rickets, with cupping and widening of the physes (Fig. 117.2).
- *Osteogenesis imperfecta ("brittle bone disease")* (Fig. 117.3)
  - Can be a difficult diagnosis to make.
  - OI has been mapped to two locations on two different genes (7 and 17) coding for collagen Type I.
  - The majority of cases are new mutations; there is often no family history.

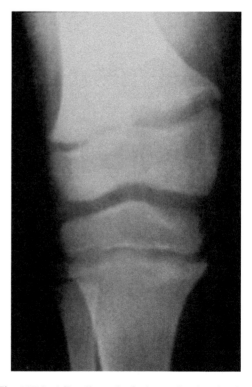

Fig. 117.2 A/P radiograph of a knee, showing the characteristic physeal widening and cupping of rickets

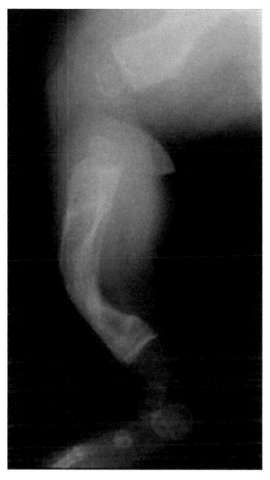

Fig. 117.3 A lateral radiograph of the tibia of a child with OI, showing deformity secondary to multiple fractures

– The diagnosis of OI may take weeks to months. There have been cases of the parents of children with undiagnosed OI suspected of child abuse. However, our mandate as physicians is to err on the side of protecting the child.
– Some child abuse experts maintain that children with OI and other chronic illnesses are more likely to be abused than others, but the literature does not support or refute this claim.

Treatment

• Fractures secondary to child abuse typically occur in very young children and can generally be managed nonoperatively.

Reporting

• Reporting is mandated for physicians.
• No liability attaches to an erroneous report made in good faith.
• A report cannot be retracted once made.
• A multidisciplinary approach to reporting, including the input of a child abuse physician, is helpful.
• The trend in many states is to maintain the family unit through investigation and intervention.

Conclusion

• Child abuse is a clinical diagnosis made on the basis of the history, physical, and radiographic findings.
• No long bone fracture pattern is pathognomonic of abuse; it is impossible to tell by looking at an isolated X-ray whether or not a child was abused.
• Transverse long bone fractures are more common than spiral fractures in cases of abuse.
• Know the high- and low-specificity fractures for abuse.
• Know the indications for imaging, particularly skeletal surveys.

– There are wide variations in phenotype and gene expressivity.
– Only about ½ of patients have blue sclerae or dentinogenesis imperfecta.
– Skin biopsy for fibroblast culture and DNA testing are helpful when positive: Fibroblast culture has a 15% false-negative rate. DNA testing has a 5% false-negative rate.
– Bone mineral density (DEXA) scans are becoming a useful adjunct in diagnosing OI: BMD is almost always decreased in patients with OI and continues to decrease as they get older. The recommendation is therefore to get sequential DEXA scans, 4–6 months apart.

- Consider doing a metabolic workup in all cases of suspected abuse.
- A multidisciplinary approach to the diagnosis and reporting of suspected abuse is helpful.

References

1. Baldwin KD, Scherl SA. Orthopedic aspects of child abuse. Instr Course Lect. 2013;62:399–403.
2. Green M, Haggerty RJ. Physically abused children. In: Green M, Haggerty RJ, editors. Ambulatory pediatrics. Philadelphia: WB Saunders; 1968. p. 285–9.
3. Harper NS, Eddleman S, Lindberg DM, Ex SI. The utility of follow-up skeletal surveys in child abuse. Pediatrics. 2013;131(3):e672–8. Epub 2013/02/13.
4. Kempe C, Silverman FN, Steele BF. The battered child syndrome. JAMA. 1962;181·17–24.
5. King J, Diefendorf D, Apthorp J, Negrete VF, Carlson M. Analysis of 429 fractures in 189 battered children. J Pediatr Orthop. 1988;8(5):585–9.
6. Lindberg DM, Shapiro RA, Laskey AL, Pallin DJ, Blood EA, Berger RP, et al. Prevalence of abusive injuries in siblings and household contacts of physically abused children. Pediatrics. 2012;130(2):193–201. Epub 2012/07/11.
7. Child Maltreatment 2013. Department of Health and Human Services, Administration for Children and Families. Washington, DC. http://www.acf.hhs.gov/sites/default/files/cb/cm2013.pdf. Accessed at: 18 Sept 2015.

Legg-Calve-Perthes

118

Evan Sheppard and Reed Estes

Background

- An avascular event that affects the capital femoral epiphysis
- Bilateral in 10–12%
- Most prevalent in kids 3–8 years of age
- More common in boys

Anatomy

- Primary blood to the head comes from two anastomotic arterial rings in the femoral neck.
- Medial and lateral femoral circumflex arteries form the extracapsular ring:
  – Medial circumflex contributes the most.
- The major arterial supply to the head is the lateral segment of the arterial ring (medial circumflex).
- This vessel courses through a narrow passage that is constricted in children younger than 8 years old.
- There is an intracapsular ring that has been found to be incomplete more often in boys than in girls.

Pathogenesis

Coagulation-Controversial

- Kids with hemoglobinopathies commonly have AVN.
- AVD also seen in kids with leukemia, lymphoma, thrombocytopenic purpura, and hemophilia.
- Increase in blood viscosity has been reported in Perthes disease.
- The most common clotting disorder is resistance to activated protein C.
- Thought that there is a venothrombotic event in the femoral head that causes venous hypertension and hypoxic bone death.

Arterial

- Angiographic studies have shown obstruction of the superior capsular arteries of the femoral head during the first 5 months of symptoms.
- Revascularization occurs as the disease progresses.
- Studies have shown that multiple infarcts are needed to cause disease.

Venous

- Normally venous drainage flows though the medial circumflex vein.

E. Sheppard, MD • R. Estes, MD (✉)
Department of Surgery, Division of Orthopedic Surgery, University of Alabama at Birmingham, Birmingham, AL, USA
e-mail: aestes@uabmc.edu

© Springer International Publishing AG 2017
A.E.M. Eltorai et al. (eds.), *Orthopedic Surgery Clerkship*, DOI 10.1007/978-3-319-52567-9_118

- In patients with Perthes disease, there is increased venous pressure in the femoral neck and associated venous congestion in the metaphysis.

Classification Systems

Waldenstrom Classification

- Initial stage → ossific nucleus is smaller, radiolucencies appear in the metaphysis, and there is medial joint space widening.
- Fragmentation → varying patterns of lucency; pillars of the femoral head demarcate:
  - Represents revascularization with bone resorption
- Reossification → new bone appears in the femoral head:
  - Can last up to 18 months
- Healed/remodeling → the femoral head is fully reossified and remodels, and the acetabulum also remodels.

Lateral Pillar (Herring) Classification (Only Done in Fragmentation Stage)

- Group A → no density change and no loss of height
- Group B → density change and central pillar collapse height loss less than 50%
- Group B/C → thin lateral pillar and borderline height loss
- Group C → more than 50% height loss

Catterall Classification

- Group I → anterior portion of the epiphysis is affected.
- Group II → more of the anterior segment is involved and central sequestrum is present.
- Group III → most of the epiphysis is involved.
- Group IV → all of the epiphysis is involved.

Stulberg Classification

- Group I → the femoral head is normal.
- Group II → the femoral head is round.
- Group III → the femoral head is ovoid; the acetabulum matches the head.
- Group IV → the femoral head is flattened more than 1 cm on weight-bearing areas; the acetabulum is also flat.
- Group V → the femoral head collapses; the acetabulum is not flattened.

Usefulness

- Lateral pillar
  - Lateral pillar classification and age at the time of onset of the disease strongly correlate with the outcome in patients with Perthes disease.
  - Patients who are over the age of 8.0 years at the time of onset and have a hip in the lateral pillar B group or B/C border group have a better outcome with surgical treatment than they do with nonoperative treatment.
  - Group B hips in children who are less than 8.0 years of age at the time of onset have very favorable outcomes unrelated to treatment.
  - Group C hips in children of all ages frequently have poor outcomes, which also appear to be unrelated to treatment.

Physical Exam

- Limp (Trendelenburg gait) with pain in the hip, thigh, or knee:
  - Gets worse with physical activities, better with rest
  - Occasional night pain
- Limited range of motion of the affected hip:
  - Especially abduction and internal rotation
- When the hip is flexed, the leg may go into obligatory external rotation.

Imaging

- Delay in bone age relative to the patient's age is the most commonly observed abnormality.
- Radiologic pause → delayed growth of the triquetrum and lunate with normal growth of the capitate and hamate.
- See pillar classification above.
- Sagging rope sign:
  - Radiodense line overlying the proximal femoral metaphysis.
  - The edge of the rope is the anterior portion of the large femoral head.
- Physeal changes:
  - Premature closure
- Acetabular changes.

- Operative
  - Groups B and B/C in whom disease started after their eighth birthday
- Surgical options
  - Varus osteotomy of the femur
    - Shortens the femur and alters the abductor mechanics
    - Results in abductor limp
  - Pelvic osteotomy
    - Hip stiffness
    - Combined femoral and pelvic osteotomies
  - Indications are changing as use of magnetic resonance imaging and blood flow studies are shedding a new light on this condition.

Treatment

- Non-op (observation, activity restriction, physical therapy)
  - Patients with onset before their 8th birthday
  - Group A and C patients with onset after their eight birthday

Suggested Readings

1. Tachdjian MO, et al. Congenital coxa vara Tachdjian's pediatric orthopedics. 4th ed. Philadelphia: Saunders/Elsevier; 2008. 897–901. Print.
2. Herring JA, Kim HT, Browne R. Legg-Calve-Perthes disease. Part II: prospective multicenter study of the effect of treatment on outcome. J Bone Joint Surg Am. 2004;86-A(10):2121–34.

Cerebral Palsy

M. Wade Shrader

Overview of Cerebral Palsy (CP)

- Incidence: 2–4 per 1000 live births
- Static encephalopathy: static (not worsening) brain lesion, but the musculoskeletal effects of CP can worsen with growth and disability
- Risk factors
- Prematurity
- Perinatal anoxia
- Multiple births
- Perinatal infections
- Placental complications

Diagnosis

- Usually made by delay in making typical developmental milestones
- MRI: may be ordered and typically shows periventricular leukomalacia
- Negative predictive factors:
- Children not sitting independently by age 2 typically do not walk independently.
- Children not walking by age 7 typically do not walk.

Classification

Anatomic

- Diplegic – affecting mostly the lower extremities (although the upper extremities can be impaired)
- Hemiplegic – affecting only one side
- Quadriplegic – affecting both upper and lower extremities and also will variably affect the trunk and head control and balance

Neurological

- Spastic
- Hypotonic
- Mixed
- Dystonic
- Athetoid/choreatic
- Gross motor functional classification system: a functional classification system that has been demonstrated to be reliable and useful to determine surgical treatment (Fig. 119.1)

Clinical Features

- Spasticity.
- Developmental delay: a combination of spasticity, developmental delay, and skeletal growth leads to progressive musculoskeletal deformities.

M. Wade Shrader, MD
Department of Orthopedic Surgery, Children's of Mississippi, University of MS Medical Center, Jackson, MS, USA
e-mail: mshrader@umc.edu

© Springer International Publishing AG 2017
A.E.M. Eltorai et al. (eds.), *Orthopedic Surgery Clerkship*, DOI 10.1007/978-3-319-52567-9_119

GMFCS E & R between 6th and 12th birthday: Descriptors and illustrations

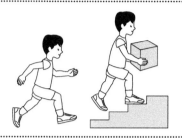

GMFCS Level I

Children walk at home, school, outdoors and in the community. They can climb stairs without the use of a railing. Children perform gross motor skills such as running and jumping, but speed, balance and coordination are limited.

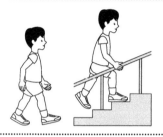

GMFCS Level II

Children walk in most settings and climb stairs holding onto a railing. They may experience difficulty walking long distances and balancing on uneven terrain, inclines, in crowded areas or confined spaces. Children may walk with physical assistance, a hand-held mobility device or used wheeled mobility over long distances. Children have only minimal ability to perform gross motor skills such as running and jumping.

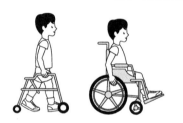

GMFCS Level III

Children walk using a hand-held mobility device in most indoor settings. They may climb stairs holding onto a railing with supervision or assistance. Children use wheeled mobility when traveling long distances and may self-propel for shorter distances.

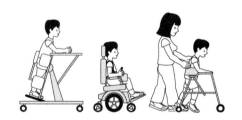

GMFCS Level IV

Children use methods of mobility that require physical assistance or powered mobility in most settings. They may walk for short distances at home with physical assistance or use powered mobility or a body support walker when positioned. At school, outdoors and in the community children are transported in a manual wheelchair or use powered mobility.

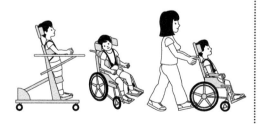

GMFCS Level V

Children are transported in a manual wheelchair in all settings. Children are limited in their ability to maintain antigravity head and trunk postures and control leg and arm movements.

GMFCS descriptors: Palisano et al. (1997) Dev Med Child Neurol 39:214–23
CanChild: www.canchild.ca

Illustrations Version 2 © Bill Reid, Kate Willoughby, Adrienne Harvey and Kerr Graham, The Royal Children's Hospital Melbourne ERC151050

Fig. 119.1 Caption

GMFCS E & R between 12th and 18th birthday: Descriptors and illustrations

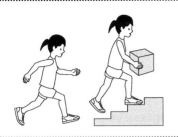

GMFCS Level I

Youth walk at home, school, outdoors and in the community. Youth are able to climb curbs and stairs without physical assistance or a railing. They perform gross motor skills such as running and jumping but speed, balance and coordination are limited.

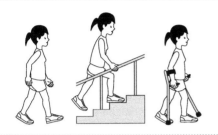

GMFCS Level II

Youth walk in most settings but environmental factors and personal choice influence mobility choices. At school or work they may require a hand held mobility device for safety and climb stairs holding onto a railing. Outdoors and in the community youth may use wheeled mobility when traveling long distances.

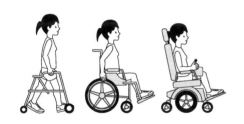

GMFCS Level III

Youth are capable of walking using a hand-held mobility device. Youth may climb stairs holding onto a railing with supervision or assistance. At school they may self-propel a manual wheelchair or use powered mobility. Outdoors and in the community youth are transported in a wheelchair or use powered mobility.

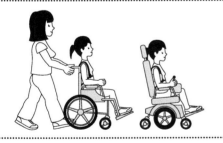

GMFCS Level IV

Youth use wheeled mobility in most settings. Physical assistance of 1–2 people is required for transfers. Indoors, youth may walk short distances with physical assistance, use wheeled mobility or a body support walker when positioned. They may operate a powered chair, otherwise are transported in a manual wheelchair.

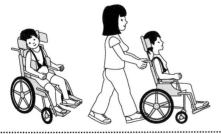

GMFCS Level V

Youth are transported in a manual wheelchair in all settings. Youth are limited in their ability to maintain antigravity head and trunk postures and control leg and arm movements. Self-mobility is severely limited, even with the use of assistive technology.

GMFCS descriptors: Palisano et al. (1997) Dev Med Child Neurol 39:214–23
CanChild: www.canchild.ca

Illustrations Version 2 © Bill Reid, Kate Willoughby, Adrienne Harvey and Kerr Graham, The Royal Children's Hospital Melbourne   ERC151050

Fig. 119.1 (continued)

- Muscle tightness.
- Joint contracture.
- Skeletal deformities.
- Negative symptoms.
- Poor coordination.
- Poor balance.
- Muscle weakness.
- Poor sensation especially proprioception.

Nonoperative Treatment

- Medication: typically used to treat spasticity and muscle spasm.
- Baclofen: can be delivered orally (with more sedation) or through intrathecal pump.
- Anti-drooling medicine.
- Typical seizure medications.
- Artane for dystonia.
- Bracing: in general, bracing of the lower extremities can improve ambulation function and decrease risk of contracture progression.
- AFO: most common brace prescribed and may be solid, hinged, or posterior leaf spring.
- Ground reaction AFO: anterior mold/strap to cause knee extension moment in stance, to counter crouch gait.
- KAFO: less commonly used in GMFCS Levels III and IV, compared to that in spina bifida.
- TLSO: may use soft back brace to improve functioning, but has not been shown to decrease rate of spine deformity progression.
- Physical therapy/occupational therapy.

Operative Treatment

Spasticity Management: Typically Done by Neurosurgery to Decrease Spasticity

- Intrathecal baclofen pump – reversible, relatively high complication rate, but most complications are minor; usually in pts with GMFCS Levels III–IV function; its causal effects on scoliosis is debatable, but probably does not cause increased rate of spine deformity.

- Selective dorsal rhizotomy – permanent transection of dorsal nerve rootlets to decrease reflex arc and decrease spasticity, usually in pts with GMFCS Levels II–III function, and more clear causal relationship to increase rate of spine deformity after procedure.

Hip: Progressive Neuromuscular Hip Dysplasia Is Common in CP

- May lead to increased pain in adolescence and adulthood and lower quality of life
- Progressive subluxation product of imbalance of spastic and weak muscles, skeletal growth, and developmental delay
- Radiographic diagnosis: increased Riemer's index of >30% on AP pelvis
- Early Rx: Botox, PT, and bracing, but that has been demonstrated with a randomized trial to only delay surgical Rx
- Early operative Rx: in patients less than 4 years old, may treat with soft tissue surgery only (adductor/proximal hamstring lengthening and abduction bracing)
- Definitive operative Rx: varus derotation osteotomy (VDRO) and ± pelvic osteotomy
- Salvage treatment: for hips that are painful with degenerative joint disease. Either proximal femoral resection (PFR) at the level of the lesser trochanter or a combination of proximal valgus osteotomy and Girdlestone (femoral head resection)

Spine: Deformity Very Common in GMFCS Levels IV and V (Almost 90%)

- Scoliosis: long-sweeping neuromuscular curves
  - Negatively affects seating balance and restrictive lung disease.
  - Progressive curves, even after maturity.
  - PSF is a treatment for progressive curves; several studies have confirmed improvement in QoL scores s/p PSF.

- Spondylolisthesis
  - 15% prevalence in CP (compared to 6% in gen population)
  - Higher risk after SDR

Lower Extremity: Rotational Abnormalities Very Common

- Negatively affect gait in GMFCS Levels I, II, and III
- Internal tibia torsion, external tibia torsion, and femoral anteversion
- Diagnosed with careful physical exam, motion analysis laboratory, or CT rotational scanogram (or more recently, EOS)
- Treatment: long-bone rotational osteotomy (often with concurrent procedures)

Foot

- Equinovarus: common in both diplegia and hemiplegia and needs flexible deformities for ST procedures to be effective.
  - Gastrocnemius recession: recommended instead of percutaneous TAL to decrease risk of overlengthening in some centers
  - Split AT transfer: supination in swing phase
  - Split PT transfer: dynamic varus at rest
  - Osteotomies: consider for more rigid deformity
    - Calcaneus: slide, lateral closing wedge
    - Cuboid: lat column shortening
    - Cuneiform: med column lengthening
- Equinovalgus: common in both diplegia and quadriplegia.
  - Gastroc recession: as above
  - Lateral column lengthening
  - Talonavicular arthrodesis: along with LC lengthening for more severe deformity
  - Subtalar arthrodesis
  - Triple arthrodesis: for most severe deformities
- Hallux valgus: traditional HV procedures do not work in setting of spasticity. MTP arthrodesis is recommended.

Upper Extremity

- Hemiplegia: need appropriate sensation (proprioception) and cognition to participate in postoperative rehab to make UE function improve.
  - Green's transfer (FCU to ECRB)
  - Thumb-in-palm correction
- Quadriplegia: surgery more for hygiene and personal care (dressing).
  - Wrist arthrodesis with proximal row carpectomy
  - Thumb CMC arthrodesis
  - Elbow flexor release
- SEMLS: single-event multilevel surgery.
- Single surgical procedure correcting all significant deformities.
- In contradistinction to correcting deformities stepwise, yearly, i.e., "the birthday syndrome."
- Single rehabilitation period.
- SEMLS has been demonstrated with RCT to improve outcomes and gait scores.

Suggested Reading

1. Dabney KW, Miller F. Cerebral palsy. In: Abel MF, editor. Orthopedic knowledge update: pediatrics. 3rd ed. Rosemont: American Academy of Orthopedic Surgeons; 2006. p. 93–109.
2. Flynn JM, Miler F. Management of hip disorders in patients with cerebral palsy. J Am Acad Orthop Surg. 2002;10(3):198–209.
3. Karol LA. Surgical management of the lower extremity in ambulatory children with cerebral palsy. J Am Acad Orthop Surg. 2004;12(3):196–203.
4. Graham KG, Selber P. Musculoskeletal aspects of cerebral palsy. J Bone Joint Surg Br. 2003;85(20):157–66.
5. McCarthy JJ, D'Andrea LP, Betz RR, Clements DH. Scoliosis in the child with cerebral palsy. J Am Acad Orthop Surg. 2006;14(6):367–75.
6. Narayanan UG, Fehlings D, Weir S, Knights S, Kiran S, Campbell K. Initial development and validation of the Caregiver Priorities and Child Health Index of Life and Disabilities (CPCHILD). Dev Med Child Neurol. 2006;48(10):804–12.
7. Palisano R, Rosenbaum P, Walter S, Russell D, Wood E, Galuppi B. Development and reliability of a system to classify gross motor function in children with cerebral palsy. Dev Med Child Neurol. 1997;39(4):214–23.

8. Rodda JM, Graham HK, Nattrass GR, Galea MP, Baker R, Wolfe R. Correction of severe crouch in gait in patients with spastic diplegia with use of multilevel orthopedic surgery. J Bone Joint Surg Am. 2006;88(12):2653–64.

9. Stout JL, Gage JR, Schwartz MH, Novacheck TF. Distal femoral extension osteotomy and patellar tendon advancement to treat persistent crouch gait in cerebral palsy. J Bone Joint Surg Am. 2008;90(11):2470–84.

Spina Bifida

120

Rajiv J. Iyengar, J. Mason DePasse, and Alan H. Daniels

Overview

- Incidence of isolated spina bifida is around 3 per 10,000 live births [1].
- Etiology is multifactorial.
  - Medications: valproic acid, carbamazepine, and methotrexate
  - Chromosomal abnormalities: trisomies 13 and 18
  - Single-gene mutations
  - Maternal folate deficiency
  - Maternal diabetes
  - Family history
- Up to 70% of cases can be prevented with maternal folate supplementation.
- 20–70% of patients have concomitant IgE-mediated latex allergy.
  - Can result in anaphylaxis.
  - Important to use non-latex-containing gloves in OR.

R.J. Iyengar, BS
Warren Alpert Medical School, Brown University, Providence, RI, USA

J. Mason DePasse, MD (✉)
Department of Orthopaedic Surgery, Division of Pediatric Surgery, Warren Alpert Medical School of Brown University, Providence, RI, USA
e-mail: jmdepasse@gmail.com

A.H. Daniels, MD
Department of Orthopedic Surgery, Warren Alpert Medical School, Brown University, Providence, RI, USA

Classification

- Spina bifida occulta
  - Vertebral arch defect with confined meninges and neural elements
- Meningocele
  - Vertebral arch defect with meninges protruding, no neural elements within the herniated sac
- Myelomeningocele
  - Vertebral arch defect with meninges and neural elements in protruding sac
- Rachischisis
  - Exposed neural elements without soft tissue coverage

Diagnosis

- Elevated maternal serum alpha-fetoprotein (AFP) in the second trimester
- Amniocentesis
  - AFP and acetylcholinesterase concentrations
- Ultrasound
  - Characterize leg and foot movement
  - Spine deformities
  - Look for associated Chiari II malformation

Initial Treatment

- Surgical closure of defect within 48 h of birth
- In utero operation

A.E.M. Eltorai et al. (eds.), *Orthopedic Surgery Clerkship*, DOI 10.1007/978-3-319-52567-9_120

– Urodynamic and leg function outcomes similar to postpartum operation
– Lower incidence of hindbrain herniation and hydrocephalus

Spine Deformities [3]

• Scoliosis
  – Thoracic-level myelodysplasia has 100% rate of scoliosis.
  – Rapidly progressive scoliosis may indicate a tethered cord, evaluated with an MRI.
  – Treat with anterior spinal fusion and posterior spinal fusion with pelvic fixation.
  – Bracing usually ineffective.
• Kyphosis
  – Kyphectomy with fusion and posterior instrumentation
  – Check shunt function prior to kyphectomy

Pathologic Fractures

• Often confused with infection secondary to swelling and warmth
• Most common near the hip and knee secondary to osteopenia in long bones
• Treat with short period of immobilization in well-padded splint

Hip Disorders

• Dislocation is most common with defects at L3 due to active hip flexors and adductors and deficient abductors.
• Abduction contracture: treat with Ober-Yount procedure—proximal division of fascia lata and distal iliotibial band release.
• Flexion contracture: if greater than 40 degrees, may perform anterior hip release with tenotomies.

Knee Deformities

• Weak quadriceps may be treated with a KAFO, knee-ankle-foot orthosis.

• Significant flexion contractures: treat with hamstring lengthening vs. supracondylar extension osteotomy.
• Extension contracture: treat with serial casting until knee flexion is great enough to allow for sitting or ambulating.

Foot Deformities [2]

• Clubfoot
  – Very common in myelodysplasia.
  – Very rigid, insensate foot.
  – Treat with serial casting or posteromedial-lateral release if casting fails (higher failure rate than for idiopathic clubfoot).
  – High recurrence rate: nonfunctioning tendons should be resected rather than lengthened (i.e., posterior tibial tendon).
• Foot dorsiflexion deformity: treat with posterior transfer of the anterior tibial tendon.

Prognosis

• Depends on the level of the defect
  – L4 root particularly important for ambulation-given contributions to the femoral nerve (innervating quadriceps muscles) and deep peroneal nerve (innervating tibialis anterior)
  – L3 or above—likely wheelchair bound
  – L5 or below—generally good prognosis for independent ambulation

References

1. Mitchell LE, et al. Spina bifida. Lancet. 2004;364(9448):1885–95.
2. Beaty JH, Canale ST. Orthopedic aspects of myelomeningocele. J Bone Joint Surg Am. 1990;72(4):626–30.
3. Karol LA. Orthopedic management in myelomeningocele. Neurosurg Clin N Am. 1995;6(2):259–68.

Charcot-Marie-Tooth Disease

121

Matthew A. Varacallo, Ettore Vulcano,
Alexander J. Kish, Tonya W. An, and Amiethab A. Aiyer

Introduction

Background

- Hereditary motor and sensory neuropathies (HMSNs) describe a group of inherited disorders manifesting as progressive peripheral neuropathies.
- CMT is the most common HMSN and comprises types I and II (CMT-I and CMT-II).

The original version of this chapter was revised. An erratum to this chapter can be found at https://doi.org/10.1007/978-3-319-52567-9_159

M.A. Varacallo, MD (✉)
Department of Orthopaedic Surgery,
Hahnemann University Hospital,
245 N. 15th Street, M.S. 420, Philadelphia, PA, USA
e-mail: matt.varacallo@tenethealth.com

E. Vulcano, MD
Orthopedics, Mount Sinai Health System,
New York, NY, USA

A.J. Kish, MD
Department of Orthopaedic Surgery,
University of Maryland Medical Center,
Baltimore, MD, USA

T.W. An
Orthopedics Cedars-Sinai Medical Center,
Los Angeles, CA, USA

A.A. Aiyer
Department of Orthopaedic Surgery,
University of Miami, Miami, FL, USA

Epidemiology

- Incidence ranges from 1 in 1100 to 2500.

Genetics and Inheritance

- Multiple types and inheritance patterns identified
- Autosomal dominant most common type (CMT-I)
  - Duplication on chromosome 17 (70% of cases)
  - Codes for peripheral myelin protein (PMP 22)
- Autosomal recessive and X-linked forms (e.g., CMT-II, CMT-X)

Pathophysiology

General CMT Hallmarks

- Motor milestones achieved at a normal age.
- Peripheral motor neurons predominantly involved and sensory deficits variable.
- Distal aspect extremities affected most.
  - Peroneus brevis (PB)
  - Tibialis anterior (TA)
  - Hand/foot intrinsics
- Deforming forces.
  - Tibialis posterior (PT)
  - Peroneus longus (PL)
- Disorder is symmetric and slowly progressive.

- Lower limb areflexia.
- Hand involvement lags behind the lower extremity and rarely needs treatment.

CMT-I

- Demyelinating condition leading to slowed nerve conduction velocity
- Onset in the first or second decade of life

CMT-II

- Wallerian degeneration
  - Process by which the myelin and axoplasm of a nerve is degraded by phagocytes distal to the injured segment
- Onset in the second decade of life or later

Orthopedic Manifestations

Cavovarus Foot

- Deformity progression
  - Plantar-flexed first ray is the initial deformity (weak TA vs strong PL).
  - Hammer/claw toes.
  - Denervation of foot intrinsics and weak ankle dorsiflexion (DF).
  - Toe extensors recruited to compensate for weak DF.
  - Cavus deformity: weak tibialis anterior overpowered by peroneus longus.
  - Hindfoot varus: weak peroneus brevis overpowered by tibialis posterior.
- Clinical presentation
  - Lateral foot pain/callus
  - Frequent ankle sprains
  - Difficulty with stairs
- Exam pearls
  - Coleman block test:
    ∘ Evaluates hindfoot flexibility.
    ∘ Block placed under the heel and lateral foot allowing the great toe to hang free.
    ∘ Rigid hindfoot will not correct to neutral and has treatment implications (see below).
  - Gait: foot drop occurs during swing phase.

Hip Dysplasia

- Controversial: thought to be secondary to subtle weakness in the proximal musculature
- Rarely seen in newborns
- Typically present in adolescence with pain and/or gait abnormalities

Scoliosis

- Up to 37% of adolescents with CMT and females at higher risk
- Curves similar to adolescent idiopathic scoliosis except
  - Increased incidence of thoracic kyphosis and right-sided curves

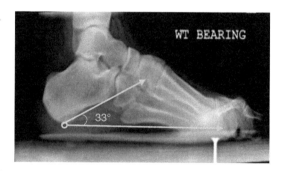

Fig. 121.1 The calcaneal pitch angle is calculated on the weight-bearing lateral radiograph of the foot. The *first line* is drawn along the inferior border of the calcaneus (calcaneal inclination axis), and the *second line* is drawn parallel with the supporting surface (normal <30°)

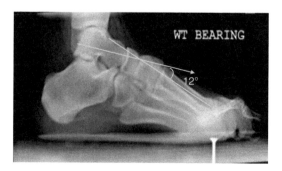

Fig. 121.2 The lateral talo-first metatarsal angle (Meary's angle) is calculated on the weight-bearing lateral radiograph of the foot. It is the angle between the long axes of the first metatarsal and the talus (normal is 0°)

Diagnostic Workup

- 80–90% of all patients with CMT can be diagnosed by a blood test for the known mutations.
- Referral to neurologist based on clinical suspicion.
- Low nerve conduction velocities with prolonged distal latencies in peroneal, ulnar, median nn.
- Radiographs: evaluate standing AP/lateral weight-bearing films of the foot and ankle
  - Findings include an increased calcaneal pitch angle (normal <30°) (Fig. 121.1) and a positive/increased lateral talo-first metatarsal (Meary's angle) (normal 0°) (Fig. 121.2).

Treatment

Cavovarus Foot

- Conservative measures tried first
  - Stretching/strengthening modalities
    ◦ Focus on peroneals, tibialis anterior
  - Orthotics
    ◦ Flexible deformity (i.e., a normal Coleman block test)
    ◦ Lateral forefoot and heel posts with recess for first ray
    ◦ Ankle-foot orthosis (AFO) for foot drop
- Surgical management
  - No established guidelines addressing appropriate age for surgery.
  - Evaluation for gastrocnemius/soleus tightening to determine if surgical lengthening is necessary.
  - Flexible deformity:
    ◦ Tibialis posterior transfer to dorsum of foot improves foot drop.
    ◦ Peroneus longus to brevis transfer.
    ◦ Plantar fascia release.
  - Rigid deformity (i.e., abnormal Coleman block test):
    ◦ First metatarsal dorsiflexion osteotomy
    ◦ Calcaneal valgus producing osteotomy

Claw Hallux

- Conservative measures tried first
- Jones procedure: extensor tendon transferred into the metatarsal neck
  - Often combined with IP fusion to avoid mallet toe (overpowering FHL)

Hip Dysplasia

- If asymptomatic leave alone/observe
- May require osteotomy (proximal femur or pelvic) depending on disease progression

Scoliosis

- Bracing rarely effective
- Posterior spinal fusion for deformity progression

Suggested Readings

1. Podeszwa DA. Disorders of the peripheral nervous system. In: Herring JA, et al., editors. Tachdijan's pediatric orthopedics. 5th ed. Philadelphia: Saunders, Elsevier Inc.; 2014.
2. Yagerman SE, et al. Pediatric orthopedic conditions in Charcot-Marie-Tooth disease: a literature review. J Curr Opin Pediatr. 2012;24(1):50–6.

Duchenne Muscular Dystrophy

122

David Johannesmeyer and Reed Estes

Background

- Epidemiology
  - Incidence between 2 and 3 per 10,000 live male births [1, 2]
- Genetics
  - X-linked recessive disease caused by the absence of the protein dystrophin.
  - Dystrophin stabilizes the muscle cell membrane and links actin to the extracellular matrix.
  - 20–30% of diagnoses are due to new mutations [2].
- Pathophysiology
  - Characterized by progressive loss of muscle mass and function with fibrofatty tissue replacing muscle.
  - The absence of dystrophin makes muscle cell membranes more permeable, preventing cellular regeneration and leading to progressive loss of muscle.
  - The absence of dystrophin also affects amount of dystrophin-associated proteins.
- Associated Conditions
  - Scoliosis
    - Up to 95% develop scoliosis [1, 2]

- Equinovarus feet
- Cardiopulmonary issues
- Increased risk of fractures secondary to decreased bone mineral density
- Prognosis
  - Often deceased by age 20, usually due to loss of respiratory musculature. However, if full-time ventilatory support is provided, patient can live much longer [2].
  - Corticosteroid treatment has the potential to improve outcomes.

Presentation and Evaluation

- Symptoms
  - Begin showing signs of disease early in life
  - Stop walking in the second decade
- History
  - Family history is important, but rarity of disease can make it elusive.
  - Have a delay in obtaining motor skills but typically walk by age 24 months.
  - Boys often noted early to be clumsy, to have a wide-based gait, to never run, to be unable to keep up with peers, and to be unable to climb stairs.
- Physical exam
  - Shoulder and pelvic girdle weakness occurs first.
  - Pseudohypertrophy of calves (connective tissue infiltration of calves)

D. Johannesmeyer, MD • R. Estes, MD (✉)
Department of Surgery, Division of Orthopedic Surgery, University of Alabama at Birmingham, Birmingham, AL, USA
e-mail: djohannesmeyer@gmail.com; reede44@uab.edu; reed.estes@gmail.com

© Springer International Publishing AG 2017
A.E.M. Eltorai et al. (eds.), *Orthopedic Surgery Clerkship*, DOI 10.1007/978-3-319-52567-9_122

– Stand with increased lumbar lordosis and walk with a wide-based gait to improve stability.
– Gower's sign: stand up by walking hands up the legs.
– Generally retain reflexes until muscles become too weak to respond.
– Large scoliotic curve that is rapidly progressive (up to 2 degrees per month) due to weakness of trunk and paraspinal musculature.
  ○ Most critical orthopedic manifestation
• Special testing
– Creatine kinase (CK): increased (particularly >5000 units/L), though should be taken during subsequent visits as other muscle injury can produce elevations [2].
– DNA analysis.
– Muscle biopsy for absolute diagnosis.
– Electromyography indicates myopathy.
– Radiography for scoliosis.
  ○ Screening should begin at age 10 with regular x-rays.
  ○ Note large C-shaped curve with the apex in the thoracolumbar region.

Differential Diagnosis

• Becker's muscular dystrophy: follow the same clinical course as Duchenne's but on a delayed course
• Emery-Dreifuss dystrophy
• Limb girdle dystrophy
• Spinal muscular dystrophy
• Dermatomyositis

Treatment

• General
– Primarily based on patient comfort.
– Necessitates a multidisciplinary approach, which includes therapy, orthotic devices, and orthopedic interventions.
  ○ Will eventually require a power wheelchair in addition to other adaptive devices

– Corticosteroids may delay loss of muscle strength and function but can have significant side effects.
– Require diligent pulmonary care with nightly ventilation.
– Soft tissue releases may prolong ambulation.
• Scoliosis
– Not amenable to nonsurgical treatment (i.e., bracing).
– Treat with early posterior spinal instrumentation and fusion early when Cobb angles are noted >20 degrees in order to prevent pulmonary and cardiac dysfunction.
– Should have a cardiac work-up prior to surgery.
– Require higher number of fusion levels than idiopathic scoliosis patients.
– High risk of pulmonary insufficiency following surgery.
– Patients undergoing surgery ultimately have a significantly enhanced quality of life.
• Equinovarus foot
– Treat initially with heel cord stretching and ankle-foot orthoses while sleeping to prevent equinus deformity.
– Treat with tendo-Achilles lengthening versus resection and consider posterior tibialis tendon transfer to dorsum of foot and toe flexor tenotomies if persistent deformity.
• Joint contractures
– Stretching and physical therapy are first-line treatment with knee-ankle-foot orthoses used to keep the knee from developing flexion contractures and to aid in standing.
– Can offer hamstring lengthenings at the expense of further weakening.
• Fractures: treat aggressive with early return to weight-bearing to prevent progressive motor weakness

References

1. Karol LA. Scoliosis in patients with Duchenne muscular dystrophy. J Bone Joint Surg Am. 2007;89(1): 155–62.
2. Sussman M. Duchenne muscular dystrophy. J Am Acad Orthop Surg. 2002;10:138–51.

Arthrogryposis

David Johannesmeyer and Reed Estes

Background

- Includes a group of unrelated diseases characterized by multiple congenital pathologic joint contractures resulting in significant limitations to range of motion
- Epidemiology and etiology
  - Occurs in approximately 1/3000 births [1].
  - Fetal akinesia (decreased fetal movements).
  - Other causes include oligohydramnios, hyperthermia, teratogens, and dysfunction of anterior horn cells.

Pathophysiology

- Multifactorial.
  - Often related to abnormalities in skeletal musculature
  - Also often related to neurologic abnormalities, particularly involving anterior horn cells
- Amyoplasia is the most common, characterized by replacement of skeletal muscle with fibrous tissue and fat.

D. Johannesmeyer, MD • R. Estes, MD (✉)
Department of Surgery, Division of Orthopedic
Surgery, University of Alabama at Birmingham,
Birmingham, AL, USA
e-mail: reede44@uab.edu; reed.estes@gmail.com

Prognosis

- Long-term function and outcomes related to family support, education, and encouragement of independence with little relation between deformity and ultimate function

Presentation and Evaluation

General

- Typically normal intelligence, no dysmorphic facial features, and no sensory deficits, though deep tendon reflexes often diminished or absent.
- All four-limb involvement in 84% of patients [1, 2].
- Joints will have limited range of motion with a firm end point.
- Decrease in overall muscle mass.
- Lack normal skin creases around joints with skin dimples often noted over the extensor surfaces of joints.

Upper Extremity

- Contractures characterized by internal rotation and adduction of the shoulders, extension of elbows, flexion and ulnar deviation of wrist, and flexed fingers with adducted thumbs

Spine

- About 30% have neuromuscular scoliosis with a stiff C-shaped curve [2].
- Curves are often progressive.

Lower Extremity

- Contractures characterized by hip external rotation, flexion and abduction, knee flexion (more common) or extension, and foot deformities, including rigid equinovarus (most common) or congenital vertical talus.
- Hips are frequently dislocated (up to 30% of patients) [2].
- Foot deformities are frequently rigid.

Treatment

General

- Goal of treatment to improve independence in activities of daily living.
- Early physical therapy and casting may improve contractures, though recurrence is common.
- Adaptive devices, such as those for eating and writing.
- Surgical treatment starts with soft tissue releases; tendon transfers are considered (though patients often lack functioning muscles) and then osteotomies once the patient nears maturity.
  - Osteotomies do not improve the overall arc of range of motion.

Upper Extremity Disorders

- Shoulder internal rotation rarely causes functional issues.
- Elbow extension contractures.
  - Treatment consideration should be to leave one elbow flexed and the other extended to give patient ability to get a hand to both their mouth and perineum.

- Can perform triceps lengthening or triceps transfer to biceps in addition to a posterior elbow capsulotomy.
- Hand and wrist contractures.
  - Flexor carpi ulnaris is often only functioning wrist muscle and therefore can transfer to wrist extensors to improve grip and move wrist to neutral position.

Spine

- Often resistant to bracing and can increase relentlessly.
- Perform posterior spinal instrumentation and fusion to prevent progression and consider additional anterior fusion in larger and stiffer curves.
- Pseudoarthrosis is frequent (up to 30%) following fusion [2].

Hip Disorders

- Compensate for flexion contractures with excessive lumbar lordosis.
- Surgical treatment indicated in patients with >45 degree flexion contracture.
- Hip dislocations often require open reduction and possible femoral shortening osteotomy.
- Reducing hips may lead to decrease range of motion.

Knee Disorders

- Early intervention necessary in setting of >30 degree flexion contractures.
- Bracing children who can walk delays further surgery and reduces number of surgical interventions.
- Surgical intervention starts with soft tissue releases, including capsulotomies and lengthening of the hamstrings (flexion contractures) and quadriceps (extension contractures) tendons.
- Care must be taken in the posterior knee to avoid injury to sciatic nerve and popliteal

artery with posterior dissection and aggressive correction of knee flexion.

- Supracondylar femur osteotomy and distal femoral hemiepiphysiodesis can be done to correct residual or recurrent contractures.

Foot Disorders

- Clubfoot
  - Ponseti casting first line but rigidity of feet often leads to recurrence.
  - Often require aggressive soft tissue releases with tendon releases with long-term casting and bracing.
  - Relapses following soft tissue releases require bony procedures, including talec-

tomy (with calcaneocuboid joint fusion), triple arthrodesis, or the use of a framed external fixator.

- Congenital vertical talus
  - Initial treatment with casting
  - Surgical treatment is used in setting of recurrence and includes anterior tibialis transfer to the neck of talus, subtalar fusion, or triple arthrodesis.

References

1. Bamshad M, Heest V, Ann E, Pleasure D. Arthrogryposis: a review and update. JBJS. 2009;91-A(4):41–6.
2. Bernstein RM. Arthrogryposis and amyoplasia. J Am Acad Orthop Surg. 2002;10:417–24.

Achondroplasia

124

David Johannesmeyer and Reed Estes

Background

- Most common cause of disproportionate dwarfism and most common skeletal dysplasia
- Epidemiology
  - Incidence of 1/30,000 live births annually [3]
- Genetics
  - Autosomal dominant
    ∘ Sporadic mutation in >80% of cases, increasing with advanced paternal age [1]
  - Mutation of fibroblast growth factor receptor 3 (FGFR3) on chromosome 4P [2]
    ∘ Leads to abnormal chondroid production by chondroblasts
    ∘ Affects the proliferative zone during enchondral bone formation, leading to shortened long bones
- Associated conditions
  - Lumbar stenosis
  - Thoracolumbar kyphosis and lumbosacral lordosis
  - Foramen magnum stenosis: associated with higher mortality in infants, leading to brainstem compression

D. Johannesmeyer, MD • R. Estes, MD (✉)
Department of Surgery, Division of Orthopedic Surgery, University of Alabama at Birmingham, Birmingham, AL, USA
e-mail: reede44@uab.edu; reed.estes@gmail.com

∘ Most often initially presents with respiratory difficulty and apnea [1]
- Otolaryngeal problems in up to 90% of patients [3]
- Hydrocephalus

Presentation and Evaluation

Symptoms

- Delayed motor milestones with normal intelligence
- Subjective weakness, numbness, paresthesias, and claudication-type symptoms as early as in adolescence

Physical Exam

- Orthopedic characteristics
  - The first sign is rhizomelic patterning (disproportionate limb shortening).
    ∘ Average height 52" for men and 49" for women [2]
  - Spine.
    ∘ Excessive lumbosacral lordosis (up to 80% prevalence) and thoracolumbar kyphosis (11% in older patients) [1, 3]

- Thoracolumbar kyphosis most pronounced in younger patients, though typically resolves when child begins walking. If persistent, it can further worsen hyperlordosis.
- Hyperlordosis results from excessive anterior pelvic tilt, leading to prominent abdomen and buttocks and likely increasing the risk of symptoms from spinal stenosis.
  - Neurologic evaluation for spinal stenosis (present in up to 89% of patients) [3]
- Upper extremity.
  - Trident hands (extra space between the third and fourth digits)
  - Fingertips only reach top of greater trochanter of the femur.
  - Elbow flexion contractures often related to distal humerus deformity can lead to radial head subluxation.
- Lower extremity.
  - Genu varum (bowed legs)
    - Often asymptomatic but can cause pain, loss of function, waddling gait, and knee instability
  - Decreased tibial external torsion, increased femoral and acetabular anteversion, and knee hyperextension
- Non-orthopedic characteristics: frontal bossing and midface hypoplasia

Radiographic Work-Up

- Plain radiographs.
  - Narrowing of the interpedicular distance from L1 to L5 on the anteroposterior (AP) lumbar spine x-ray
  - Short pedicles (leads to hyperlordosis) and thoracolumbar vertebral wedging
  - Squared iliac wings with pelvis being wider than it is deep ("champagne glass pelvis")
  - Flared metaphyses of long bones

- CT or MRI recommended to screen for foramen magnum stenosis – stenosis may cause fatal brainstem compression.
- MRI also indicated with concerns for spinal stenosis.

Further Testing

- Chorionic villus sampling or amniocentesis can offer a prenatal diagnosis [2].

Treatment

- Foramen magnum stenosis
  - Require treatment in first 2 years of life though can present later
  - Involves decompression of foramen magnum and upper cervical laminectomy
- Spine
  - Thoracolumbar kyphosis tends to resolve.
    - Can prevent with supported sitting with firm backed devices in young child.
    - Brace child if vertebral wedging and fixed kyphosis >30 degrees develops.
    - Posterior spinal instrumentation and fusion offered in persistent kyphosis. Anterior fusion may be indicated with kyphosis >50 degrees in hyperextension radiographs.
  - Hyperlordosis: treatment indications are unclear.
  - Spinal stenosis: approximately 25% of patients require surgery for spinal stenosis.
    - Indications include progressive symptoms, including claudication and loss of urinary function, unchanged after conservative measures with activity modification and anti-inflammatories.
    - Treated with posterior spinal instrumentation and fusion with decompression of neural elements

- Upper extremity: generally nonoperative
- Lower extremity
  - Genu varum: generally surgical treatment, which includes corrective osteotomies in the proximal tibia and fibula or hemiepiphysiodeses
- Limb lengthening: controversial
  - Must weigh risks of complications and length of treatment (whether injections with growth hormone or surgical lengthening) with benefits of procedure

References

1. Carter CW, Sharkey MS. Contemporary management of the pediatric patient with achondroplasia. OKOJ. 2014;12(10):1.
2. Richette P, Bardin T, Stheneur C. Achondroplasia: from genotype to phenotype. Joint Bone Spine. 2008;75:125–30.
3. Shirley ED, Ain MC. Achondroplasia: manifestations and treatment. J Am Acad Orthop Surg. 2009;17(4): 231–41.

Dana Olszewski

Spondyloepiphyseal Dysplasia (SED)

- Genetics: AD (but random mutation in 50% of cases)
  - COL2A1 on Chromosome 12.
  - Advanced paternal age increases risk.
- Presentation: atlantoaxial instability - > cervical myelopathy
  - Respiratory difficulty
  - Myopia or retinal detachment
  - Coxa vara
  - Short stature
  - Kyphoscoliosis
  - Genu valgum
  - Lumbar lordosis
  - Flattened facies
- Imaging: c spine (instability)
  - TL spine (platyspondyly, kyphoscoliosis, increased lumbar lordosis, partial fusion of spinal ossification centers).
  - AP pelvis (coxa vara).
  - MRI c spine if myelopathy symptoms are present.
- Treatment:
  - Nonop: PT/OT, ophthalmologist, bracing for scoliosis, pulmonology

- Op: posterior atlantoaxial fusion (aa instability >8 mm or myelopathy), PSIF (> 50 degrees), valgus intertrochanteric osteotomy (coxa vara <100 degrees or if progressive)

Multiple Epiphyseal Dysplasia (MED)

- Genetics:
  - Type I – AD COMP
  - Type II – AD Type IX collagen
- Presentation: short limbs and stature
  - Waddling gait
  - Valgus knees - > early OA
  - ** Normal spine
- Imaging: c spine flexion/extension films
  - AP pelvis (bilateral epiphyseal defects)
  - BLE alignment (genu valgum, double layer patella, epiphyseal defects)
  - Hand and feet (short metacarpals and metatarsals, respectively)
- Treatment:
  - Nonop: NSAIDs and therapy
  - Op: Hemiepiphysiodesis or osteotomies for genu valgum THA for arthritis

Diastrophic Dysplasia

- Genetics: AR sulfate transport protein (DTDST gene on Chromosome 5)

D. Olszewski, MD, MPH
Childrens Orthopaedics of Atlanta, Atlanta, GA, USA
e-mail: olszewskimd@gmail.com

© Springer International Publishing AG 2017
A.E.M. Eltorai et al. (eds.), *Orthopedic Surgery Clerkship*, DOI 10.1007/978-3-319-52567-9_125

- Presentation: rhizomelic shortening
  - Cleft palate
  - Cauliflower ears
  - Hitchhikers thumb
  - Cervical kyphosis
  - Scoliosis
  - Genu valgum
  - Skewfoot
  - Clubfeet
- Imaging: AP and lateral c spine and TL spine
  - BLE alignment films
- Treatment:
  - Cauliflower ears – compressive bandages.
  - Occipital-cervical fusion for atlantoaxial instability.
  - Posterior cervical fusion for cervical kyphosis – many cases resolve spontaneously.
  - TL fusion for kyphoscoliosis.
  - Casting and possible releases for clubfeet.
  - LE osteotomies for progressive valgus deformity.

Cleidocranial Dysplasia

- Genetics: AD with a RUNX2/CBFA-1
- Presentation: proportionate dwarfism
  - Clavicle dysplasia/aplasia
  - Wormian bones
  - Frontal bossing
  - Coxa vara
  - Shortened middle phalanges long through small fingers
  - Delayed eruption of permanent teeth

- Imaging: AP chest (clavicle absence or shortening)
  - AP pelvis (coxa vara)
- Treatment: most problems are observed.
  - Coxa vara can be treated with an intertrochanteric osteotomy when neck shaft angle <100 degrees.

Suggested Reading

1. Anthony S, Munk R, Skakun W, and Masini M. Multiple epiphyseal dysplasia. J Am Acad Orthop Surg. 2015;23:164–72; published ahead of print February 9, 2015, doi:10.5435/JAAOS-D-13-00173.
2. Beals R, Sauser DD. Nontraumatic disorders of the clavicle. J Am Acad Orthop Surg. 2006;14:205–14.
3. Cole WG. Genetics and pediatric orthopedics. J Pediatr Orthop. 1999;19(3):281–2.
4. Crossan JF, Wynne-Davies R, Fulford GE. Bilateral failure of the capital femoral epiphysis: bilateral perthes disease, multiple epiphyseal dysplasia, pseudoachondroplasia, and spondyloepiphyseal dysplasia congenita and tarda. J Pediatr Orthop. 1983;3(3):297–301.
5. Diamond LS. A family study of spondyloepiphyseal dysplasia. J Bone Joint Surg Am. 1970;52(8):1587–94.
6. Murphy MC, Shine IB, Stevens DB. Multiple epiphyseal dysplasia. J Bone Joint Surg Am. 1973;55(4):814–20.
7. Rimoin DL, Rasmussen IM, Briggs MD, Roughley PJ, Gruber HE, Warman ML, Olsen BR, Hsia YE, Yuen J, Reinker K, et al. A large family with features of pseudoachondroplasia and multiple epiphyseal dysplasia: exclusion of seven candidate gene loci that encode proteins of the cartilage extracellular matrix. Hum Genet. 1994;93(3):236–42.
8. Wills B, Dormans JP. Nontraumatic upper cervical spine instability in children. J Am Acad Orthop Surg. 2006;14:233–45.

126

Howard Y. Park and Anthony A. Scaduto

Marfan's Syndrome:

- Connective tissue disorder (defective fibrillin) manifesting in the heart/aorta (mitral/aortic valve prolapse, aortic dissection), chest wall deformity (pectus carinatum/excavatum), lungs (spontaneous pneumothorax), eyes (superior lens dislocation), dural ectasia, spine, and long bones
  - Incidence: 1/10,000
  - Genetics: Autosomal dominant (AD) mutation in *fibrillin-1 (FBN1) gene* → defective folding of glycoprotein integral to extracellular matrix
  - Physical exam pearls: *Wrist sign* (thumb/small finger overlap when wrapped around contralateral wrist), *thumb sign* (fist over thumb reveals distal thumb beyond the ulnar border), and *hyperextensibility of joints*

H.Y. Park, MD
Orthopedic Surgery,
UCLA Medical Center, 1250 16th Street,
Suite 2100A, Santa Monica 90404, CA, USA
e-mail: howardypark@mednet.ucla.edu

A.A. Scaduto, MD (✉)
Department of Orthopaedic Surgery,
Orthopaedic Institute for Children/UCLA,
403 West Adams Blvd, Los Angeles, CA 90007, USA
e-mail: tscaduto@mednet.ucla.edu

- Orthopedic: Arachnodactyly, degenerative disk disease, dural ectasia, osteoarthritis, ligamentous laxity, pes planus, scoliosis, and protrusio acetabuli
  - Scoliosis – 63% incidence in Marfan's syndrome [1]
    - Bracing (17% success in Marfan's) [2] ineffective compared to AIS (45–75% success) [3]
    - The minority (12%) develop scoliosis requiring surgery [1]
    - Imaging → *MRI of spine to assess for dural ectasia*
  - Prior to surgery, *cardiac evaluation*

Ehlers-Danlos Syndrome:

- Group of *connective tissue disorders (collagen)* manifesting with the heart/aorta (valve disease, aortic root dilation), GI (hiatal hernia, anal prolapse), soft tissue symptoms (*hyperelastic skin*), and early arthritis
  - Prevalence: 1:2500–5000
  - Genetics: Common types include *COL5A* and *COL3A* mutations
  - Physical exam pearls: Fragile, hyperelastic skin with ligamentous laxity and *chronic pain* (can be misdiagnosed as hypochondriasis)
  - Orthopedic: Sprains/dislocations/hyperextension of joints, kyphosis/scoliosis

A.E.M. Eltorai et al. (eds.), *Orthopedic Surgery Clerkship*, DOI 10.1007/978-3-319-52567-9_126

○ Physical therapy and orthotics for joint stability and pain control
○ Joint fusions
○ Scoliosis surgery for kyphoscoliosis
– Prior to surgery, *cardiac evaluation*

Neurofibromatosis (NF):

• Group of inherited conditions: NF1, NF2, and schwannomatosis → NF1 most common with orthopedic issues (covered below)
  – Incidence: 1:3500
  – Genetics: AD mutation of *NF1* gene on *chromosome 17q21*
    ○ *Neurofibromin* protein deficient
  – Diagnosis: NIH criteria of "cardinal clinical features" [4]
    ○ *Café au lait spots (flat, tan pigments on skin)*, neurofibromas, freckling in axilla/ inguinal region, optic glioma, Lisch nodules (iris hamartomas), sphenoid dysplasia, first-degree relative affected
  – Physical exam: See above, anterolateral bowing of the tibia, hemihypertrophy
  – Orthopedic manifestations:
    ○ Scoliosis in 20%: Dystrophic and non-dystrophic
      – Dystrophic – thoracic kyphoscoliosis and vertebrae/rib abnormalities
        • Operate early
        • High rates of pseudarthrosis → perform ASF + PSF to reduce pseudarthrosis rate
      – Non-dystrophic – brace and surgery if progressive/large
      – *MRI* for dural ectasia and spinal neurofibroma
    ○ *Anterolateral tibial bowing* in 10% of NF1 patients
      – Prone to fracture and develop pseudarthrosis
      – Surgery possible for fixation of fractures and bone grafting → amputation if recalcitrant to fixation and grafting

Mucopolysacharide (MPS) Disorders:

• Family of six *lysosomal metabolism deficiencies* leading to *glycosaminoglycan accumulation*
  – Combined incidence: 1/25000
  – Genetics: Autosomal recessive lysosomal enzyme deficiencies (except Hunter: X-linked recessive)
  – *Bone marrow transplant* has increased lifespans of MPS disorders
  – Orthopedic manifestations:
    ○ *Cervical stenosis* (myelopathy symptoms), *occipitocervical instability* (may need fusion), dwarfism, thoracolumbar kyphosis, scoliosis, hip dysplasia, genu valgum, carpal tunnel syndrome
  – Classic types include:
    ○ MPS I – Hurler syndrome (dermatan sulfate accumulates)
    ○ MPS II – Hunter Syndrome (dermatan/ heparan sulfate)
    ○ MPS III – Sanfilippo syndrome (heparin sulfate)
    ○ MPS IV – Morquio syndrome (keratan sulfate)

Down's Syndrome:

• Syndrome with mental retardation, cardiac defects, and Down's faces
  – Incidence: 1/1000 births
  – Genetics: Trisomy 21
  – Ligamentous laxity and hypotonia causes orthopedic manifestations:
    ○ C1-C2 instability → *flexion-extension cervical radiographs* to assess stability prior to intubation and some advocate for prior to contact sports
      – Cervical fusion if ADI >10 mm or symptomatic
    ○ *Patellofemoral instability/dislocation*
    ○ Hip subluxation/dislocation
    ○ Scoliosis and spondylolisthesis
    ○ Pes planus

Prader-Willi Syndrome:

- Rare disorder marked by hypotonia, aggressive behavior, and *overconsumption leading to obesity*
  - Incidence: 1/25,000 births
  - Genetics: Chromosome 15 partial deletion
  - Physical exam pearls: Obesity, almond-shaped eyes, *weak cry*
  - Orthopedically, assess for hip dysplasia and scoliosis
    - Pes planus, genu valgum, and leg length difference also manifest

Turner Syndrome:

- Incidence: 1/2000–5000 females at birth
- Genetics: 45 XO – female missing an X chromosome
- Sexual infantilism – will not have menses

- Physical exam pearls: Short stature, webbed neck, low-set ears, and signs of coarctation of the aorta (differential blood pressure in arms vs. legs)
- Orthopedic manifestations: Short fourth metacarpal, scoliosis, and osteoporosis (no estrogen)

References

1. Sponseller PD, Hobbs W, Riley LH, Pyeritz RE. The thoracolumbar spine in Marfan syndrome. J Bone Joint Surg Am. 1995;77(6):867–76.
2. Sponseller PD, Bhimani M, Solacoff D, Dormans JP. Results of brace treatment of scoliosis in Marfan syndrome. Spine (Phila Pa 1976). 2000;25(18):2350–4.
3. Rowe DE, Bernstein SM, Riddick MF, Adler F, Emans JB, Gardner-Bonneau D. A meta-analysis of the efficacy of non-operative treatments for idiopathic scoliosis. J Bone Joint Surg Am. 1997;79(5):664–74.
4. Gutmann DH. The diagnostic evaluation and multidisciplinary management of neurofibromatosis 1 and neurofibromatosis 2. JAMA J Am Med Assoc. 1997;278(1):51. doi:10.1001/jama.1997.03550010065042.

127

Juvenile Idiopathic Arthritis

Amit Momaya and Reed Estes

Juvenile Idiopathic Arthritis (JIA)

- Autoimmune arthritis lasting more than 6 weeks in a child younger than 16 years of age
- Diagnosis of exclusion
- Affects 294,000 children in the USA
- Pathogenesis
  - Multifactorial – genetic and environmental
  - HLA genes associated with various subtypes of JIA

Common Symptoms

- Morning stiffness that may improve throughout the day, limp, joint effusion, limited activity secondary to pain, and intermittent flares with periods of remission

Subtypes

Systemic-Onset Arthritis
- Symptoms: rash, spiking fevers, acute presentation

A. Momaya, MD • R. Estes, MD (✉)
Department of Surgery, Division of Orthopedic Surgery, University of Alabama at Birmingham, Birmingham, AL, USA
e-mail: reede44@uab.edu; reed.estes@gmail.com

- Lab abnormalities: anemia, leukocytosis, thrombocytosis, elevated liver enzymes
- Affects males and females equally
- Must rule out infection
- Worst prognosis of JIA subtypes

Oligoarticular Arthritis
- Most common JIA subtype
- Affects four or fewer joints in the first 6 months of disease (the knee is the most commonly affected joint)
  - Patients often present with limp
- Large joint involvement
- Female to male ratio 3:1
- 15–20 % of patients have uveitis
  - Refer for ophthalmologic evaluations to help prevent complications including vision loss

Polyarticular RF-Positive Arthritis
- Arthritis affecting five or more joints during the first 6 months of disease
- Small joints (hand/wrist) affected
- Females > males

Polyarticular RF-Negative Arthritis
- Similar to polyarticular RF positive but tend to have fewer joints involved
- Better functional outcomes

© Springer International Publishing AG 2017
A.E.M. Eltorai et al. (eds.), *Orthopedic Surgery Clerkship*, DOI 10.1007/978-3-319-52567-9_127

Psoriatic Arthritis

- Asymmetric arthritis affecting both large and small joints
- Psoriatic skin plaques
- Radiographic findings: "pencil in cup" shape in the finger
- May develop iritis
  - Should undergo slit lamp evaluations every 6 months

Enthesitis-Related Arthritis

- Differentiated by the presence of inflammation at the tendon insertion sites in the bone.
- Generally males older than 8 years of age.
- Most are HLA-B27 positive.
- Patients with enthesitis-related arthritis may develop ankylosing spondylitis, reactive arthritis, or enteropathic arthropathy.

Undifferentiated Arthritis

- Those children who do not meet the criteria for one of the subtypes above or fit into more than one category

Complications

- Iridocyclitis
  - Occurs in 15–20 % of patients with JIA and can lead to blindness
  - Need referral for ophthalmologic screenings with a slit lamp
- Growth disturbances
  - Chronic arthritis can lead to limb length discrepancies.
- Joint damage, osteoporosis, and psychological issues

Treatment

- The goal is to implement therapy early.
  - Multimodal – physical, pharmacological, and psychological

Pharmacological Therapies

- Nonsteroidal anti-inflammatory drugs are first line.
  - Ibuprofen, naproxen, or indomethacin
  - Cox-2 inhibitors if significant gastrointestinal side effects
- Disease-modifying antirheumatic drugs (DMARDs).
  - Slow the radiological progression of the disease
  - Two-thirds of children require DMARDs
- Biologic agents.
  - Monoclonal antibodies, soluble cytokine receptors, and receptor antagonists
- Intra-articular corticosteroids.

Surgical Therapies

- Arthroscopic versus open synovectomy
- Epiphysiodesis and osteotomy for limb length discrepancy and deformity
- Arthrodesis/arthroplasty for adults with end-stage arthritis

References

1. Espinosa M, Gottlieb B. Juvenile idiopathic arthritis. Pediatr Rev. 2012;33(7):303–13.
2. Gowdie PJ, Tse SM. Juvenile idiopathic arthritis. Pediatr Clin North Am. 2012;59(2):301–27.
3. Weiss JE, Ilowite NT. Juvenile idiopathic arthritis. Pediatr Clin North Am. 2005;52(2):413–42, vi.

Shoulder and Elbow Deformities

128

Howard Y. Park and Anthony A. Scaduto

Brachial Plexopathy of Birth Stretching injuries of brachial plexus during difficult delivery:

- Incidence: 1–4/1000 births.
- *Vast majority recover within the first 2 months:*
  - If not recovered by 3 months, considerable risk of long-term deficit possibly indicating surgery
- Risk factors: large size, multiparous pregnancy, prolonged labor, and difficult delivery:
  - *Horner's syndrome* a very poor prognosticator
- Preganglionic injury (avulsions from cord) will not spontaneously recover.
- Erb's palsy (C5, 6) → Axillary, suprascapular, musculocutaneous, and radial nerves affected:

- *Waiter's tip* – adducted, internally rotated shoulder, elbow extended, and wrist flexed
- Very good prognosis
- *Klumpke's palsy* (C8, T1) → Median and ulnar nerves affected:
  - Deficits of muscles controlling hands
  - *Claw hand* – extended wrist and MCP and flexed IP joints
  - Poor prognosis
- *Total plexus palsy* (all roots):
  - Full, flaccid paralysis with sensory loss
  - Very poor prognosis
- Treatment – Dependent upon the type of palsy seen:
  - Monitor for the first 3 months with passive ROM by the parent/therapist:
    - If biceps function returns → observe until age 2.
    - If no biceps function and no Horner's syndrome → observe for additional 3 months.
    - If no biceps function and Horner's syndrome → microsurgery [1].
  - Microsurgery nerve repair, nerve grafting, and nerve transfer.
  - Corrective surgeries for glenohumeral dislocations and shoulder, forearm, elbow, and hand contractures.

H.Y. Park, MD
Department of Orthopedic Surgery,
UCLA Medical Center, 1250 16th Street, Suite 2100A, Santa Monica, CA 90404, USA
e-mail: howardypark@mednet.ucla.edu

A.A. Scaduto, MD (✉)
Department of Orthopaedic Surgery,
Orthopaedic Institute for Children/UCLA,
403 West Adams Blvd, Los Angeles, CA 90007, USA
e-mail: tscaduto@mednet.ucla.edu

Sprengel's Deformity Development failure of the shoulder to descend from the neck leading to high scapula:

- Associated with *Klippel-Feil syndrome*, congenital scoliosis, rib anomalies, and spina bifida
- Often can have *omovertebral bone* between the cervical spine and scapula
- Incidence left > right, although can be bilateral:
  - 75% of cases are female.
- Physical exam pearls: high, rotated scapula (inferior angle pointing medially) and decreased abduction/forward elevation of the shoulder due to decreased scapulothoracic motion
- Surgery indicated if functional deficits:
  - Surgery preferred earlier (age 4–8) to decrease risk of nerve injury when altering scapular position at older ages

Congenital Radioulnar Synostosis Developmental failure of radius/ulna to divide:

- Majority proximal as division of forearm occurs distal to proximal:
  - The other form is distal to the proximal radial epiphysis.
- 60% bilateral.
- Males > females.
- Genetics: Mostly sporadic, autosomal dominant transmission seen in certain regions and sex chromosomal duplication also seen.
- *Presents with limited pronation/supination.*
- Detected in late childhood when functional impairments become evident.
- Treatment is mostly observation unless functional deficit:
  - Surgery utilized to place the forearm in rotation of maximum function (slight pronation)
  - Cannot simply excise synostosis as *recurrence* is likely

Post-traumatic Cubitus Varus/Valgus

- Varus/valgus deformities of the elbow resulting from distal humerus fractures (supracondylar fractures, lateral/medial condyle fractures, distal humerus physeal separation):
  - Cubitus varus commonly the result of *malunion*
  - Cubitus valgus commonly the result of *lateral physeal growth arrest*
- Cubitus varus (*gunstock deformity*) is the most common complication of the most common pediatric elbow injury, supracondylar humerus fracture:
  - Result of malunion – medial tilt coronally, extension sagittally, and internally rotated in horizontal plane.
  - Function is rarely limited, but cosmetic deformity can be severe.
- Cubitus valgus can lead to a *tardy ulnar nerve palsy*:
  - Slow, progressive paralysis of ulnar nerve
  - Can be present years after injury
- Treatment:
  - Observation and reassurance, especially if cosmetic concern is low.
  - Supracondylar corrective osteotomy for after skeletal maturity:
    - Lateral closing-wedge, dome rotational, step-cut lateral closing-wedge osteotomies for cubitus varus
    - Osteotomies associated with significant complication rates
  - Cubitus valgus tardy ulnar nerve palsies may be addressed with nerve transposition.

Reference

1. Smith NC, Rowan P, Benson LJ, Ezaki M, Carter PR. Neonatal brachial plexus palsy. Outcome of absent biceps function at three months of age. J Bone Joint Surg Am. 2004;86-A(10):2163–70.

John M. Stephenson, Allen Borne,
and Theresa Wyrick

Pediatric Trigger Thumb (Fig. 129.1)

Overview

- Estimated incidence of 1 in 2000 children.
- Bilateral in 25–30% of children.
- Often referred to as "congenital"; however screening of newborns has not found this to be present at birth.
- Occurs ten times more commonly than trigger finger.

Anatomy

- Thickening of the FPL at the A1 pulley
- "Notta's" nodule may be felt in this area of tendon thickening

Classification

- Proposed by Sugimoto:
  - Stage 1 – "tumor type" (nodule present but no catching)
  - Stage 2 – active triggering
  - Stage 3 – lacks active IP extension, but can be passively corrected
  - Stage 4 – "rigid type" (fixed flexion deformity with no passive correction)

Evaluation

- History:
  - Often discovered incidentally
  - Not associated with injury
  - Typically not associated with pain, unless passively extended
- Physical examination:
  - Observe for a fixed IP deformity either in flexion (most common) or extension.
  - Palpate for Notta's nodule at the MP flexion crease.
  - Palpate for triggering.
  - Passive extension may be tried, but pain will occur if forcefully extended.
  - The absence of a flexion crease can represent absent FPL or symphalangism.
- Associated syndromes are not commonly observed with trigger thumb.
- Imaging is not commonly done as this is largely a clinical diagnosis.

J.M. Stephenson, MD (✉) • A. Borne, MD
T. Wyrick, MD
Department of Orthopaedic Surgery,
University of Arkansas for Medical Sciences,
Little Rock, AR, USA
e-mail: johnmstep@gmail.com

A.E.M. Eltorai et al. (eds.), *Orthopedic Surgery Clerkship*, DOI 10.1007/978-3-319-52567-9_129

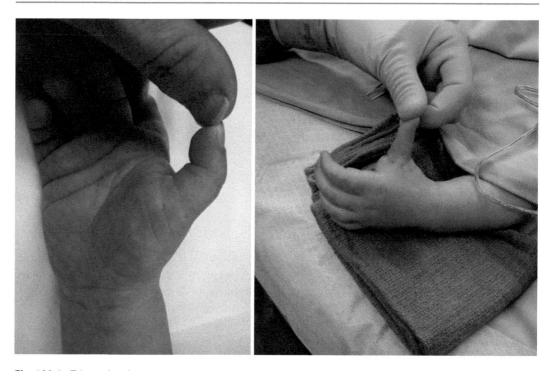

Fig. 129.1 Trigger thumb

Treatment

Nonsurgical
- There is no harm in a short period of observation (approximately 6 months), and this is recommended up to age 3 or 4.
- Some advocate for earlier release if fixed contracture or bilateral.
- Family preference often determines how long the condition is observed.

Surgical
- Transverse incision in the metacarpophalangeal joint flexion crease.
- Only the skin is incised as the digital nerves are directly underneath the skin with the radial digital nerve being most at risk.
- Clearly identify the A1 pulley and release it longitudinally.
- Observe for restoration of IP hyperextension and no locking or triggering.
- Do not release the oblique pulley to prevent resultant tendon bowstringing.

Clinodactyly

Overview

- Defined as angulation with apex radial/ulnar located distal to the MP joint.
- Angulation greater than 100 is considered abnormal.
- Incidence has been reported up to 20%.
- Autosomal dominant transmission occurs in some cases with variable penetrance.
- Males tend to be more commonly affected.
- Differentiated from Kirner's deformity in which deviation occurs in more than one plane and is typically isolated to the small finger distal phalanx.
- Can be acquired due to trauma to physis.

Anatomy

- The small finger is the most common with an apex ulnar deformity.

- The deformity is often due to the middle phalanx having a more trapezoidal shape.
- Other digits may have more deformity causing problems with function.

Classification

Proposed by Cooney
- Simple: deformity of the middle phalanx less than 450 angulation
- Simple complicated: deformity of the middle phalanx greater than 450 angulation
- Complex: deformity of bone and soft tissue less than 450 with associated syndactyly
- Complex complicated: deformity of bone and soft tissue greater than 450 with associated polydactyly or macrodactyly

Evaluation

History
- Often noted at birth
- Can demonstrate progressive compensatory contracture

Physical Examination
- Measure the degree of clinical deformity.
- Carefully evaluate for other associated hand conditions or joint contractures.

Associated Syndromes
- Rubinstein-Taybi:
  - Short stature, learning difficulties, facial anomalies, and broad thumb and great toe
  - Increased risk of cancer
  - Autosomal dominant vs. spontaneous mutation
  - Increased anesthetic risk
- Cenani-Lenz syndactyly:
  - Syndactyly resembles Apert syndrome.
  - Shortening of radius and ulna.
  - Can be associated with abnormal fusion/phalanx development.
  - Associated kidney abnormalities.

Imaging
- Plain radiographs can demonstrate abnormal C-shaped physis or a fusion causing a bracketed epiphysis and an associated "delta phalanx."
- Advanced imaging is not required.

Treatment

Nonsurgical
- Treatment is not necessary for most digits.
- Splinting is not effective.

Surgical
- Indicated for severe deformities or those that interfere with function.
- Closing or opening wedge osteotomies.
- Epiphyseal bracket resection and fat grafting.
- Stiffness can result; thus surgery should be avoided for purely cosmetic reasons.

Camptodactyly

Overview

- Flexion contracture of the PIP joint.
- Can be progressive.
- Not frequently associated with pain.
- Some cases are autosomal dominant with variable expressivity and penetrance.
- Less than 1% of the population.

Anatomy

- Multiple structures around the PIP joint have been known to cause this clinical picture:
  - Skin and subcutaneous tissue contractures
  - Ligamentous anomalies
  - Musculotendinous anomalies
  - Bone/joint anomalies
- Most common anomalies are in the FDS/FDP relationship, lumbricals, or interossei.

Classification

- Type I: appears in infancy with males > females
- Type II: appears in preadolescence with females > males
- Type III: severe deformity, often multiple digits and bilateral extremities, and syndromic associations

Evaluation

History
- Determine age of presentation.
- Inquire about progression.
- Evaluate for other associated anomalies.

Physical
- Measure the degree of contracture.
- Determine if flexible vs. fixed.

Associated Syndromes
- Craniofacial disorders
- Short stature (such as mucopolysaccharidosis)
- Multiple chromosomal alterations

Imaging
- Plain radiographs to evaluate primary or compensatory bone abnormalities.
- Advanced imaging is not required.

Treatment

Nonsurgical
- Most often treated conservatively and includes stretching/splinting program.
- Contractures under 400 are generally not associated with a functional deficit, and nonsurgical treatment is recommended.
- Static vs. dynamic splinting may help to reduce the degree of contracture and prevent progression.
- Splinting has been recommended from 8 to 18 h per day with continuation with growth of the child.

Surgical
- Indicated in only severe or progressive deformities that have not improved despite appropriate nonsurgical treatment.
- Typical procedure involves addressing all possible abnormal structures:
  - Z-plasty with possible full-thickness skin graft
  - Tendon release/transfers
  - Joint release
- Stepwise approach until acceptable correction can be obtained.
- Associated bony changes typically have a worse prognosis.

Syndactyly (Fig. 129.2)

Overview

- Fusion (failure to separate) of the skin, soft tissue, and/or bone.
- Isolated syndactyly has an incidence of 1 in 2000.
- 50% are bilateral.
- Family history is reported up to 40%.
- Autosomal dominant with variable expressivity and penetrance.
- Male/female ratio approximately 2:1.
- The most common is the long/ring finger and then the ring/small finger.

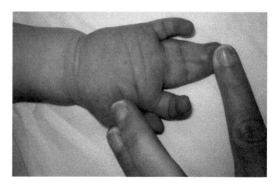

Fig. 129.2 Syndactyly

Anatomy

- Digits are formed from the mesodermal layer.
- Apoptosis separates the digits from distal to proximal.
- Apical ectodermal ridge is important in this regulated process.
- Lateral digital sheet is thickened and runs through across the syndactylous bridge.
- Digital neurovascular bundle may bifurcate more distally.

Classification

- Complete: web space extends to fingertips.
- Incomplete: web space terminates short of the fingertips.
- Simple: soft tissue connections only.
- Complex: bony connections and associated skeletal anomalies.
- Complex complicated: accessory bones within the syndactylous bridge.

Evaluation

History
- Inquire about associated family history.
- Assess child's progressive development.
- Assess for other associated syndromes.

Physical
- The entire body should be examined (head, chest, feet).
- Evaluate the range of motion of the affected digits.
- Examine the nail/nail fold involvement.
- Observe the child's ability to grasp and hold.

Associated Syndromes
- Acrosyndactyly:
  - Fenestration (sinus tract) is proximal to the distal fusion mass.
  - Associated with constriction ring syndrome.
- Apert syndrome:
  - Combination of craniofacial anomalies with complex hand/foot syndactyly.
  - Mutation of FGFR2.
  - Other extremity findings include glenohumeral as well as radiocapitellar anomalies.
- Poland syndrome:
  - Disruption of blood flow in the subclavian artery
  - Shortened webbed digits with associated ipsilateral chest wall anomalies involving the pectoralis muscles

Imaging
- Plain radiographs to determine the bony involvement.
- MRI or ultrasound can help to define anomalous tendon and neurovascular anatomy, not typically necessary.

Treatment

Nonsurgical
- Recommended only for mild, incomplete forms.
- Some complex syndactylous digits are not amenable to reconstruction.

Surgical
- Goal is separation of digits before child starts school.
- Staged release of multiple digit involvement due to risk of neurovascular compromise (one side of a digit at a time).
- Local skin flaps will usually be insufficient to cover, so full-thickness skin graft is almost always needed.
- Multiple flaps/configurations have been described.
- The most common complication is "web creep" (distal migration of the surgically reconstructed web space with growth).

Symphalangism (Stiff Interphalangeal Joints)

Overview

- A term describing a rare congenital anomaly characterized by failure of interphalangeal joint development and fusion

Anatomy

- Longitudinal bone or fibrous fusion across interphalangeal joints
- Proximal interphalangeal joint most commonly affected

Classification

Flatt and Wood
- True symphalangism – digits have normal length, and there are no other skeletal abnormalities.
- Symphalangism associated with symbrachydactyly – digits are short/stiff.
- Symphalangism with associated anomalies.

Based on Type of Ankylosis
- Grade I – fibrous symphalangism
- Grade II – cartilaginous symphalangism
- Grade III – bony symphalangism

Evaluation

- History: stiff fingers or toes.
- Physical: stiff fingers, no active motion, and 10/20 degrees passive motion:
  - Absence of flexion/extension creases
  - Proximal interphalangeal joint abnormal and other joints with motion
- Associated syndromes: Apert syndrome and Poland syndrome.
- Imaging: X-rays may show fused phalanges or joint space.

Treatment

- Nonsurgical: classically the treatment for children with little functional deficit
- Surgical:
  - Classically of little success:
    - Arthroplasty had poor results; joint preservation had repeat ankylosis.
  - Arthrodesis in flexion – option for difficulty with grip/grasp.
  - Soft tissue release (dorsal capsule, dorsal half collateral ligaments) at a young age has shown early encouraging results in Grades I and II.

Symbrachydactyly (Fused Short Fingers)

Overview

- A term describing a spectrum of deficiencies beginning with short middle phalanges extending to the absence of central rays and finally the absence of the entire hand

Anatomy

- Displays features of undergrowth and failure of differentiation and formation. Central rays are often the most abnormal. Thought to be a transverse deficiency (differentiating from cleft hand's longitudinal deficiency) and mesodermal in nature.

Classification

Blauth and Gekeler
- Short finger type
- Cleft hand type
- Monodactylous type
- Peromelic type

Yamauchi: Focuses on the Number of Phalanges Missing

- Triphalangia – all four fingers have three phalanges.
- Diphalangia – one finger missing one or more phalanges.
- Monophalangia – finger or fingers with only one phalange.
- Aphalangia – all three phalanges are missing in a digit.
- Ametacarpia – the absence of a metacarpal bone.
- Acarpia – the absence of the distal forearm, usually with rudimentary digits.
- Forearm amputation type.

Evaluation

- History: congenital hand deformity/deficiency.
- Physical: spectrum of deformity based on severity. Evaluate for short middle phalanges and overall function. Central rays most affected as severity increases. Evaluate for proximal enabling structures that may be used for reconstruction.
- Associated syndromes: Poland syndrome and unilateral hand hypoplasia with the absence of shoulder girdle muscles.
- Imaging: X-ray determines the presence or absence of phalanges, metacarpals, and carpal bones:
  - Mild cases – the middle phalanx reduced in size or absent

Treatment

- Nonsurgical: observation if function is adequate in mild forms.
- Surgical:
  - Variable based on degree of suppression. Severe forms may benefit from free toe transfer if no thumb or fingers for prehension.

- Short finger types (mild): function usually excellent:
  - Web deepening for incomplete syndactyly
  - Free phalangeal bone graft possible if skeletally deficient with adequate soft tissues
- Oligodactic (few fingers) type:
  - Web deepening.
  - Metacarpal osteotomy to improve prehension of the thumb and small finger.
  - Free toe transfers (to increase number of digits) may improve grasp of large or heavy objects.
- Monodactylic (single finger):
  - Free toe transfer is an option.
- Peromelic (short limb):
  - Reconstruction difficult due to lack of proximal structures

Macrodactyly

Overview

- Describes an uncommon congenital or developmental large digit

Anatomy

- Both soft tissue and bone elements are enlarged, and there is fatty infiltration of the nerve.
- Most common: isolated anomaly with lipofibromatosis of the proximal nerve
- Etiology unknown, thought to be nerve related
- Usually unilateral, multiple affected digits can occur, index being the most common.

Classification: Flatt

- Type I – Gigantism and lipofibromatosis
- Type II – Gigantism and neurofibromatosis

- Type III – Gigantism and digital hyperostosis (periarticular osteochondral masses, nodular involvement of digits)
- Type IV – Gigantism and hemihypertrophy (all digits involved)

Evaluation

- History: Congenital deformity or developing in the first few years. May be static or progressive (continued disproportionate growth of affected digit). Digits often stiffen with growth. May present with compressive neuropathy. Can be disfiguring with social stigma.
- Physical: affected radial digits deviate radially, ulnar digits deviate ulnarly, and two digits deviate away from each other.
- Associated syndromes: neurofibromatosis, syndactyly, Klippel-Trenaunay-Weber syndrome, and lipofibromatous hamartoma of the median nerve
- Imaging:
  - X-rays show enlarged skeleton with advanced bone age and osteoarthritic changes.
  - Angiography – one digital artery enlarged.

Treatment

- Very difficult to treat due to progressive and diffuse nature. Multiple procedures may be necessary with unsatisfactory results.
- Nonsurgical: compressive bandaging.
- Surgical:
  - Limiting growth – artery ligation, digital nerve stripping/resection, and epiphysiodesis
  - Correcting deviation – closing-wedge physeal resection
  - Debulking the digit – fat resection and narrowing and shortening of bone via a variety of techniques
  - Ray amputation

Polydactyly

Overview

- Congenital malformation of the hand with extra (supernumerary) digits

Classification

Preaxial: Thumb Duplication
- Wassel classification:
  - Type I – Bifid distal phalanx
  - Type II – Duplicated distal phalanx
  - Type III – Bifid proximal phalanx
  - Type IV – Duplicated proximal phalanx (most common)
  - Type V – Bifid metacarpal
  - Type VI – Duplicated metacarpal
  - Type VII – Triphalangia

Postaxial: Small Finger Duplication
- Type A – well-developed digit
- Type B – rudimentary and pedunculated digit
- Central – extra digit within the borders of the hand

Evaluation

History
- Preaxial – more common in white individuals, most are unilateral and sporadic, without systemic problems (Fig. 129.3)
- Postaxial – frequently autosomal dominant, more common in African Americans
- Central – uncommon compared to pre- and postaxial, may be hidden within syndactyly (synpolydactyly)

Physical
- Preaxial – widening of nail plate in type I:
  - Asses thumb function, bony elements, and joint stability.

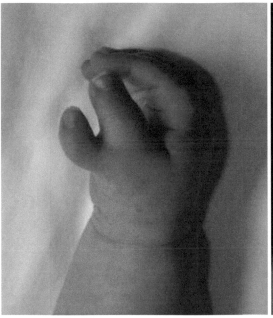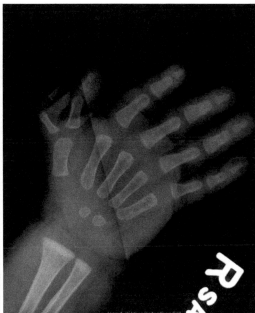

Fig. 129.3 Thumb duplication

– Not true duplication, neither digit com-
  pletely normal, a.k.a. "split thumb."
- Postaxial – rudimentary or well-formed digit
  on ulnar hand.
- Central – may involve webbing, synpolydactyly.
- Associated syndromes:
  – Grebe's chondrodysplasia – central
    polydactyly
  – Ellis-van Creveld syndrome – dwarfism
    and well-formed postaxial polydactyly
- Imaging: X-rays assist in defining the extent
  of duplication; cartilaginous connections may
  not be identified.

Treatment

Nonsurgical
- Preaxial – subtle types I and II with common
  nail and well aligned
- Postaxial – Type B: tying at the base of digit in
  nursery (may have residual bump/neuroma)

- Central:
  – Fully formed digit with normal function
    does not require removal.
  – Synpolydactyly with complex connections
    may have little functional benefit from sur-
    gical reconstruction.

Surgical
- Preaxial – goal is to create the best aligned and
  functional thumb possible using portions of
  each thumb component (size, alignment, joint
  stabilization, balanced motor function, nail
  plate).
  – Types II, IV, and VI – resection requires
    joint stability with:
    ∘ Preservation/reconstruction of collateral
      ligaments
  – Types I and II – distinct components:
    ∘ Ablation of smaller thumb, collateral
      ligament transfer, and centralization of
      extensor tendon
    ∘ Bilhaut-Cloquet procedure:

(i) Wedge resection of central portions of the bone and nail with approximation of border components

(ii) Inconsistent results

- Types III and IV – selection of dominant thumb and ablation of lesser thumb:
  ○ Retain ulnar thumb if equal to preserve ulnar collateral ligament.
  ○ May require phalangeal osteotomy for alignment, tendon centralization, and transfer of thenar intrinsics with osteoperiosteal sleeve.
- Types V and VI – similar principles:
  ○ Added complexity of intrinsic reconstruction
  ○ Z-plasty of wcb space
- Type VII – similar principles:
  ○ Extra joint may be treated with chondrodesis at a joint with least motion.
  ○ "Spare parts" surgery if elements needed from each thumb.
- Postaxial – Type A: operative resection with transfer of ulnar collateral ligament and abductor digiti quinti to the adjacent finger.
- Central:
  - Fully formed, limited motion – ray resection
  - Synpolydactyly – difficult to teat:
    ○ Separation and reduction of polydactyly, may need osteotomy for alignment

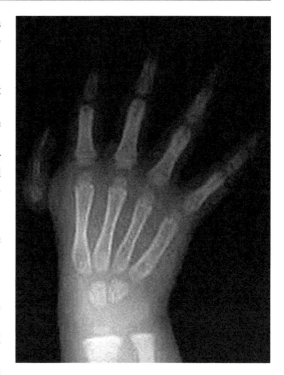

Fig. 129.4 Thumb hypoplasia

Thumb Hypoplasia (Fig. 129.4)

Overview

- Congenital underdevelopment of the thumb ranging in severity from a slightly smaller thumb to complete thumb absence.
- Considered a part of the spectrum of radial longitudinal deficiency (see below) – other organ systems may be affected.
- Workup should include musculoskeletal examination, renal ultrasound, cardiac examination with echocardiogram, spine radiographs, and complete blood count.
- Can be seen in isolation or in conjunction with radial longitudinal deficiency and may be bilateral.

Classification: Modified Blauth (Describes Severity of the Hypoplasia and Guides Treatment)

- I – minor hypoplasia, stable thumb, good function, and often unnoticed until child is older (no treatment needed)
- II – narrow first web space, ulnar collateral ligament insufficiency, and thenar muscle hypoplasia (treatment options: first web space deepening/release, UCL reconstruction, tendon transfer for thumb opposition)
- III – similar findings as II above plus extrinsic tendon and muscle abnormalities (extensor pollicis longus, flexor pollicis longus) and bone deficiency (further subdivided):
  - IIIA – stable carpometacarpal joint (treatment option includes reconstruction options seen above for type II)
  - IIIB – unstable carpometacarpal joint (reconstruction of the existing thumb is not recommended; pollicization of the index finger is considered (i.e. moving the index finger with tendons, nerves, and

blood vessels into the position of the thumb))
- IV – floating thumb (pouce flottant) (excise floating thumb; consider pollicization based on family preferences)
- V – absent thumb (surgical treatment option is pollicization) (Soldado F et al.)

Radial Club Hand (a.k.a. Radial Longitudinal Deficiency)

- Underdevelopment or the absence of the radius and radial structures in the forearm, wrist, and hand ranging from mild to severe
- May be seen with shortened forearm which can be severe and/or lack of active elbow flexion (Fig. 129.5)

Classification: Bayne and Klug

- Type 1 – short distal radius with present epiphysis and slight radial deviation of the hand, often associated with thumb hypoplasia
- Type 2 – hypoplastic radius with more significant radial deviation at the wrist
- Type 3 – partial absence of the radius, most frequently proximal radius absent, the hand radially deviated, and the wrist unsupported
- Type 4 – complete absence of the radius (James et al.)

Associated Anomalies

- Thrombocytopenia-absent radius (TAR)   low platelet count.
- Vertebral, anal, cardiac, tracheoesophageal, renal, and limb abnormalities (VACTERL) association.
- Holt-Oram syndrome – cardiac problems including ventriculoseptal defects (VSD) or conduction problems.
- Fanconi anemia – aplastic anemia.
- Cardiac anomalies – commonly septal defects.
- Spinal or lower extremity musculoskeletal anomalies.
- Workup should include musculoskeletal examination, cardiac examination with echocardiogram, complete blood count, renal ultrasound, and spine radiographs (Goldfarb et al.).

Treatment

- Early nonsurgical treatment – stretching and splinting in the infant is recommended to stretch the tightened radial structures and is often guided by occupational therapists.
- Surgical treatment:
  - Surgery can provide improvement in appearance and function, but good function is also seen in patients who do not have surgical management.
  - Surgical options – the presence of active elbow flexion is thought to be a prerequisite

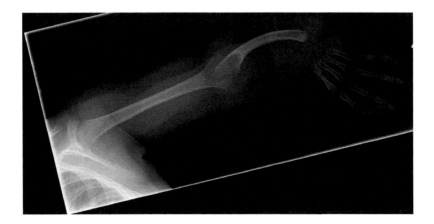

Fig. 129.5 Radial club hand

for surgical treatments on the forearm/wrist:

- ○ Ulnocarpal arthrodesis (fusion)
- ○ Soft tissue procedures to first stretch the tight radial tissue through external distraction followed by tendon transfer to rebalance the wrist: – Recurrence of radial deviation can be seen postoperatively.
- ○ Ulnar lengthening for the foreshortened forearm
- ○ Radial lengthening in less severe cases (Abzug et al.) (Hung et al.)

Madelung Deformity

- Deformity of the wrist usually seen in patents aged 8 to 14 years
- More commonly seen in females
- Can be associated with Leri-Weill dyschondrosteosis – a mesomelic dwarfism

Clinical Presentation

- Gross deformity of the wrist is often seen with the prominence of the relatively long ulna at the wrist.
- In the presence of associated short stature, Leri-Weill dyschondrosteosis should be suspected.
- Changes in range of motion and pain can be seen in addition to the clinical deformity.

Etiology

- Typically associated with the presence of a Vickers ligament which is a shortened abnormal volar radioulnar ligament originating from the metaphysis rather than from the normal epiphysis.
- This ligament creates a tether to normal growth across the volar ulnar portion of the distal radius.
- With growth, the resulting increase in volar tilt and radial inclination is seen in the distal radius.

Treatment

- Depends on age and severity of the deformity at presentation.
- Guided growth allows younger patients with less severe deformities to correct with growth:
  - Release of Vickers ligament – untethering of the volar ulnar portion of the distal radius
  - +/− stapling of part of the physis to restrict growth in the unaffected portions of the distal radius to allow deformity to correct and prevent worsening
- For more skeletally mature patients with more severe deformity, the patient's symptoms must be taken into account – if symptomatic, then surgery can be considered:
  - Surgical dome-shaped corrective osteotomy of the radius can be considered to correct bony deformities.
  - Ulnar shortening osteotomy can be done in patients with severely relatively long ulnas (ulnar positive variance) and ulnar-sided wrist pain (Kozin et al.).

Further Reading

1. Abzug JM, Kozin SH. Radial longitudinal deficiency. J Hand Surg. 2014;39:1180–2.
2. Baek G, et al. Classification and surgical treatment of symphalangism in interphalangeal joints of the hand. Clin Orthop Surg. 2012;4(1):58–65.
3. Bates S, et al. Reconstruction of congenital differences of the hand. Plast Reconstr Surg. 2009;124 (Suppl):128e.
4. Bauer A, Bae D. Pediatric trigger digits. J Hand Surg Am. 2015;40(11):2304–9;Goldfard C. Congenital hand anomalies: a review of the literature, 2009–2012. J Hand Surg. 2013;38A:1854–9.
5. Goldfarb CA, Wall L, Manske PR. Radial longitudinal deficiency: the incidence of associated medical and musculoskeletal conditions. J Hand Surg. 2006;31A:1176–82.
6. Green's Operative Hand Surgery-6th ed. Edited by: Wolfe, Hotchkiss, Pederson, Kozin. Elsevier, Philadelphia PA. Chapters 39–43.

7. Hung LK, et al. Congenital hand anomalies: principles of management. J Hand Surg. 2002;2:204–24.

8. Hutchinson D, Sullivan R. Rubinstein-Taybi syndrome. J Hand Surg. 2014;40:1711–2.

9. James MA, McCarroll R, Manske PR. The spectrum of radial longitudinal deficiency: a modified classification. J Hand Surg. 1999;24A:1145–55.

10. Kozin SH, Zlotolow DA. Madelung deformity. J Hand Surg. 2015;40:2090–8.

11. Soldado F, Zlotolow DA, Kozin SH. Thumb hypoplasia. J Hand Surg. 2013;38A:1435–44.

Genu Varum

Michael R. Ferrick

Definition

- Bowlegs. Apex of the angle between the femur and tibia at the knee points away from midline of the body.

Etiology

Physiologic: Most Common Form Seen in Young Childhood

- Normal "variant" of growth
- Resolves spontaneously with growth
- No treatment needed, just parental reassurance

Blount's Disease: Unique Growth Disturbance Medial Aspect Proximal Tibia

- Early onset (infantile)
  - Obese, early walker
  - Lateral thrust of knee during stance phase of gait cycle

M.R. Ferrick, MD
Department of Orthopaedic Surgery, SUNY Buffalo,
Women and Children's Hospital of Buffalo,
Amherst, NY, USA
e-mail: mferrick@buffalo.edu

- Significant distortion/deformation of proximal tibial epiphysis, physis, and metaphysis
  - Langenskiold's classification correlates with both maturity and severity of process
  - Later/most severe stage bone bar across medial physis causing further increase in varus
- Late onset (adolescent)
  - Obese
  - Often have limb length discrepancy in unilateral cases
  - Less distortion of joint/epiphysis than that seen in persistent infantile form
  - Treatment surgical
    - Hemiepiphysiodesis
    - Osteotomy

a. Skeletal Dysplasias (Such as Achondroplasia or Metaphyseal Chondrodysplasia)
b. Metabolic bone disease (e.g., rickets or renal disease)
c. Trauma
  i. Fracture causes acute deformity
  ii. Injury causes partial growth disturbance at physis (growth plate)
d. Focal fibrocartilaginous dysplasia
  i. Unique defect of proximal tibial metaphysis consisting of fibrocartilaginous tissue, results in varus deformity of the tibia

A.E.M. Eltorai et al. (eds.), *Orthopedic Surgery Clerkship*, DOI 10.1007/978-3-319-52567-9_130

Significance of Genu Varum

- Malalignment predisposes joint to degenerative osteoarthritis
  - Varus causes increased pressure in medial aspect of joint leading to increased wear and degeneration of medial compartment of knee
- Pain/joint dysfunction from uneven joint loading/abnormal mechanics
- Cosmetic – less of an issue than (a) or (b)

Evaluation

Clinical Examination

- Gait pattern
  - Lateral thrust of knee indicates lateral ligament incompetence
  - Antalgic limp indicates pain
- Standing alignment
  - Measure distance between knees with ankles together
  - Goniometer to measure varus angle between femur and tibia
- Supine non weight bearing alignment

Radiologic Imaging

- Standing hips to ankles x-ray
  - Mechanical axis of lower extremity (Fig. 130.1)
    ◦ Line from center of femoral head to center of knee (*not* down shaft of the femur)
    ◦ Line from the center of the knee to the center of the ankle
    ◦ Mechanical axis of lower extremity is an angle between those two lines – should be 0 or 180° (straight line)
  - MAD (mechanical axis deviation) (Fig. 130.2)
    ◦ Line straight from center femoral head to center ankle
    ◦ MAD is the distance from that line to the center of the knee – should be 0 mm

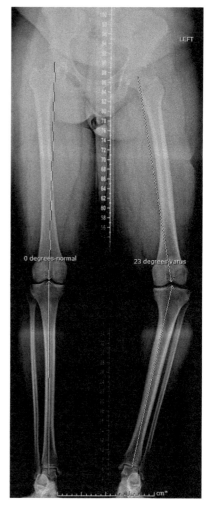

Fig. 130.1 Mechanical axis of the leg. Right normal 0°, left varus 23°

  - Drennan's metaphyseal-diaphyseal angle (MDA). Used for infant, predictive of whether benign physiologic varus or pathologic early-onset Blount's disease (Fig. 130.3)
    ◦ <11° almost always physiologic and varus resolves
    ◦ >11° increased chance of pathologic Blount's disease
- Dedicated hip, knee, or ankle x-rays depending on location of any symptoms
- MRI in rare situations to evaluate knee meniscus, hip labrum, cartilage, and ligamentous tissues

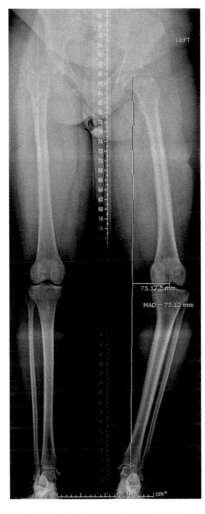

Fig. 130.2 Mechanical axis deviation (*MAD*)

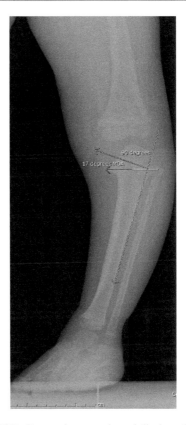

Fig. 130.3 Drennan's metaphyseal-diaphyseal angle (*MDA*)

Treatment

- Observation – especially in under 2 years old, typically with physiologic varus which will resolve on own
- Correction of any metabolic bone disease (rare in the USA) with medical treatment
- Bracing – used in early onset/infantile Blount's less than age 4
  - Daytime upright knee-ankle-foot orthosis (KAFO) with hinged knee and wide band directing the knee away from varus
  - Nighttime supine A frame brace that pulls the knees toward a bar between the legs – correcting varus
- Hemiepiphyseodesis

  - Surgical manipulation of one side of growth plate
    - Placement of two-hole plate straddling growth plate which serves as a hinge/tether on the one side of growth plate.
    - Older techniques involve directly scraping out or ablating growth plate or placement of a staple straddling growth plate on one side.
- Osteotomy – cutting bone and correcting malalignment
  - Varus corrected acutely at time of surgery and fixed with pins, plate/screws, or external fixation, slight overcorrection desirable
  - Varus corrected gradually with external fixation device which is adjusted in small increments multiple times daily to allow gradual new bone tissue formation and healing

Suggested Reading

1. Herring JA, et al. Disorders of the leg. In: Herring JA, editor. Tachdjian's pediatric orthopedics. Philadelphia: Saunders Elsevier; 2008. p. 973–96.
2. Brooks WC, Gross RH. Genu varum in children: diagnosis and treatment. J Am Acad Orthop Surg. 1995;3(6):326–35.
3. Birch JG. Blount disease. J Am Acad Orthop Surg. 2013;21(7):408–18.
4. Saran N, Rathjen KE. Guided growth for the correction of pediatric lower limb angular deformity. J Am Acad Orthop Surg. 2010;18(9):528–36.

Genu Valgum

131

Paul Esposito

Normal Growth and Development

- Bow legs or genu varum is present in most children at birth.
- Bow legs are most noticeable at 6 months of age and then decrease to approximately neutral at about 18 months of age:
  - There is some racial and familial variation, and bow legs can persist beyond 18 months of age and still be normal. Increasing or worsening bowing is never normal and requires further evaluation including standing X-rays to exclude metabolic, congenital, or developmental bone problems:
    - ○ Clinically measure the distance between the femoral condyles with the ankles opposed (intercondylar distance).
- Genu valgum typically starts developing at about age 18 months and reaches its maximum by 4 years and gradually decreases by 11 years of age:
  - Clinically measure the distance between the ankles with the knees opposed (intermalleolar distance).
- Normal development is typically symmetrical genu valgum.

P. Esposito
Department of Orthopaedic Surgery, University of Nebraska Medical Center, Children's Hospital and Medical Center, Omaha, NE, USA
e-mail: pesposito@childrensomaha.org

- Internal rotation from increased femoral anteversion can exaggerate the appearance of normal genu valgum.
- Pes planus, typical up to age 5, can also exaggerate apparent clinical genu valgum. Conversely, excessive genu valgum can cause apparent pes planus (flatfeet).

Indications for Further Evaluation in Young Children

- Progressive asymmetrical angular deformity.
- The child falling off the growth charts in terms of height and/or weight with increasing angular deformity.
- Child with obvious metabolic disease with increasing deformity.
- Associated abnormalities with progressive deformity such as multiple hereditary exostosis or syndromes such as nail-patella.
- Painful progressive deformity.
- Patellar subluxation or maltracking.
- Be sure to look at the whole child! Problems frequently don't arise in isolation.

X-Ray Evaluation

- The standard is a full-length standing AP from the hips to the ankles on the same cassette.
- The mechanical and anatomic axis should be measured (Fig. 131.1).

© Springer International Publishing AG 2017
A.E.M. Eltorai et al. (eds.), *Orthopedic Surgery Clerkship*, DOI 10.1007/978-3-319-52567-9_131

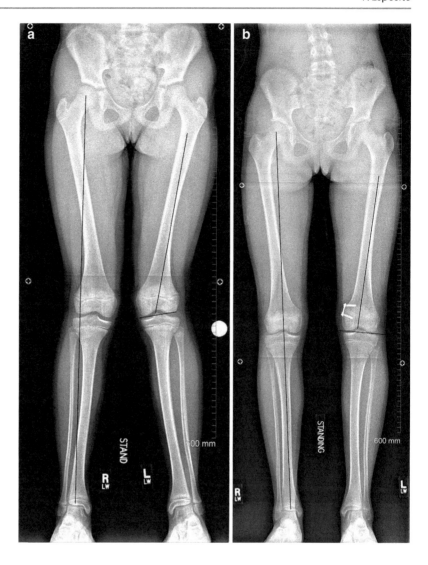

Fig. 131.1 (**a**) (19°) An 11-year- and 4-month-old with well-controlled vitamin D resistant rickets. Mechanical axis is measured on the right and should be through the center of the knee. Distal femoral angle should be less than a few degrees of negative valgus. (**b**) (3°) Same child at age 13 + 5. The eight plate has been removed on the right when she achieved correction. Because the deformity was more severe on the left, it took longer for the hemiepiphysiodesis to correct, and thus, the plate was left in longer/mechanical axis, and distal femoral angle is now corrected on both sides

Metabolic Bone Disease

- May be manifested by decreasing growth, pain, or signs of systemic illness.
- Genetic rickets or vitamin D deficiency is frequently apparent on the plain radiograph.
- Congenital causes of metabolic bone disease frequently lead to progressive varus, while acquired diseases such as renal insufficiency with the onset occurring after age 18 months will lead to progressive valgus.
- Laboratory studies including BUN and creatinine as well as calcium, phosphorus, alkaline phosphatase, and vitamin D may be indicated.
- Treatment of the underlying disease is paramount and orthopedic treatment is typically supportive, and any surgery is withheld until the primary disease is controlled. Medical treatment can lead to at least partial resolution of deformity with growth. Well inadequate treatment may cause recurrent deformity following corrective surgery.
- Orthopedic treatment addresses any deformity which does not resolve with primary treatment of the disorder.

Trauma

- Proximal tibial metaphyseal fracture known as the Cozen fracture can lead to asymmetrical progressive valgus for up to 18 months post-injury in young children even with perfect fracture reduction and casting:
  - Initial treatment is correction of any valgus and education of the parents of the risk of progressive valgus.
  - Deformity may gradually diminish over many years.
  - Growth modulation known as hemiepiphysiodesis can be used for patients not improving over time (Fig. 131.1a, b).

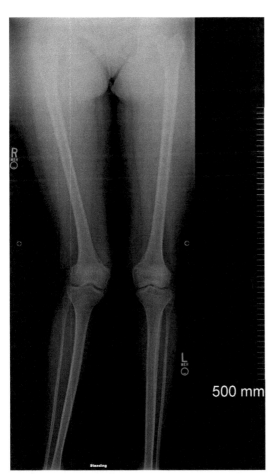

500 mm

Fig. 131.2 Several years post-fracture distal femur in Africa. Presumed to have asymmetrical growth arrest. Skeletally mature individuals require osteotomies to correct deformity and may also require lengthening

- Malunion of fractures, typically distal femurs, may require correction and may also require surgical procedures to equalize leg length (Fig. 131.2).

Genu Valgum Secondary to Bone Lesions

- The most common lesion is osteochondromatosis (multiple hereditary exostoses).
- Fibrous lesions can also lead to genu valgum either primarily or secondary to pathologic fracture.

Obesity

- Can cause progressive genu valgum in children and adolescents.
- This can lead to lateral overload with lateral compartment osteochondritis dissecans (Fig. 131.3a, b):
  - Younger children can be treated with hemiepiphysiodesis, but mature individuals may require osteotomy.
- Beware of associated disorders such as diabetes, contralateral Blount disease, and slipped capital femoral epiphysis.

Adolescent Genu Valgum

- More commonly otherwise normal tall thin children growing rapidly
- Can be seen in connective tissue disorders such as osteogenesis imperfecta or Marfan syndrome

Treatment Options

- In children with significant remaining growth, hemiepiphysiodesis is the most benign effective treatment:
  - Guided growth ("eight plates"), staples, and percutaneous screws most commonly used now for hemiepiphysiodesis rather than permanent, destructive hemiepiphysiodesis.

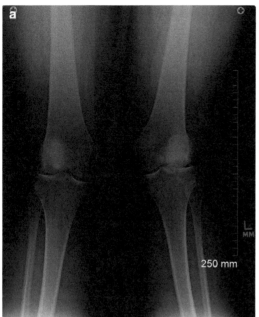

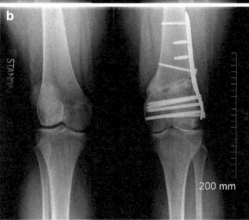

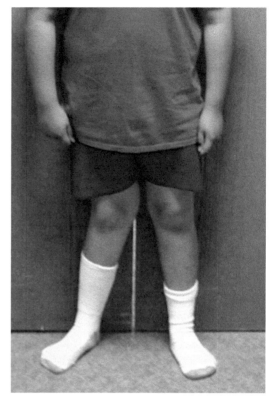

Fig. 131.4 Posttraumatic distal femoral valgus. Note that this causes significant stress on the medial ankle and foot

than hemiepiphysiodesis so early diagnosis and treatment are vital (Fig. 131.4).

Fig. 131.3 (**a**) A 16-year-old female with severe obesity and secondary genu valgum. Note on the left-side osteochondritis dissecans of the lateral femoral condyle and bilateral osteophytes. Failure to correct this severe deformity may well lead to degenerative arthritis. (**b**) Three months post-osteotomy to correct distal femoral deformity. Osteochondritis dissecans healing

- – Plates or staples are left in place until the mechanical axis is slightly overcorrected as there can be some "rebound" back to valgus if they have remaining growth.
- Osteotomies are necessary if the patient is skeletally mature:
  - – This is a much more substantial procedure, with a much higher risk of complications

Suggested Reading

1. Davids JR, Fisher R, Lum G, Von Glinski S. Angular deformity of the lower extremity in children with renal osteodystrophy. J Pediatr Orthop. 1992;12(3):291–9.
2. Heath CH, Staheli LT. Normal limits of knee angle in white children--genu varum and genu valgum. J Pediatr Orthop. 1993;13(2):259–62.
3. Hennrikus W, Pylawka T. Patellofemoral instability in skeletally immature athletes. J Bone Joint Surg Am. 2013;95(2):176–83.
4. Jackson DW, Cozen L. Genu valgum as a complication of proximal tibial metaphyseal fractures in children. J Bone Joint Surg Am. 1971;53(8):1571–8.
5. Kang S, Kim JY, Park SS. Outcomes of hemiepiphyseal stapling for genu valgum deformities in patients with multiple hereditary exostoses: a comparative study of patients with deformities of idiopathic cause. J Pediatr Orthop. 2015.

6. McCarthy JJ, Kim DH, Eilert RE. Posttraumatic genu valgum: operative versus nonoperative treatment. J Pediatr Orthop. 1998;18(4):518–21.

7. Sabharwal S, Zhao C. The hip-knee-ankle angle in children: reference values based on a full-length standing radiograph. J Bone Joint Surg Am. 2009;91(10):2461–8.

8. Stevens PM. Guided growth for angular correction: a preliminary series using a tension band plate. J Pediatr Orthop. 2007;27(3):253–9.

9. Tuten HR, Keeler KA, Gabos PG, Zionts LE, MacKenzie WG. Posttraumatic tibia valga in children. A long-term follow-up note. J Bone Joint Surg Am. 1999;81(6):799–810.

10. Voloc A, Esterle L, Nguyen TM, Walrant-Debray O, Colofitchi A, Jehan F, et al. High prevalence of genu varum/valgum in European children with low vitamin D status and insufficient dairy products/calcium intakes. Eur J Endocrinol. 2010;163(5):811–7.

Lower Extremity Rotational Deformities

132

Dominic J. Gargiulo

Internal Tibial Torsion (ITT)

I. Presentation
   A. Intoeing
      (i) Usually noticed once child reaches walking age.
      (ii) Child may trip over own feet.
II. Physical Exam
   A. Assess in prone position (Fig. 132.1)
      (i) Thigh-foot angle
         1. Angle formed between lines bisecting the foot and thigh.
         2. Normal is from 0 to −10° during childhood and 15° at maturity.
         3. > −15 may be abnormal.
      (ii) Transmalleolar angle (Fig. 132.2)
         1. Removes foot pathology (metatarsus adductus/clubfoot) from exam
III. Treatment
   A. Observation
      (i) Most children externally rotate to physiologic angle by age 6 years.
      (ii) Bracing and orthotics are not indicated.
   B. Operative intervention
      (iii) Derotation tibial osteotomy.

D.J. Gargiulo, DO
Pediatric Orthopedics, Children's Hospital New Orleans, New Orleans, LA, USA
e-mail: dgargi@lsuhsc.edu

   (iv) > Age 8 years with internal tibial torsion >20° should only be done for significant functional limitation.

External Tibial Torsion (ETT)

I. Presentation
   A. Outtoeing.
   B. May be associated with decreased physical performance.
   C. Associated with early degenerative disease, knee pain, osteochondral defects, and patellar instability.
   D. Natural history is for the lower extremity to continue to externally rotate, worsening the problem as the child matures.

II. Physical Exam
   A. Assess in prone position
      (i) Thigh-foot angle
         1. Angle formed between lines bisecting the foot and thigh.
         2. Normal is from 0 to −10° during childhood.
         3. Average at 8 years of age is 10° external (−5–30 is normal range).
      (ii) Transmalleolar angle
         1. Removes foot pathology (metatarsus adductus/clubfoot/pes valgus) from exam

© Springer International Publishing AG 2017
A.E.M. Eltorai et al. (eds.), *Orthopedic Surgery Clerkship*, DOI 10.1007/978-3-319-52567-9_132

Fig. 132.1 Thigh-foot angle

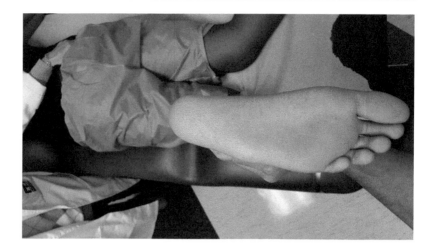

Fig. 132.2 Trans-malleolar angle

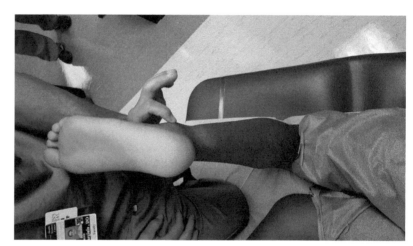

III. Treatment
  A. Observation
    (i) Natural history is for the lower limb to externally rotate so usually worsens as child grows.
  B. Tibial Derotational Osteotomy
    (ii) Indicated in children >8 years old with angle >30–40 external

Femoral Anteversion (Internal Femoral Torsion)

I. Presentation
  A. Intoeing.
  B. Kissing kneecaps.
  C. "W" sit (Fig. 132.3).

D. More common in females.
E. Packaging disorder/intrauterine positioning.
  (i) May be associated with metatarsus adductus
  (ii) Congenital muscular torticollis
  (iii) Developmental dysplasia of the hip
F. Average anteversion at birth is 30–40° and decreases to 10–15° at maturity.

II. Physical Exam
  A. Test in hip motion in *prone* position with knees flexed to 90°
    (i) Feet fall to table with increased internal rotation of hip >70° (normal is 20–60°)
    (ii) Trochanteric prominence test (Fig. 132.4)

Fig. 132.3 "W" sit

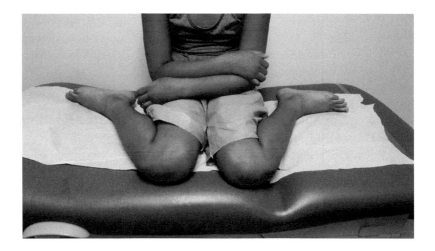

Fig. 132.4 Greater
troch prominence test

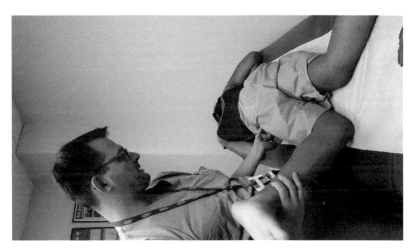

1. Estimate anteversion by palpating when greater troch is most prominent while internally rotating hip.

III. Imaging

A. X-rays usually not helpful.

B. CT or MRI scan may be helpful to assess femoral anteversion.

IV. Treatment

A. Most cases resolve by 10 years of age.

B. Bracing not indicated.

C. Femoral derotational osteotomy (rare).

(i) Indicated in severe cases <10° of external hip rotation

Femoral Retroversion (External Femoral Torsion)

I. Presentation

A. Outtoeing.

B. Kneecaps rotate externally.

C. Patient may prefer to sit cross-legged.

D. May increase risk of slipped capital femoral epiphysis.

II. Physical Exam

A. Test in hip motion in *prone* position with knees flexed to 90°

(i) Feet cross easily with increased external rotation of the hip <20° (normal is 20–60°).

    (ii) Trochanteric   prominence   test (Fig. 132.4).

       1. Estimate retroversion by palpating when greater troch is most prominent while internally rotating hip.

III. Imaging

   A. X-rays usually not helpful.

   B. CT or MRI scan may be helpful to assess femoral version.

IV. Treatment

   A. Most cases will progress until 10 years of age and may be associated with hip/knee pain and early degenerative changes.

   B. Bracing not indicated.

   C. Femoral derotational osteotomy.

    (iii) Indicated in severe cases

Suggested Readings

1. Staheli L. Practice of pediatric orthopedics. 2nd ed. Philadelphia: Lipincott Williams & Wilkins; 2006. p. 77–103.
2. Tolo S. Master techniques in orthopedic surgery; pediatrics. Philadelphia: Lipincott Williams & Wilkins; 2008. p. 110–9.

Limb Deficiency

133

Alexander J. Kish, Ettore Vulcano, Matthew A. Varacallo,
Tonya W. An, and Amiethab A. Aiyer

Epidemiology [1–3]

- Estimated incidence at 3–8:10,000 in the USA varies throughout the world.
- Precise causes of deficiencies mostly unknown but speculated as environmental factors, hypoperfusion/embolic events, or genetic factors.
- Thalidomide is only pharmaceutical proven to be directly related to limb deficiency although others are suspected.
- Gene mutations can be syndromic or a point mutation. Examples are Turner's syndrome, autosomal dominant longitudinal tibial deficiency, or thrombocytopenia with absent radius (TAR mutation).
- Acquired deficiencies represent around one-third of all pediatric limb deficiencies and are comprised of both traumatic amputations and systemic diseases such as malignancy.

Embryology [4, 5]

- Upper and lower limb buds begin to develop during the third week of gestation in a proximal to distal fashion with the upper limb bud becoming visible around 24 days of gestation and the lower limb bud becoming visible at 28 days of gestation.
- Three signaling centers control limb development: the apical ectodermal ridge, the zone of polarizing activity, and the Wingless-type (Wnt) signaling center and mutations or insults to these centers are proposed as causing limb anomalies.
- It is important to realize that limb development coincides with organ development and patients with deficient limbs should be evaluated for organ damage as well.

Classification

- Generally, congenital limb deficiencies fit into one of seven categories as defined by the International Federation of Societies for Surgery of the Hand:

The original version of this chapter was revised.
An erratum to this chapter can be found at
https://doi.org/10.1007/978-3-319-52567-9_159

A.J. Kish, MD (✉)
Department of Orthopaedic Surgery, University of
Maryland Medical Center, Baltimore, MD, USA
e-mail: alexanderjkish@gmail.com

E. Vulcano, MD
Orthopedics, Mount Sinai Health System,
New York, NY, USA

M.A. Varacallo, MD
Department of Orthopaedic Surgery,
Hahnemann University Hospital,
245 N. 15th Street, M.S. 420, Philadelphia, PA, USA

T.W. An
Orthopedics Cedars-Sinai Medical Center,
Los Angeles, CA, USA

A.A. Aiyer
Department of Orthopaedic Surgery,
University of Miami, Miami, FL, USA

© Springer International Publishing AG 2017
A.E.M. Eltorai et al. (eds.), *Orthopedic Surgery Clerkship*, DOI 10.1007/978-3-319-52567-9_133

- Failure of formation
- Failure of differentiation
- Duplication
- Overgrowth
- Undergrowth
  ○ Congenital constriction band syndrome
  ○ Generalized skeletal abnormality

Lower Extremity Conditions

Tibial Deficiency [6]

- Longitudinal deficiency with varying degrees of tibial remnant acquired in an autosomal dominant inheritance pattern.
- Often has knee contractures and a rigid foot in equinovarus.
- Surgical management consists of knee disarticulation if no tibia present, a Syme/Boyd amputation or Browne procedure.
- Tibial hemimelia only inherited limb deficiency.

Fibular Deficiency [7]

- Commonly associated with anteromedial bowing, associated with other orthopedic limb deficiencies (lesser ray deficiencies, tarsal coalition).
- Most common congenital long bone deficiency.
- Treatment goals are to restore foot and ankle function, and options include epiphysiodesis and limb-lengthening procedures.

Proximal Femoral Focal Deficiency [8, 9]

- Spectrum of deficiencies including absent hip joint, absent femur, short femur, or femoral neck pseudoarthrosis.
- Fifty percent are associated with other orthopedic conditions.
- Wide spectrum of nonsurgical and surgical options that rely heavily on prosthesis to preserve ambulation.

Upper Extremity Conditions

Radial Deficiencies [5]

- Longitudinal deficiency of the radius (radial clubhand) is related to a mutation in the sonic hedgehog gene.
- Usually associated with the absence of the thumb and is bilateral in 50–75% of cases.
- Highly associated with systemic conditions like TAR, Holt-Oram syndrome, Fanconi's anemia, VACTERL and VATER syndrome.
- Conservative management includes stretching of tightened radial sided structures, while operative management consists of hand centralization before 18 months of age.

Ulnar Deficiencies

- Less common than radial deficiencies.
- Not associated with systemic conditions, but often radial sided abnormalities are present as well as other orthopedic deficiencies, confounding the diagnosis.
- Characterized by unstable elbow joint.
- Surgical treatments vary, but the goal is to stabilize elbow joint while preserving thumb function. Options include radial head resection to create a one-bone forearm, syndactyly release, and digital rotation osteotomies.

Central Deficiencies [5]

- The index, middle, and long fingers develop at different intervals from the thumb and little finger.
- Cleft hand is categorized as typical or atypical. Typical cleft hand results from fusion of digital rays while atypical cleft hand results from necrosis of mesenchymal tissue during development.
- The usual presentation is the absence of phalanges with preserved metacarpals for typical cleft hand and results in a V-shaped deformity due to fusion of the bones. Atypical cleft hand is missing the phalanges but usually has preservation of the metacarpals without fusion so the deformity is shaped in a U fashion.

Syndactyly [5]

- Abnormal interconnection between digits
- More common than other upper extremity deformities and tends to run in families.
- Complicated syndactyly is associated with systemic conditions like Apert syndrome, the abnormally early fusion of skull bones, or Poland syndrome, the underdevelopment or absence of chest musculature with webbing of the fingers.

References

1. McGurik C, Westgate M, Holmes L. Limb deficiencies in newborn infants. Pediatrics. 2001;108(4):E64.
2. Kallen B, Rahmani TM-Z, Winberg J. Infants with congenital limb reduction registered in the swedish register of congenital malformations. Teratology. 1984;29:73–85.
3. McCarroll HR. Congenital anomalies: a 25-year overview. J Hand Surg [Am]. 2000;25:1007–37.
4. Wolpert L. Vertebrate limb development and malformations. Pediatr Res. 1999;46:247–54.
5. Kozin S. Upper-extremity congenital anomalies. J Bone Joint Surg Am. 2003;85:1564–76.
6. Kalamchi A, Dawe RV. Congenital deficiency of the tibia. J Bone Joint Surg Br. 1985;67(4):581–4.
7. Oberc A, Sulko J. Fibular hemimelia - diagnostic management, principles, and results of treatment. J Pediatr Orthop B. 2013;22(5):450–6.
8. Manner H, Radler C, Ganger R, Grill F. Dysplasia of the cruciate ligaments: radiographic assessment and classification. J Bone Joint Surg Am. 2006;1988(1):130–7.
9. Westberry D, Davids J. Proximal focal femoral deficiency (PFFD): management options and controversies. Hip Int. 2009;19(Suppl 6):S18–25.

Limb Length Discrepancy (LLD)

134

Dominic J. Gargiulo

Presentation

- Usually asymptomatic
- Clinical assessment of LLD
  - Measure from anterior superior iliac spine to medial malleolus (Fig. 134.1).
  - Block testing: place block under short leg until pelvis level.
  - Examine for flexion contractures of the ankle/knee/hip which can distort measurements (common in cerebral palsy).

Causes

Congenital Disorders

- Hemihypertrophy
- Skeletal dysplasia
- Proximal femoral focal deficiency
- Developmental dysplasia of the hip

Physeal Disruption

- Infection
- Trauma
- Tumor

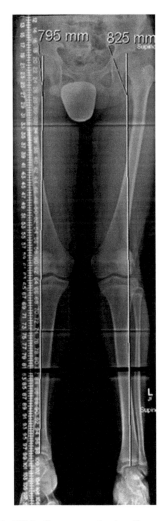

Fig. 134.1 Clinically measure leg lengths

D.J. Gargiulo, DO
Orthopedic Department, Louisiana State University
School of Medicine, New Orleans, LA, USA
e-mail: dgargi@lsuhsc.edu

Normal Physiology

- 2 cm LLD occurs in up to 2/3 of the general population.

Classification

Static LLD

- Secondary to malunion of a fracture (tibia or femur)

Progressive LLD

- Secondary to physeal arrest (e.g., trauma, infection, tumor)
- Congenital
  - Absolute discrepancy increases proportionally.

Imaging

Scanogram

- Measure the left and right femur and tibia; document differences in each bone.

CT Scan

- Useful in children with flexion contractures

Left Hand for Bone Age

- Determine difference between skeletal age and chronologic age.

Estimation of LLD at Skeletal Maturity

- Generally assumed that males grow until age 16 and females until 14 (bone age by hand X-ray)

Estimation

- Proximal femur 3 mm/year
- Distal femur 9 mm/year
- Proximal tibia 6 mm/year
- Distal tibia 5 mm/year

Multiplier Method

- Prediction based on multiplying current LLD by a factor specific for age and sex
- Most accurate with congenital LLD

Treatment

Nonoperative

- Shoe lift <2 cm LLD at maturity

Operative

- Shorten longer leg via epiphysiodesis
  - 2–5 cm projected LLD
  - Time with bone age and estimated growth (mm/year) remaining
- Limb lengthening of short side via osteotomy and Taylor Spatial Frame
  - >5 cm projected LLD.
  - Lengthening can be combined with shortening of other side.
- Physeal bar excision
  - Bar usually due to disruption of physis, e.g., trauma or infection
  - Can perform if bar is <50% of physis, 2 years of predicted growth remaining

References

1. Staheli, Lynn. Practice of pediatric orthopedics 2nd. Philadelphia: Lipincott Williams & Wilkins, 2006:96-100
2. Tolo S. Master techniques in orthopedic surgery; pediatrics. Philadelphia: Lipincott Williams & Wilkins; 2008. p. 303–11.

Pseudarthrosis of the Tibia

135

Maegen Wallace

Pseudarthrosis of the Tibia

- Rare pediatric diagnosis
  - Challenging to manage
    - Often difficult to achieve union
    - Also difficult to maintain union and keep the patient functional

Etiology

Several Theories Proposed [1]

- Intrauterine trauma
- Birth fracture
- Generalized metabolic disease
- Vascular malformation

Anatomy

- Anterolateral bowing of the tibia [1]
  - 6% of patients with neurofibromatosis (NF) type I develop tibial deformity.
  - 55% of cases of anterolateral bowing and pseudarthrosis are associated with NF.

M. Wallace, MD
Department of Orthopaedic Surgery, University of
Nebraska Medical Center/Omaha Children's
Hospital, 8200 Dodge Street, Omaha,
NE 68114-4113, USA
e-mail: mawallace@childrensomaha.org

Pathology [2]

- Thickened periosteum with cuff fibrous tissue
- Abnormal, cellular fibrovascular tissue [3] with paucity of vascular ingrowth
- Felt to be a disease of the periosteum more than a disease of the local bone itself

Classification

- Descriptive, does not guide management and not predictive of outcomes

Boyd [3]

- Type I: born with anterior bowing and tibial defect
- Type II: born with anterior bowing and hourglass constriction of the tibia. Fracture commonly before age 2, often associated with NF
- Type III: bone cyst at the junction of the proximal 2/3 and lower 1/3 of the tibia resulting in fracture
- Type IV: sclerotic area with near complete obliteration of the medullary canal
- Type V: dysplastic fibula with pseudarthrosis of the fibula and/or tibia
- Type VI: intraosseous neurofibroma

A.E.M. Eltorai et al. (eds.), *Orthopedic Surgery Clerkship*, DOI 10.1007/978-3-319-52567-9_135

Andersen [4]

- Cystic
- Dysplastic
- Clubfoot
- Sclerotic

Crawford [5]

- Type I (Non-dysplastic): anterolateral bowing with increased bone density
- Type II-A (Dysplastic): anterolateral bowing with increased medullary canal width
- Type II-B (Dysplastic): anterolateral bowing with cystic lesion, post fracture
- Type II-C (Dysplastic): anterolateral bowing with fracture, cysts, or frank pseudarthrosis

Clinical Features/Presentation

- Anterolateral bowing of the tibia (Fig. 135.1a, b)
  - May be noted at birth
  - Foot inverted or medially displaced
- Short limb (Fig. 135.1c)
- Fracture

Treatment [1, 6]

Goals

- Obtain union
- Maintain union
- Minimize angular deformity
- Equalize leg lengths

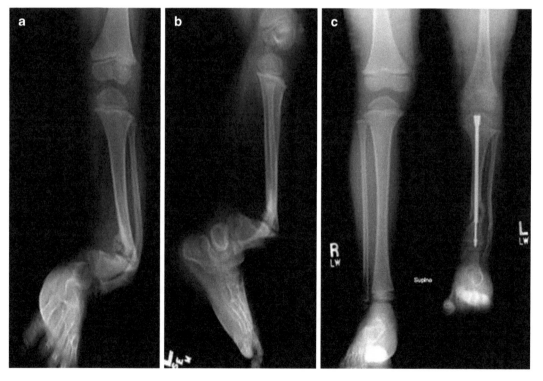

Fig. 135.1 (a) AP X-ray of a 3-year-old child with untreated left tibial pseudarthrosis. Note the lateral bowing. (b) Lateral X-ray of a 3-year-old child with untreated left tibial pseudarthrosis. Note the anterior bowing. (c) X-ray bilateral lower extremities of the same child 1 year after resection of the pseudarthrosis site, iliac crest autografting with telescoping nail insertion. Note the delay in union of the tibia and the significant leg length discrepancy that is present at the age of 4

Brace Once Deformity Identified

- Prevent or delay fracture
- Wear at all times when weight bearing
- Continue until skeletally mature

Principles of Surgical Intervention

- Resect pseudarthrosis; including bone and diseased periosteum.
- Deformity correction.
- Biologic bone/compression at pseudarthrosis site.
- Stable fixation.
- Literature suggests union rate >80% can be obtained with the following surgical approaches.
- Treatment can be each of the following listed below independently or multiple options in the same surgical sitting.

Intramedullary Stabilization

- First-line surgical treatment
- Consider telescoping nails based on patient's age and growth remaining (Fig. 135.1c)
- Consider placement of an IM rod across ankle and subtalar joints, increases stabilization of distal fragment
  - Pay attention to position of the ankle before passing rod so the patient will be able to ambulate with a plantigrade foot.
  - Monitor position of nail as patients grow and consider pushing the nail across the joint before it becomes intra-articular to try and decrease damage to the joint.

Free Vascularized Fibula Graft

- Can utilize contralateral fibula with vascular pedicle or ipsilateral fibula if bone is normal
- Fibula placed into the gap created by resection of the pseudarthrosis
- Fixation of graft with screw, plates, or IM nailing

Circular Frame (Ilizarov) Technique [7]

- Allows compression at the pseudarthrosis site after resection
- Allows gradual correction of angular deformities
- Allows lengthening of the tibia proximally via corticotomy when leg length discrepancy is present
- Union varies from 50 to 90%

Bone Morphogenetic Protein -7

- Supplement at pseudarthrosis site at time of surgery
- Randomized controlled trial [8]
  - 20 patients
  - Half received BMP-7, intramedullary Kirschner wire fixation, and autologous bone grafting
  - Half received intramedullary Kirschner wire fixation and autologous bone grafting
  - No difference in time to union
  - At 5-year follow-up no difference between groups

Amputation

- Discuss this potential early with parents.
- Good option when union not achieved after three procedures.
- Consider when >5 cm leg length discrepancy.
- Deformed foot with poor function.

Complications

- Frequent during treatment of this complex disease process
- Deformity
- Refracture
- Leg length discrepancy
- Poor function

References

1. Vander Have KL, Hensinger RN, Caird M, et al. Congenital pseudarthrosis of the tibia. J Am Acad Orthop Surg. 2008;16:228–36.
2. Ippolito E, Corsi A, Grill F, et al. Pathology of bone lesions associated with congenital pseudarthrosis of the leg. J Pediatr Orthop B. 2000;9:3–10.
3. Boyd HB. Pathology and natural history of congenital pseudarthrosis of the tibia. Clin Orthop Relat Res. 1982;166:5–13.
4. Andersen KS. Radiological classification of congenital pseudarthrosis of the tibia. Acta Orthop Scand. 1973;44:719–27.
5. Crawford AH. Neurofibromatosis in children. Acta Orthop Scand Suppl. 1986;218:1–60.
6. Pannier S. Congenital pseudarthrosis of the tibia. Orthop Traumatol Surg Res. 2011;97:750–61.
7. Grill F, Bollini G, Dungl P, et al. Treatment approaches for congenital pseudarthrosis of tibia: results of the EPOS multicenter study. European paediatric orthopedic society (EPOS). J Pediatr Orthop B. 2000;9:75–89.
8. Das SP, Ganesh S, Pradhan S, et al. Effectiveness of recombinant human bone morphogenetic protein-7 in the management of congenital pseudoarthrosis of the tibia: a randomised controlled trial. Int Orthop. 2014;38:1987–92.

Foot Deformities

James Reagan and Viorel Raducan

Clubfoot (Congenital Talipes Equinovarus)

Epidemiology [1, 3]

- Common congenital anomaly of the foot; about 1 in 1000 live births
- More common in males
- 50% have bilateral involvement
- Likely has genetic cause
- Possible link to PITX1 gene, a transcription factor involved in limb development
- Associated conditions: diastrophic dysplasia, arthrogryposis, prune-belly syndrome, tibial hemimelia, and myelomeningocele [3].

The Deformity (CAVE) [1, 2]

- **C**avus.
- Forefoot **a**dductus and supination.
- Hindfoot **v**arus and **e**quinus.

J. Reagan, MD
Marshall Orthopaedics, 1600 Medical Center Dr. Suite G500, Huntington, WV 25701, USA

V. Raducan, MD (✉)
Marshall University,
1 John Marshall Dr, Huntington, WV 25755, USA
e-mail: raducan@marshall.edu

- The talus is deformed at the neck with medial and plantar deviation; the calcaneus is also internally rotated, and there is medial displacement of the navicular and cuboid bones as well [1, 2].
- Shortened and contracted soft tissues contribute to the deformity.

Clinical Evaluation

- Assess rigidity of deformity
- Examine for possible associated conditions
- Classifications [2]
  - Pirani.
  - Dimeglio.
  - Both are based on physical examination findings and require no imaging.
  - Both allow providers to follow maintenance of correction or recurrence over time.

Radiographic Evaluation [4]

- Radiographs are generally unnecessary in the diagnosis.
- Dorsiflexion lateral radiograph (Turco view) demonstrates small talocalcaneal angle (normal is 25–50°) with flat talar head.
- AP radiograph has a talocalcaneal angle <20° (normal kite angle is 30–55°) and a negative

© Springer International Publishing AG 2017
A.E.M. Eltorai et al. (eds.), *Orthopedic Surgery Clerkship*, DOI 10.1007/978-3-319-52567-9_136

639

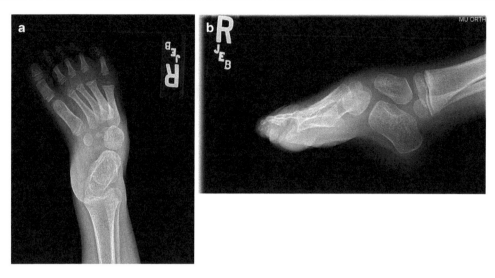

Fig. 136.1 AP and lateral radiographs of a right clubfoot, (**a**) and (**b**), respectively

talus-first metatarsal (MT) angle owing to forefoot adduction.
- Hindfoot parallelism is demonstrated on AP and lateral views (Fig. 136.1a, b).

Treatment

- Nonoperative
  - Initial treatment of choice for most clubfeet
  - Ponseti casting
- General
  - Involves weekly gentle manipulation and serial casting.
  - Successful in over 90% of cases in children 2 years or younger, but optimal start time is as early as possible.
  - Recurrence rates range from 10 to 30%, but most are amenable to repeat casting.
  - The Ponseti method.
- Treatment (5–6 casts) [2]
  - Order of correction is CAVE.
  - Supinate the forefoot and dorsiflex the first MT.
  - Abduct the forefoot around the head of talus.
  - Gradually decrease amount of supination and increase abduction.
  - Final cast is forefoot in neutral, maximally abducted, and dorsiflexed about 15°.

- Percutaneous Achilles tenotomy is typically done before final cast to prevent rocker bottom deformity.
- Can also add an anterior tibialis transfer to regimen if necessary, usually done for residual dynamic supination.
- Maintenance [1, 2]
  - Bracing with a foot abduction orthoses is critical to final success.
  - Denis Browne bars.
  - Worn 23 h/day for 3 months and then while sleeping for 3 years.
  - The most important factor to prevent recurrence is adherence to bracing regimen.
- Operative [1, 3, 4]
  - Generally reserved for rigid or resistant clubfeet.
  - Tendon transfer, Achilles lengthening, or limited posterior release often done for recurrence after casting.
  - Extensile posteromedial and posterolateral soft tissue release with tendon lengthenings at 6–9 months.
  - In older children (3–10 years), bony work such as a medial column lengthening or lateral column shortening osteotomy may be indicated.
  - For those over 10 years old, triple arthrodesis or talectomy may be necessary as salvage procedures.

Complications

- Recurrence
- Rocker bottom deformity
- Persistent supination – treat with anterior tibialis transfer laterally [3]
- Dorsal bunion

Pes Cavus Foot

Introduction

- Key pathology – plantar flexion of the first ray; all other changes are secondary and determined by it [2].
- Elevated longitudinal arch.
- Hindfoot is commonly in varus.
- Two thirds are associated with neurologic disorders to include polio, cerebral palsy, Friedreich ataxia, Charcot-Marie-Tooth disease, and spinal dysraphism [1, 2].
- Neurologic workup is mandatory in these children.

Clinical evaluation

- Symptoms include pain, fatigue, and instability.
- Must assess hindfoot flexibility:
  - Flexible deformities – heel corrects to neutral on Coleman block test.
  - Rigid deformities do not correct on Coleman block test.
- Assess muscular imbalance that may lead to the deformity.
- Detailed neurologic exam is necessary.

Radiographic Evaluation (Fig. 136.2) [2]

- AP and lateral standing radiographs.
- On lateral, Meary angle (talus – first MT angle) is apex dorsal, but in normal state these two are collinear.
- Hibb angle (calcaneus – first MT angle) is normally >150°, but in cavus foot this angle steadily decreases as the deformity worsens.
- MRI and other studies of neuraxis may be warranted to determine etiology.

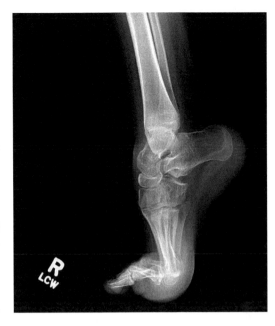

Fig. 136.2 Lateral radiograph demonstrating a cavus foot

Treatment [1, 2]

- Rarely responsive to nonoperative treatment.
- Surgical plan must transfer tendons to balance muscles, osteotomy for fixed deformity.
- Flexible deformities are more amenable to procedures addressing soft tissues:
  - Plantar fascia release to address elevated arch
  - Tendon transfers to address plantar-flexed first ray
- Rigid deformities require bony work:
  - Rigid varus – calcaneal osteotomy
  - Multiple MT extension osteotomies
  - Triple arthrodesis reserved as salvage for rigid deformities in skeletally mature

Congenital Vertical Talus

Introduction [2, 3]

- Navicular is dislocated dorsolaterally on the head of talus.
- Hindfoot equinovalgus and anterior soft tissue contractures.

- Rare condition that is mostly sporadic and bilateral in 50% of cases.
- Associated with a variety of disorders including trisomies, arthrogryposis, myelomeningocele, sacral agenesis, and diastematomyelia [2].
- Investigation of neuraxis with MRI is indicated in these patients.

- Talonavicular joint is irreducible in true vertical talus.
- Oblique talus [2]:
  - Similar condition that reduces and corrects with plantar flexion
  - Amenable to conservative management with casting and arch support

Clinical Evaluation (Fig. 136.3a) [1, 2]

- Limited/absent plantar flexion.
- Rigid convex plantar surface with abducted and dorsiflexed forefoot and hindfoot equinovalgus.
- May have dorsal dislocation of cuboid as well.
- Achilles and anterior foot soft tissue contractures are typically present.
- Talar head is palpable at medial aspect of midfoot.
- Awkward "peg-leg" gait with limited push off strength.

Radiographic Evaluation [1]

- AP and lateral radiographs in neutral position.
- Addition of forced plantar flexion view is diagnostic:
  - Long axis of talus is not collinear with the first MT; line passes below first the MT (Fig. 136.3b).
  - Navicular and cuneiforms not ossified in infancy, and so dislocation must be inferred from alignment.

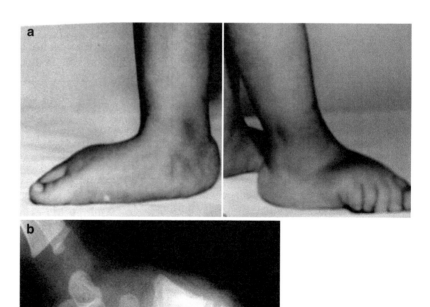

Fig. 136.3 Clinical photograph and lateral plantarflexion radiograph demonstrating congenital vertical talus, (**a**) and (**b**), respectively

Treatment [1, 4]

- Surgery is the rule.
- A period of corrective casting preoperatively may assist in stretching tight structures for later surgery.
- Before 2 years old is optimal timing.
- Surgery involves releasing or lengthening tight soft tissue structures and realignment of osseous structures.
- With increasing age, correction may require naviculectomy, subtalar arthrodesis, or triple arthrodesis.
- Newer procedures utilizing casting and limited minimally invasive surgical techniques show promise for future treatment of congenital vertical talus.

Juvenile Hallux Valgus (Bunion)

Introduction [2, 3]

- Lateral deviation of the great toe with medial prominence of the first MT head.
- Usually caused by increased intermetatarsal angle.
- Apex of deformity is medial at first MTP joint.
- As the deformity progresses, flexor tendons and the sesamoid complex sublux laterally.
- More common in females and often associated with flatfoot.
- Often bilateral and familial.

Clinical Evaluation

- Most are asymptomatic but may cause pain with certain footwear.
- Pain may come from medial MT head prominence or the second toe overlapping the laterally deviated great toe.
- Look for associated flatfoot deformity.
- Be aware of neurologic causes in the atypical patient with unilateral disease and no family history.

Radiographic Evaluation (Fig. 136.4) [2]

- Standing AP and lateral radiographs
- Hallux valgus angle (HVA)
- Intermetatarsal angle (IMA)
- Distal metatarsal articular angle (DMAA)
- Assess first MTP joint congruity – typically congruent in children

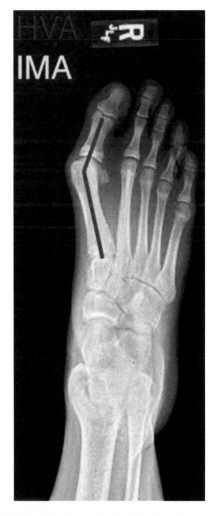

Fig. 136.4 AP radiograph of a right foot demonstrating juvenile hallux valgus and pictorial representation of HVA and IMA angles

Treatment [1, 2, 4]

- Nonoperative
  - Mainstay of treatment in children
  - Shoe wear modification with wide toe box
  - Arch supports
  - Possible role of night splinting
- Operative
  - Only indicated with pain not manageable by conservative measures.
  - Recurrence of the deformity is common in growing patients.
  - If possible, surgery should be delayed until the end of growth.
  - Surgery includes distal soft tissue realignment (McBride procedure), MT or first cuneiform osteotomy, and attention to correcting the DMAA.
  - Long oblique osteotomy ("scarf") can correct IMA and DMAA.
  - Complications of surgical treatment include recurrence, overcorrection, and hallux varus.

Metatarsus Adductus

Introduction [1, 3]

- Adduction of forefoot relative to midfoot and hindfoot
- Common cause of intoeing in children
- Up to 10–15% have concomitant developmental dysplasia of the hip (DDH)
- Also associated with congenital clubfoot
- 85% resolve spontaneously

Clinical Evaluation [2]

- Can be classified as mild, moderate, or severe based on flexibility:
  - Normal – Heel bisector line falls between the second and third toes.
  - Mild – Forefoot can be abducted beyond midline.
  - Moderate – Forefoot can be abducted to midline.

- Severe – Forefoot is rigid and cannot be abducted at all.
- Transverse crease on medial border of foot is seen in more rigid cases.
- Enlargement of web space between the first and second toes.
- Skewfoot (serpentine foot) – metatarsus adductus with addition of hindfoot valgus and midfoot lateral subluxation:
  - Some flexible forms may be treated nonoperatively, but many require surgery.

Treatment [1, 2]

- Mild deformities typically resolve without treatment.
- Moderate to severe deformities are initially treated with serial stretching and casting.
- Surgical indications include:
  - Severe deformities that fail conservative management
  - Pain
  - Objectionable appearance
  - Difficulty in fitting shoes
- Surgical options:
  - 2–4 years old – tarsometatarsal soft tissue releases
  - >4 years old – bony procedures:
    - Multiple MT osteotomies
    - Lateral column (cuboid) shortening and medial column (cuneiform) lengthening osteotomies
- Skewfoot – May require calcaneal, midfoot, and multiple MT osteotomies to achieve acceptable correction depending on flexibility of deformities [1].

Flatfoot (Pes Planus)

Flexible Flatfoot (FFF) [5]

Introduction [2, 3]
- Common condition in children
- Decrease in longitudinal arch of the foot that is present only in stance

- Commonly associated with valgus hindfoot alignment
- Oftentimes familial
- Associated with other lower extremity rotational deformities, ligamentous laxity, and high BMI

Clinical evaluation [5]
- Evaluate for other lower extremity anomalies.
- Evaluate for generalized ligamentous laxity.
- Assess flexibility of hindfoot.
- Heel cord contracture may contribute to deformity or be secondary to the deformity.
- FFF should revert to normal position in a non-weight-bearing state or when rising on toes, with reestablishment of longitudinal arch and the hindfoot tipping into varus [2].
- Assess muscle strength and range of motion in lower extremity.

Radiographic Evaluation [1]
- Lateral radiograph mimics vertical talus, but plantar flexion lateral demonstrates a line through long axis of talus that passes through or above first MT axis.
- May see hindfoot in equinus with decreased calcaneal pitch.
- Look for talonavicular or navicular – first cuneiform sag.
- Look for signs of tarsal coalition (unnecessary in asymptomatic/painless FFF).

Treatment [1, 5]
- If asymptomatic, observation is best as most cases spontaneously resolve with time.
- If symptomatic (pain), try conservative measures first:
  - Arch support
  - Shoe modifications – stiffer soles
  - Heel cord stretching regimen
  - Can relieve symptoms but do not correct deformity
- If disabling pain refractory to conservative measures, then may consider operative management [4]:

- Calcaneal lengthening osteotomy – sacrifices some subtalar motion
- Heel cord lengthening

Tarsal Coalition/Peroneal Spastic Flatfoot (PSFF) [5]

Introduction [1, 2]
- Rigid flatfoot deformity with minimal subtalar motion.
- PSFF is most commonly caused by a tarsal coalition, which is a fibrous, cartilaginous, or bony connection between two or more tarsal bones due to a failure of segmentation.
- PSFF can also be caused by arthritis, bone lesions, or trauma.
- Calcaneonavicular (CN) and talocalcaneal (TC) coalitions are fairly common and together comprise 90% of all tarsal coalitions [1].
- Frequently familial and bilateral in 50%.
- CN coalitions become symptomatic in children 8–12 years old.
- TC coalitions become symptomatic in children 12–16 years old.
- Associated conditions include fibular hemimelia, clubfoot, and Apert syndrome.

Clinical Evaluation [1, 2, 5]
- Symptoms appear by early adolescence and include calf pain (due to peroneal spasticity) and aching foot pain near the area of coalition.
- Progressive valgus hindfoot, arch collapse, and decreased subtalar motion ensue.
- Pain often is aggravated by activity and alleviated with rest.
- Little to no subtalar motion on exam.
- Hindfoot does not invert into normal varus position on toe rise, and arch does not reconstitute.
- Look for associated conditions.

Radiographic Evaluation [1]

- CN coalition
  - "Anteater" sign on lateral radiograph – elongated anterior process of calcaneus attaching to navicular.
  - Coalition is best seen on an oblique radiograph (Fig. 136.5).
- TC coalition
  - C sign on lateral radiograph – outline of talar dome going around inferior margin of sustentaculum tali (Fig. 136.6a)
  - Talar beaking on lateral radiograph
  - Irregular middle facet on Harris heel radiograph

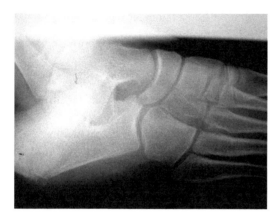

Fig. 136.5 Oblique radiograph demonstrating calcaneonavicular coalition

- Bone scan, computed tomography, and MRI may prove useful if negative radiographs but strong suspicion
  - MRI is most sensitive.
  - CT is good for measuring cross-sectional area of TC coalition (Fig. 136.6b).

Treatment [1, 2, 5]

- Nonoperative
  - If asymptomatic, observation is reasonable.
  - Goal is relief of pain and restoration of motion.
    Initial treatment involves activity modification, NSAIDS, shoe inserts, and immobilization in short leg walking cast or orthoses.
- Operative
  - Resection of coalition
    ○ Commonly successful in restoring motion.
    ○ Contraindicated if significant degenerative arthritis exists.
    ○ With TC coalitions, resection is an option if <50% of the posterior facet is involved; if >50%, arthrodesis is preferred [1].

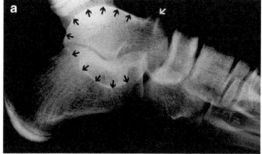
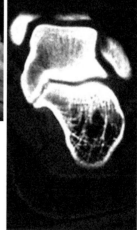

Fig. 136.6 Lateral radiograph and coronal CT demonstrating talocalcaneal coalition, (**a**) and (**b**), respectively

- Arthrodesis (subtalar or triple)
- Osteotomies to improve alignment (calcaneal lengthening osteotomy)

References

1. Kasser JR. The foot. In: Morissy RT, et al., editors. Lovell & winter's pediatric orthopedics. 6th ed. Philadelphia: Lipincott Williams & Wilkins; 2006 .Electronic Text

2. Herring JA, et al. Disorders of the foot. In: Herring JA, editor. Tachdjian's pediatric orthopedics. 4th ed. Philadelphia: Elsevier; 2008 .Electronic Text

3. Milbrandt TA, ct al. Pediatric orthopedics. In: Miller MD, et al., editors. Review of orthopedics. 6th ed. Philadelphia: Elsevier; 2012. p. 255–84.

4. Kelly DM. Congenital anomalies of the lower extremity. In: Canale ST, et al., editors. *Campbell's operative orthopedics*. 12th ed. Philadelphia: Elsevier; 2013. p. 980–1016.

5. Bauer K, et al. "What's new in pediatric flatfoot?". J Pediatr Orthop. 2015;PAP:1–5.

Idiopathic Scoliosis

Brien Rabenhorst

Definition

- Spinal curvature in the coronal plane of >10°:
  - No syndromic, congenital, or neuromuscular causes
- Scoliosis is a three-dimensional deformity: coronal, sagittal, and axial (rotation) planes.

Classifications

- Infantile: Age 0–3
- Juvenile: Age 3–10
- Adolescent: Age 11–17

Epidemiology

Tendencies

- Infantile
  - Affects males > females
  - Most commonly left thoracic curve
- Juvenile
  - Affects females > males

B. Rabenhorst, MD
University of Arkansas for Medical Sciences,
Little Rock, Arkansas, USA
e-mail: bmrabenhorst@uams.edu

- Most commonly right-sided thoracic curve
- Adolescent [4]
  - Most common type
  - Affects females > males
  - Most commonly a right thoracic curve with hypokyphosis of the thoracic spine

Etiology

- No specific gene has been identified as the cause of idiopathic scoliosis:
  - Likely multifactorial with possible influences from hormones, brain stem, and proprioception
- A higher incidence has been observed in patients with a family history of scoliosis.

Diagnosis

History

- School screenings:
  - Performed by specialty-trained nurses in elementary and middle schools
- Parents or patient notices a change in appearance:
  - Usually an asymmetric waist or protrusion of one side of the back on forward bending

© Springer International Publishing AG 2017
A.E.M. Eltorai et al. (eds.), *Orthopedic Surgery Clerkship*, DOI 10.1007/978-3-319-52567-9_137

Physical Exam

- Shoulder and pelvic balance (Fig. 137.1):
  - Unequal limb length may result in pelvic tilt and resemble scoliosis.
- Truncal asymmetry.
- Skin exam – Café au lait spots, axillary freckling, dimples, or hairy patches on the back can point to other causes for scoliosis, i.e., neurofibromatosis and spina bifida occulta.
- Look for hyperlaxity and arachnodactyly consistent with connective tissue disorder.
- Motion and flexibility of the spine in flexion/extension/lateral bending.
- Adam's forward bending test and scoliometer readings (Figs. 137.2 and 137.3):
  - The patient will bend forward to touch their toes.
  - Look for prominence in the scapula, ribs, and lumbar areas.
  - Scoliometer measures the amount of rotation of the spine at a given level.

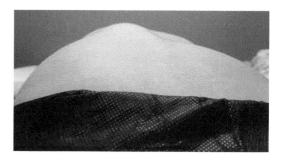

Fig. 137.2 Adam's forward bending test: *Left lumbar* prominence is better visualized

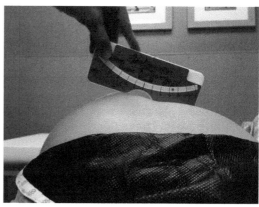

Fig. 137.3 Scoliometer reading: Across prominence to measure rotation

- Strength:
  - Examine both upper and lower extremities in all muscle groups.
- Sensation:
  - Examine all dermatomal distributions in upper and lower extremities.
- Reflexes:
  - Including biceps, triceps, brachioradialis, patella, Achilles, abdominal reflex
  - Upper motor neuron signs including Babinski and Hoffman's sign

Imaging

- Standing PA and lateral view radiographs that include shoulders and entire pelvis
- Bend films
  - Demonstrate the flexibility of spinal curves and can help dictate surgical planning in patients with multiple curves

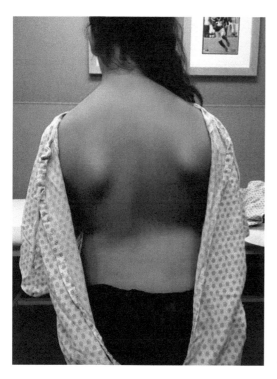

Fig. 137.1 Standing posterior view of 13 female with scoliosis: Examiner must visualize entire back. Note *right shoulder* elevation and *left lumbar* prominence

- Cobb angle [3] (Fig. 137.4)
  - Method of measuring spinal curvature on radiographs.
  - A line is drawn parallel to the superior end-plate of the most superior end vertebra with maximum tilt and another line at the inferior endplate of the most inferior end vertebra maximally tilted.
- Risser stage
  - Radiographic sign from AP pelvis that characterizes stage of growth by calcification of the apophysis of the iliac wings:
    - Stage 0: No ossification noted
    - Stages 1–4: 25-50-75-100% – capping of iliac wing
    - Stage 5: Complete ossification and fusion of apophysis

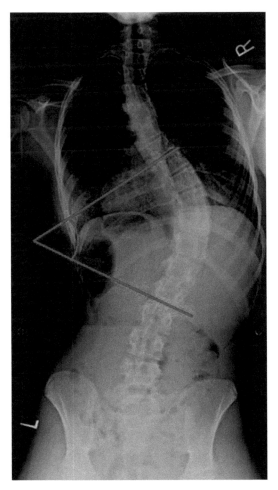

Fig. 137.4 PA spine with pelvis standing: Cobb measurement of thoracic curve demonstrated

- Risser 0–2 represent significant growth remaining.
- Risser 3–5 represent end of peak growth phase.
- MRI
  - Indicated in atypical curves, abnormal neurological findings, rapidly progressive curves, and patients less than 10 years with a surgical grade curve

Classification Systems

- Lenke classification [2] – evaluates three deformity characteristics
  - Coronal plane deformity (curve pattern)
  - Sagittal plane deformity of the thoracic spine (hyper/hypokyphosis)
  - Degree of lumbar spine deviation from the midline

Treatment

Infantile

- Observation for curve of <25°
- Bracing/surgical treatment for a progressive curve >25° with significant growth remaining
  - Casting and bracing both play an important role in preventing curve progression.
  - Surgical treatment must allow for growth to enable the thoracic cavity and lungs to develop via growing construct ("growing rods").

Juvenile

- Observation for curve of <25°
- Bracing for a curve 25–45°
  - Compliance is the most important factor in treatment with bracing (>12–18 h per day).
  - Bracing will not correct the curve; goal is to prevent progression.
- Surgical treatment with fusion and instrumentation for curves >50°
  - If significant growth remains, a growing rod/growth guidance construct may be

utilized until majority of spinal growth is completed.

- Anterior/posterior spinal fusion with instrumentation.
- Posterior spinal fusion with instrumentation.

Adolescent

- Observation for curve of <25° or a skeletally mature patient with a curve <50°
- Bracing for a curve 25–45° with significant growth remaining [1, 5]
  - Compliance is the most important factor in treatment with bracing (>12–18 h per day).
  - Bracing will not correct the curve; goal is to prevent progression.
- Surgical treatment with fusion and instrumentation for curves >50°
  - Posterior spinal fusion with instrumentation (most common)
  - Anterior release/fusion/instrumentation
  - Thorascopic fusion/instrumentation

Complications

Untreated Progressive Scoliosis

- Cardiopulmonary failure
- Degenerative changes of the spine
- Pain
- Cosmetic deformity
- Spinal imbalance

Posterior spinal fusion

- Infection
- Neurologic injury

- Spinal/shoulder imbalance
- Curve progression
- Crankshaft
  - Twisting of the spine through the fusion mass
  - Due to continued anterior growth
  - Seen in patients with significant growth remaining who undergo posterior spinal fusion, usually less than 10 years old
- Implant failure
  - Screw pullout
  - Rod fracture
- Pseudoarthrosis
  - Presents with late pain, progressing deformity, implant failure
  - If symptomatic, requires revision
- Superior mesenteric artery (SMA) syndrome
  - Resembles bowel obstruction
  - Results when correction of scoliosis stretches the SMA as it crosses over the duodenum
  - Treated with NG tube and fluids

References

1. Katz DE, Herring JA, Browne RH, Kelly DM, Birch JG. Brace wear control of curve progression in adolescent idiopathic scoliosis. J Bone Joint Surg Am. 2010;92:1343–52.
2. Lenke LG, Betz RR, Harms J, Bridwell KH, Clements DH, Lowe TG, Blanke K. Adolescent idiopathic scoliosis: A new classification to determine extent of spinal arthrodesis. J Bone Joint Surg Am. 2001;83:1169–81.
3. Morrissy RT, Goldsmith GS, Hall EC, et al. Measurement of the Cobb angle on radiographs of patients who have scoliosis. Evaluation of intrinsic error. J Bone Joint Surg Am. 1990;72:320–7.
4. Rogala EJ, Drummond DS, Gurr J. Scoliosis: incidence and natural history. A prospective epidemiological study. J Bone Joint Surg Am. 1978;60:173–6.
5. Weinstein SL, Dolan LA, Wright JG, et al. Effects of bracing in adolescents with idiopathic scoliosis. N Engl J Med. 2013;369:1512–21.

Neuromuscular Spine Deformity

138

John P. Lubicky

Definition

- NSD is a spinal deformity associated with/or caused by an associated NMD.
- Commonly seen in DMD, CP, MM SMA, Friedrich ataxia, CMT, and post-SCI.
- NSD incidence and severity usually parallels that of the NMD.
- NSD may be mainly scoliotic, mainly kyphotic or lordotic, or a combination of coronal and sagittal deformity.

Etiology and Natural History

- NSD is caused by trunk muscle weakness, spasticity, or imbalance.
- Not all patients with NMD develop NSD.
- Treatment of the underlying NMD can prevent or mitigate the severity of NSD
- (steroids in DMD, special diets, or supplements in certain muscle diseases).
- Treatment of the underlying NMD can worsen the course of NSD (baclofen pump in
- CPs, improper surgical treatment of spinal injury in SCI).

J.P. Lubicky, MD
Department of Orthopaedics, West Virginia
University, PO Box 9196, Morgantown,
WV 26506, USA
e-mail: jlubicky@hsc.wvu.edu

- Rapid growth is usually associated with rapid progression.
- Severity of the NMD (GMFSC) usually parallels severity of the NSD.
- With increased NSD severity problems like poor sitting posture, respiratory compromise pressure sores occur.

Clinical Presentation

- Nonambulatory child with a NMD having difficulty sitting with or without pressure
- sores or respiratory compromise or an ambulatory child with increasing NSD.
- GMFSC is useful in predicting natural history and how NSD will impact patient.
- Physical exam.
  - Note patient status: alertness, communication ability, and general overall condition
  - Note curve pattern, flexibility, presence or absence of pelvic obliquity, and presence of pressure areas/sores
  - Check U and LEs for contractures and function

Imaging

- Radiographs
  - Upright (standing or sitting) front and lateral views
  - Side bending/hyperextension views as needed

A.E.M. Eltorai et al. (eds.), *Orthopedic Surgery Clerkship*, DOI 10.1007/978-3-319-52567-9_138

- CT: for specific cases. 3D reconstructions useful in severe deformities
- MRI: primarily used in patients with documented spinal cord disease (e.g., Chiari I, MM, MM)

Treatment

Nonoperative

- Bracing
  - Not definitive treatment for progressive deformity
  - Used in slim patients with flexible curves to prove trunk alignment and improve sitting and only when up and about
  - Cannot/should not be used in obese patients or those with stiff curves

- Molded wheelchair inserts – cannot control deformity
- Halo traction: may be used before bracing or surgery to improve correction

Operative

- Non-fusion – Std strategy: posterior spinal "growing rods"
  - Rib or spine based, +/– to pelvis (Fig. 138.1)
- Fusion – goals balanced spine over level pelvis
  - Std: PSF/PSSI +/– to pelvis (Fig. 138.2)
    - ASF/PSSI (or VCR) for severe, stiff NSD (Fig. 138.3)
    - ASF/ASSI for selected cases (Fig. 138.4)
    - ASF/PSSI hybrid (Fig. 138.5)
    - Revision for failed prior surgery (Fig. 138.6)

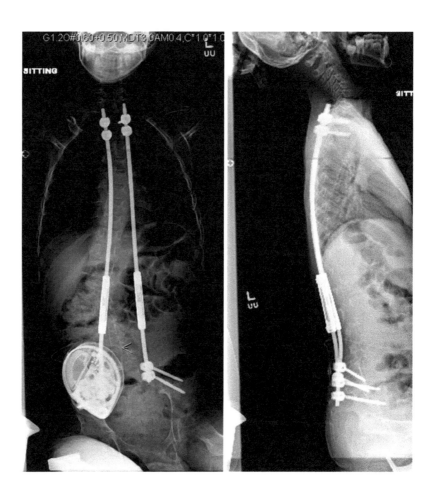

Fig. 138.1 Posterior spinal "growing rods" in a boy with CP unable to be braced b/c of pulmonary issues

Fig. 138.2 Teenage boy with CP: curve progression after BP PSF/PSSI to the pelvis

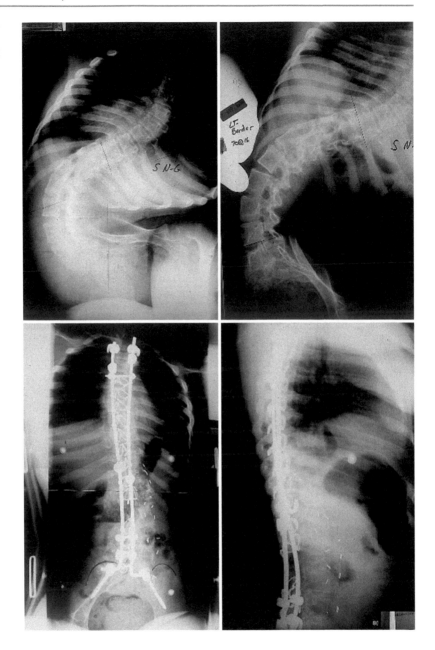

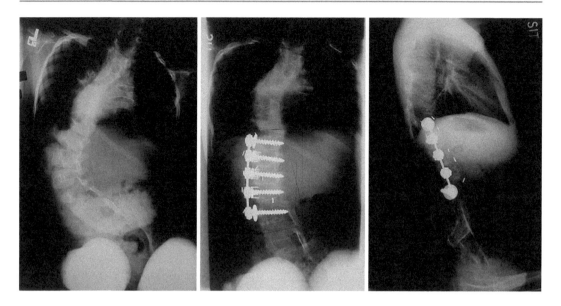

Fig. 138.3 Teenage girl with polio (two-stage, two level vertebrectomy, ASF/PSF with PSSI, and allograft)

Fig. 138.4 Young child with MM and bad skin on the back (single-stage ASF/ASSI with the rib and allograft)

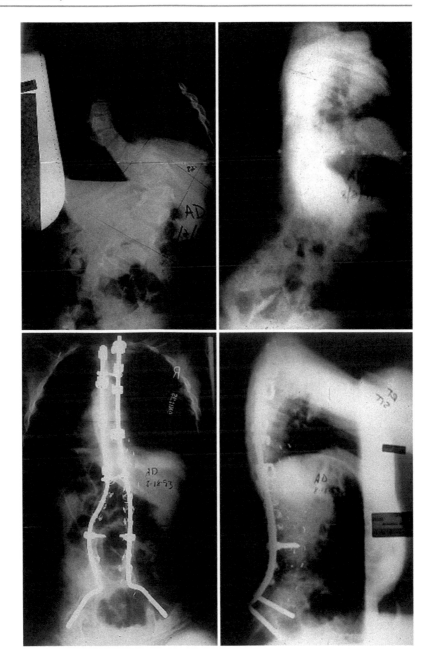

Fig. 138.5 Teenage boy
with MM ASF/PSF/PSSI
(hybrid)

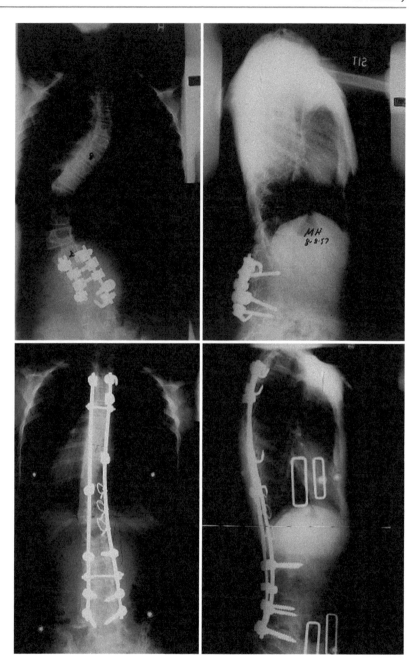

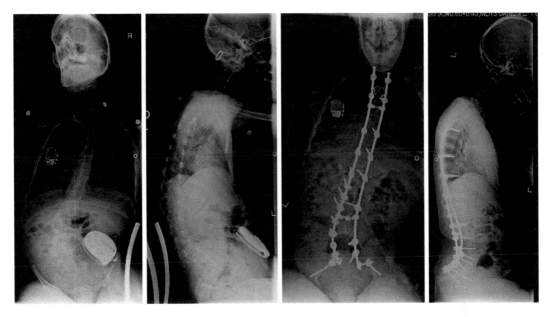

Fig. 138.6 Young paraplegic girl with scoliosis after surgically treated SI/SCI (HWR, revision PSSI, PSF, and allograft)

Prerequisites for Surgery

- Control of comorbidities: maximize nutrition, clear pulmonary issues, control seizures, heal pressure sores, and treat UTIs

Complications

- Overall higher incidence than in AIS
- Infection risk: (highest in MM) prophylactic antibiotics
  - Consider vancomycin in those with MRSA hx
  - Wound infection –aggressive I and D + antibiotics
- Instrumentation failure – avoid inappropriate constructs, revise for early loss of correction or malpositioned implants
- Respiratory issues: aggressive pulmonary care and mobilization
- Nutrition – ensure calorie intake (N-J or G tube)
- Pressure sores – avoid with proper positioning and mobility

The treatment of NSD is still controversial with even ethical issues involving GMFSC IV and V patients. However, caregiver questionnaires indicate a high degree of satisfaction with the surgical treatment. The purpose of the surgery is to improve the quality of life for the patient and the caregivers and not to cure the NMD. Proper selection and management of surgical patients will minimize complications and improve outcomes.

References

(Students are encouraged to peruse these textbook chapters which have extensive bibliographies)

1. Chan G, Spiegel DA: Drummond DS. Surgical treatment of flaccid neuromuscular scoliosis. In: Bridwell KH, DeWald RL editors. The textbook of spinal surgery. 3rd edn. Philadelphia: Lippincott,Williams & Wilkins; 2011.
2. Lubicky JP. Neuromuscular scoliosis. In: Heary RF, Albert TJ, editors. Spinal deformities: the essentials. New York: Thieme Medical Publishers; 2014.

3. Luhman SJ. Introduction/state of the art in the care of paralytic and neuromuscular scoliosis. In: Bridwell KH, DeWald L, editors. The textbook of spinal surgery. 3rd edn. Philadelphia: Lippincott, Williams & Wilkins; 2011.

4. McPartland TYG, Emans JB. Paralytic scoliosis and the spastic patient. In: Bridwell KH, DeWald, RL. editors. The textbook of spinal surgery. 3rd edn. Philadelphia: Lippincott, Williams & Wilkins; 2011.

Dana Lycans, LeeAnne Torres, and Viorel Raducan

Overview

- Prevalence 1–4%. True incidence/prevalence difficult to ascertain due to many congenital spine anomalies going unrecognized [3].
- Generally, curve has a sharper angle over a shorter segment and is more resistant to conservative treatment than idiopathic curves (Fig. 139.1).

Causes [3]

- Spontaneous (most common)
- In utero exposure (alcohol, valproate, diabetes)
- Genetic

D. Lycans, MD • L. Torres, MD
Department of Orthopaedic Surgery, Marshall University/Cabell Huntington Hospital, Huntington, WV, USA

V. Raducan, MD (✉)
Marshall University, 1 John Marshall Dr, Huntington, WV 25755, USA
e-mail: raducan@marshall.edu

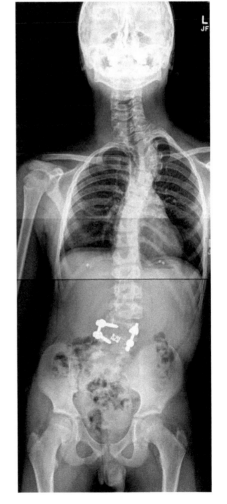

Fig. 139.1 Example of congenital scoliosis in a child

© Springer International Publishing AG 2017
A.E.M. Eltorai et al. (eds.), *Orthopedic Surgery Clerkship*, DOI 10.1007/978-3-319-52567-9_139

Associated Conditions (Up to 61%)

- Can occur along with cardiac defects (20%), genitourinary defects (20%), and spinal cord malformations such as diastematomyelia or tethered cord (21–37%)
- VACTERL syndrome, Klippel-Feil syndrome, and Alagille syndrome

Prognosis

- Progress rapidly during rapid growth (spine grows most rapidly during the first 5 years of life).
- Rate of progression depends on the type of vertebral anomaly:
  - Fused ribs indicate higher risk of progression.
- Significant curves can affect the development of the thoracic cavity and lungs leading to early morbidity/mortality through decreased lung capacity.

Classification (Figs. 139.2 and 139.3)

Failure of Formation [1, 3]

- Full hemivertebra, semi-segmented hemivertebra, unsegmented hemivertebra, unincarcerated hemivertebra, and wedge vertebra

Failure of Segmentation [1, 3]

- Block vertebra (bilateral bony bars)
- Bar body (unilateral bony bar)

Mixed [3]

- Unilateral unsegmented bar with contralateral hemivertebra (fastest progression)

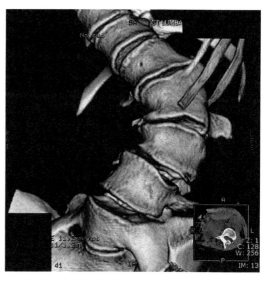

Fig. 139.3 3D CT reconstruction demonstrating wedge vertebra

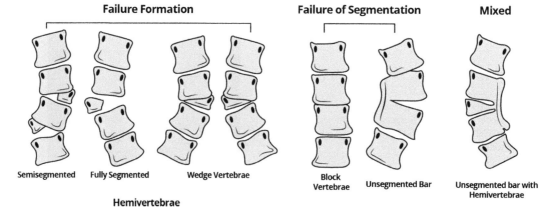

Fig. 139.2 Classification of congenital scoliosis. Adapted from Orthobullets.com

Natural History [2]

- Progresses with age.
- With kyphotic deformity, more rapid progression with failure of formation anomaly.
- With scoliosis deformity, more rapid progression with failure of segmentation anomaly.
- Significant progression can lead to impaired development of the thoracic cavity leading to thoracic insufficiency syndrome, decreased lung volumes, and early morbidity/mortality [2]:
  - In kyphosis deformity, higher risk of neurologic compromise in addition to pulmonary function

Treatment

Nonoperative [2, 3]

- Observation – indicated only for small curves to document the presence or absence of progression
- Bracing – not effective in congenital spinal deformity

Operative [2, 3]

- Indications: curve progression, onset of neurological deficit, and decreased pulmonary function
- Goals:
  - Stop progression
  - Correct deformity/reestablish physiological alignment
- Challenge: growth preservation (spine/thorax/lungs)
  - Congenital deformities occur during the period of maximum growth velocity/critical period of thorax/lung growth and maturation.
- Techniques:
  - In situ posterior fusion – indicated in older patients (girls >10 years old and boys >12 years old) with progression, neurologic deficits, or declining respiratory function

- Anterior/posterior fusion – indicated in [1] younger patients who have had progression, neurologic deficits, or declining respiratory function or [2] mixed anomaly
  - Fusion anteriorly prevents crankshaft phenomenon, which is a continued growth of the anterior column in the setting of posterior fusion leading to increased lordosis of the spine:
- Growth preservation techniques
  - Growing rods – helps control rate of progressive while still allowing for growth while awaiting final fusion:
    - Requires repeat surgeries to lengthen construct every 6–8 months.
    - Newer technologies use magnets outside the body for construct lengthening.
  - VEPTR (vertical expanding prosthetic titanium rib) – initially indicated in thoracic insufficiency syndrome (TIS), but now indications expanded to scoliosis even without TIS. Allows chest wall expansion theoretically improving the respiratory function.

Complications from Surgery [3]

- Crankshaft phenomenon – continued anterior spinal growth in the presence of posterior growth arrest (fusion) resulting in increased deformity
- Infection
- Neurologic deficit – highest incidence in surgery for congenital spinal deformity, especially kyphosis
- Specific to growth preservation techniques:
  - Wound dehiscence
  - Infection
  - Reason: multiple surgeries/bulky implants in small patients
- Growth arrest – fusion at early age – short trunk/small thorax with secondary restrictive pulmonary syndrome/insufficiency

References

1. Weiss HR, Moramarco M. Congenital scoliosis (Mini-review). Curr Pediatr Rev. 2016;12(1):43–7.
2. Gard S, Johnson C. Early-onset scoliosis. In: Song K, editor. Orthopedic knowledge update pediatrics. 4th edn. Rosemont: American Academy of Orthopedic Surgeons; 2011. p. 243–57.
3. Emans J. Congenital scoliosis. In: Morrissy R, Weinstein SL, editors. Lovell & winter's pediatric orthopedics. 6th edn. Philadelphia: Lippincott Williams & Wilkins; 2006.

Scheuermann's Kyphosis

140

John P. Lubicky

Introduction/Definitions

- SK – abnormally increased kyphosis of the thoracic and thoracolumbar spine with apical vertebral wedging. (Normal range of T kyphosis is 20–45° measured on standing radiographs.)
- Described by Scheuermann in 1921 – rigid angular kyphosis.
- Sorenson criteria (three apical vertebrae at 5° of wedging) in the sagittal plane (Fig. 140.1)
- Most common structural cause of hyperkyphotic deformity in adolescence.
- Incidence is 0.4–8.3% of the population.
- Males > females.
- Those affected are taller and heavier than normal controls.

Etiology and Pathologic Anatomy

- Mechanical factors – tight and thick anterior longitudinal ligament – tethers growth and causes deformity
- Abnormal enchondral ossification (imbalance of the collagen/cartilage/bone matrix)
- Vascular abnormalities

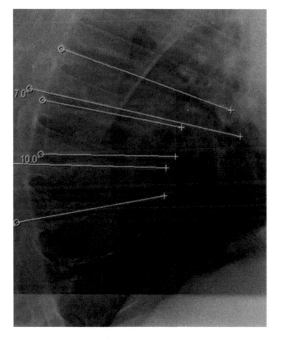

Fig. 140.1 Cone down lateral radiograph of the apical vertebrae of a kyphotic patient demonstrating the vertebral body wedging

- Osteoporosis
- Hueter-Volkmann effect – deformity begins as postural round back > increased pressure on anterior physis > asymmetric growth > increased kyphosis > vicious cycle
- "Unloading" affected vertebra (bracing) reverses process
- Schmorl's nodes, herniation of disc into vertebral bodies
- Familial – exact heredity – not established

J.P. Lubicky, MD
Department of Orthopaedics, West Virginia University, PO Box 9196, Morgantown, WV 26506, USA
e-mail: jlubicky@hsc.wvu.edu

© Springer International Publishing AG 2017
A.E.M. Eltorai et al. (eds.), *Orthopedic Surgery Clerkship*, DOI 10.1007/978-3-319-52567-9_140

Presentation

- Develops in adolescence.
- Families notice round back which worsens with increased growth rate.
- Sometimes only found at PE for sports or annual examination.
- +/− complaints of pain (at apex or lumbar) without radiation
- +/− complaints of low stamina, SOB
- PE – slumped shoulders, increased kyphosis – increased with forward bending:
  - ^ lumbar lordosis, +/− forward head thrust.
  - Evaluate stiffness while prone doing active hyperextension of chest and shoulders off table.
  - Observe any cutaneous lesions (may indicate other diagnosis).

Natural History

- Risk of continued progress – unclear (osteoporotic compression fractures – later in life increased deformity)
- With age – +/− pain, limited trunk ROM and strength, and respiratory insufficiency
- Symptoms – usually worse with large curves (> 75°)
- PROs – assess HRQOL:
  - SRS 22 (Lonner) – scores in SK pts < AIS and nl controls (in pain, self-image, mental health domains)
  - Neurologic deficit d/t deformity – very uncommon

Imaging

- Standing PA and lateral radiographs – gold std
- Measure sagittal and coronal curves and vertebral wedging (Fig. 140.1)
- Note Schmorl's nodes and end plate and disc abnl
- EOS (EOS Imaging, Paris, France) – more information – less radiation

- Assess flexibility with cross table lateral with bump beneath the apex
- MRI and CT reserved for specific indications

Differential Diagnoses

- Postural round back
- Congenital kyphosis
- Syndromic spine deformity
- SK Type II – affects T-L and L spine – uncommon:
  - Usually a painful condition
  - Loss of LL and kyphosis at T-L jct
  - Vertebral end plate abnl and Schmorl's nodes
  - Rx, PT, rest, and NSAIDS; surgery, unlikely

Treatment

Nonoperative

- Bracing – gold std – less effective in curves >70°:
  - Must be skeletally immature – ring apophyses – open
  - Milwaukee brace – most efficacious/least accepted
  - TLSO
  - Perhaps a period of corrective casting before bracing
  - Brace "unloads" wedged vertebral physes by correcting curve – lasting correction with reversal of wedging requires 12–18 months full time – wean
- PT/exercise – not effective alone
  - Used in conjunction with bracing

Operative

- Goals – prevent progression, restore spinal alignment, and relieve pain
- Indications – curves >70° in mature and immature pts
- Correction goal – restore kyphosis into normal range:

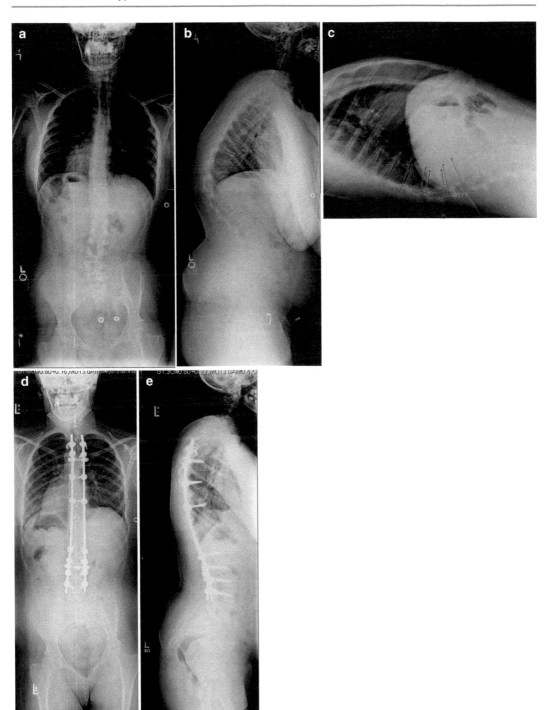

Fig. 140.2 Teenage boy with kyphotic deformity with the apex at the T-L junction associated with minimal scoliosis. Cross table lateral radiograph done with a bump under the apex demonstrates correctability AP and lateral radiographs after PSF/PSSI and Ponte osteotomies. Adolescent with T-L apex SK, (**a, b**) – pre-op radiographs; (**c**) – cross table lateral radiograph with apex on a bump; (**d, e**) – post-op radiographs after PSF/PSSI + Ponte osteotomies

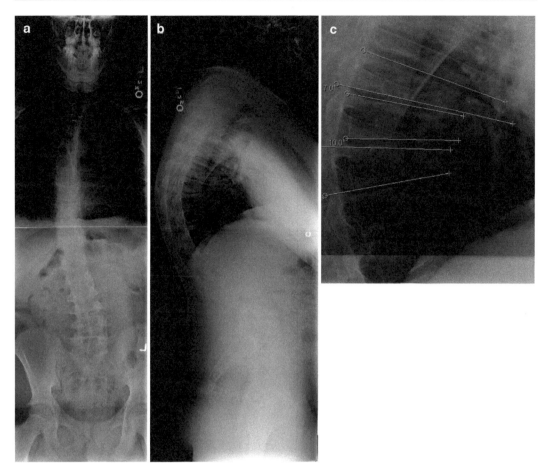

Fig. 140.3 Teenage boy with a kyphotic deformity with the apex midthoracic associated with a mild scoliosis. Cone down lateral radiograph demonstrating the vertebral wedging. PA and lateral radiographs after PSF/PSSI and Ponte osteotomies. Adolescent with T-L apex SK, (**a, b**) – pre-op radiographs; (**c**) – cross table lateral radiograph with apex on a bump; (**d, e**) – post-op radiographs after PSF/PSSI + Ponte osteotomies

Fig. 140.3 (continued)

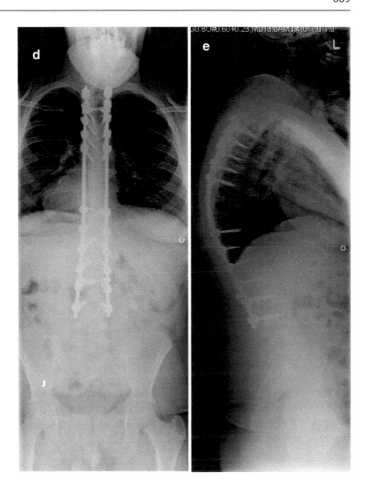

- Evaluate stiffness with cross table lateral radiograph with bump beneath the apex.
- Many techniques have been described:
  - Preliminary halo tx; staged ASF/PSF with or without intervening
  - Halo tx; same day ASF/PSF; PSF only with or without
  - Osteotomies (Fig. 140.2)
  - PSF/PSSI with Ponte osteotomies and bone graft – gold std (Fig. 140.3)
  - Correct choice of UIV and LIV – critical: UIV well above the apex into lordotic transition and LIV no higher than the first lordotic disc

- Segmental instrumentation – all hooks, all screws, or hybrids – okay; all screws except hooks at UIV – best
- Implants at every level – not necessary and expensive
- Cantilever and compression forces to correct
- Neuromonitoring – essential and std of care
  - Can see transient changes in signals
  - Usually not associated with SCI or other deficit
- Complications – infection, neurologic injury, and instrumentation failure

Summary

- Patients with SK can be offered both nonoperative and operative treatment for their deformities. Compliance issues in those treated with a brace can be significant barriers to a successful nonoperative treatment. Even the ability to obtain a Milwaukee brace may be daunting. With powerful and stable spinal instrumentation, excellent correction of the deformity can be achieved in those with large curves. Significant complications of the surgery can occur. Proper patient selection should be exercised by evaluating the curve size, the skeletal maturity, and physical demands with the natural history, i.e., chronic compensatory changes in spinal alignment, pain, and potential pulmonary issues.

Reference

(Students are encouraged to peruse the collection of classic papers included in the bibliographies on the following textbook chapters)

1. Boachie-Adjei O. Scheuermann's Kyphosis. In: DeWald RL, editor. Spinal deformities: the comnprehensive text. New York: Thieme Medical Publishers; 2003. p. 777–86.

Pediatric Cervical Spine Conditions

141

Michael Heffernan and Viral Patel

Abbreviations

ADI	Atlantodens interval
AP	Anteroposterior
CT	Computer tomography
LAT	Lateral
MRI	Magnetic resonance imaging
SAC	Space available for spinal cord

Pseudosubluxation in Cervical Spine

Introduction

In children up to 8 years of age, there can be anterior displacement of C2 relative to C3 which is seen on the lateral cervical spine radiograph. At first glance, it may appear pathologic; however, it

M. Heffernan, MD (✉)
Orthopedic Department, Children's Hospital Of New Orleans, Louisiana State University, New Orleans, LA, USA
e-mail: mheff1@lsuhsc.edu

V. Patel, MD
Orthopedic Department, Gillette Children's Hospital, University of Minnesota, St. Paul, MN, USA
e-mail: drpviralr@yahoo.com

is most frequently a benign condition called pseudosubluxation.

Incidence

- It is more common at the C2–C3 level and less commonly seen at C3–C4.
- Cattell et al. reported on 161 normal children and found 9% had pseudosubluxation between C2 and C3 [1].
- Shaw et al. looked at 108 children after polytrauma and found 22% of children had pseudosubluxation between C2 and C3 [2].

Etiology

- There are many hypotheses with no definitive etiology.
- Most texts agree that there is a different facet angle in childhood compared to adults associated with disco-ligamentous laxity and larger skull size seen in children.

Investigation

- Anteroposterior (AP) and lateral (LAT) radiographs of the cervical spine

© Springer International Publishing AG 2017
A.E.M. Eltorai et al. (eds.), *Orthopedic Surgery Clerkship*, DOI 10.1007/978-3-319-52567-9_141

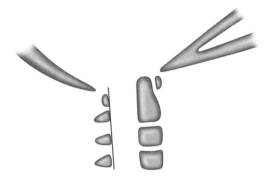

Fig. 141.1 Lateral view of the upper cervical spine on plain radiograph showing the Swischuk line

- Swischuk et al. performed radiographic study to differentiate between physiologic and

  pathologic displacement.

- Swischuk line – It is a line drawn from the anterior cortex of the posterior arch of C1 to the anterior cortex of the posterior arch of C3 [3] (Fig. 141.1).

In physiologic subluxation, this line should pass	In pathologic subluxation, this line
through the anterior cortex of the posterior arch of	passes in front of the anterior cortex
C2 or at most 1mm in front of the anterior cortex.	≤ 2mm.

Treatment

- No treatment is required for this condition.

Atlantoaxial Instability

Introduction

- Atlantoaxial instability is associated with or precipitated by other congenital craniocervical anomalies. Therefore, it is important to review atlantoaxial instability on imaging in patients with other craniocervical anomalies in pediatric patients.

Pathoanatomy

- Articulation between C1 and C2 is the most mobile part in the cervical spine. The normal cervical spine can have 90° of lateral rotation on each side, of which the C1–C2 joint contributes 50%. There is a limited degree of flexion and extension that is present at this joint (normally about 10° of extension and 5° of flexion).
- The ligaments stabilizing craniocervical junction also stabilize the C1–C2 vertebrae. Ligaments of craniocervical junction are as follows:
  - Posterior atlanto-occipital membrane
  - Tectorial membrane
  - Transverse ligament, cruciate ligament (superior and inferior crus), and accessory atlantoaxial ligament
  - Apical ligament and alar ligament
  - Atlanto-dental ligament
  - Anterior atlanto-occipital ligament
- As mentioned cervico-cranial junction is a highly mobile part of the cervical spine, which has a complex ligamentous stabilizing system.

Etiology

- Idiopathic
- Traumatic
- Congenital
  - Os odontoideum
  - Atlanto-occipital fusion
  - Klippel-Feil syndrome
- Ligamentous laxity
  - Down syndrome
  - Marfan syndrome
  - Ehler-Danlos syndrome
- Associated with other anomalies
  - Congenital scoliosis
  - Spondyloepiphyseal dysplasia
  - Osteogenesis imperfect
  - Neurofibromatosis

Clinical Features

- Most patients develop symptoms in their third to fourth decade due to increased ligament laxity and degenerative changes associated with age [4].
  - History of neck trauma, neck pain, and torticollis
  - Quadriparesis
  - Symptoms of spinal cord compression [5, 6]
    - Muscle weakness
    - Ataxia
    - Wasting
    - Spasticity
    - Hyperreflexia
  - Symptoms of cranial nerve compression
    - Tinnitus
    - Earaches
    - Dysphasia
    - Poor phonation
  - Symptoms of posterior column compression in the spinal cord
    - Alteration in deep pain
    - Change in vibratory sensation
    - Loss of proprioception
  - Symptoms from compression of vertebral artery [4]
    - Dizziness
    - Syncope
    - Mental deterioration
    - Seizure
  - Symptoms specific for pediatric patients [7]
    - Generalized weakness
    - Lack of physical endurance
    - Frequent falling
    - Child asking to be carried
  - Signs and symptoms from compression of brain stem [8, 9]
    - Decrease in vital capacity and chronic alveolar hypoventilation
    - Depressed gag and cough reflexes

Investigation

- Radiography of cervical spine – anteroposterior, lateral, flexion, and extension views and an odontoid view. In traumatic instability, standard flexion and extension views are hazardous.
  - Atlantodens interval (ADI): This is a space between the anterior aspect of the dens and the posterior aspect of the anterior ring of C1. It is seen in lateral view. More than 4–5 mm indicates instability in pediatric patient and more than 3 mm indicates instability in adult patient. ADI is of limited value in chronic instability like congenital, rheumatoid, Down syndrome and other ligamentous laxity conditions (Figs. 141.2, 141.3, and 141.4).
  - Space available for spinal cord (SAC): This is a space between the posterior aspect of the dens and the nearest posterior bony structure (Figs. 141.2, 141.3, and 141.4). Cord compression never occurs if it is ≥18 mm, cord compression is possible between

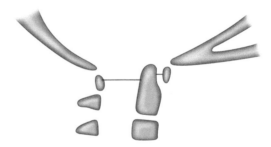

Fig. 141.2 Lateral view of the upper cervical spine on plain radiograph showing normal atlantodens interval (*ADI*) and space available for spinal cord (*SAC*)

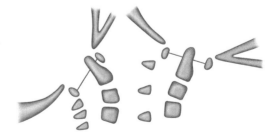

Fig. 141.3 Lateral view of the upper cervical spine with flexion and extension views. *Left side image*, extension of the cervical spine with ADI and SAC is normal as dens and posterior arch of C2 provides bony block for further subluxation in extension. *Right side image*, flexion of the cervical spine with increased ADI and decreased SAC due to instability

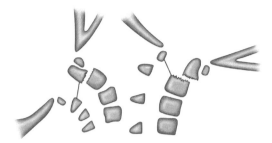

Fig. 141.4 Lateral view of the upper cervical spine on plain radiograph with flexion and extension view with atlantoaxial instability with traumatic nonunion, os odontoideum. Both flexion and extension views show that ADI remains normal in both the views, but SAC is decreased in both views

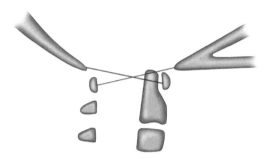

Fig. 141.5 Lateral view of the upper cervical spine on plain radiograph showing two lines which is used to determined power ratio

15 and 17 mm, and cord compression occurs if it is ≤14 mm [4].

- Power ratio: This is determined by the length of the two lines. One line is from basion to the posterior arch of the atlas and other line is from opisthion to the anterior arch of the atlas, and then length of the first line is divided by the second line. Ratio >1 is diagnostic of the atlanto-occipital anterior translation and <0.55 is diagnostic of posterior translation [10] (Fig. 141.5).
- CT and MRI of cervical spine – usually dynamic (flexion and extension) views on CT and MRI are more helpful than static ones. They are useful to determine:
  - Bony anomalies of the spine [7]
  - Compression on the spinal cord [11, 12]
  - Ligament integrity, especially transverse atlantal ligament and alar ligament [13]

- Rule of third by Steel: the area of the vertebral canal at C1 can be divided into three parts. One part is occupied by the dens, second part occupied by the spinal cord, and third part is a "safe zone space" which allows dens displacement without any neurological compromised [13].
- Vertebral arteriography: this is useful in the patient who presents with the vertebral artery compression symptoms.
- Somatosensory-evoked potential: useful for patients for whom a detailed neurological examination is always difficult.

Treatment

- ADI 4–5 mm:
  - If patient remain symptomatic, then restrict high-risk activities with close follow up.
- ADI 6–7 mm:
  - Needs MRI and CT scan for evaluation of neurological compromise.
  - Asymptomatic patients need restriction of high-risk activities and close follow-up.
  - Symptomatic patients need surgical stabilization of atlantoaxial instability.
- ADI 10 mm or more:
  - Both symptomatic and asymptomatic patients need surgical stabilization of atlantoaxial instability.
- Surgical stabilization of the atlantoaxial instability can be done using sub-laminar wires, C1–C2 transarticular screws, and C1–C2 posterior screws. This may also require decompression of the spinal cord. The choice of the surgical procedure depends on the individual patient's and surgeon's preference [14, 15].

Atlantoaxial Instability in Down Syndrome

- Atlantoaxial instability in Down syndrome is first described in 1961 by Spitzer et al.
- It occurs approximately 10–20% of children with Down syndrome.
- It usually occurs in more than one level and also more than one plane in the cervical spine.

- Atlanto-occipital instability is also common in Down syndrome.
- A direct correlation between neurological symptoms and atlantoaxial instability in Down syndrome has not been established yet.
- You may accept ADI up to 10 mm in asymptomatic patients with Down syndrome.

Atlantoaxial Rotatory Subluxation

Etiology

- It occurs when C1–C2 motion becomes abnormal.
- Can occur spontaneously or following minor trauma.
- Can also occur after URI due to inflammation of the adjacent soft tissue in the neck and is called Grisel syndrome [16].
- Hyperemic calcification of the atlas can cause loosening of the transverse ligament and allows subluxation [17].
- Synovial joint fringes of C1–C2 joint become inflamed and act as an obstruction [18].
- Can occur with one or both alar ligament disruption with intact transverse ligament [19].
- Synovial joint meniscal-like fold can impinge on lateral C1–C2 joint causing subluxation as well [20].
- But main pathology is laxity of the ligament and joint capsule is present in all cases.

Classification

- Fielding and Hawkins Classification of the atlantoaxial rotatory subluxation [21]
- Type I – Rotatory displacement without anterior shift
  - Most common type.
  - Primary occurs in child.
  - Usually not associated with neurological injury.
- Type II – Rotatory displacement with an anterior shift of C1 on the C2 less than 5 mm
  - Less common type
  - Greater risk for the neurological injury

- Type III – Rotatory displacement with an anterior shift of C1 on the C2 more than 5 mm
  - Rare type and usually associated with neurological injury
- Type IV – Rotatory displacement with posterior shift
  - Rare type and usually associated with neurological injury.
  - Anterior shift is considered pathological if it is more than 3 mm in adult and more than 4 mm in pediatric patient.

Clinical Features

- Patient's head tilted on one side and rotated to the opposite side with neck slightly flexed (cock-robin deformity).
- In the acute setting can be associated with axial neck pain and pain in the movement of the neck.
- On long-standing cases, plagiocephaly and facial flattening may develop on the side of the tilt.

Investigation

- AP, lateral, and odontoid views
  - On odontoid view, the lateral mass on one side looks wider and nearer to the dens, while in the opposite side, lateral mass looks narrower and further away.
  - In lateral view, lateral mass looks wedged in front of the dens.
- CT scan with head rotated to the right and left
  - To assess the rotation of C1 on C2 when patient's head is rotated to the right and left
- MRI of the cervical spine
  - Utilized to assess pathologic compression of the spinal cord in the setting of neurologic deficit

Treatment

- Philip and Hensinger postulated the treatment plan of the atlantoaxial rotatory subluxation [22].
- Atlantoaxial subluxation is less than 1 week:
  - Immobilization in soft collar.
  - Analgesics.

- Bed rest for 1 week.
- Closed follow-up

- If reduction of subluxation is not achieved, than hospitalization of pateint with halter traction and muscle relaxants.
- Atlantoaxial subluxation is more than 1 week but less than 1 month:
  - Hospitalization
  - Cervical traction in head halter
  - Muscle relaxants
  - Analgesics

- Achieve reduction and see for the anterior shift or displacement.

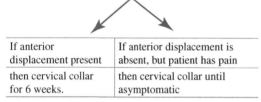

If anterior displacement present	If anterior displacement is absent, but patient has pain
then cervical collar for 6 weeks.	then cervical collar until asymptomatic

- Atlantoaxial subluxation is more than 1 month:
  - Hospitalization
  - Skeletal cervical traction
  - Muscle relaxants
  - Analgesics

- Achieve reduction and cervical collar for 6 weeks.
- Indication for the surgical intervention [23]:
  - Neurological deficit
  - Anterior displacement
  - Failure of conservative treatment
  - Recurrence of deformity
  - Fixed deformity
  - Subluxation more than 3 months

Anomalies of Odontoid (Dens)

Introduction

- Congenital anomalies of odontoid are very rare.
- Usually detected as incidental finding after trauma or when patients present with some symptoms.
- Exact incidence is unknown, but aplasia is very rare and mostly incidental finding.

Types

It can be divided in three types (Fig. 141.6):

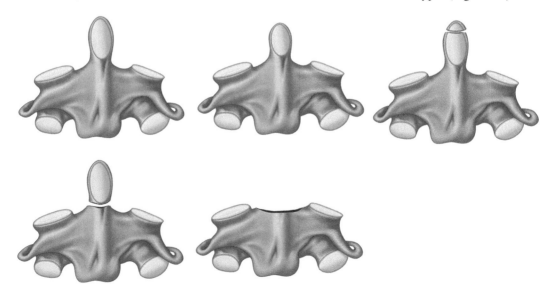

Fig. 141.6 Types of anomalies of odontoid: (**a**) normal, (**b**) hypoplastic, (**c**) ossiculum terminale, (**d**) os odontoideum, (**e**) aplasia

- Aplasia
  - Complete absence of odontoid
- Hypoplasia
  - Partial development of the odontoid and varies from peg-like projection to almost normal size
- Os odontoideum
  - Oval or round ossicle with smooth sclerotic margin and separated from the body of C2 by a transverse gap

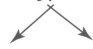

Orthotopic	Dystopic
Located at normal position of densLocated near to the occiput or in area of foramen magnum	

Embryology

- Odontoid is developed from mesenchyme of the first C1 sclerotome [24–26].
- Vestigial disc between C1 and C2 forms synchondrosis, and this looks like the epiphyseal line present between the body of axis and odontoid on X-rays. This epiphyseal line is present in almost all 3-year-old patients and 50% of 4-year-old patients. If still present at age 6, this epiphyseal line is considered abnormal [27, 28].
- Apex or tip of the odontoid develops from most caudal part of the occipital sclerotome or proatlas. This ossification center is called ossiculum terminale. It appears at the age of 3 years and fuses by 12 years.
- If ossiculum terminale persists after the age of 12, then it is called as ossiculum terminale persistent, and it has no clinical importance as it seldom causes instability and symptoms.

Etiology

- Idiopathic
- Familial or congenital [29, 30]

- Os odontoideum in identical twins without any evidence of trauma
- Acquired [6, 31–33]
  - Trauma (most common)
  - Infection
  - Osteonecrosis after halo pelvic traction [34]
- Associated with syndromes [35–37]
  - Down syndrome
  - Klippel-Feil syndrome
  - Morquio syndrome
  - Spondyloepiphyseal dysplasia

Pathogenesis

- The free ossicle of os odontoideum appears to be fixed with C1 arch and moves like one unit with C1 arch in flexion and extension movement of the neck.
- If there is instability present between C1 and C2 vertebrae due to os odontoideum, then it reduces the space available for spinal cord (SAC), but there is no change in ADI as the ossicle move with C1 arch (Figure 141.4).
- Instability is predominantly present in flexion and extension, but may present as grossly unstable in all directions [31, 38, 39].

Clinical Features

The average age of diagnosis is approximately 20 years [33].

- Symptoms from local irritation of C1–C2 joint [39, 40]
  - Neck pain
  - Torticollis
  - Headache
- Symptoms of spinal cord compression [39]
  - Episode of transient paresis after trauma
  - Complete myelopathy
  - Weakness
  - Loss of balance
  - Proprioceptive disturbances
  - Sphincter disturbances

- Symptoms of vertebral artery compression [25, 38, 41]
  - Seizures
  - Syncope
  - Vertigo
  - Mental disorientation
  - Visual disturbances

There is no cranial nerve involvement as the spinal cord affects below the level of foramen magnum.

Investigation

Investigation is done in the form of imaging.

- Plain X-ray cervical spine with anteroposterior, lateral neutral, lateral flexion, lateral extension, and open mouth view
- CT scan of the cervical spine with flexion and extension
  - Helpful to distinguish from fracture and in the case of multiple anomalies
- MRI of the cervical spine with flexion and extension of the neck
  - Helpful in seeing spinal cord compression, abnormal cord signal, and myelopathy and assessing space available for spinal cord (SAC)

Finding in imaging according to types of anomalies of odontoid:

- Agenesis
  - Slight depression between two superior articular facet of axis in open mouth view or on CT scan
- Hypoplasia
  - The most common type is peg-like odontoid projecting beyond the level of superior articular facet joint of axis.
- Os odontoideum
  - The free ossicle (oval or round) is about half the size of the odontoid with smooth sclerotic margins.
  - Usually it is confused with the following:
    ○ Traumatic nonunion [6, 33]

○ Acute fracture (usually fracture line is thin irregular and below the level of superior articular facet of axis)
○ Neurocentral synchondrosis in child younger than 5 years

- Finding of instability
  - Atlantodens interval (ADI)
    ○ More than 3 mm in adult and more than 4–5 mm in child
  - Space available for spinal cord (SAC)
    ○ Less than 14 mm
  - Sagittal plane rotation angle
    ○ More than 20°
  - Instability index [maximum SAC - minimum SAC + maximum SAC x 100(%)]
    ○ More than 40%

Prognosis

- Prognosis is good if the patient presents with mechanical symptoms like neck pain, headache, and torticollis or with transient neurological symptoms.
  - Prognosis is bad if the patient presents with progressive neurologic deficit.

Treatment

- In os odontoideum, the atlantoaxial joint is abnormal and can subluxate or dislocate with trivial trauma causing severe upper cervical spinal cord injury and on rare occasions death [39].

The patient with minor symptoms can be treated with cervical traction or immobilization.

- Prophylactic operative stabilization of asymptomatic patients with the instability of <5 mm is controversial [39, 42, 43].
- Indication of surgery:
  - Neurological involvement

- Instability of more than 5–10 mm posteriorly or anteriorly
- Progressive instability
- Persistent neck complaints
- Patients who require surgery need a CT angiogram to see vertebral artery anatomy and C1–C2 anatomy as anomalies of C1 are increased with os odontoideum [31]. The patient with the neurologic deficits needs skull traction before surgery to achieve reduction and allow recovery of spinal cord irritation by compression.

Surgical plan can be decided with the following flowchart:

Klippel-Feil Syndrome (Congenital Synostosis of Cervical Vertebrae)

Introduction

- In 1912, Klippel and Feil recognized this syndrome and described its clinical and pathological aspect [44].
- Their description included all manners of congenital fusion of the cervical vertebrae, whether it involves two segments, congenital block vertebrae, or the whole cervical spine.
- Male predominance (M/F, 1.5:1).
- Between 20 and 30 days of gestational age, paraxial mesoderm undergoes segmentation from cephalad to caudal.

- Each segment is called a somite.

- These somites are further divided into sclerotomes, myotomes, and dermatomes.

- The caudal portion of one sclerotome fuses with the cephalad portion of the sclerotome below to form vertebral body.

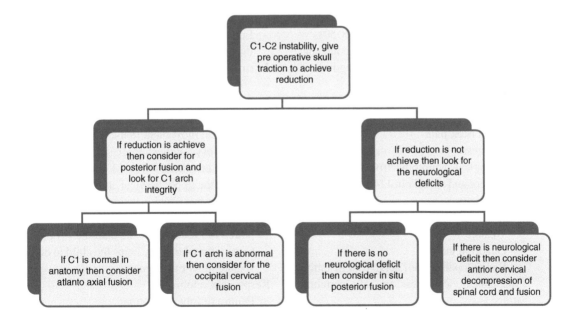

Etiology

- It is theorized that it results from disruption of the normal segmentation process during the third to eighth week of gestation.
- In a small subset of patients, this condition is inherited [45–48].
- Pedigree analysis explains specific genetic anomalies associated with this syndrome:
  - Heritable paracentric inversion of chromosome 8
  - Pax 1, Pax 9, and HOX
- Sometimes it is associated with the fetal alcohol syndrome [49].

Clinical Features

- Classic triad of clinical features:
  - Limitation of neck motion (most consistent finding) [50, 51]
  - Short neck
  - Low posterior hairline
- Range of motion can be compensated for due to hypermobility of unfused segments which caused near normal cervical range of motion.
- Less than 20% have fascial asymmetry, torticollis, or webbing of the neck (extreme case of webbing of the neck is called pterygium colli) [48, 50].
- Symptoms usually occur at the second and third decade of life at the unfused segment of the cervical spine [48, 51, 52].
  - Mechanical symptom from irritation of hypermobile joint capsule and ligaments
    ◦ Axial neck pain
    ◦ Stiffness
  - Neurological symptoms from irritation of nerve root and spinal cord [48, 53–55]
    ◦ Spasticity
    ◦ Hyperreflexia
    ◦ Weakness
    ◦ Quadriplegia
    ◦ Radiculopathy from nerve root irritation
  - Mechanical compression of vertebral artery
    ◦ Syncope
    ◦ Emboli
    ◦ Ischemic episode

Associated Anomalies

- Scoliosis
  - 60–70% of cases
  - Usually more than 15° Cobb's angle
  - May be associated with hemivertebra and may occur in the thoracic and lumbar spine as well
  - Needs entire spine radiograph to diagnose
- Renal anomalies
  - 30% of cases
  - Most common is unilateral absence of the kidney
  - Other anomalies are malrotation of the kidney, horseshoe kidney, ectopic kidney, and hydronephrosis of the kidney due to ureteropelvic obstruction
  - Needs ultrasound or intravenous pyelogram to diagnose [50]
- Cardiovascular anomalies
  - 4–14% of cases.
  - VSD is the most common anomaly.
  - May be associated with other congenital heart diseases.
- Deafness [56–59]
  - 30% of cases.
  - It may be conductive, sensorineural, or both.
  - Needs audiometric testing.
  - Earlier testing is better; otherwise, patient may develop some speech problem.
- Mirror motions (synkinesis)
  - 20% of cases.
  - Paired movement of the hand.
  - Unable to move one hand without similar reciprocal movement in the other hand.
  - In autopsy studies, there is presence of incomplete decussation of the pyramidal tract in the upper cervical cord.
  - In electromyography, patient with Klippel-Feil syndrome has electrically detectable paired motion in opposite extremity [60].
  - Occupational therapy helps the child to dissociate mirror movement.
- Respiratory anomalies
  - Failure of lobe formation
  - Ectopic lung
  - Restriction of lung function by scoliosis, rib fusion, or deformed costovertebral joints

- Sprengel deformity [48, 50, 55, 61]
  - 15–35% of cases
  - Unilateral or bilateral
  - Can cause decrease shoulder mobility
- Upper extremity anomalies
  - Syndactyly
  - Hypoplastic thumb
  - Supernumerary digit
  - Hypoplasia of the upper extremity

Classification

- Feil classification
  - Type I – lock fusion of all cervical and upper thoracic vertebrae
  - Type II – fusion of one or two pairs of cervical vertebra
  - Type III – cervical fusion in combination with lower thoracic and lumbar vertebrae
- Samartzis et al. classification [62]:
  - Type I – single-level fusion
  - Type II – multiple noncontiguous fusion
  - Type III – multiple contiguous fusion

Pattern of Cervical Fusion with Poor Prognosis (Fielding and Hensinger et al.)

- Pattern I – fusion of C2–C3 with occipitalization of the atlas.
- Pattern II – long fusion below C2 with abnormal occipitocervical junction.
- Pattern III – single open interspace between two fused segments.
- The first two patterns put stress on C1–C2, and the last pattern puts stress on open interspace between fused segments.

Investigation

- Plain radiograph
  - Cervical spine – anteroposterior, lateral, flexion, extension, and odontoid views
  - Entire spine – anteroposterior and lateral
- CT scan in flexion and extension

- MRI in flexion and extension
- Findings on imaging:
  - Fusion of cervical vertebrae is a hallmark of Klippel-Feil syndrome.
  - Other findings are widening and flattening of vertebral bodies, increase space available for the spinal cord, and absence of disc space.
  - Hemivertebra and fusion of posterior elements are also common.
  - Narrowing of the spinal canal due to degenerative changes at hypermobile segment is late finding.
  - Posterior spina bifida is common and present in 45% of cases.
  - Complete absences of posterior elements associated with fixed hyperextension and enlarged foramen magnum are also present and called as iniencephaly [63].
  - In young child narrowing of disc is not appreciable because unossified endplates give a false impression of disc space.

Treatment

- Patient with minimal involvement can expect normal active life without any treatment.
- Patient with high-risk pattern should restrict activity that put stress on the cervical spine.
- Neurologic injury and even death that can occur after minor trauma from disruption of hypermobile segment have been reported [48, 55].
- For symptomatic patients:
  - Mechanical symptoms
    ◦ Traction
    ◦ Cervical collar
    ◦ Analgesics
  - Neurological symptoms
    ◦ Surgical stabilization of the segment
    ◦ Surgical decompression of the spinal cord if it is present
  - Sprengel shoulder
    ◦ Surgical correction
  - Short neck and webbed neck
    ◦ Z-plasty and muscle resection can change contour of the neck and shoulder and can make the neck long [64].

- Scoliosis
  - Closed follow-up in the clinic
  - Bracing
  - Vertical expandable prosthetic titanium rib placement
  - Surgical correction fixation and fusion of the spine

Mass becomes maximal size at 1-2 month	If fails to disappear than muscle becomes permanently
and then remain same or disappear at 1 year.	fibrotic and develop torticollis

Congenital Muscular Torticollis (Wry Neck)

Introduction

- Usually discovered in the first 6–8 weeks of life
- The deformity caused by sternocleidomastoid muscle contracture with the head tilted toward the involved side and the chin rotated toward the other side
- More common on the right side
- Caused by the fibromatosis of the sternocleidomastoid muscle and either whole muscle becomes fibrotic or localized to the clavicular attachment of the muscle

Etiology

- Etiology is yet to be determined and unclear.
- But clinical studies suggest that it is due to difficult labor [65].
- It may represent the intrauterine or perinatal compartment syndrome in the sternocleidomastoid muscle [65].
- Various hypotheses of the cause of torticollis include malposition in utero, birth trauma, infection, and vascular injury to muscle.
- There may be increased risk of associated musculoskeletal disorder like:
- Metatarsal adductus
- Dysplastic disease of the hip (present in 7–20% of cases)
- Talipes equinovarus
- Sometimes, mass present on sternocleidomastoid muscle either is palpable at birth or usually appears during the first 4 weeks of age [66].

Differential Diagnosis

- Atlantoaxial rotatory subluxation
- Atlanto-occipital fusion
- Congenital odontoid anomalies
- Basilar impression
- Congenital C1 anomalies
- Klippel-Feil syndrome

Clinical Features

- Complains of head tilted toward the affected side and face toward opposite side.
- On clinical examination, compare the ear distance from the shoulder on both side, and on the affected side, the distance should be smaller than the non-affected side.
- Mass in the sternocleidomastoid muscle may be visible or palpable.
- Sternocleidomastoid muscle may feel tight and rigid on palpation.
- If deformity becomes worse, then patient may compensate with elevation of the shoulder and flattening of the face on the affected side.
- Resolution before 1 year may allow remodeling of the facial asymmetry.

Investigation

- US can be done to see mass and to see the sternocleidomastoid muscle [67].
- Radiograph of cervical spine to rule out bony anomalies or CT scan can be done to further work up possible bony abnormalities [68, 69].

Treatment

- Below 1 year –conservative treatment [66, 70, 71]
  - Parent should inform to stretch the sterno-cleidomastoid muscle by manipulating child's head manually during feeding, clothing, and diaper change.
  - Physical therapy is also an important component of treatment at this age.
- Prognostic factor for success of conservative treatment
  - Minimal initial rotation
  - Age less than 1 year at the presentation
  - Lack of tight palpable band
  - Mass in affected sternocleidomastoid muscle
- After 1 year
  - Mild deformity and age below 4 years – unipolar release of sternocleidomastoid muscle
  - Moderate to severe deformity and age more than 6 years – bipolar release of sternocleidomastoid muscle
- Indication of surgical treatment [72]
  - More than 1 year of age at presentation
  - Limitation of more than 30° in neck motion

Basilar Impression

Introduction

- It is deformity of the base of the skull and around foramen magnum.
- In 1939 Chamberlain first recognized this condition having clinical significance [73].
- Basilar impression is invagination of the upper cervical spine into the foramen magnum and tip of the odontoid migrate cephalad in the foramen magnum.

Types and Etiology of Basilar Impression

There are two types of basilar impression:

- Primary basilar impression

- It is congenital anomaly usually associated with the below-mentioned congenital abnormalities:
  - Atlanto-occipital fusion
  - Hypoplasia of the atlas
  - Bifid posterior arch of the atlas
  - Odontoid abnormalities
  - Klippel-Feil syndrome
  - Goldenhar syndrome [74]
- Secondary basilar impression
  - It is secondary to the other condition that causes softening of the bony structures of the base of the skull. And in the later life, weight of the head approaches more toward the ground, and the cervical spine remains in the same position:
    - Osteogenesis imperfecta (more common in types III and IV than in type I)
    - Osteochondrodysplasias
    - Osteomalacia
    - Rickets
    - Paget disease
    - Renal osteodystrophy
    - Rheumatoid arthritis
    - Neurofibromatosis
    - Ankylosing spondylitis
- Basilar impression is also associated with Arnold-Chiari malformation and syringomyelia [75–77].

Clinical Features

- If it is pure basilar impression, usually patients present with sensory and motor symptoms like weakness and paresthesia and headache and pain in the nape of the neck [76]. Even if this condition is congenital, most of the patient develops symptoms in their second and third decade because of increased ligament laxity and instability with age and decreased tolerance to compression of the spinal cord and vertebral arteries [76, 78].
- If associated with Chiari malformation, then it also presents with cerebellar and vestibular symptoms:
  - Unsteadiness of gait
  - Dizziness

– Nystagmus (vertical or lateral nystagmus)
- Symptoms with lower cranial nerve impingement, which comes from the medulla oblongata like V, IX, X, and XII like tinnitus, earaches, dysphasia, and poor phonation [76].
- Symptoms from blockage of aqueduct of Sylvius:
  – Increased intracranial pressure
  – Hydrocephalus
- Symptoms from compression of vertebral artery:
  – Dizziness
  – Syncope
  – Mental deterioration
  – Seizures
- It is also associated with the short neck, asymmetry of the face, and torticollis, but this is not specific with the basilar impression and can be present with other conditions of the cervical spine in pediatric patients.

Investigation

- Plain X-ray of the upper cervical spine with anteroposterior (AP), lateral (LAT), and odontoid view (Fig. 141.7).
  – It is very difficult to find the posterior lip of the foramen magnum, so Chamberlain line and McRae line are very difficult to define on plain X-rays. But McGregor line is easy to define on X-rays. If the tip of the odon-

toid is >4.5 mm above, McGregor line is considered as abnormal finding. But McGregor line depends on the hard palate, and sometimes patient may have high arched palate, facial abnormalities, and cranio-vertebral anomalies that make it difficult to review plain X-rays.
  – In AP view, Fischgold and Metzger (digastric) line extends between two digastric grooves (junction of the medial aspect of mastoid process at the base of the skull), and the line normally passes 10.7 mm above the odontoid tip and 11.6 mm above the atlanto-occipital joint.

- CT scan and MRI of the upper cervical spine.
- Normal measurement for CT scan and MRI is as follows:
  – Tip of odontoid should be 1.2 mm below Chamberlain line.
  – Tip of odontoid should be 0.9 mm below McGregor line.
  – Tip of odontoid should be 4.6 mm below McRae line.
- MRI also allows us to identify neural compression and presence of other pathological findings. Functional MRI obtained with cervical spine in flexion and extension gives an idea about the dynamic compression.

Treatment

- Many patients with basilar impression have no neurological symptoms, and some have minimal symptoms with no sign of progressive neurological involvement; these patients can be observed and need closed follow-up for neurology examination.
- Conservative treatment for symptomatic basilar impression has not been successful. Treatment of symptomatic patients requires multidisciplinary approach, and it includes orthopedics, neurosurgeon, neurologist, and radiologist and also for the symptomatic patients.
  – Hydrocephalus from aqueductal stenosis, if present, must be addressed first with the ventricular shunting before any other surgeries [80].

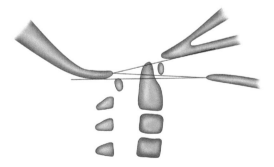

Fig. 141.7 Lateral view of the upper cervical spine with lower cranium showing three lines. (1) Chamberlain line is from the posterior lip of the foramen magnum to the dorsal margin of the hard palate. (2) McGregor line is from the upper surface of the posterior edge of the hard palate to the caudal part of the occipital curve of the skull [79]. (3) McRae line is from the posterior lip to the anterior lip of the foramen magnum

– Try to realign the cervical spine and decompress the neural elements by head position and halo traction and then do pain X-ray or MRI to check decompression and realignment.

If patient respond to the alignment then	If patient no respond to the alignment then
do suboccipital craniotomy and upper cervical	do anterior decompression by resecting ante-
laminectomy and occipitocervical arthrodesisrior atlas, odontoid, distal clivus and then	posterior decompression and fusion

References
Pseudosubluxation in Cervical Spine

1. Cattell HS, Filtz DL. Pseudosubluxation and other normal variation in cervical spine in children. J Bone Joint Surg Am. 1965;47-A:1295–309.
2. Shaw M, Burnett H, Wilson A. Pseudosubluxation of C2 on C3 in polytraumatized children – prevalence and significance. Clin Radiol. 1979;54:377–80.
3. Swischuk LE. Anterior displacement C2 in children: physiologic or pathologic. Radiolog. 1977;122:759–63.

Atlantoaxial Instability

4. Greenberg AD. Atlantoaxial dislocation. Brain. 1968;91:655.
5. Bharucha EP, Dastur HM. Craniovertebral anomalies (a report on 10 cases). Brain. 1964;87:469.
6. McRae DL. Bony abnormalities in the region of the foramen magnum: correlation of the anatomic and neurologic findings. Acta Radiol. 1953;40:335.
7. Perovic NM, Kopits SE, Thompson RC. Radiologic evaluation of the spinal cord in congenital atlanto-axial dislocation. Radiology. 1973;109:713.
8. Ali MM, Russell N, Awada N, et al. Acraniocervicalmalforma- tion presenting as acute respiratory failure. J Emerg Med. 1996;14:569–72.
9. Reddy KR, Rao GS, Devi BI, et al. Pulmonary function after surgery for congenital atlantoaxial dislocation. J Neurosurg Anesthesiol. 2009;21:196–201.
10. Parfenchuck TA, Bertrand SL, Powers MJ, et al. Posterior occipitoatlantal hypermobility in down syndrome: an analysis of 199 patients. J Pediatr Orthop. 1994;14:305.

11. Dickman CA, Mamourian A, Sonntag VK, et al. Magnetic reso- nance imaging of the transverse atlan-tal ligament for the evalu- ation of atlantoaxial insta-bility. J Neurosurg. 1991;75:221–7.
12. Gupta V, Khandelwal N, Mathuria SN, et al. Dynamic magnetic resonance imaging evaluation of cranio-vertebral junction abnormalities. J Comput Assist Tomogr. 2007;31:354–9.
13. Steel HH. Anatomical and mechanical considerations of the atlanto-axial articulations. J Bone Joint Surg Am. 1968;50:1481.
14. Ahmed R, Trynelis VC, Menezes AH. Fusions at the craniover- tebral junction. Childs Nerv Syst. 2008;24:1209–24.
15. Kumar R, Kalra SK, Mahapatra AK. A clinical scoring system for neurological assessment of high cervical myelopathy: Mea- surements in pediatric patients with congenital atlantoaxial dislocations. Neurosurgery. 2007;61:987–94.

Atlantoaxial Rotatory Subluxation

16. Mezue WC, Taha ZM, Bashir EM. Fever and acquired torticollis in hospitalized children. J Laryngol Otol. 2002;116:280–4.
17. Watson-Jones R. Spontaneous hyperaemic dislocation of atlas. Proc R Soc Med. 1931;25:586.
18. Coutts MB. Atlantooccipital Subluxations. Arch Surg. 1934;29:297.
19. Firrani-Gallotta G, Luzzatti G. Sublussazione laterale e sublussazione rotatorie dell atlante. Arch Orthop Trauma Surg. 1957;70:467.
20. Kawabe N, Hirotani H, Tanaka O. Pathomechanism of atlanto-axial rotatory fixation in children. J Pediatr Orthop. 1989;9:569.
21. Fielding JW, Hawkins RJ. Atlantoaxial rotatory fixa-tion (fixed rotatory subluxation of the atlantoaxial joint). J bone Joint surg. 1977;59A:37.
22. Phillips WA, Hensinger RN. The management of rota-tory atlantoaxial subluxation in children. J Bone Joint Surg. 1989;71A:664.
23. Fielding JW, Hawkins RJ, Ratzan S. Fusion for atlan-toaxial instability. J Bone Joint Surg. 1976;58A:400.

Anomalies of Odontoid (Dens)

24. Macalister A. Notes on the development and varia-tions of the atlas. J Anat Physiol. 1983;27:519.
25. Shapiro R, Youngsberg AS, SLGR. Thedifferentialdiag-nosis of traumatic lesions of the occipito-atlanto-axial segment. Radiol Clin North Am. 1971;3:505.
26. Sherk HH, Nicholson JL. Ossiculum terminale and mongolism. J Bone Joint Surg Am. 1969;51:957.
27. Cattell HS, Filtzer DL. Pseudosubluxation and other normal variations in the cervical spine in children. J Bone Joint Surg Am. 1965;47:1295.

28. Fielding JW. The cervical spine in the child. Curr Pract Orthop Surg. 1973;5:31.
29. Kirlew KA, Hathout GM, Reiter SD, et al. Os odontoideum in identical twins: perspectives on etiology. Skeletal Radiol. 1993;22:525–7.
30. Phillips PC, Lorentsen KJ, Shropshire LC, et al. Congenital odontoid aplasia and posterior circulation stroke in childhood. Ann Neurol. 1988;23:410–3.
31. Fielding JW, Hensinger RN, Hawkins RJ. Os odontoideum. J Bone Joint Surg Am. 1980;62:376.
32. Sankar WN, Wills BP, Dorman JP, Drummond DS. Os odontoideum revisted: the case for a multifactorial etiology. Spine. 2006;31:979.
33. Wollin DG. The os odontoideum: separate odontoid process. J Bone Joint Surg Am. 1963;45:1459.
34. Tredwell SJ, O'Brien JP. Avascular necrosis of the proximal end of the dens: a complication of halopelvic distraction. J Bone Joint Surg. 1975;57A:332.
35. Burke SW, French HG, Roberts JM, et al. Chronic atlanto-axial instability in down syndrome. J Bone Joint Surg Am. 1985;67:1356–60.
36. Hensinger RN. Osseous anomalies of the craniovertebral junc- tion. Spine. 1986;111:323.
37. Spitzer R, Rabinowitch JY, Wybar KC. A study of the abnor- malities of the skull, teeth, and lenses in mongolism. Can Med Assoc J. 1961;84:567–72.
38. Fielding JW, Hawkins RJ, Ratzan SA. Spine fusion for atlanto- axial instability. J Bone Joint Surg Am. 1976;58:400.
39. Klimo Jr P, Kan P, Rao G, et al. Os odontoideum: presentation, diagnosis, and treatment in a series of 78 patients. J Neurosurg Spine. 2008;9:332–42.
40. Gwinn JL, Smith JL. Acquired and congenital absence of the odontoid process. Am J Roentgenol Radium Ther Nucl Med. 1962;88:424.
41. Rowland LP, Shapiro JH, Jacobson HG. Neurological syn- dromes associated with congenital absence of the odontoid process. Arch Neurol Psychiatry. 1958;80:286.
42. Garber JN. Abnormalities of the atlas and axis vertebrae, congenital and traumatic. J Bone Joint Surg Am. 1964;46:1782.
43. Minderhoud JM, Braakman R, Penning L. Os odontoideum: clinical, radiological and therapeutic aspecs. J Neurol Sci. 1969;89:521.

Klippel-Feil Syndrome (Congenital Synostosis of Cervical Vertebrae, Brevicollis)

44. Klippel M, Feil A. Un cas d'absence des vertèbres cervicales avec cage thoracique remontant jusqu'a la base du crane. Nouv Icon Salpet. 1912;25:223.
45. Clarke RA, Kearsley JH, Walsh DA. Patterned expression in familial Klippel-Feil syndrome. Teratology. 1996;53:152–7.
46. Clarke RA, Singh S, McKenzie H, et al. Familial Klippel-Feil syndrome and paracentric inversion inv(8)(q22.2q.23.3). Am J Hum Genet. 1995;57:1364–70.
47. Gunderson CH, Greenspan RH, Glaser GH, et al. Klippel-Feil syndrome: genetic and clinical re-evaluation of cervical fusion. Medicine. 1967;46:491–511.
48. Gray SW, Romaine CB, Skandalakis JF. Congenital fusion of the cervical vertebrae. Surg Gynecol Obstet. 1964;118:373.
49. Schilgen M, Loeser H. Klippel-Feil anomaly combined with fetal alcohol syndrome. Eur Spine J. 1994;3:289–90.
50. Hensinger RN, Lang JR, MacEwen GD. The Klippel-Feil syn- drome: a constellation of related anomalies. J Bone Joint Surg Am. 1974;56:1246.
51. Ulmer JL, Elster AD, Ginsberg LE, et al. Klippel-Feilsyndrome: CT and MRI of congenital abnormalities of cervical spine and cord. J Comput Assist Tomogr. 1993;17:215–24.
52. Pizzutillo PD, Woods MW, Nicholson L. Risk factors in the Klippel-Feil syndrome. Orthop Trans. 1987;11:473.
53. Erskine CA. An analysis of the Klippel-Feil syndrome. Archives of Pathology. 1946;41:269–81.
54. Illingworth RS. Attacks of unconsciousness in association with fused cervical vertebrae. Arch Dis Child. 1956;31:8.
55. Shoul MI, Ritvo M. Clinical and roentgenological manifesta- tions of the Klippel-Feil syndrome (congenital fusion of the cervical vertebrae, brevicollis): Report of eight additional cases and review of the literature. AJR Am J Roentgenol. 1952;68:369.
56. Jalladeau J. Malformations congénitales associées syndrome de Klippel-Feil. Thèse de Paris. 1936.
57. McLay K, Maran AG. Deafness and the Klippel-Feilsyndrome. J Laryngol Otol. 1969;83:175.
58. Palant DI, Carter BL. Klippel-Feil syndrome and deafness. Am J Dis Child. 1972;123:218.
59. Stark EW, Borton TE. Hearing loss and the Klippel-Feil syn- drome. Am J Dis Child. 1972;123:233.
60. Baird PA, Robinson GC, Buckler WS. Klippel-Feil syndrome. Am J Dis Child. 1967;113:546.
61. Forney WR, Robinson SJ, Pascoe DJ. Congenital heart disease, deafness, and skeletal malformations: a new syndrome? J Pediatr. 1966;68:14.
62. Samartzis D, Kalluri P, Herman J, et al. The role of congenitally fused cervical segments upon the space available for the cord and associated symptoms in Klippel-Feil patients. Spine. 2008;33:1442–50.
63. Sherk HH, Shut L, Chung S. Iniencephalic deformity of cervical spine with Klippel-Feil anomalies and congenital elevation of the scapula. J Bone Joint Surg Am. 1974;56:1254.
64. McElfresh E, Winter R. Klippel-Feil syndrome. Minn Med. 1973;56:353.

Torticollis (Wry Neck)

65. Davids JR, Wenger DR, Mubarak SJ. Congenital muscular tor- ticollis: sequela of intrauterine or perinatal compartment syn- drome. J Pediatr Orthop. 1993;13:141–7.
66. Ling CM, Low YS. Sternomastoid tumor and muscular torticol- lis. Clin Orthop. 1972;86:144.
67. Chan YL, Cheng JC, Metreweil LC. Ultrasonography of con- genital muscular torticollis. Pediatr Radiol. 1992;22:356–60.
68. Brougham DI, Cole WG, Dickens DR, et al. Torticollis due to a combination of sternomastoid contracture and congenital vertebral anomalies. J Bone Joint Surg Br. 1989;71:404.
69. Slate RK, Posnick JC, Armstrong DC, et al. Cervical spine subluxation associated with congenital muscular torticollis and craniofacial asymmetry. Plast Reconstr Surg. 1993;91:1187.
70. Coventry MB, Harris LE. Congenital muscular torticollis in infancy: some observations regarding treatment. J Bone Joint Surg Am. 1959;41:815.
71. MacDonald C. Sternomastoid tumor and muscular torticollis. J Bone Joint Surg Br. 1969;51:432.
72. Canale ST, Griffin DW, Hubbard CN. Congenital muscular tor- ticollis: long-term follow-up. J Bone Joint Surg Am. 1982;64:810.

Basilar Impression

73. Chamberlin WE. Basilar Impression (Platybasia): a bizarre developmental anomaly of the occipital bone and upper cervical spine with striking and misleading neurological manifestation. Yale J Biol Med. 1939;11(487)

74. Gosain AK, McCarthy JG, Pinto RS. Cervicovertebral anomalies and basilar impression in Goldenhar syndrome. Plast Reconstr Surg. 1994;93:498–506.
75. Bassi P, Corona C, Contri P, et al. Congenital basilar impression: correlated neurological syndromes. Eur Neurol. 1992;32:238–43.
76. De Barros MC, Faria W, Ataide L, et al. Basilar impression and Arnold-Chiari malformation: a study of 66 cases. J Neurol Neurosurg Psychiatry. 1968;1:596.
77. Kohno K, Sakaki S, Nakamura H, et al. Foramen Magnum decompression for syringomyelia associated with basilar impression and chiari I malformation: Report of three cases. Neurol Med Chir. 1991;31:715–9.
78. Samartzis D, Kalluri P, Herman J, et al. Superior odontoid migration in Klippel-Feil patient. Eur Spine J. 2007;16:1489–97.
79. McGregor M. The significance of certain measurements of the skull in the diagnosis of basilar impression. Br J Radiol. 1948;21:171.
80. Sawin PD, Menezes AH. Basilar Invagination in osteogenesis imperfecta and related osteochondral dysplasisas: medical and surgical management. J Neurosurg. 1997;86:950–60.

John P. Lubicky

Introduction

- Spondylolisthesis – slipping of one vertebra on another most commonly at L5-S1
- Spondylolysis – defect/fracture of the pars interarticularis also most frequent at L5 (Fig. 142.1)
- Spondylolisthesis: First described by Herineaux, an obstetrician, in 1782 – discovered spondyloptosis blocking the birth canal

- Kilian – in 1852 – coined the term.
- Neugebauer, in 1888, recognized the lytic type.
- Robert, the 1800s – cadaver studies sequentially severing posterior ligamentous elements and pars to demonstrate how slipping occurs.
- Descriptions based on anatomic dissections before radiography.

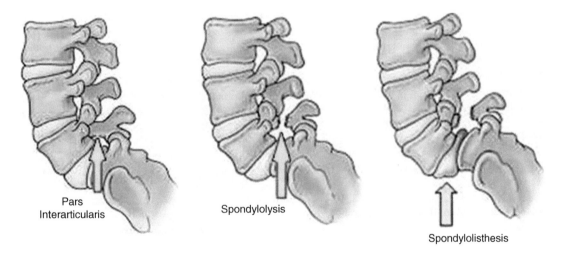

Pars Interarticularis

Spondylolysis

Spondylolisthesis

Fig. 142.1 Illustration of the status of the pars from intact to lysis to lysis with slip

J.P. Lubicky, MD
Department of Orthopaedics, West Virginia University, Morgantown, WV 9196, USA
e-mail: jlubicky@hsc.wvu.edu

© Springer International Publishing AG 2017
A.E.M. Eltorai et al. (eds.), *Orthopedic Surgery Clerkship*, DOI 10.1007/978-3-319-52567-9_142

- Radiography allowed diagnosis on live patients and revealed different types and severity of slips necessitating a classification system.
- Newman and Wiltse – first comprehensive classification – (Table 142.1)
  ○ Weakness was not differentiating enough difference between dysplastic and lytic types – different natural history
- Marchetti and Bartolozzi classification (Table 142.2)
  ○ Two broad groups: developmental and acquired
  ○ Developmental type – high and low dysplasia – bad actor
    • Dysplasia of the components of the L-S junction
    • Underdeveloped facets, poor disc bond – hook-clasp concept of stability
    • Remodeling of sacral dome
    • Lysis of pars – not essential

Table 142.1 Newman – Wiltse classification

I	Dysplastic	A: facet with axial orientation B: facet with sagittal orientation
II	Isthmic	A: lysis B: elongation C: fracture
III	Degenerative	
IV	Post-traumatic	
V	Pathologic	
VI	Postsurgical	

Table 142.2 Marchetti-Bartolozzi classification

Developmental	Acquired
High dysplastic	Traumatic
With lysis	Acute fracture
With elongation	Stress fracture
	Postsurgical
	Direct
	Indirect
Low dysplastic	Pathologic
With lysis	Local
With elongation	Systemic
	Degenerative
	Primary
	Secondary

Etiology and Risk of Slippage

Developmental Type: Dysplasia of the Formation of the L-S Junction

- Abnormality allows gravity to displace the spine because of incompetent anatomic structures
- Displacement can be severe > spondyloptosis – L5 in front of the sacrum
- May be familial – potential genetic component

Acquired Type: Most Common (Lytic Type), Essential Component – Pars Defect

- Defect provides point of disconnection of the posterior elements of L5 with the sacrum and pelvis from the spine above.
- The spine can "rock" on the L5-S1 disc.
- Not a bad actor; maximal amount of slip not severe and reaches maximum in adolescence.

Risk Factors for Further Slip

- Patient characteristics – age, heredity, and pathology
- Classification – developmental vs acquired – different natural history
- Anatomy – integrity of the hook and clasp, disc bond, sacral doming, and slip angle
- Spinopelvic relationship – described by radiographic parameters as measured on standing lateral C-T-L radiographs that include the hip joints (Fig. 142.2)
- Pelvic incidence – specific for each individual – constant relationship
  - Sum of pelvic tilt and sacral slope
  - Should be within 10° of lumbar lordosis
- Patients with high PI and SS – "shear" force across L-S junction – set up for "unbalanced spine" described as + imbalance – lean forward with or without knee flexion
- Patients with low PI and SS – posterior compression at L-S junction, "nutcracker" – tend to be "balanced" (six types described)
- High slip angle – most important factor for further slip – basically a kyphotic relationship between L5 and S1 (Fig. 142.3)

Fig. 142.2 Demonstration of a severe developmental spondylolisthesis with typical rounding of the top of the sacrum seen on the lateral and the axial view of the slipped L5 sometimes called the "Inverted Napoleon's Hat" sign

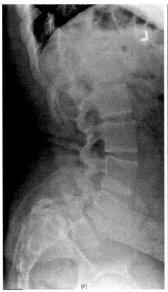
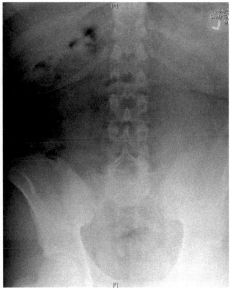

Presentation

- Presenting complaints – back pain +/– deformity; +/– history of recent injury; +/– history of leg pain
- Activities associated with repeated back hyperextension (gymnastics, FB, diving, etc), abnormality of gait
- Pain – activity related and usually without sciatica
- Physical exam – may appear normal, or + spinal imbalance, gait abnormality, tight hamstrings, limited ROM, abnormal stance (jump position), abnormal appearance of back (L-S step-off), and appearance of shortened trunk

Diagnosis

- Conventional radiography
- Standing long PA and lateral C-T-L plain radiographs to include the hips
- Standing spot lateral L-S spine to include the hips (Fig. 142.3)
- Oblique L-S spine images – usually unhelpful – needless radiation
- Measure spinopelvic parameters and amount of slip and assess global balance
  - Nuclear imaging – three-phase technetium bone scan with SPECT imaging
    - Assesses metabolic activity in pars

- Advanced imaging – CT without contrast
  - Best to demonstrate the anatomy (unfortunately done recumbent, do standing if technology available)
  - MRI without contrast
  - Best to evaluate disc, nerve roots, and thecal sac
  - May demonstrate metabolic activity in the pars – signal change

Treatment

Spondylolysis

- Determine acuity – + bone scan – chance to heal pars
- If bone scan + LSO for at least 3–6 months evaluate healing on radiograph or CT > gradually wean from brace > PT for core strengthening > slowly resume activities
- If bone scan cold – treat symptomatically with or without LSO (no natural endpoint for bracing in this scenario), PT, NSAIDs, resume activities when symptoms resolved or tolerable
- If symptoms recur or never resolve consider:
  - Pars repair (best for lysis above L5) no more than G 1-associated slip
  - P-L fusion with instrumentation (Fig. 142.4)

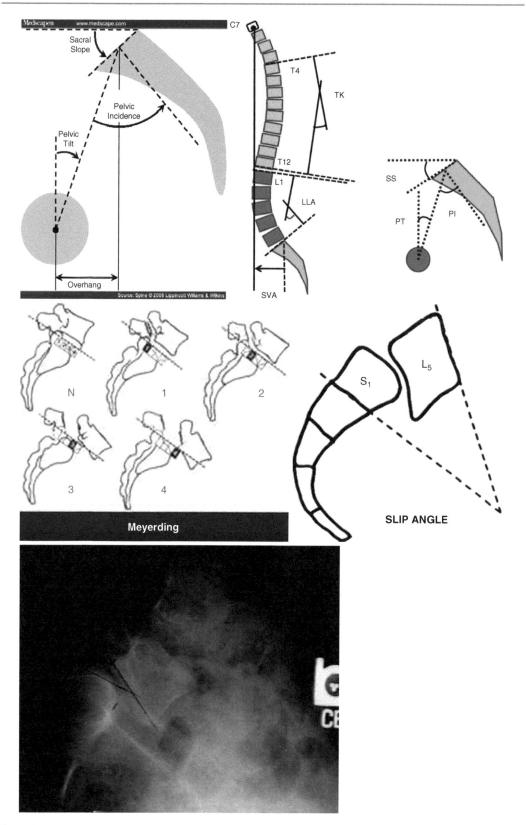

Fig. 142.3 Illustration of the various spino-pelvic parameters

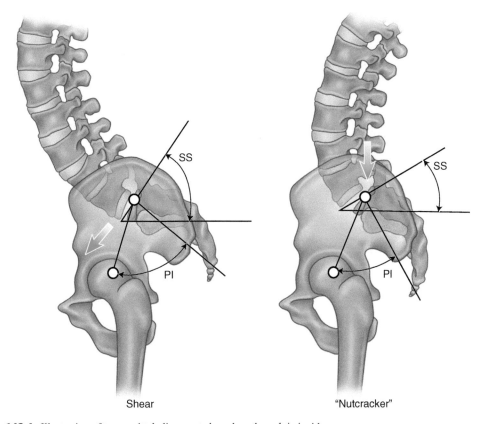

Shear   "Nutcracker"

Fig. 142.4 Illustration of two sagittal alignments based on the pelvic incidence

Spondylolisthesis

- Nonoperative treatment (mainstay): activity modification, PT, and NSAIDs
  - May have asymptomatic periods interspersed with symptomatic ones
- Surgical treatment – P-L fusion in situ – gold standard
  - Traditionally no instrumentation but not now
  - Options: P-L fusion with instrumentation – when overall balance is good
    - May supplement usual construct with ASF. PLIF TLIF or transsacral bone graft and/or cage
    - Reduction – more complicated and neuro risky
      - Goal is to realign, not 100% reduction
      - Requires 360 fusion with instrumentation
    - Vertebrectomy (Gaines procedure)
    - For spondyloptosis – usually two stages (Figs. 142.5 and 142.6)
      - Technically very difficult and tedious
      - >50% risk of some neuro deficit postoperative
      - Completely realigns the spine
    - Neuromonitoring is essential for all options – cauda equina
    - Syndrome described after P-lL fusion in situ

Summary

- Spondylolysis and spondylolisthesis are diagnosis contradictions because symptoms in patients carrying these diagnoses can be so disparate. There seem to be few absolute indications for any kind of treatment, especially

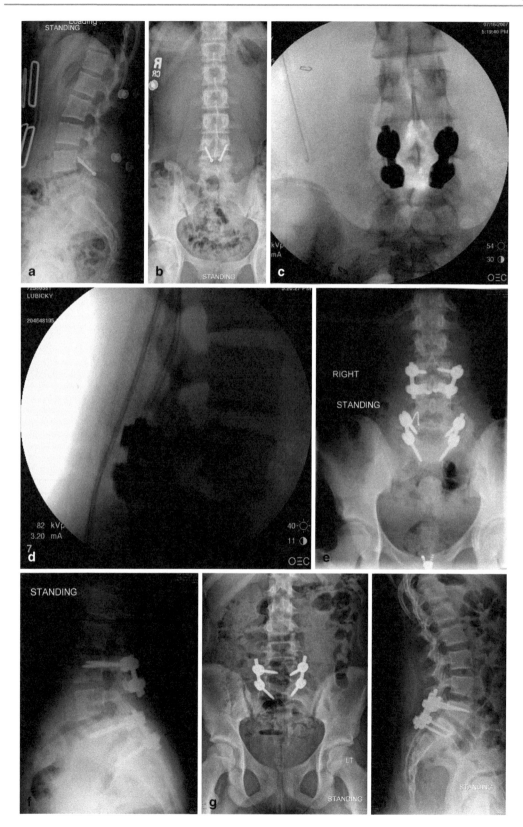

Fig. 142.5 (**a**, **b**) Buck pars repair. (**c**, **d**) pedicle screw/sublaminar hook repair. (**e**, **f**) 1 level pars reapir & L5-S1 PL fusion. (**g**, **h**) L5-S1 PL fusion

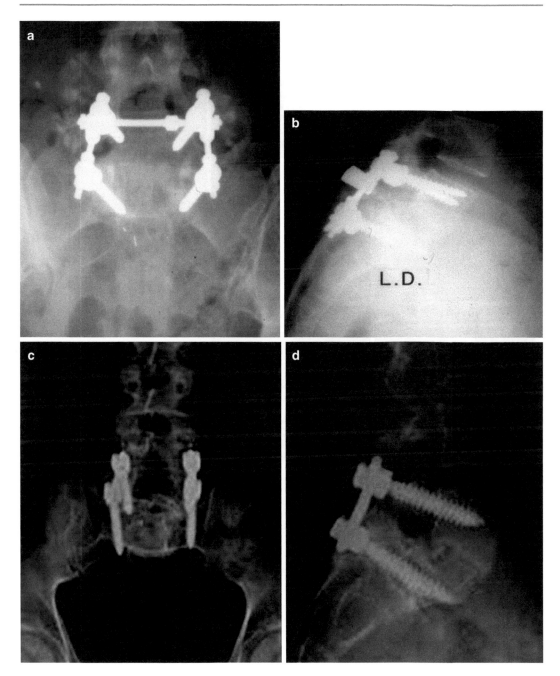

Fig. 142.6 (a–f) listhesis reductions using different implants a interbody structural supports. (g–i) spondyloptosis treated with Gaines procedure

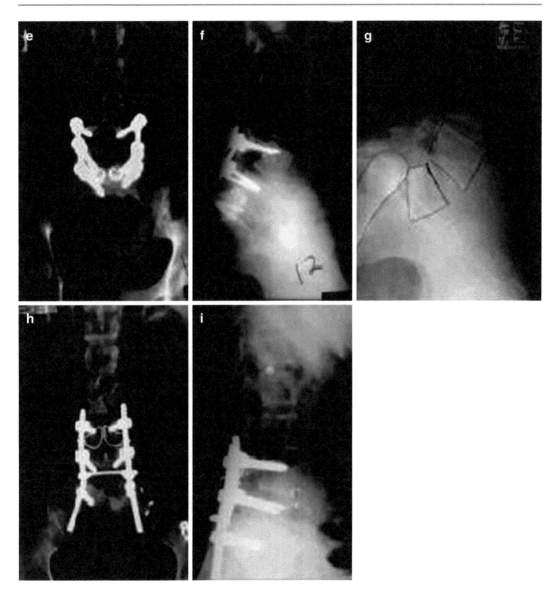

Fig. 142.6 (continued)

surgery. Neurologic deficit (uncommon) and severe deformity that interferes with function may qualify. Surgery for the relief of back pain is always problematic and often unreliable. An uneventful operation without complications evaluated by the usual radiographic may seem perfect. Yet the PRO may be poor. This and the fact that some patients with even severe slips may be asymptomatic is a treatment conundrum.

Reference

(Students are encouraged to peruse the extensive collection of classic papers included in the bibliographies of the following textbook chapters)

1. Shah SA, Shafa E. Scheuermann's Kyphosis. In: Heary RF, Albert TJ, editors. Spinal deformities: the essentials. 2nd edn. New York: Thieme Medical Publishers; 2014. p. 163–74.

Pediatric Spine Trauma

143

J. Mason DePasse, Craig P. Eberson,
and Alan H. Daniels

Spine Trauma Evaluation

- Suspect spine trauma in high-energy injuries, head injuries, or multiple abdominal injuries.
- Use a pediatric backboard – the high head/neck ratio in children may result in cervical hyperflexion when on a standard backboard.
- Perform a thorough neurologic exam.
  - If deficits are present, check for spinal shock by checking the bulbocavernosus reflex.

Imaging

- Begins with plain films of the affected area of the spine.
- Any detected fracture mandates imaging of the entire spine and advanced imaging.
- Low-dose CT or MRI should also be performed in the setting of high clinical suspicion, head injuries, altered mental status, or inability to cooperate with exam.

J.M. DePasse, MD (✉) • C.P. Eberson, MD
Department of Orthopedic Surgery, Division of
Pediatric Surgery, Warren Alpert Medical School of
Brown University, Providence, RI, USA
e-mail: jmdepasse@gmail.com

A.H. Daniels, MD
Department of Orthopedic Surgery, Division of Spine
Surgery, Warren Alpert Medical School of Brown
University, Providence, RI, USA

- May perform flexion and extension plain films to check for occult ligamentous injury.

Upper Cervical Spine Trauma

Occipitocervical Dissociation or Atlanto-occipital Dissociation

- Very high mortality.
- Young children at highest risk due to a larger head/neck ratio, smaller occipital condyles, and ligamentous laxity.
- Common measurements used to make the diagnosis, such as Power's ratio or Harris' rule of 12, may be ineffective.
- Treated with surgical stabilization and immobilization in a halo.

Occipital Condyle Fractures

- Rare in children, though CT should be performed in patients with basilar skull fractures or head injuries with neck pain
- Three types:
  - Type 1 – comminuted impaction fracture
  - Type 2 – condyle fracture with associated basilar skull fracture
  - Type 3 – alar ligament avulsions
- Most treated with cervical orthosis

© Springer International Publishing AG 2017
A.E.M. Eltorai et al. (eds.), *Orthopedic Surgery Clerkship*, DOI 10.1007/978-3-319-52567-9_143

- Occipitocervical fusion or halo immobilization for unstable type 3 fractures

Atlas or C1 Ring Injuries

- May fail through the bone or synchondrosis:
  - Posterior synchondrosis closes at 3 years of age, while neurocentral synchondrosis closes at 7 years.
  - Fractures through the synchondrosis are difficult to appreciate.
- Type:
  - Anterior or posterior arch fracture
  - Burst or "Jefferson" fracture, bilateral anterior, and posterior arch fractures from axial load
  - Lateral mass fracture
- Stability determined by the transverse atlantal ligament (TAL):
  - May evaluate TAL on open-mouth odontoid view or CT scan.
  - Rule of Spence – if lateral masses displaced more than 6.9 mm (8 mm with radiographic magnification), then TAL is disrupted, and fractures are unstable.
  - Displacement of the lateral masses >2 mm relatively to the superior articular facet of the axis is concerning in adults, but in children younger than 4, a "pseudo-spread" is commonly seen.
- Treated with a cervical orthosis, Minerva cast, or halo vest if stable or halo traction if unstable:
  - Fusion required if instability persists

Atlantoaxial Rotatory Subluxation (AARS)

- Fixed rotational deformity of C1 on C2 with loss of motion and pain:
  - Patients present with head tilted to one side and rotated toward the other.
- May follow minor trauma, an upper respiratory infection (Grisel syndrome) or an ENT procedure.
- Differentiate from congenital torticollis:
  - No pain in congenital torticollis.
  - Torticollis is passively correctable.

- In torticollis, sternocleidomastoid tight on side contralateral to chin deviation, while in AARS, sternocleidomastoid tight on ipsilateral side as an attempt to correct deviation.
- Types:
  - Unilateral rotation of C1 without displacement
  - Anterior displacement of one lateral mass by 3–5 mm and deficiency of TAL
  - Anterior displacement of both lateral masses by 5 mm and deficiency of the TAL and secondary ligaments
  - Posterior displacement due to an injury to the dens
- May evaluate with lateral skull radiograph, open-mouth odontoid, or dynamic CT.
- Treatment depends on duration of symptoms:
  - Less than 1 week – soft collar, anti-inflammatories, and physical therapy
  - Greater than 1 week – halter traction and muscle relaxants
  - Greater than 1 month – halo traction and bracing
  - Greater than 3 months or irreducible – posterior fusion

Odontoid or Dens Fractures

- Most commonly through the synchondrosis at the base of the odontoid, Salter-Harris I fractures
  - Synchondrosis fuses at 6 years of age, so fractures usually before 6
- Likely from sudden deceleration and forced head flexion
- Spinal cord injury more common than in adults
- Treated with closed reduction in extension followed by a halo or Minerva cast

Os Odontoideum

- Hypoplastic dens separate from the C2 vertebral body with smooth cortical margins.
- Unclear if developmental abnormality or nonunion after trauma.

- May be asymptomatic, cause pain, cause myelopathic symptoms, or cause intracranial symptoms from vertebrobasilar ischemia.
- Instability can be seen on flexion and extension radiographs.
- Surgical fusion followed by halo immobilization required for neurologic symptoms or instability.

Traumatic Spondylolisthesis, also Called "Hangman's Fracture"

- Bilateral pars fracture caused by hyperextension and axial load
- Neurologic injury rare, as this widens the canal
- Often associated with child abuse
- Anterolisthesis of C2 on C3 seen on radiographs, but must be differentiated from persistent synchondrosis or congenital arch defect
- Treated with closed reduction with neck extension and placement of a halo or Minerva cast

Lower Cervical Spine Trauma

- More common in adolescents as their spine approaches maturity

Ligamentous Injuries

- Usually in children younger than 8
- Caused by flexion and distraction
- Diagnosed with radiography or MRI
- Treated with immobilization in a hard collar or halo
- Fusion required for persistent instability

Compression Fractures Are Failure of the Anterior Column or Anterior Vertebral Body

- Caused by flexion and axial loading.
- Must be differentiated from incomplete ossification of anterior vertebral body

- Treated with hard collar if stable, surgical fusion required if unstable from injury to the posterior ligamentous complex.
- Burst fractures include failure of the anterior and middle columns, often with retropulsion of fracture into the spinal canal.
- Treated with a hard collar or halo in patients without neurologic symptoms or decompression and fusion if symptoms are present.

Facet Dislocations

- Bilateral or unilateral
  - Unilateral facet dislocations missed frequently on plain radiographs.
- May cause radiculopathy (more common with unilateral) or significant spinal cord injury (more common with bilateral).
- Prereduction MRI performed if the patient is obtunded or unable to cooperate.
- Reduction with Gardner-Wells tongs or a halo and hanging weights.
- Surgical fixation should be considered following reduction.

Thoracolumbar Spine Trauma

Commonly Caused by Inappropriate Seat Belt Use

- Tends to lie over the abdomen in small children, causing hyperflexion of the spine in deceleration.
- Lap belts should always lie over the pelvis.

Denis Three-Column Classification

- Anterior column consists of the anterior longitudinal ligament and anterior two thirds of the vertebral body.
- Middle column consists of the posterior one third of the vertebral body, intervertebral disc, and posterior longitudinal ligament.
- Posterior column consists of posterior elements of the osseous spine.

Compression Fractures

- Most common thoracolumbar injury in pediatric spine trauma
- Caused by flexion and axial compression
- Failure of the anterior column only
- Treated with 6–8 weeks of bracing in a thoracolumbosacral orthosis (TLSO)

Burst Fractures

- Caused by axial load
- Thoracic fractures more likely to cause neurologic injury due to tighter canal
- Stability assessed by kyphotic deformity, lamina fracture, and posterior ligamentous injury
- Treated with 6–8 weeks of bracing in a TLSO or hyperextension cast if stable and instrumentation with or without decompression and fusion if unstable

Flexion-Distraction Injuries (Chance Injuries)

- May be purely boney, purely ligamentous, or a mix
- Treated with 8 weeks of TLSO immobilization if the injury is boney and the fracture is reduced or surgical stabilization with instrumentation if purely ligamentous

Apophyseal Fractures

- Unique to children with open physes, typically under 10
- Separation of the vertebral apophysis from the spongiosa of the vertebral body
- Analogous to adult disc herniation, as the apophysis herniates into the canal
- Treated with 8 weeks of TLSO immobilization and anti-inflammatories if no neurologic symptoms but may require decompression if symptoms are present

Spinous and Transverse Process Fractures

- Isolated fractures may be treated with pain control.
- Lower lumbar transverse process fractures may be associated with unstable pelvic fractures.

Cauda Equina Syndrome

- The spinal cord ends at L3 in newborns and then migrates to L1 in adults.
- Injury to the neural elements caudal to the cord may cause cauda equina syndrome.
- Bilateral lower extremity weakness, perianal and perigenital numbness, loss of bowel control, and urinary retention
- Treated with emergent decompression

Spinal Cord Injury

- Relatively rare in the pediatric population.
  - Most occur in the cervical spine
- Neurologic prognosis is better than in adults, but development of scoliosis secondary to neurologic injury is common, especially in younger children.
- Spinal cord injury without radiographic abnormality (SCIWORA):
  - Defined as traumatic myelopathy without evidence of vertebral column disruption on radiography or CT scans.
  - More common in children younger than 8 years.
  - Believed to be caused by ligamentous laxity allowing displacement of the cord without boney injury.
  - May present with complete or incomplete spinal cord injury.
  - MRI should be obtained to determine degree of soft tissue and neural injury.
  - Treated with bracing for 7–10 days if symptoms resolve within 24 h or 3 months for persistent symptoms.
    - May require surgical stabilization if ligamentous injury is present.

Part VI

Systemic Conditions

Septic Arthritis

Erik Bowman and Justin Siebler

Definition

- An infection within a native joint space that is a surgical emergency affecting people of all ages [1]

Location in Order of Occurrence

- Knee (~50%)
- Hip
- Shoulder
- Elbow
- Ankle
- Sternoclavicular joint
- IV drug users [1]

Mechanism of Infection

Hematogenous

- Transient bacteremia leading to seeding of the joint through the capillary-synovial membrane [2].

E. Bowman, MD • J. Siebler, MD (✉)
Department of Orthopaedic Surgery and
Rehabilitation, University of Nebraska Medical
Center, Omaha, NE, USA
e-mail: jsiebler@unmc.edu

Adjacent Osteomyelitis

- Direct intra-articular spread of metaphyseal osteomyelitis
- Can occur in all joints where the metaphysis is intracapsular
  - The metaphysis of the knee is extra-articular and, therefore, unlikely to spread to the joint.
  - Most commonly occurs in hip osteomyelitis [1, 5].

Pathogens

- *Staphylococcus aureus* (~60% of cases)
- *Streptococcus* species
- Gram-negative organisms
- Special considerations
  - IV drug users
    - Most common is *S. aureus*, but highly associated with *Pseudomonas*
  - Young, sexually active preceded by fever, chills, rash, and migratory arthritis
    - *Neisseria gonorrhoeae*
  - Children
    - < 6 weeks
      - Group B strep
      - Group A strep
      - Gram-negative rods
    - > 6 weeks
      - Most commonly *S. aureus*
    - < 5 years

A.E.M. Eltorai et al. (eds.), *Orthopedic Surgery Clerkship*, DOI 10.1007/978-3-319-52567-9_144

- Increasing incidence of Kingella
- Incidence of *Haemophilus influenzae* B decreasing due to HIB vaccine
  - Surgically related septic arthritis
    ○ *Staphylococcus aureus* still the most common.
    ○ Normal skin floras are occasional causes (may require alternate detection methods).
      - *P. acnes* (shoulder)
      - *S. epidermis* (prosthetic joint infections) [1, 3, 4]

Pathophysiology

Cellular Mechanism of Injury

- Proteolytic enzymes (matrix metalloproteinases) released from polymorphonuclear leukocytes causes cartilage destruction within 8 h.
- Irreversible cartilage damage after 8 h [1, 3, 5].

Presentation (Red Hot Swollen Joint)

Symptoms

- Fever often present (but not always)
- Pain localized to joint
- Refusal to bear weight or lift with affected extremity

Physical Examination

- Inability/refusal to actively move joint/extremity
- Erythema about the joint
- Joint effusion (difficult to appreciate in hip and shoulder)
- Inability to tolerate joint passive ROM

Differential Diagnosis

- Transient synovitis in children
- Crystalopathy in adults [6]

  - Gout
  - Pseudogout
- Acute inflammatory arthropathy in adults and children [2, 5]

Imaging

Radiographs

- Often normal
- Effusion/widened joint space
- Delayed presentations
  - Periosteal elevation or cortical thickening
  - Loss of joint space

MRI

- Indicated if concern for the bone involvement
- Will demonstrate effusion
- Not necessary for diagnosis and not routinely ordered [4, 5, 9]

Laboratory Studies

CBC

- Nonspecific. Only 50% of adults have a leukocytosis.
- Blood cultures.

ESR and CRP

- CRP most commonly elevated.
- ESR may remain normal in very acute presentations, typically elevated [8].

Criteria for Predicting Septic Arthritis and Distinguishing Transient Synovitis in Children

- Three out of four have a 93% probability of septic arthritis.
  - WBC > 12 K
  - Fever >38.5 C

- ESR > 40
- Inability to bear weight [7]

Joint Aspiration

- Required for diagnosis.
- Especially indicated when presentation and laboratories are equivocal but concern is high for septic arthritis.
- Attempt should be made to avoid aspiration through cellulitic skin; however, do not avoid aspiration if this is not possible [1, 9, 10].
- Fluid studies.
  - Cell differential (no one value is absolutely diagnostic)
    ○ > 50–75% PMN is suspicious.
    ○ > 95% very likely infectious.
  - Cell count (no one value is absolutely diagnostic)
    ○ <50,000 WBC, unlikely infection.
    ○ 50,000 – ~75,000 WBC can be infectious or inflammatory.
    ○ >75,000 WBC, more than likely infectious.
  - Gram stain
    ○ Gram stain is often negative.
    ○ Considered diagnostic if positive.
  - Culture and sensitivities
    ○ Guides antibiotic treatment [3, 9, 10]
  - Crystal examination [6]
    ○ Gout – negative birefringent
    ○ Pseudogout – positive birefringent

Treatment (Surgical Emergency)

- Emergent surgical drainage (debridement) and irrigation of joint open or arthroscopically to reduce bacterial load, toxin levels, and PMN proteases.
  - It is possible to have crystals in a joint and also have an acute infection.
  - Intraoperative cultures are routinely sent.
  - Surgical drain often left in place.
  - May require repeat debridement and irrigation [1, 2, 9].

- Empiric antibiotic coverage postoperatively with transition to culture-specific antibiotic(s) when sensitivities are complete.
  - Ideally given after joint aspiration/cultures to increase probability of detecting organism.
  - Typically cover *S. aureus* and gram-negative rods. However, dependent on hospital/local bacterial biome.
    ○ Nafcillin/oxacillin (MSSA) or vancomycin (MRSA) + third-generation cephalosporin
  - If suspect *N. gonorrhoeae*
    ○ Large doses of PCN or third-generation cephalosporin
  - If suspect *Pseudomonas* (IV drug user)
    ○ Add antipseudomonal [2]
- Length and route of antibiotic administration varies depending on severity/duration of infection, bacteria isolated, and patient's health/immune status.
  - Typically 2–6 weeks of intravenous antibiotics.
- Outcome is multifactorial but influenced by time to surgery.

References

1. Mazurek Michael T, Paul J Girard. American Academy of Orthopedic Surgery: orthopedic knowledge update: Trauma 4. Ch. 15, Section 2 162–165.
2. Goodman SB, Chou LB, Schurman DJ. Management of pyarthrosis. In: Chapman MW, editor. Chapman's orthopedic surgery. 3rd edn. Philadelphia: Lippincott Williams & Wilkins; 2001. p. 3561–75.
3. Esterhai Jr JL, Ruggiero V. Adult septic arthritis. In: Esterhai Jr JL, Gristina AG, Poss R, editors. Musculoskeletal infections. Park Ridge: American Academy of Orthopedic Surgeons; 1992. p. 409–19.
4. Bernstein J. Musculoskeletal medicine. Park Ridge: American Academy of Orthopedic Surgeons; 2003. p. 131–4.
5. Salava JK, Springer B. Orthopedic knowledge update 11. Park Ridge, Il: American Academy of Orthopedic Surgeons, 2014. p. 293–5.
6. Eggebeen AT. Gout: an update. Am Fam Physician. 2007;76(6):801–8.
7. Luhmann SJ, Jones A, Schootman M, Gordon JE, Schoenecker PL, Luhmann JD. Differentiation between septic arthritis and transient synovitis of the

hip in children prediction algorithms. J Bone Joint Surg Am 2004;86(5):956–62.

8. Greidanus NV, Marsri BA, Garbuz DS, et al. Use of erythrocyte sedimentation rate and C-reactive protein level to diagnose infection before revision total knee arthroplasty: a prospective evaluation. J Bone Joint Surg Am. 2007;98(7):1409–16.

9. Boyer MI. AAOS comprehensive orthopedic review. Rosemont: American Academy of Orthopedic Surgeons; 2014. p. 1327–35.

10. Montgomery NI, Rosenfeld S. Pediatric Osteoarticular infection update. J Pediatr Orthop 2015;35(1):74–81.

Osteomyelitis

Noah Porter and Justin Siebler

Definition

- Infection of the bone, osteomyelitis is a complex disease with heterogeneous presentation across the skeleton in patients of all ages [1].

Pathophysiology

Mechanism of Infection: Three Common Etiologies

- Hematogenous seeding during bacteremia. Most common etiology for metaphyseal involvement of long bones [6]
- Contiguous spread from involvement of adjacent soft tissue abscess, wounds, or septic arthritis
- Direct inoculation secondary to trauma or surgical inoculation

Inflammatory Response [2]

- Local host response with cascade of pro-inflammatory cytokines and leukocyte recruit-ment, potential negative effect on perfusion and architecture of the local bone.
- Sequestrum – necrotic bone secondary to disrupted endosteal and/or periosteal blood supply serves as nidus for continued infection.
- Involucrum – sclerotic new bone formation about sequestrae, visible by plain radiography in cases of chronic osteomyelitis.

Host Risk Factors [1]

- Increased risk of osteomyelitis with systemic comorbidities that suppress the immune system and decrease systemic neurovascular supply:
  - Diabetes mellitus
  - Cardiovascular disease
  - Immunosuppression medications
  - Smoking
  - Systemic infections
- Local factors:
  - Chronic wounds
  - Trauma that disrupted local vascular and the lymphatic system
  - Previous surgery or radiation

Microbiology

- Hematogenous osteomyelitis more likely to be monomicrobial, with contiguous spread and direct inoculation more likely polymicrobial [3].

N. Porter, MD • J. Siebler, MD (✉)
Department of Orthopaedic Surgery and Rehabilitation,
University of Nebraska Medical Center, Omaha,
NE, USA
e-mail: jsiebler@unmc.edu

© Springer International Publishing AG 2017
A.E.M. Eltorai et al. (eds.), *Orthopedic Surgery Clerkship*, DOI 10.1007/978-3-319-52567-9_145

- *Staphylococcus aureus* species are most common across all cases and ages. Coagulase-negative *Staphylococcus*, aerobic gram-negative bacilli, *Enterococcus*, and streptococcal species are also prevalent.
- Biofilm formation via quorum sensing and glycocalyx production present significant challenge for host response and antibiotic therapy.

Pediatric Skeleton [6]

- Metaphyseal bone with non-anastomosing capillary loops and venous sinusoids, turbulent flow, and lack of phagocytic lining cells.
- Vascular configuration may predispose to seeding during bacteremia, resulting in spread of infection to capillaries, through cortex, or across physis and adjacent articular surfaces.

Clinical Presentation

- Thorough history and physical exam is of paramount importance, including past medical, surgical, and social history. Details of treatment and culture which result from any past infectious process should be obtained.

Symptoms

- Constitutional symptoms of fever, chills, malaise, and weight loss are nonspecific but represent systemic involvement [7].
- Reports of pain are variable, often gradual onset with dull pain. Involvement of adjacent joints may lead to presentation as septic arthritis.
- Any history of trauma, laceration, or other skin disruption must be noted.

Signs

- Cardinal signs of inflammation (erythema, hyperthermia, swelling) are also nonspecific and may not be present in chronic cases [7].

- Drainage with the presence of sinus tract requires further investigation.
- Local soft tissue breakdown and ulceration, especially in high-risk patients (vasculopathy, neuropathy) about bony prominences.

Diagnosis

- *History* and physical exam are the keystones to establishing diagnosis, with additional testing as confirmation, and to help guide treatment.

Imaging

- Plain radiography:
  - Likely normal in acute disease
  - In chronic disease, erosive changes, sequestrum, and involucrum are seen.
- CT is helpful for anatomic localization, determination of bony destruction, classification, and preoperative planning.
- MRI is useful to evaluate local soft tissue involvement, particularly in cases involving the axial skeleton, abscesses, and ulcers about bony prominences.
- Scintigraphy is nonspecific; however, it may detect multiple infectious foci [1].

Laboratory

- WBC is often normal in chronic cases; leukocytosis may be present in acute cases or those associated with significant soft tissue involvement.
- ESR and CRP are nonspecific but often elevated in the absence of clear symptoms or exam findings. These may be used to monitor response to treatment, with CRP trending downward prior to ESR.

Culture and Histologic Evaluation

- Positive culture obtained via sterile technique remains gold standard [1].

- Superficial swabs of ulcers and draining wounds are often polymicrobial and are typically not useful/diagnostic of deeper bacterium.
- Multiple deep tissue samples should be obtained as biopsies and handled appropriately prior to culture.
- Histologic evaluation may reveal acute and/or chronic inflammation, bone necrosis, and new bone formation.

Differential Diagnosis

- Soft tissue infection – cellulitis, abscess, and myositis
- Joint involvement – gout, toxic synovitis, septic arthritis, and bursitis
- Noninfectious skeletal conditions – Charcot arthropathy, fracture, malignancy, and osteonecrosis

Classification [4]

- Several classification schemas exist with temporal or prognostic basis.
- Cierny-Mader (Table 145.1)
  - Stages disease and guides treatment based on location, bony involvement, and host status
- Lew-Waldvogel
  - Etiologic classification based on timing and mechanism

Table 145.1 Cierny-Mader staging system for long bone osteomyelitis

Classification	Description
Anatomic type	
Stage I	Medullary osteomyelitis
Stage II	Superficial osteomyelitis
Stage III	Localized osteomyelitis
Stage IV	Diffuse osteomyelitis
Physiological class	
A host	Normal host
B host	Systemic, local, or systemic/local compromise
C host	Treatment worse than disease

Adapted from Mader et al. [4]

Treatment – goal of eradicating local infection, limiting local and systemic morbidity, and recurrence of disease

Surgical Treatment

- Necessary to debride any devitalized bone, necrotic soft tissue, and continued nidus for infection. Medical therapy alone will not cure osteomyelitis [1].
- Debridement and irrigation:
  - Contaminated wounds require meticulous evaluation of the skin, soft tissue, muscle, and bone involvement with debridement of all devitalized and contaminated tissue.
  - Cases of chronic osteomyelitis may require resection of large segments with advanced reconstructive techniques (Ilizarov, Masquelet) required to restore stability and function.
  - Often require plastic surgical soft tissue reconstruction procedures for coverage of the bone.
  - Amputation (depending on the location of the infection) is sometimes preferred by the patient and/or recommended by the surgeon.
  - Regarding open fractures leading to osteomyelitis:
    ○ Immediate administration of parenteral antibiotics decreases the rate of infection.
    ○ Debate exists regarding recommended time to debridement. However, quality of debridement in terms of removing all foreign material and nonviable tissue is paramount.
    ○ Ideal composition and volume of irrigate is unknown.

Medical Therapy [5]

- Antibiotics
  - In a hemodynamically stable host, empiric therapy should be withheld until cultures have been obtained.

– Broad-spectrum empiric therapy including B-lactam antibiotics and vancomycin is common; however, it should be based on local antibiogram.
– Therapy is tailored based on laboratory identification and speciation from tissue samples and in vitro susceptibilities.
– Total duration of therapy required is controversial, with organism-specific intravenous treatment of 4–6 weeks most common.
• Hyperbaric oxygen
– Has been proposed to facilitate oxygen-dependent killing from native immune response and anaerobic organisms

Complications

Local

• Despite appropriate medical and surgical treatment, local recurrence rates approximately 3–25%.
• Soft tissue compromise and pathologic fracture related to trauma and comorbidities.

Marjolin's Ulcer/Squamous Cell Carcinoma

• Malignant transformation of chronic sinus tracts has been documented [7].

• Histopathologic examination of chronic wounds and those with delayed healing should be considered.

Systemic

• Bacteremia, sepsis, bacterial endocarditis, venous thromboembolism, and anemia of chronic disease

References

1. Berbari EF, Steckelberg JM, Osmon DR. Osteomyelitis. In: Mandell GL, Bennett JE, Dolin R, editors. Principles and practice of infectious diseases. 6th ed. Philadelphia: Elsevier; 2005.
2. Lew DP, Waldvogel FA. Osteomyelitis. Lancet. 2004;364:369.
3. Rubin RJ, Harrington CA, Poon A, et al. The economic impact of *Staphylococcus aureus* infection in New York City hospitals. Emerg Infect Dis. 1999;5:9–17.
4. Mader JT, Shirtliff M, Calhoun JH. Staging and staging application in osteomyelitis. Clin Infect Dis. 1997;25:1303–9.
5. Ostermann PA, Seligson D, Henry SL. Local antibiotic therapy for severe open fractures. A review of 1085 consecutive cases. J Bone Joint Surg Br. 1995;77:93–7.
6. Harik NS, Smeltzer MS. Management of acute hematogenous osteomyelitis in children. Expert Rev Anti Infect Ther. 2010;8:175–81.
7. Flynn JM. OKU 10: orthopedic knowledge update. Rosemont: American Academy of Orthopedic Surgeons; 2011.

Necrotizing Fasciitis

146

Justin Siebler and Darin Larson

Description

- Rare, but potentially fatal bacterial infection of the soft tissues.
  - Spreads rapidly and characterized by necrosis of the fascial planes, subcutaneous fat, and surrounding tissue [1, 2].
  - Can cause systemic toxicity, loss of limb or life.
  - Mortality rates have declined in recent decades, but still remain 25–35%.

Pathophysiology

- Typically, but not always, follows an injury causing disruption of the skin barrier
  - May be minor (insect bites, abrasions, injection sites, splinters) or major (surgical incisions, burns, penetrating trauma, blunt trauma) insults to the skin and underlying tissues [3]
  - Can occur in the absence of a wound
- May involve any body part, but most commonly found in the extremities [4].

J. Siebler, MD (✉) • D. Larson, MD
Department of Orthopaedic Surgery and Rehabilitation,
University of Nebraska Medical Center,
Omaha, NE, USA
e-mail: jsiebler@unmc.edu

- Risk factors
  - Diabetes mellitus is the most common (up to 60% of cases).
  - IV drug use, alcohol abuse, smoking, or any other condition that causes immunosuppression (liver cirrhosis, cancer, kidney disease, chronic corticosteroid use, etc.).
  - Approximately 50% of cases develop in patients with no known risk factors.

Microbiology

- Three groups based on Gram stain and culture results [5]
  - Type 1 (most common): polymicrobial; non-group A *Streptococcus*, anaerobes, *Enterobacteriaceae*.
    ◦ More common in immunocompromised patients
  - Type 2: Group A β-hemolytic *Streptococcus* with or without *Staphylococcus aureus*
    ◦ Typically seen in previously healthy patients
    ◦ More common in the extremities
    ◦ Can cause NF within 24 h after surgery
    ◦ Recent increases of NF caused by MRSA
  - Type 3: Marine bacteria (*Vibrio* spp., *Aeromonas* spp., and *Shewanella* spp.)

© Springer International Publishing AG 2017
A.E.M. Eltorai et al. (eds.), *Orthopedic Surgery Clerkship*, DOI 10.1007/978-3-319-52567-9_146

Presentation

- May be mimic cellulitis in early stages
  - Maintain high index of suspicion for patients with swelling, erythema, and pain out of proportion.
  - Erythema and skin induration may rapidly migrate (1+ cm/h).
  - Skin may appear normal in early stages while the infection tracks subcutaneously.
- Later findings: bullae, necrosis of the skin and underlying soft tissues, and subcutaneous crepitus
  - Necrosis of fascia and superficial soft tissues can result in gray, watery, foul-smelling "dishwater" pus, as seen at time of debridement.
- Unreliable findings: fever and altered mental status
- Late findings: acute renal failure, acute respiratory distress syndrome, and septic shock

Diagnosis

- Primarily a clinical diagnosis
- Laboratory tests or radiologic evaluation may aid in diagnosis
  - Should never delay treatment to obtain labs or imaging.
  - Subcutaneous gas seen on radiographs is a late finding.
- Laboratory risk indicator for necrotizing fasciitis (LRINEC) described by Wong et al. Table 146.1.
  - Summative scoring system of abnormal serum laboratory values
    ∘ CRP, WBC, hemoglobin, sodium, creatinine, and blood glucose
    ∘ As the number of these abnormal laboratory values increases, the possibility of NF increases

Treatment

- Combination of thorough surgical debridement and empiric intravenous broad-spectrum antibiotics are required for limb salvage and survival.

- Time to initial debridement is most important factor influencing mortality. Surgical incisions are left open (not closed primarily) at first debridement.
- May require multiple debridements in the operating room; daily reevaluations are important.
- Cannot be managed by antibiotics alone; empiric antibiotics should be started as soon as cultures are obtained, followed by culture-specific intravenous antibiotics.
- Patients must receive adequate fluid resuscitation and proper nutrition.
- Incisions may be closed following resolution of the infection.
  - Skin grafts are commonly required.
- Amputation may be necessary in up to 15% of cases.
- Increasing number of immunosuppressed patients and the higher incidence of multiresistant pathogens represent a challenge for treatment.
- Notable complications: nosocomial infection, respiratory failure, acute renal failure, cardiac arrest, and late amputation.

Table 146.1 Laboratory risk indicator for necrotizing fasciitis

Laboratory value	Point value
C-Reactive protein, mg/L	
≥150	4
Total white cell count, per mm³	
15–25	1
>25	2
Hemoglobin, g/dL	
<11	2
11–13.5	1
Sodium, mmol/L	
<135	2
Creatinine, μmol/L	
>141	2
Glucose, mmol/L	
>10	1

A total point value greater than or equal to 6 should raise suspicion; greater than or equal to 8 is strongly predictive of necrotizing fasciitis (Adapted from Wong et al. [6])

Pearls

- The single most important variable influencing mortality is time to surgical debridement.
- A high degree of clinical suspicion is necessary to avert potentially disastrous consequences.
  - Nonspecific symptoms, the extremely fulminant progression, the need for treatment on an emergency basis, as well as the extended and repeated necessary operations create a combination of factors that are often limb or life threatening [3].
- The diagnosis of necrotizing fasciitis should be considered for any individual who has unexplained limb pain and elevated laboratory values, especially, but not exclusively, if that person has diabetes mellitus or chronic liver disease Table 146.1.

References

1. Bellapianta JM, et al. Necrotizing fasciitis. J Am Acad Orthop Surg. 2009;17(3):174–82.
2. Sarani B, et al. Necrotizing fasciitis: current concepts and review of the literature. J Am Coll Surg. 2009;208(2):279–88.
3. Siebler J. Necrotizing Fasciitis. Presentation. University of Nebraska Medical Center, Omaha: NE. 2015.
4. Wang KC, Shih CH. Necrotizing fasciitis of the extremities. J Trauma. 1992;32(2):179–82.
5. Tsitsilonis S, et al. Necrotizing fasciitis: is the bacterial spectrum changing? Langenbecks Arch Surg. 2013;398(1):153–9.
6. Wong CH, et al. The LRINEC (Laboratory Risk Indicator for Necrotizing Fasciitis) score: a tool for distinguishing necrotizing fasciitis from other soft tissue infections. Crit Care Med. 2004;32(7):1535–41.

Rheumatoid Arthritis

Sylwia Sasinowska and Bobby Kwanghoon Han

Overview [1]

- Rheumatoid arthritis (RA) affects 0.5–1% of the adult population, and women are affected two to three times more than men.
- Genetic factors contribute to disease susceptibility and 1.5-fold higher risk of developing RA in first-degree relatives of rheumatoid arthritis patients as compared with the general population.
- Environmental factors also contribute to RA risks. Smoking increases the risk of developing anti-cyclic citrullinated peptide (CCP) antibody positive RA.

Pathogenesis [1]

- The synovium of the joints is the primary site of inflammation (synovitis) in RA. Chronic synovial inflammation leads to encroachment of hypertrophied synovium (pannus) over the bone and cartilage, which causes joint destruction.
- Synovitis is caused by autoimmunity which involves T and B lymphocytes, macrophages, synovial fibroblasts, and a network

of cytokines including tumor necrosis factor (TNF) and interleukin-6 (IL-6).
- Rheumatoid factor (RF) is an autoantibody directed against the Fc portion of an immunoglobulin.
- Anti-cyclic citrullinated peptide (CCP) antibodies are autoantibodies directed against citrullinated peptides. Citrullination is the conversion of arginine into citrulline in peptides and is catalyzed by peptidylarginine deiminases (PADIs) which are expressed at high levels in inflamed rheumatoid synovium [2].

Classification Criteria

- 2010 American College of Rheumatology/ European League Against Rheumatism (ACR/ EULAR) criteria [3]:
  - Joint involvement (number and size of involved joints)
  - Serology (presence of rheumatoid factor (RF) or anti-cyclic citrullinated peptide (CCP) antibody)
  - Acute phase reactants (elevation of erythrocyte sedimentation rate (ESR) or C-reactive protein (CRP))
  - Duration of symptoms
- 1987 American College of Rheumatology (ACR) criteria [4] – need at least four of these criteria present for at least 6 weeks:
  - Morning stiffness for at least 1 h
  - Arthritis of three or more joints

S. Sasinowska, MD • B.K. Han, MD (✉)
Division of Rheumatology, Cooper University
Hospital, Camden, NJ, USA
e-mail: han-kwanghoon@cooperhealth.edu

© Springer International Publishing AG 2017
A.E.M. Eltorai et al. (eds.), *Orthopedic Surgery Clerkship*, DOI 10.1007/978-3-319-52567-9_147

- Arthritis of hand joints
- Symmetric arthritis
- Rheumatoid nodules
- Serum rheumatoid factor (RF)
- Radiographic changes

Evaluation [4]

- History:
  - The onset of symptoms is usually insidious, occurring over weeks to months.
  - Classically presents with symmetrical polyarthritis, which may lead to pain, swelling, stiffness, and weakness in multiple joints.
  - Small synovial joints of hands (wrists, metacarpophalangeal (MCP) joints, proximal interphalangeal (PIP) joints) and feet (metatarsophalangeal (MTP) joints) are affected most frequently. Larger joints (ankles, knees, elbows, shoulders) are also affected. Distal interphalangeal (DIP) joints and thoracolumbar spine are spared.
  - Morning joint stiffness lasts more than an hour.
  - Patients with RA may have extraarticular manifestations including rheumatoid nodules, keratoconjunctivitis sicca, scleritis, serositis, interstitial lung disease, anemia, peripheral nerve entrapment neuropathy, and vasculitis.

- Physical examination:
  - Tenderness and swelling of the affected joints are observed.
  - Fusiform swelling around proximal interphalangeal (PIP) joints may be seen in early stages.
  - Deformities of the joints occur in advanced disease, and hand deformities include ulnar deviation of the fingers at the metacarpophalangeal (MCP) joints, dorsal subluxation of the metacarpophalangeal (MCP) joints, hyperextension of the proximal interphalangeal (PIP) joints (swan neck deformities), and hyperflexion of the proximal interphalangeal (PIP) joints (boutonniere deformities) (Fig. 147.1).
  - Median nerve entrapment neuropathy (carpal tunnel syndrome) can result from synovitis in the wrist.
  - Dorsal subluxation of the toes at the metatarsophalangeal (MTP) joints in the feet is commonly seen.
  - Knee involvement may result in joint effusion and herniation of synovium posteriorly into the popliteal fossa, creating Baker's cyst.
- Laboratory tests:
  - Rheumatoid factor (RF) is an antibody directed against the Fc portion of IgG and associated severe joint disease and extraarticular involvement.

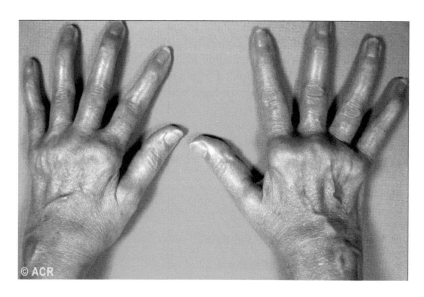

Fig. 147.1 Synovitis and subluxations of the metacarpophalangeal joints in advanced rheumatoid arthritis. Early "swan neck" deformities, interosseous muscle atrophy, and wrist swelling are also present

- Anti-cyclic citrullinated peptide (CCP) antibody is directed against citrullinated peptides and is associated with greater risks of joint erosion and radiographic progression [5].
- The above serology tests aid in confirming a diagnosis of RA and, however, should not be used as the only criterion for diagnosis because they may be falsely present in healthy population or may be both absent in about 20% of RA patients (seronegative RA).
- Inflammatory markers including erythrocyte sedimentation rate (ESR) or C-reactive protein (CRP) may correlate with ongoing inflammation.
- Imaging:
  - Plain radiograph findings include periarticular osteopenia, marginal joint erosion, joint subluxations, and joint space narrowing (Fig. 147.2).
  - Ultrasonography and magnetic resonance imaging (MRI) are more sensitive for detecting synovitis and joint erosion and, however, are not routinely used.

Treatment [6]

- Conventional disease-modifying antirheumatic drugs (DMARDs)
  - First-line treatment to control inflammation and inhibit disease progression.
  - Early treatment with DMARDs is important to prevent permanent joint damages.
  - Include methotrexate, leflunomide, hydroxychloroquine, and sulfasalazine
  - Targeted therapies (biologic agents):
    ◦ Advanced treatment for patients who have inadequate response to conventional DMARDs or severe disease.
    ◦ Biologic agents are substances made from a living organism or its products. Currently approved biologic agents for RA include tumor necrosis factor (TNF) inhibitor, interleukin-6 (IL-6) inhibitor, T cell costimulation inhibitor, and B cell depletion therapy.
    ◦ Janus kinase (JAK) inhibitor is a small molecule drug targeting JAK which is involved in signal transduction of pro-inflammatory cytokines.

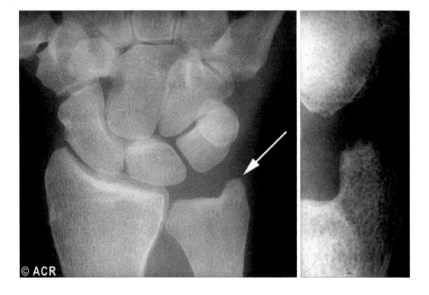

Fig. 147.2 Irregularity of the tip of the ulnar styloid process resulting from erosive change (*arrow*) in rheumatoid arthritis

- Anti-inflammatory agents:
  ◦ Adjunct therapy for symptomatic relief
  ◦ Include nonsteroidal anti-inflammatory drugs (NSAIDs) and glucocorticoids

References

1. Waldburger JM, Firestein GS. Rheumatoid arthritis. B. epidemiology, pathology, and pathogenesis. In: Klippel J, et al., editors. Primer on the rheumatic diseases. 13th ed. New York: Springer; 2008. p. 122–32.
2. Chang X, et al. Localization of peptidylarginine deiminase 4 (PADI4) and citrullinated protein in synovial tissue of rheumatoid arthritis. Rheumatology. 2005;44:40–50.
3. Aletaha D, et al. 2010 Rheumatoid arthritis classification criteria: an American College of Rheumatology/European League Against Rheumatism collaborative initiative. Arthritis Rheum. 2010;62:2569–81.
4. O'Dell JR, et al. Rheumatoid arthritis. In: Imboden JB, et al., editors. Current rheumatology diagnosis & treatment, vol. 15. 3rd ed. New York: The McGraw-Hill Companies; 2013. p. 139–55.
5. Avouac J, et al. Diagnostic and predictive value of anti-cyclic citrullinated protein antibodies in rheumatoid arthritis: a systematic literature review. Ann Rheum Dis. 2006;65:845–51.
6. West SG, O'Dell JR. Rheumatoid arthritis. In: West SG, et al., editors. Rheumatology secrets, vol. 15. 3rd ed. Philadelphia: Hanley & Belfus; 2015. p. 107–17.

Crystalline-Induced Arthropathies

148

Jenna Cooley and Bobby Kwanghoon Han

Overview [1–4]

- Gouty arthritis is a common inflammatory arthritis and occurs in 2–3% of the adult population. The prevalence rises with advancing age. Gouty arthritis is more common in men and may occur in women after menopause [5].
- Gouty arthritis has significantly increased over the last 20 years due to diet, metabolic syndrome including obesity, and increasing use of diuretics or low-dose aspirin.
- Calcium pyrophosphate dihydrate (CPP) deposition disease primarily occurs in the elderly.

Pathogenesis [1, 2, 4, 6–8]

- In gouty arthritis, monosodium urate (MSU) crystals are deposited in the joints and soft tissues as a result of hyperuricemia over years. MSU crystals may trigger inflammation by activating innate immunity including macrophages and neutrophils.
- Hyperuricemia is defined as a serum uric acid level > 6.8–7.0 mg/dL in males and >6.0 mg/dL in females and could be caused by overproduction of urate (10%), underexcretion of urate (90%), or a combination of both. However, majority of people with hyperuricemia do not develop clinical gout.
- Predisposing risk factors for gouty arthritis include chronic kidney disease, medications (diuretics, low-dose aspirin, cyclosporine), alcohol, purine-rich diet, metabolic syndrome, fructose, hematologic malignancy, and inherited enzyme defects.
- Calcium pyrophosphate dihydrate (CPP) crystal deposition is associated with increased age, osteoarthritis, a history of joint injury, and certain metabolic diseases including hyperparathyroidism, hemochromatosis, hypomagnesemia, and hypophosphatasia.

Evaluation

History [1–3]

- In the beginning, gouty arthritis usually presents as rapid-onset, inflammatory arthritis in joints of lower extremities including metatarsophalangeal (MTP) joints of big toes, ankles, or knees and resolves within 7–10 days.
- In some patients, multiple joints including joints of upper extremities are involved.
- After the initial episode, gouty arthritis flares may occur intermittently and become more frequent as time passes by.

J. Cooley, DO • B.K. Han, MD (✉)
Division of Rheumatology, Cooper University
Hospital, Camden, NJ, USA
e-mail: bobbyhan@hotmail.com

© Springer International Publishing AG 2017
A.E.M. Eltorai et al. (eds.), *Orthopedic Surgery Clerkship*, DOI 10.1007/978-3-319-52567-9_148

- Chronic gouty arthritis may develop after recurrent episodes of acute gouty arthritis without appropriate treatments.

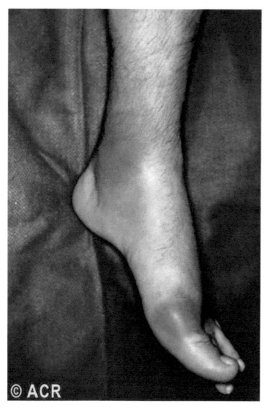

Fig. 148.1 Acute gouty arthritis involving the base of the big toe and ankle

- Calcium pyrophosphate dihydrate (CPP) deposition disease could present as acute arthritis usually involving knees or wrists. Some patients may develop into chronic CPP deposition disease.

Physical Examination [1, 3]

- The joints affected by gouty arthritis are exquisitely tender, swollen, warm, and erythematous, and inflammation may extend into surrounding soft tissues (Fig. 148.1).
- Chronic gouty arthritis may cause joint deformities.
- Deposits of monosodium urate (MSU) crystals in soft tissues are called tophi. Tophi may accompany chronic gouty arthritis, and common locations for tophi include the olecranon bursa or digits of the hands and feet (Fig. 148.2).

Laboratory Tests [1, 3, 6, 7]

- Diagnosis of crystal-induced arthropathies is made by aspirating synovial fluid from affected joints and visualizing crystals in the fluid under polarized light microscopy.
- Monosodium urate crystals are needle-shaped, negatively birefringent crystals, and calcium

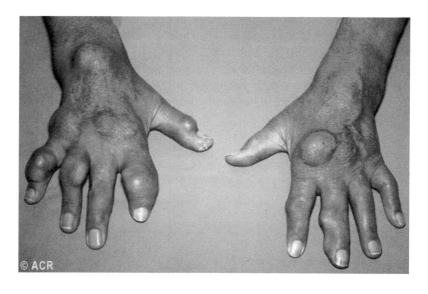

Fig. 148.2 Multiple tophi affecting the wrists and several finger joints in chronic tophaceous gout

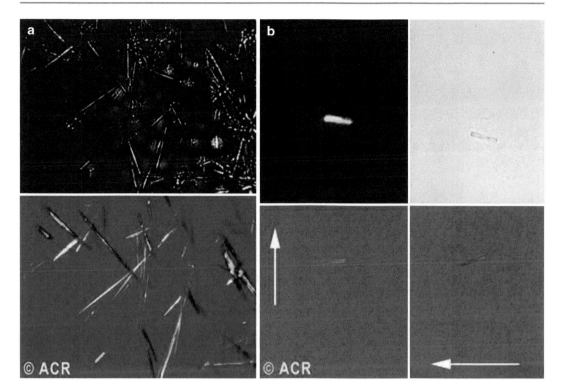

Fig. 148.3 Polarized light microscopy findings of monosodium urate (MSU) crystals (**a**) which are needle-shaped and negatively birefringent and calcium pyrophosphate dihydrate (CPP) crystals (**b**) engulfed by a leukocyte which are rhomboid shaped and positively birefringent

pyrophosphate (CPP) crystals are rhomboid shaped and positively birefringent (Fig. 148.3).

- Increased leukocyte count of 2000–100,000 cells/mm^3 in the synovial fluid is commonly seen, which suggests inflammation.
- Elevated serum uric acid levels is helpful but not specific in diagnosing gouty arthritis.
- Elevated serum inflammatory markers including erythrocyte sedimentation rate (ESR) and/or C-reactive protein (CRP) may be seen.

Imaging [1–4]

- Plain radiographs of advanced gouty arthritis may show joint erosions (appear as "punched out" lesions with overhanging edges, AKA "rate bite" erosions), joint space narrowing, and tophi. Periarticular osteopenia seen in rheumatoid arthritis is absent (Fig. 148.4).
- Ultrasonography of gouty arthritis may show superficial, hyperechoic band above the cartilage in joints termed as "double contour sign." Tophi appear as nonhomogeneous material that is surrounded with an anechoic rim.
- Radiographs of CPP disease may show chondrocalcinosis which is calcifications within articular cartilage or fibrocartilage of the joints. Common sites for chondrocalcinosis include menisci of knees and triangular fibrocartilage of wrists (Fig. 148.5).

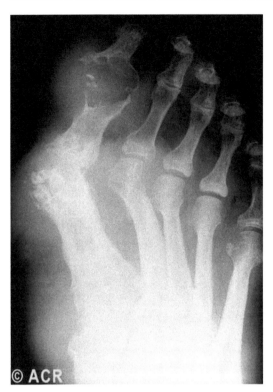

Fig. 148.4 Radiograph of advanced gout showing tophi in the proximal and distal phalanges of the great toe and erosion with overhanging margin of bone

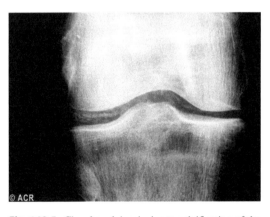

Fig. 148.5 Chondrocalcinosis due to calcification of the menisci and articular cartilage in knee radiograph

Treatment [1–7]

Management of Acute Gouty Arthritis

- Relief of acute pain and inflammation
- Nonsteroidal anti-inflammatory drugs (NSAIDs) including indomethacin, glucocorticoids, and colchicine
- Intraarticular glucocorticoids injection
- IL-1 inhibitors including Kineret

Uric Acid-Lowering Agents

- Prevention of recurrence or progression of gouty arthritis by gradually eliminating monosodium urate (MSU) crystals from the joints.
- Xanthine oxidase inhibitors (allopurinol, febuxostat) are mainstay of urate-lowering therapy.
- URAT-1 inhibitor (lesinurad)
- Pegloticase
- Used along with daily colchicine or NSAIDs which suppresses crystal-induced inflammation
- Avoidance of excessive alcohol use and purine-rich diet intake including red meat (including organ meat), shell fish, and fructose.
- Treatments of acute CPP deposition disease are similar to those of gout. There are no proven treatments to eliminate calcium-containing crystals from the joints.

References

1. Janson R. Gout. In: West S, et al., editors. Rheumatology secrets, vol. 45. 3rd ed. Philadelphia: Hanley & Belfus; 2015. p. 337–44.
2. Murphy F. Calcium pyrophosphate deposition disease. In: West S, et al., editors. Rheumatology secrets, vol. 46. 3rd ed. Philadelphia: Hanley & Belfus; 2015. p. 346–50.
3. Burns CM, et al. Gout. In: Imoden J, et al., editors. Current diagnosis and treatment in rheumatology, vol. 44. 3rd ed. New-York: McGraw-Hill; 2013. p. 332–8.

4. Alderman JS, et al. Pseudogout. In: Imoden J, et al., editors. Current diagnosis and treatment in rheumatology, vol. 45. 3rd ed. New-York: McGraw-Hill; 2013. p. 339–43.
5. Zhu BJ, et al. Prevalence of gout and hyperuricemia in the US population. Arthritis Rheum. 2011;63: 3136–41.
6. Burns CM, et al. Clinical features and treatment of gout. In: Firestein GS, Budd RC, et al. Kelley's text-book of rheumatology. 9th ed. Philadelphia: Elsevier Saunders; 2013. p. 94–5, 1533–1576.
7. Edwards NL, et al. Gout. In: Klippel JH, et al., editors. Primer on the rheumatic diseases, vol. 12. 13th ed. New York: Springer; 2008. p. 241–62.
8. McCarthy G. Pseudogout. In: Klippel JH, et al., editors. Primer on the rheumatic diseases, vol. 13. 13th ed. New York: Springer; 2008. p. 263–9.

Fibromyalgia

Chad S. Boomershine

Diagnosis

1990 American College of Rheumatology (ACR) Classification Criteria [1]

- Developed to identify subjects for research studies, later applied to clinical diagnosis but 2010 and 2011 diagnostic criteria have largely supplanted it (see below)
- Requires widespread pain (axial plus upper and lower segment plus left- and right-sided pain) for 3 months or more in combination with pain to palpation at 11 or more of the 18 specific tender point sites
- Eighteen tender points located bilaterally at suboccipital muscle insertions, midpoint of upper border of trapezius, above medial border of scapular spines, upper outer quadrant of buttocks, anterior aspect of intertransverse space of C5-7, second costochondral junctions, 2 cm distal to lateral epicondyles, posterior to trochanteric prominence, medial fat pad proximal to joint line in knees [2]
- Tender points palpated using thumb pad applying 4 kg pressure for 4 seconds

2010 ACR Diagnostic Criteria [3]

- Developed specifically for clinical diagnosis and also to provide a symptom severity scale
- Diagnosis requires all three of the following conditions be met:
  - Widespread pain index (WPI) ≥7 and symptom severity (SS) scale score ≥ 5 or WPI 3–6 and SS scale score ≥ 9.
    - WPI is total number of areas in which patient has had pain over the last week including the chest, abdomen, upper back, lower back, and neck and bilateral body areas including the shoulder girdle, upper arm, lower arm, hip, upper leg, lower leg, and jaw.
    - SS scale score is a 0–12 score which is the sum of the severity of symptoms of fatigue, waking unrefreshed, and cognitive symptoms over the past week each on a 0–3 scale where 0 = no problem and 3 = a severe, pervasive, continuous, life-disturbing problem plus the number of general somatic symptoms as determined by the physician where 0 = no symptoms and 3 = a great deal of symptoms.
  - Symptoms have been present at a similar level for at least 3 months.
  - The patient does not have a disorder that would otherwise explain the pain.
    - This provision makes fibromyalgia a diagnosis of exclusion.

C.S. Boomershine, MD, PhD
Rheumatology and Immunology, Vanderbilt University, Nashville, TN, USA
e-mail: fibromd1@gmail.com

© Springer International Publishing AG 2017
A.E.M. Eltorai et al. (eds.), *Orthopedic Surgery Clerkship*, DOI 10.1007/978-3-319-52567-9_149

○ Must perform thorough evaluation to rule out other disorders.

○ If other disorders found, disorder should be successfully treated, and then patient should be reassessed for fibromyalgia if pain persists.

Modification to the ACR 2010 Fibromyalgia Diagnostic Criteria (Fig. 149.1) [4]

• Developed to allow for use of 2010 ACR Diagnostic Criteria utilizing a patient self-report questionnaire without the requirement for an examiner.
• Diagnosis using Modification analogous to 2010 Criteria except physician assessment of number of general somatic symptoms replaced by number of the following symptoms occurring during the previous 6 months: headaches, pain or cramps in the lower abdomen, and depression.
• Patients cannot self-diagnose; diagnosis must be made by a clinician.

Pathophysiology [5]

• Fibromyalgia is primarily a neurologic disorder.
  – Pain results from neurochemical imbalances that lead to "central amplification" of pain characterized by allodynia and hyperalgesia.
    ○ Fibromyalgia patients have lower levels of neurotransmitters important for descending inhibitory pain pathways including serotonin and norepinephrine.
    ○ Fibromyalgia patients have higher levels of neurotransmitters involved in ascending excitatory pain pathways including glutamate and substance P.
  – Functional MRI studies have shown that fibromyalgia patients have increased activity in brain areas involved in pain processing.
• Baseline endogenous opioid activity in fibromyalgia patients is increased.
• Endogenous opioid levels are increased.
• Opioid receptor binding is decreased.

Please check (√)Yes or No to indicate whether or not you have had PAIN or TENDERNESS in each area OVER THE PAST WEEK.								
Right Side	Yes (1)	No (0)	Trunk	Yes (1)	No (0)	Left side	Yes (1)	No (0)
Jaw			Neck			Jaw		
Shoulder			Upper Back			Shoulder		
Upper Arm			Chest			Upper Arm		
Lower Arm			Abdomen			Lower Arm		
Hip/Buttock			Low Back			Hip/Buttock		
Upper Leg			OFFICE USE ONLY:			Upper Leg		
Lower Leg			Widespread Pain Index (WPI) (0-19)____			Lower Leg		

Circle the number that best indicates the severity of each symptom OVER THE PAST WEEK 0 = No Problem; 1 = Slight or Mild Problem: Generally Mild or Intermittent; 2 = Moderate: Considerable Problem, Often Present and/or at a Moderate Level; 3 = Severe: Pervasive, Continuous, Life-disturbing problem.				
SYMPTOM	No problem	Slight/Mild	Moderate	Severe
Fatigue or Tiredness Through the Day	0	1	2	3
Waking Up Tired or Unrefreshed	0	1	2	3
Trouble Thinking or Remembering	0	1	2	3

Please check (√) Yes or No to indicate whether or not you have experienced any of the following symptoms OVER THE PAST 6 MONTHS.		
SYMPTOM	Yes (1)	No (0)
Pain or cramps in the lower abdomen		
Depression		
Headache		
Symptom Severity (SS) Scale (0-12)____ FM Diagnosed if WPI ≥7 and SS ≥5 or WPI 3-6 and SS ≥ 9		

Fig. 149.1 Modified ACR 2010 fibromyalgia diagnostic criteria (Adapted from Wolfe et al. [4])

- This explains why opioids are typically not effective and not recommended for treating fibromyalgia pain.

Presentation

- In addition to widespread pain, fibromyalgia patients typically present with multiple other problematic symptoms that can be recalled using the FIBRO mnemonic.
  - F = Fatigue, Fog (cognitive difficulty), and poor physical Function
  - I = Insomnia (difficulty with all aspects of sleep: initiation, maintenance and restoration)
  - B = Blues (depression and anxiety symptoms)
  - R = Rigidity (muscle stiffness)
  - O = Ow! (widespread pain)
- In addition to FIBRO symptoms, fibromyalgia patients tend to present with other central sensitivity syndromes including systemic exertion intolerance disease (previously chronic fatigue syndrome), irritable bowel syndrome, chronic low back pain, migraine, restless legs syndrome, temporomandibular dysfunction syndrome, and multiple chemical sensitivity [6].

Treatment [6]

- Effective fibromyalgia management requires an individualized regimen of pharmacologic and nonpharmacologic treatments that address not only pain but all associated FIBRO symptoms [6].
- Nonpharmacologic treatments include stretching, graduated aerobic and resistance exercise, education, and psychological, physical, and manual therapies.
  - Combining education and aerobic and resistance exercise is superior to the use of these modalities in isolation.

Pharmacologic Therapies

Anticonvulsants

- Pregabalin is FDA approved for managing fibromyalgia.
  - Recommend starting with a low dose (25–50 mg) at night.
  - Increase as needed and tolerated up to 225 mg twice daily.
- Gabapentin has been shown to improve fibromyalgia symptoms.
  - Recommend starting with a low dose (100–300 mg) at night.
  - Increase as needed and tolerated up to 800 mg three times daily.
  - Sustained-release preparations can limit side effects and permit once-daily dosing.
- Combining pregabalin or gabapentin with serotonin and norepinephrine reuptake inhibitors (SNRIs) has been shown to improve efficacy and reduce side effects.
- Topiramate may be helpful particularly in patients with migraines and/or obesity.
  - Recommend starting with low dose (25–50 mg) at night.
  - Increase as needed and tolerated up to 200 mg twice daily.
  - Sustained-release preparations can limit side effects and permit once-daily dosing.

Antidepressants

- Duloxetine is FDA approved for managing fibromyalgia.
  - Available in 20, 30, and 60 mg capsules, may be taken morning or night
  - Fibromyalgia approved dosing up to 60 mg per day, may increase up to 120 mg per day if needed and tolerated
- Milnacipran is FDA approved for treating fibromyalgia.
  - Available as 12.5, 25, 50, and 100 mg tablets
  - Recommend starting 12.5 mg once daily with food since frequently causes nausea
  - FDA-approved dosing 50–100 mg twice daily
- Other SNRIs such as venlafaxine, desvenlafaxine, and levomilnacipran are also reasonable options.
- Fluoxetine or paroxetine can be helpful since they have SNRI activity.
  - Start with low dose (10–20 mg) once daily.
  - If used as monotherapy, typically need to use high doses (60 mg/day paroxetine,

80 mg/day fluoxetine) that are usually not well tolerated.

- Combining with tricyclic antidepressants (TCAs) can allow for efficacy at lower doses with fewer side effects (see below).
- Newer highly serotonin-selective drugs are typically not helpful for fibromyalgia pain but can help depression and anxiety symptoms.
- TCAs can be helpful including nortriptyline, amitriptyline, and desipramine.
  - Start low dose (10–25 mg) at night.
  - Consider nortriptyline or desipramine first since amitriptyline causes more severe anticholinergic side effects (e.g., dryness, constipation).
  - Effectiveness of TCAs can be increased by combining with fluoxetine or paroxetine.
- Bupropion reduces pain by inhibiting neuronal uptake of norepinephrine and dopamine.
  - Recommend starting at low dose (37.5–75 mg) in the morning.
  - Can increase up to 450 mg per day.
  - Typically avoid night-time dosing or 24 h preparations since they can cause or worsen insomnia.
- Serotonergic 5-HT1A receptor agonists including buspirone, vilazodone, and vortioxetine are alternatives if patients don't tolerate other antidepressants.

Muscle Relaxers

- Cyclobenzaprine is a TCA that has demonstrated efficacy in fibromyalgia
  - Recommend starting with low dose at night (5–10 mg).
  - Can be increased up to 30 mg per day.
  - Sustained-release preparation allows for once-daily dosing.

Tramadol

- While traditional opioids should be avoided, tramadol has been recommended for fibromyalgia treatment since it combines SNRI and mu-opioid agonist activities.
- 1–2 tramadol/acetaminophen 37.5/325 mg tablets taken four times daily have been shown

to improve pain, stiffness, and work interference in fibromyalgia patients.

- Also available as single-ingredient 50 mg immediate-release and 24 h extended-release tablets up to 300 mg.
- Maximum per day dosing 400 mg.

Medications to Avoid

- Benzodiazepines should be avoided since they can worsen nonrestorative sleep and cognition and have high addiction potential.
- Opioids other than tramadol should typically be avoided since they can paradoxically worsen pain by increasing central sensitization.
  - Due to increased central sensitization, patients can become dependent on opioids as discontinuation can dramatically worsen pain.
  - Opioids should be tapered off very slowly in fibromyalgia patients.
- Steroids are typically not helpful and should not be used as primary therapy.
- Nonsteroidal anti-inflammatory drugs (NSAIDs) are not helpful for the majority of patients and should not be used first line.

References

1. Wolfe F, et al. The American college of rheumatology 1990 criteria for the classification of fibromyalgia. Arthritis Rheum. 1990;33(2):160–72.
2. Okifuji A, et al. A standardized manual tender point survey. I. Development and determination of a threshold point for the identification of positive tender points in fibromyalgia syndrome. J Rheumatol. 1997;24(2):377–83.
3. Wolfe F, et al. The American college of rheumatology preliminary diagnostic criteria for fibromyalgia and measurement of symptom severity. Arthritis Care Res. 2010;62(5):600–10.
4. Wolfe F, et al. Fibromyalgia criteria and severity scales for clinical and epidemiological studies: a modification of the ACR preliminary diagnostic criteria for fibromyalgia. J Rheumatol. 2011;38:1113–22.
5. Boomershine CS. Fibromyalgia: the prototypical central sensitivity syndrome. Curr Rheumatol Rev. 2015;2(11):131–45.
6. Boomershine CS. The FIBRO system: a rapid strategy for assessment and management of fibromyalgia syndrome. Ther Adv Musculoskel Dis. 2010;2(4):187–200.

Aprajita Jagpal, Surahbhi S. Vinod,
and S. Louis Bridges Jr.

Introduction

Seronegative spondyloarthritis (SpA) is a heterogenous group of diseases [7, 10, 11, 12] characterized by:

- Inflammation of axial skeleton involving spine
  and sacroiliac (SI) joints
- Peripheral inflammatory arthritis
- Association with HLA B27
- Absence of serum rheumatoid factor
  (seronegative)

Classification

- Ankylosing spondylitis (AS)
- SpA associated with psoriasis
- SpA associated with inflammatory bowel disease
- Reactive arthritis (formerly known as Reiter
  syndrome)
- Undifferentiated spondyloarthritis

A. Jagpal, MBBS • S.S. Vinod, BS
S. Louis Bridges Jr., MD, PhD (✉)
Division of Clinical Immunology and Rheumatology,
School of Medicine, University of Alabama at
Birmingham, 1720 2nd Avenue South,
Birmingham, AL 35294, USA
e-mail: lbridges@uab.edu

Clinical Features

Inflammatory Back Pain

- Located in lower back and buttock area
- Onset before the age of 40 years
- Chronic in duration (>3 months)
- Night pain
- Early morning stiffness lasting for more than
  an hour
- Pain worsens with rest and improves with
  exercise

Peripheral Arthritis and Enthesitis

- Asymmetrical and oligoarticular (<4 joints)
- Usually acute onset
- Dactylitis or sausage digits – painful inflam-
  mation of the entire digit (Fig. 150.7).
- Enthesitis (inflammation at sites of attachments
  of ligaments or tendons to bone) (Fig. 150.6).

Eye Involvement

- Anterior uveitis (Fig. 150.8) characterized by
  redness, pain, and photophobia
- Vision loss may occur if not treated promptly

© Springer International Publishing AG 2017
A.E.M. Eltorai et al. (eds.), *Orthopedic Surgery Clerkship*, DOI 10.1007/978-3-319-52567-9_150

Diagnosis

- In addition to characteristic features of the medical history and physical exam, laboratory tests and radiographs may be helpful.
- Erythrocyte sedimentation rate (ESR) and C-reactive protein (CRP) may be increased, indicating systemic inflammation, but this is not a specific finding.
- A positive genetic test for HLA-B27 supports the diagnosis of SpA, but it can be positive in normal individuals and is therefore not useful as a diagnostic test.
- Radiographs of the sacroiliac joints should be obtained to look for sacroiliitis (Fig. 150.10). If there are abnormalities, MRI or CT scan of the SI joints (Fig. 150.11) may provide confirmation and can be considered if initial radiographs are nonrevealing and clinical suspicion for SpA is high. These imaging tests have higher sensitivity than radiographs but are more expensive.
- Radiographs of the lumbosacral, thoracic, or cervical spine may be helpful if those regions of the spine are symptomatic or have limitation in range of motion.

Subtypes

Ankylosing Spondylitis

- More common in males (male to female ratio of 2–3:1) [9].
- Age of onset typically <40 years.
- Associated with HLA-B27.
- Characterized by inflammatory back pain and stiffness in the spine.
- Sacroiliitis is the most common clinical feature.
- Uveitis, enthesitis, and peripheral arthritis may also be present.
- Less common extra-articular manifestations include restrictive lung disease from chest wall stiffness, apical pulmonary fibrosis [8], aortic regurgitation, and renal disease from amyloid or related to NSAIDs.
- New bone formation (e.g., syndesmophytes (Fig. 150.5) – bony growths originating in the ligaments) may occur in response to the inflammation and can lead to spinal fusion and loss of spinal mobility.
- On physical examination, one must evaluate spinal range of motion, sacroiliac joint tenderness, and perform the Schober's test, occiput to wall distance, and FABER (Flexion, ABduction, and External Rotation) test.
- Earliest radiographic changes are erosions on the iliac side of the sacroiliac joints.
- Fusion of the SI joints occurs in advanced disease.
- In severe cases, imaging may reveal the typical "bamboo spine" appearance of the spine (Fig. 150.4) with ankylosis (fusion).
- Treatment consists of symptomatic relief with NSAIDs, exercise to maintain range of motion (ROM) and strength, and TNF inhibitors.
- Total joint replacement (e.g. hip) may be necessary for patients with severe joint space loss and refractory pain. Surgical interventions in the spine are rarely indicated.

Psoriatic Arthritis

- Inflammatory arthritis associated with psoriasis.
- Affects men and women equally.
- Seen in as many as 11 % of patients with psoriasis [5].
- In a small number of patients, arthritis can precede the onset of skin lesions.
- Typically involves axial and peripheral joints including distal interphalangeal (DIP) joints (Fig. 150.1).
- Examination should include evaluation of skin and nails in addition to musculoskeletal assessment.
- Skin changes comprise erythematous scaly plaques (Fig. 150.2), most often on extensor surfaces and in the scalp.
- Nail changes include pitting, oil drop discoloration, and onycholysis (separation of nail from its bed) (Fig. 150.1).
- Radiographs may reveal features of joint erosions, "pencil in cup deformity," and new bone formation.

- Arthritis mutilans is a severe form of psoriatic arthritis causing joint destruction and deformities.
- Treatment consists of NSAIDS and DMARDs such as methotrexate, sulfasalazine, and TNF inhibitors [2].

Spondyloarthritis with Inflammatory Bowel Disease (IBD)

- Also called enteropathic arthritis.
- Associated with inflammatory conditions of the GI tract, mainly Crohn's disease and ulcerative colitis [4].
- Peripheral arthritis can be pauciarticular or polyarticular.
- Axial arthritis mimics ankylosing spondylitis.
- Erythema nodosum and pyoderma gangrenosum can also be seen in patients with IBD.
- Treatment options are sulfasalazine, immunomodulatory agents such as 6-mercaptopurine, azathioprine (used for IBD) [3], and TNF inhibitors.
- NSAIDs may provide symptomatic relief, but should be used with caution due to potential GI adverse effects.

Reactive Arthritis

- Previously known as Reiter syndrome [13] referring to the triad of arthritis, uveitis, and conjunctivitis [14].
- This classic triad may not be always present.
- Is associated with and typically occurs after a gastrointestinal (dysentery) or genitourinary infection (urethritis).
- Implicated organisms are Chlamydia trachomatis, Chlamydia pneumonia, Yersinia, Salmonella, Shigella, and Campylobacter species [1].
- Clinical features include inflammatory back pain, acute onset peripheral asymmetric oligoarthritis, conjunctivitis, uveitis, dactylitis, and enthesitis.
- Skin lesions include keratoderma blennorrhagicum (Fig. 150.3), erythema nodosum, and circinate balanitis (lesions on glans penis).

- Often is a self-limited illness.
- NSAIDs provide symptomatic relief.

Undifferentiated Spondyloarthritis (USpA)

- Spondyloarthropathy that does not meet criteria for other subtypes.
- Majority are HLA-B27 positive.
- Treatment consists of NSAIDS, DMARDs, and TNF inhibitors.

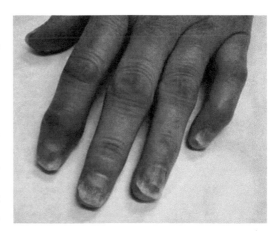

Fig. 150.1 Psoriatic arthritis. This photograph of the hand of a patient with psoriatic arthritis shows characteristic early nail separation (onycholysis), swelling, and erythema of the index and little finger distal interphalangeal joints (Reproduced with permission from Daniel Z Sands, MD, MPH)

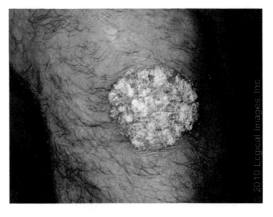

Fig. 150.2 Plaque psoriasis. An erythematous plaque with coarse scale is present on the knee of this patient with psoriasis (Reproduced with permission from: www.visualdx.com. Copyright Logical Images, Inc)

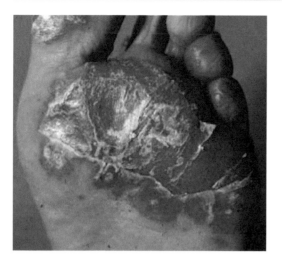

Fig. 150.3 This close-up photograph shows the erythematous, scaly plaques of keratoderma blennorrhagicum in a patient with reactive arthritis (formerly Reiter's Syndrome) (Courtesy of Filip de Keyser)

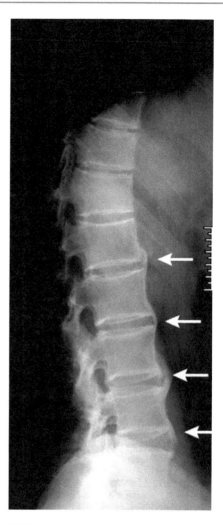

Fig. 150.5 Lateral view of the lumbar spine showing syndesmophytes. Syndesmophytes are shown in *white arrows* (Courtesy of Dr. Sheng Guang Li, PLA Hospital, China)

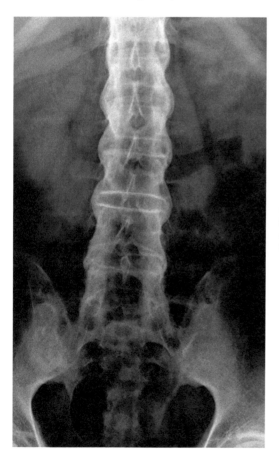

Fig. 150.4 Bamboo spine in ankylosing spondylitis. Radiograph shows continuous fusion of the lumbar spine and lateral fusion of the sacroiliac joints (Courtesy of Dr. Sheng Guang Li, PLA Hospital, China)

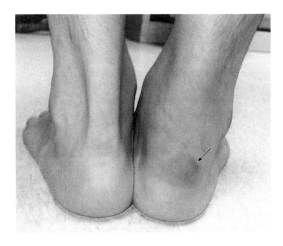

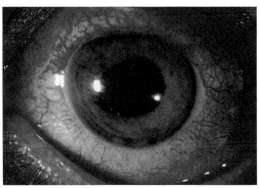

Fig. 150.8 Anterior uveitis. The irregular pupil shape is caused by inflammatory adhesion of the iris margin to the anterior lens surface superiorly (Reproduced with permission from: Trobe JD. The Physician's Guide to Eye Care, *American Academy of Ophthalmology* 1993. Copyright © 1993)

Fig. 150.6 Heel enthesitis. Right heel shows swelling at the insertion of the Achilles tendon to the calcaneus (*arrow*). This type of swelling is best examined from the back (Courtesy of James Wei, MD)

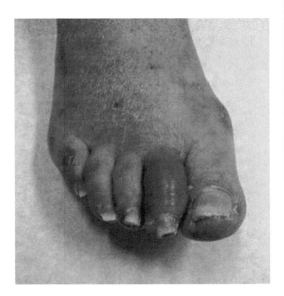

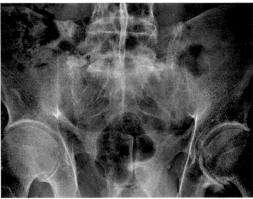

Fig. 150.9 Sacroiliitis grade 4 example 2. Bilateral grade 4 sacroiliitis with fusion of the sacroiliac joints (Courtesy of Xenofon Baraliakos, Rheumazentrum Ruhrgebiet Herne, Ruhr-Universität, Herne, Germany)

Fig. 150.7 Psoriatic arthritis. This photograph of the foot of a patient with psoriatic arthritis shows the early separation of the nails (onycholysis), swelling of the entire second toe (dactylitis), and some psoriatic skin lesions (Reproduced with permission from Daniel Z Sands, MD, MPH)

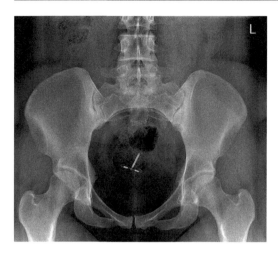

Fig. 150.10 Sacroiliitis grade 1 bilaterally. Bilateral suspicion of sacroiliitis in a female patient (grade 1 bilaterally). Intrauterine device is present. *L* left (Courtesy of Astrid van Tubergen, MD)

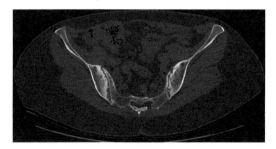

Fig. 150.11 CT scan showing bilateral, symmetrical, moderately advanced erosive arthropathy of the SI joints with associated reactive sclerosis

References

1. Ajene AN, Fischer Walker CL, Black RE. Enteric pathogens and reactive arthritis: a systematic review of Campylobacter, salmonella and Shigella-associated reactive arthritis. J Health Popul Nutr. 2013;31(3):299–307.

2. Brockbank J, Gladman D. Diagnosis and management of psoriatic arthritis. Drugs. 2002;62(17):2447–57.

3. De Keyser F, Van Damme N, De Vos M, Mielants H, Veys EM. Opportunities for immune modulation in the spondyloarthropathies with special reference to gut inflammation. Inflamm Res. 2000;49(2):47–54.

4. De Vos M. Joint involvement associated with inflammatory bowel disease. Dig Dis. 2009;27(4):511–5.

5. Gelfand JM, Gladman DD, Mease PJ, Smith N, Margolis DJ, Nijsten T, et al. Epidemiology of psoriatic arthritis in the population of the United States. J Am Acad Dermatol. 2005;53(4):573.

6. Healy PJ, Helliwell PS. Classification of the spondyloarthropathies. Curr Opin Rheumatol. 2005;17(4):395–9.

7. Kanathur N, Lee-Chiong T. Pulmonary manifestations of ankylosing spondylitis. Clin Chest Med. 2010;31(3):547–54.

8. Kidd B, Mullee M, Frank A, Cawley M. Disease expression of ankylosing spondylitis in males and females. J Rheumatol. 1988;15(9):1407–9.

9. Rudwaleit M, van der Heijde D, LandewÈ R, Akkoc N, Brandt J, Chou CT, et al. The Assessment of SpondyloArthritis International Society classification criteria for peripheral spondyloarthritis and for spondyloarthritis in general. Ann Rheum Dis. 2011;70(1):25–31.

10. Rudwaleit M, van der Heijde D, LandewÈ R, Listing J, Akkoc N, Brandt J, et al. The development of Assessment of SpondyloArthritis international Society classification criteria for axial spondyloarthritis (part II): validation and final selection. Ann Rheum Dis. 2009;68(6):777–83.

11. Sieper J, van der Heijde D, LandewÈ R, Brandt J, Burgos-Vagas R, Collantes-Estevez E, et al. New criteria for inflammatory back pain in patients with chronic back pain: a real patient exercise by experts from the Assessment of SpondyloArthritis international Society (ASAS). Ann Rheum Dis. 2009;68(6):784–8.

12. Wallace DJ, Weisman MH. The physician Hans Reiter as prisoner of war in nuremberg: a contextual review of his interrogations (1945–1947). Semin Arthritis Rheum. 2003;32(4):208–30.

13. Wu IB, Schwartz RA. Reiter's syndrome: the classic triad and more. J Am Acad Dermatol. 2008;59(1):113–21.

14. Zochling J, Smith EU. Seronegative spondyloarthritis. Best Pract Res Clin Rheumatol. 2010;24(6):747–56.

Polymyalgia Rheumatica

151

Aprajita Jagpal and S. Louis Bridges Jr.

Polymyalgia Rheumatica

Definition

- Polymyalgia rheumatica (PMR) is an inflammatory syndrome characterized by proximal muscle stiffness primarily in the neck, arms, shoulder, and hip girdle.

Epidemiology

- It is seen almost exclusively in adults aged 50 and older, and prevalence increases with advancing age [2].
- Mean age at diagnosis is 70 years [9].
- Women are affected twice as often as men.
- It most commonly affects individuals of European ethnicity, particularly of Scandinavian ancestry.

Pathogenesis

- The exact etiology of this condition is unknown [10].
- Association with HLA-DRB1*04 alleles has been reported in some studies [11].

- PMR is closely related to giant cell arteritis (GCA), a form of large vessel vasculitis. PMR occurs in ~40–50 % of patients with GCA, and GCA occurs in ~15 % of patients with PMR [7, 10].

Clinical Features

- Classic symptoms of PMR are aching, muscle pain, and stiffness in the neck, shoulder, and hip girdle [5, 6]. The pain is usually worse in the morning and lasts for more than 45 minutes.
- Patients often complain of difficulty with rising from a chair or lifting arms above the shoulders due to muscle stiffness. See Fig. 151.1.
- Distal muscle groups are typically not involved. See Fig. 151.2.
- Systemic symptoms such as malaise, fatigue, weight loss, and low-grade fever can also be seen.
- On physical examination, decreased range of motion can be appreciated in shoulders and hip joints.
- Although patients report some subjective weakness, true muscle weakness is generally absent.
- Synovitis, tenosynovitis, and peripheral edema may be present.

A. Jagpal, MBBS • S. Louis Bridges Jr., MD, PhD (✉)
Division of Clinical Immunology and Rheumatology,
School of Medicine, University of Alabama at
Birmingham, 1720 2nd Avenue South, Birmingham,
AL 35294, USA
e-mail: lbridges@uab.edu

© Springer International Publishing AG 2017
A.E.M. Eltorai et al. (eds.), *Orthopedic Surgery Clerkship*, DOI 10.1007/978-3-319-52567-9_151

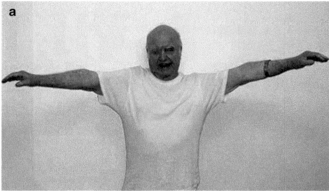
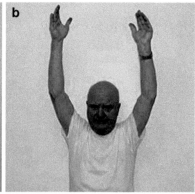

Fig. 151.1 Patient with PMR. (a) Inability to abduct actively the arms above 90° in a patient presenting with 2 weeks of proximal achiness and protracted morning stiffness. (b) Painless active abduction of the shoulders after 1 week on prednisone 10 mg/day (From Dockcn WP. Two inflammatory conditions—polymyalgia rheumatica and giant cell arteritis—share clinical connection. *The Rheumatologist.* 2013. http://www.the-rheumatologist.org/article/two-inflammatory-conditionspolymyalgia-rheumatica-and-giant-cell-arteritisshare-clinical-connection/. Copyright © 2013 American College of Rheumatology. Reproduced with permission of John Wiley & Sons Inc. This image has been provided by or is owned by Wiley. Further permission is needed before it can be downloaded to PowerPoint, printed, shared, or emailed. Please contact Wiley's permissions department either via email: *permissions@wiley.com* or use the RightsLink service by clicking on the 'Request Permission' link accompanying this article on Wiley Online Library (http://onlinelibrary.wiley.com))

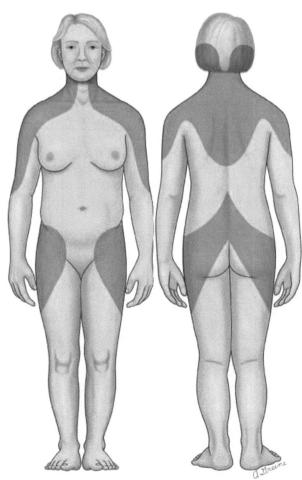

Fig. 151.2 PMR pain distribution. *Shaded areas* demonstrate the typical sites of pain in patients with PMR, including a shoulder girdle and neck pain distribution and a pelvic girdle pain distribution

Diagnosis

- There is no gold standard test to diagnose PMR. Diagnosis is made clinically based on history, examination, and laboratory data and exclusion of other diagnoses.
- Age > 50 years, typical symptoms, and elevation in erythrocyte sedimentation rate > 40 mm/h and high serum CRP levels are highly suggestive. Lab studies may also indicate normocytic anemia.
- Muscle enzymes are not elevated which helps to differentiate PMR from other myopathies.
- Radiographs of the affected areas tend to be normal; however MRI and ultrasonography may show evidence of inflammation in periarticular structures [1].
- Careful evaluation should be done to differentiate PMR from other clinical entities that may cause similar symptoms. Some examples include hypothyroidism, rheumatoid arthritis, fibromyalgia, systemic lupus erythematosus, inflammatory myopathies, statin therapy, and malignancy.

Treatment

- Polymyalgia rheumatica is characterized by prompt response to corticosteroids [3, 4]. Initial dose of prednisone 10–20 mg is usually sufficient to control symptoms. Some patients may require higher doses.
- The initial dose is maintained for 2–4 weeks, and taper is then initiated as tolerated.
- Response is measured with resolution of clinical symptoms and normalization of inflammatory markers.
- Biologic agents are generally ineffective in treating this condition.

Complications

- The disease is usually self-limited, with median duration of 11 months

- Long-term complications from PMR are rare.
- Adverse effects due to long-term prednisone use, such as hyperglycemia, impaired wound healing, infection, and osteoporosis, should be addressed appropriately.

References

1. Cantini F, Salvarani C, Olivieri I, Niccoli L, Padula A, Macchioni L, et al. Shoulder ultrasonography in the diagnosis of polymyalgia rheumatica: a case-control study. J Rheumatol. 2001;28(5):1049–55.
2. Chuang TY, Hunder GG, Ilstrup DM, Kurland LT. Polymyalgia rheumatica: a 10-year epidemiologic and clinical study. Ann Intern Med. 1982;97(5):672–80.
3. De Bandt M. Current diagnosis and treatment of polymyalgia rheumatica. Joint Bone Spine. 2014;81(3):203–8.
4. Dejaco C, Singh YP, Perel P, Hutchings A, Camellino D, Mackie S, et al. Current evidence for therapeutic interventions and prognostic factors in polymyalgia rheumatica: a systematic literature review informing the 2015 European League Against Rheumatism/American College of Rheumatology recommendations for the management of polymyalgia rheumatica. Ann Rheum Dis. 2015;74(10):1808–17.
5. Gonzalez-Gay MA, Barros S, Lopez-Diaz MJ, Garcia-Porrua C, Sanchez-Andrade A, Llorca J. Giant cell arteritis: disease patterns of clinical presentation in a series of 240 patients. Medicine (Baltimore). 2005;84(5):269–76.
6. Gonzalez-Gay MA, Pina T. Giant cell arteritis and polymyalgia rheumatica: an update. Curr Rheumatol Rep. 2015;17(2):6.
7. Gonzalez-Gay MA, Vazquez-Rodriguez TR, Lopez-Diaz MJ, Miranda-Filloy JA, Gonzalez-Juanatey C, Martin J, et al. Epidemiology of giant cell arteritis and polymyalgia rheumatica. Arthritis Rheum. 2009; 61(10):1454–61.
8. Owen CE, Buchanan RR, Hoi A. Recent advances in polymyalgia rheumatica. Intern Med J. 2015;45(11):1102–8.
9. Salvarani C, Gabriel SE, O'Fallon WM, Hunder GG. Epidemiology of polymyalgia rheumatica in Olmsted County, Minnesota, 1970-1991. Arthritis Rheum. 1995;38(3):369–73.
10. Weyand CM, Goronzy JJ. Giant-cell arteritis and polymyalgia rheumatica. N Engl J Med. 2014;371(17):1653.
11. Weyand CM, Hunder NN, Hicok KC, Hunder GG, Goronzy JJ. HLA-DRB1 alleles in polymyalgia rheumatica, giant cell arteritis, and rheumatoid arthritis. Arthritis Rheum. 1994;37(4):514–20.

Osteoporosis

Jonathan M. Karnes and Colleen Watkins

Introduction

- Definition – decrease in bone mineral density due to imbalance in cancellous bone deposition and remodeling:
  - Osteopenia and osteoporosis result from this imbalance.
  - Most commonly associated with estrogen withdrawal following menopause.
  - Other factors contributing to osteoporosis include smoking and alcohol use, glucocorticoid use, autoimmune processes, and hypogonadism.
- Osteoporosis vs. osteomalacia:
  - Osteoporosis: reduction in bone mass, no change in mineralization
  - Osteomalacia: reduction in mineralization, bone mass independent
- Areas affected – the degree of bone mineral density lost is positively correlated with intensity of regional bone remodeling:
  - Cortical bone undergoes less remodeling than cancellous bone.
  - Therefore, osteoporosis is more commonly found in areas of cancellous bone (metaphyseal bone – vertebral bodies, proximal humerus, distal radius, proximal and distal femur, proximal tibia).
  - This distribution predicts areas of most commonly injured in patients with osteoporosis.
- Importance in orthopedics:
  - Low bone mineral density predisposes patients to significant injury (hip fractures, distal radius fractures, and spine compression fractures) following relatively minor trauma.
  - Extension of life expectancy and the increased number of the elderly in the USA are leading to an increase in the total number of osteoporotic fractures treated.
  - 30-day mortality following an untreated hip fracture is greater than the 30-day mortality following an MI [1].

Describing and Measuring Osteoporosis

- Dual-energy X-ray absorptiometry (DEXA) – used to measure bone mineral density (BMD) of a patient (absolute value):
  - BMD by itself is useless; clinical value is appreciated through T- and Z-scores (Fig. 152.1)
    - Reported as standard deviations from the population mean
      - T-score compares the mean BMD *against the average value of 30-year-old men/women.*

J.M. Karnes, MD (✉) • C. Watkins, MD
Department of Orthopedics, West Virginia University, Morgantown, WV, USA
e-mail: jmkarnes@hsc.wvu.edu

© Springer International Publishing AG 2017
A.E.M. Eltorai et al. (eds.), *Orthopedic Surgery Clerkship*, DOI 10.1007/978-3-319-52567-9_152

Fig. 152.1 Illustration of how a patient's bone mineral density can be interpreted through the use of Z- and T-scores

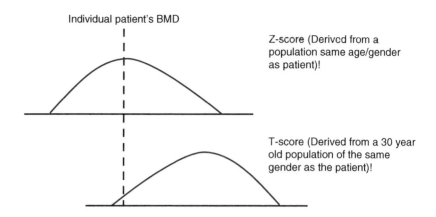

- • Z-score compares the mean BMD *against the average value for a patient's current age and gender.*
  - ◦ Osteopenia: T-score of −1 to −2.5 (1 to −2.5 standard deviations below the mean)
  - ◦ Osteoporosis: T-score of < −2.5 (>2.5 standard deviations below the mean)
- • Fracture Risk Assessment Tool (FRAX) [2]:
  - – Patient-specific data to estimate a 10-year osteoporotic hip fracture risk if untreated in 40–90-year patient
    - ◦ Previous hip fracture carries the highest risk for future hip fracture.
  - – Can be used to determine individuals that would best benefit from medical therapies (i.e., higher fracture risk would outweigh the potential side effects)

Treatment

- • Types of treatment:
  - – Medical treatment (prophylaxis) attempts to improve bone mineral density in order to protect patients against osteoporotic fractures.
  - – Surgical management (salvage) attempts to stabilize fractures and reduce pain to limit the time patients are not mobile.
- • Indications for medical treatment [3]:
  - – Postmenopausal females and men over 50 with:

- ◦ Hip or vertebral fracture
- ◦ T-score < −2.5
- ◦ T-score − 1.0 to −2.5 with a 10-year probability of hip fracture greater than 3% or a 20% or greater risk of osteoporosis-related fracture
- • Medication classes:
  - – Osteoclast inhibition
    - ◦ Bisphosphonates (mainstay of osteoporosis treatment)
      - • Nonnitrogen: induces osteoclast apoptosis
      - • Nitrogen: inhibits osteoclast ruffled border formation
    - ◦ Calcitonin
      - • Direct inhibition of osteoclast function
    - ◦ Monoclonal antibody (denosumab)
      - • Receptor activator of nuclear factor kappa-B ligand (RANKL) inhibitor
        - – RANKL stimulates osteoclast precursors to form osteoclasts; therefore, inhibition reduces number of active osteoclasts.
  - – Osteoblast stimulation
    - ◦ Parathyroid hormone analogue (teriparatide)
      - • Stimulates osteoblasts
  - – Osteoblast stimulation and osteoclast inhibition
    - ◦ Selective estrogen receptor modulators (SERMs): raloxifene
    - ◦ Vitamin D (Fig. 152.2)

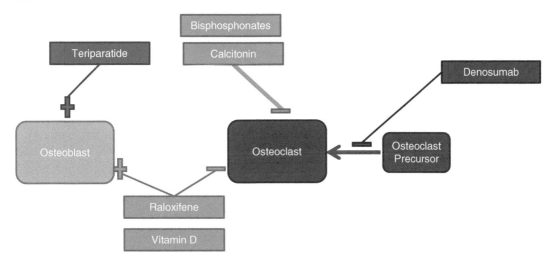

Fig. 152.2 Illustration of the mechanisms of commonly used medications in osteoporosis management

References

1. Roche JJ, Wenn RT, Sahota O, Moran CG. Effect of comorbidities and postoperative complications on mortality after hip fracture in elderly people: Prospective observational cohort study. BMJ. 2005;331(7529):1374.

2. https://www.shef.ac.uk/FRAX/tool.jsp.

3. http://nof.org/files/nof/public/content/file/917/upload/481.pdf.

Christopher Treager and Carlos Isales

Osteomalacia

Definition

Both osteomalacia (OM) and rickets are characterized by impaired bone mineralization, but the former occurs in adults and the latter in children.

Etiologies

- Nutritional – Vitamin D deficiency resulting in dietary calcium and phosphorus malabsorption. This results in secondary hyperparathyroidism, inducing further phosphate wasting, causing defective mineralization [1].
  - Common causes: Decreased sun exposure, decreased dietary vitamin D intake, malabsorption, pharmacologically induced degradation of calcifediol/calcitriol (rifampicin, isoniazid)
  - Less common causes: Reduced hydroxylation of vitamin D to 25(OH)D in the liver, due to liver disease. Reduced hydroxylation of 25(OH)D to 1,25(OH)D2 in the kidney, due to kidney disease

C. Treager • C. Isales (✉)
Regenerative Medicine, Orthopaedic Surgery,
Medical College of Georgia, CA 1004 1120 15th
Street, Augusta, GA, USA
e-mail: cisales@augusta.edu

- Tumor-induced osteomalacia (TIO) – Mesenchymal tumor overproducing FGF23, resulting in phosphaturia [2]. Tumors are often benign and slow growing and occur in the soft tissue and bone in equal amounts [3].
- Fanconi syndrome – The damage to the renal proximal tubule and proximal tubular acidosis results in phosphaturia and hypophosphatemia, thus reducing bone mineralization [4].
- Hypophosphatasia – Mutation in the ALPL gene, causing a reduced activity in tissue-nonspecific alkaline phosphatase (TNAP). This increases inorganic pyrophosphate (PPi), which is a strong mineralization inhibitor, thus leading to osteomalacia [5]. Can be autosomal dominant or recessive inheritance.
- Mineralization inhibitors – Increased intake of inhibitors, such as aluminum or fluoride.

Clinical Presentations [6]

General Presentations

- Bone pain and tenderness in the spine, ribs, pelvis, and/or lower extremities made worse with muscle strain or load-bearing activities.
- In severe cases, skeletal deformities, such as bowing or pigeon chest, can occur.
- Muscle weakness is an important but often overlooked clinical finding.
- If serum calcium levels are severely decreased, tetany and convulsions may develop.

© Springer International Publishing AG 2017
A.E.M. Eltorai et al. (eds.), *Orthopedic Surgery Clerkship*, DOI 10.1007/978-3-319-52567-9_153

Specific Considerations

- TIO often presents in adults, often in the 60s, but can present at any age. In cases with suspected TIO, the tumor may be in the subcutaneous tissue and may be palpable. However, the tumor most often can be difficult to locate, even with imaging [7].
- Hypophosphatasia has a wide range of presentations, ranging from stillborn infants with no calcification of the bone to middle age presentation of premature loss of teeth with foot and hip pain due to microfractures and/or arthritis [5].

Diagnostics

Lab Studies (See Table 153.1 for Overview of Expected Lab Results)

- Initial tests to order: CMP with alkaline phosphatase, calcium and phosphate, PTH, vitamin D study, and 24-h urinary calcium and phosphate [8].
  - If TIO is suspected, FGF23 levels should be measured.
  - If hypophosphatasia is suspected, plasma PLP (pyridoxal phosphate) and urinary phosphoethanolamine levels should be ordered.
- Expected results
  - Nutritional OM [9]
    - Elevated: Alkaline phosphatase, PTH.
    - Reduced: Serum 25(OH)D and serum calcium and phosphate. Vitamin D insufficiency, <30 ng/ml and deficiency, <20 ng/ml. OM prevalence increases at values <15 ng/ml.
    - 1,25(OH)2D levels can present as high, normal, or low in nutritional OM and are therefore not useful in diagnostics.

- TIO [8]
  - Elevated: Alkaline phosphatase, phosphaturia
  - Reduced: Serum phosphorus, 1,25(OH)2D
  - Normal: Serum calcium and PTH
- If previous serum phosphorus levels were normal, this suggests possible TIO. However, the tumor must be found to confirm diagnosis.
- Hypophosphatasia.
- Elevated: Plasma pyridoxal-5 phosphate (PLP), urinary phosphoethanolamine. Serum calcium and phosphate may be elevated.
- Reduced: Serum alkaline phosphatase. (This is a red flag for hypophosphatasia as all other etiologies of OM or rickets cause elevated alkaline phosphatase.)
  - Normal: Vitamin D and metabolites, PTH

Imaging Studies

- Imaging studies of a patient with OM can show several characteristic findings [9, 10].
  - Radiographs show less contrast and are less sharp (milk glass appearance).
  - Lumbar vertebrae may develop a biconcave, or codfish, appearance.
  - Pseudofractures (Looser zones) are narrow radiolucent lines often perpendicular to the cortical plate. Develop due to improper healing of fractures due to improper mineralization.
    - Often found in the ribs, pubic rami, outer borders of the scapula, and ends of long bones
- If TIO is suspected, whole-body imaging with octreotide SPECT should be performed. If no clear single lesion is present, then follow with a whole-body FDG PET/CT and confirm the presence of the tumor with MRI [11].

Table 153.1 Lab Studies

Labs	Nutritional rickets	Tumor-induced osteomalacia	Hypophosphatasia
Calcium	Normal–low	Normal	Normal–high
Phosphorus	Low	Low	Normal–high
Alkaline phosphatase	High	Normal–high	Low
Vitamin D	Low	Normal	Normal
PTH	Normal–high	Normal	Normal
24-hour urinary calcium	Low	Normal	Normal–high

– If multiple lesions are present or if it is in an area with high surgical morbidity, venous sampling near the tumor for FGF23 levels can be useful in confirming TIO.

Treatments

- No matter what the treatment is, proper monitoring of the patient should include [8]:
  – Urinary calcium after 1, 3, and 6 months, until urinary calcium returns to normal
  – Serum calcium to monitor for hypercalcemia
  – Serum 25(OH)D to monitor for overdosing of vitamin D
- Patients must have a daily calcium intake of at least 1000–1200 mg for children and 1500–2000 mg for adults [9, 12].

Nutritional OM
- When possible, vitamin D supplements should be used instead of the calcifediol/calcitriol due to lower cost of vitamin D. However, in the case of malabsorption or abnormal vitamin D metabolism, metabolites should be used.
- For patients with normal metabolism: 2000–4000 IU/day orally of cholecalciferol (vitamin D3) until 25(OH)D is at the proper levels. Then, a maintenance regiment of 600–800 IU/day for adults and 400 IU/day for children [9].
- Malabsorptive patients: Depending on their absorptive capability, dosages can range from 10,000–50,000 IU of cholecalciferol per day. If there is no response to this treatment, the use of vitamin D metabolites is suggested.
  – Patient monitoring is very important to ensure proper therapy and to avoid toxicity.
- Calcifediol or calcitriol can also be prescribed instead of cholecalciferol [11, 13].
  – Calcifediol: 50–100 μg/day
  – Calcitriol: 0.015–0.02 mcg/kg/day PO, with maintenance dosage of 0.03–0.06 mcg/kg/day PO

TIO
- Complete surgical removal of the tumor with wide margins if possible. Removal should

result in normalization of lab values and rapid remineralization.
- If not completely removed, phosphorus and calcitriol supplements may be necessary.
  – Phosphorus: 1–2 g/day, divided into 3–4 doses daily
  – Calcitriol: 0.015–0.02 mcg/kg/day PO, with maintenance dosage of 0.03–0.06 mcg/kg/day PO
- Proper monitoring includes serum and urine calcium, renal function, and PTH status every 3 months to prevent complications. Monitor for nephrocalcinosis.
- Fanconi syndrome
  – 5000–10,000 IU cholecalciferol/day in addition to correction of acidosis [8]
- Hypophosphatasia – Asfotase alfa available as enzyme replacement therapy. The use of vitamin D or phosphate may lead to complications such as hypercalcemia [4].
- Mineralization inhibitors – Remove the source of the mineral overdosing. Vitamin D supplementation may or may not be indicated depending on the status of the patient.

Outcome
- Signs of improvement rapid normalization of serum calcium and phosphorus, as well as urinary calcium. Alkaline phosphatase may remain elevated for a few weeks, but will eventually return to normal. Pseudofractures should heal within a year for adults and much more rapidly for children [9].

Rickets

Etiologies

Nutritional Rickets
- Inadequate intake of vitamin D and/or calcium. Typically presents between 3 months and 3 years of age. Risk factors include maternal vitamin D deficiency during pregnancy, prolonged breastfeeding, dark skin pigmentation and low sun exposure, and malabsorptive diseases.

Vitamin D-Dependent Rickets Type 1 (VDDR-1)

- Autosomal recessive mutation in the 1-alpha hydroxylase enzyme that converts 25(OH)D to 1,25(OH)D2 in the kidneys.

Hereditary Vitamin D-Resistant Rickets (HVDRR)

- Autosomal recessive mutation in the vitamin D receptor (VDR), which recognizes 1,25(OH)2D

X-Linked Hypophosphatemic Rickets (XLH)

- Most common form of heritable rickets
- Mutation in PHEX gene, leading to increased levels of FGF23, thus inducing phosphaturia and phosphate wasting [14]

Autosomal Dominant Hypophosphatemic Rickets (ADHR)

- Mutation in the FGF23 gene, resulting in elevated FGF23 levels, inducing phosphaturia and phosphate wasting

Hereditary Hypophosphatemic Rickets with Hypercalciuria (HHRH)

- Mutation in the SLC34A3 gene, encoding for a sodium phosphate cotransporter in the proximal renal tubule. Results in urinary phosphate wasting and hypophosphatemia

Clinical Presentations

General Presentations

- Decreased stature and widening and painful swelling of the epiphyseal zones.
- Bowing of the lower extremities presents as weight-bearing activity increases.
- Rachitic rosary develops due to swelling of the rib cartilage and can be felt lateral to the nipple line.

Specific Considerations

- XLH adults can experience mineralization of tendons and ligaments, as well as development of dental abscess [3].

- ADHR: Exhibits incomplete penetrance and variable age of onset. Spontaneous resolution of phosphate wasting has been documented in some cases [15].

Diagnostics

Lab Studies

- Initial tests to order: CMP including alkaline phosphatase and phosphate, PTH, vitamin D study, and 24-h urinary calcium and phosphate.
- If there is a known family history of XLH, a newborn genetic screen is indicated.
- Expected results
  - Nutritional rickets
    - Elevated: alkaline phosphatase, PTH.
    - Reduced: serum calcium and phosphorus, 25(OH)D.
    - 1,25(OH)2D may be elevated, normal, or low, so it is not useful in diagnosing nutritional rickets.
  - VDDR-1
    - Elevated: alkaline phosphatase, PTH
    - Reduced: serum calcium and phosphate, very low 1,25(OH)2D
    - Normal: 25(OH)D
  - HVDRR
    - Elevated: alkaline phosphatase, PTH, serum 1,25(OH)2D
    - Reduced: serum calcium and phosphate
  - XLH and ADHR
    - Elevated: alkaline phosphatase, phosphaturia.
    - Reduced: serum phosphorus, urine calcium.
    - Normal: serum calcium.
    - PTH may be normal or high.
  - HHRH
    - Elevated: alkaline phosphatase, 1,25(OH)2d, hypercalciuria
    - Reduced: low to very low serum phosphate
    - Normal: serum calcium

Imaging Studies

- Radiograph of the distal ulna or the metaphysis of the femur and/or tibia near the knee

is the best location to find evidence of
rickets.

- Expected findings: Widening of metaphysis, cup-shaped metaphysis, loss of definition around the epiphysis due to decreased mineralization, and Looser zones [16]

Treatments

- No matter what the treatment is, proper monitoring of the patient should include [8]:
  - Urinary calcium after 1, 3, and 6 months, until urinary calcium returns to normal
  - Serum calcium to monitor for hypercalcemia and PTH
  - Serum 25(OH)D to monitor for overdosing of vitamin D
- Patients must have a daily calcium intake of at least 1000–1200 mg for children and 1500–2000 mg for adults [9, 12].
  - Nutritional Rickets: 800–1000 IU/day PO cholecalciferol and 1000 mg/day of calcium until serum alkaline phosphate levels and skeletal deformities heal. After resolution of symptoms, vitamin D supplementation should continue at 600 IU/day [16].
  - VDDR-1: Calcitriol (0.5–1.0 mcg/day) or alphacalcidol (0.5–1.5 mcg/day), in addition to proper calcium supplementation. This treatment should continue for life along with proper monitoring.
  - HVDRR: Treatment regimen and success depend on severity of resistance to 1,25(OH)2D.
    - If some function remains in VDR, then 0.5–1.0 mcg/day calcitriol may be effective.
    - If no VDR activity, calcium infusions to normalize calcium levels have been shown to help with proper mineralization, as long as phosphorus levels are normal as well [17].
  - XLH: 20–30 nanograms/kg/day of calcitriol and 20–40 mg/kg/day of oral phosphorus divided into 3–5 dosages [14]. Surgery may also be required to repair any

skeletal deformities. Nasal calcitonin being evaluated for effectiveness.

- Treatment should continue until adulthood when the epiphyseal plates close and bone turnover declines. If an adult patient is suffering from spontaneous insufficiency fractures and undergoing orthopedic procedures and develops OM or skeletal pain, treatment should be resumed.
- ADHR: Similar treatment to XLR.
- HHRH: Phosphate supplementation alone (20–40 mg/kg/day phosphorus PO divided into 3–5 doses).
  - It is vital to ensure the diagnosis of HHRH because if calcitriol is included in the treatment for HHRH, this could result in hypercalciuria, nephrocalcinosis, and renal damage [18].

Outcomes

- Proper diagnosis and treatment should allow normal bone mineralization and growth to resume. If there has been significant damage to the skeletal structure, surgical intervention may be necessary.

References

1. Gallagher J. Vitamin D insufficiency and deficiency. In: The American Society for Bone and Mineral Research. Primer on the metabolic bone disease and disorders of mineral metabolism. 8th ed. Ames: Wiley-Blackwell; 2013. p. 624–631.
2. Kapelari K, Köhle J, Kotzot D, Högler W. Iron supplementation associated with loss of phenotype in autosomal dominant hypophosphatemic rickets. J Clin Endocrinol Metabol. 2015;100(9):3388–92.
3. Ruppe M, Jan de Beur S. Disorders of phosphate homeostasis. In: The American Society for Bone and Mineral Research. Primer on the metabolic bone disease and disorders of mineral metabolism. 8th ed. Ames: Wiley-Blackwell; 2013. p. 601–12.
4. Greenspan F, Gardner D, Shoback D. Basic & clinical endocrinology. New York: McGraw-Hill; 2011.
5. Gasque K, Foster B, Kuss P, Yadav M, Liu J, Kiffer-Moreira T, et al. Improvement of the skeletal and dental hypophosphatasia phenotype in Alpl−/− mice by

administration of soluble (non-targeted) chimeric alkaline phosphatase. Bone. 2015;72:137–47.

6. Frame B, Parfitt A. Osteomalacia: current concepts. Ann Intern Med. 1978;89(6):966–82.

7. Drezner M. Tumor-induced osteomalacia. Rev Endocr Metab Disord. 2001;2:175–86.

8. Reginato AJ, Coquia JA. Musculoskeletal manifestations of osteomalacia and rickets. Best Pract Res Clin Rheumatol. 2003;17(6):1063–80.

9. Munns CF, Shaw N, Kiely M, Specker BL, Thacher TD, Ozono K, et al. Global Consensus Recommendations on Prevention and Management of Nutritional Rickets. J Clin Endocrinol Metab. 2016;101(2):394–415.

10. Rabelink N, Westgeest H, Bravenboer N, Jacobs M, Lips P. Bone pain and extremely low bone mineral density due to severe vitamin D deficiency in celiac disease. Arch Osteoporos. 2011;6(1–2):209–13.

11. Chong W, Andreopoulou P, Chen C, Reynolds J, Guthrie L, Kelly M, et al. Tumor localization and biochemical response to cure in tumor-induced osteomalacia. J Bone Miner Res. 2013;28(6):1386–98.

12. Balvers MG, Brouwer-Brolsma EM, Endenburg S, de Groot LC, Kok FJ, Gunnewiek JK. Recommended intakes of vitamin D to optimise health, associated circulating 25-hydroxyvitamin D concentrations, and dosing regimens to treat deficiency: workshop report and overview of current literature. J Nutr Sci. 2015;4(e23):1–8.

13. Basha B, Rao D, Han Z, Parfitt A. Osteomalacia due to vitamin D depletion: a neglected consequence of intestinal malabsorption. Am J Med. 2000;108(4):296–300.

14. Carpenter T, Imel E, Holm I, Jan de Beur S, Insogna K. A clinician's guide to X-linked hypophosphatemia. J Bone Miner Res. 2011;26(7):1381–8.

15. Econs M, McEnery P. Autosomal dominant hypophosphatemic rickets/osteomalacia: clinical characterization of a novel renal phosphate-wasting disorder. J Clin Endocrinol Metabol. 1997;82(2):674–81.

16. Joiner T, Foster C, Shope T. The many faces of vitamin D deficiency rickets. Pediatr Rev. 2000;21(9): 296–302.

17. Balsan S, Garabédian M, Larchet M, Gorski A, Cournot G, Tau C, et al. Long-term nocturnal calcium infusions can cure rickets and promote normal mineralization in hereditary resistance to 1,25-dihydroxyvitamin D. J Clin Investig. 1986;77(5):1661–7.

18. Lorenz-Depiereux B, Benet-Pages A, Eckstein G, Tenenbaum-Rakover Y, Wagenstaller J, Tiosano D, et al. Hereditary hypophosphatemic rickets with hypercalciuria is caused by mutations in the sodium-phosphate cotransporter gene SLC34A3. Am J Hum Genet. 2006;78(2):193–201.

Renal Osteodystrophy

154

Phillip A. Bostian and Colleen Watkins

Pathophysiology

High-Turnover Renal Osteodystrophy

- Chronic renal disease leads to deficient electrolyte homeostasis.
- Chronic renal disease → defective 1-alpha-hydroxylase → decreased 1,25-dihydroxycholecalciferol (calcitriol, active form of vitamin D) and decreased phosphate secretion → decreased absorption of calcium from intestines → decreased serum calcium → hyperparathyroidism (hyperplasia of chief cells) → increased activation of osteoclasts and osteoblasts → increased bone turnover [1].
- Lab findings:
  - ↓ calcium
  - ↑ phosphate
  - ↑ PTH
  - ↑ alkaline phosphatase

Low-Turnover Renal Osteodystrophy

- Normal PTH levels.
- Aluminum deposition in the bone → impaired osteoblast function.
- Bony lesions are still seen even after aluminum overload is treated [2].
- Seen within 5 years following renal transplantation [3].

Clinical Findings

Adults

- Pathologic fracture
- Bone pain
- Proximal muscle weakness
- Hypocalcemia
- Heterotopic calcifications
- Vascular calcification of small and medium arteries
- Visceral calcifications (lungs, heart, kidneys, and skeletal muscle)
- Brown tumors due to hyperparathyroidism

Children [4]

- Growth retardation
- Progressive skeletal deformity:
  - Rachitic rosary

P.A. Bostian, MD (✉) • C. Watkins, MD
Department of Orthopedics, West Virginia University,
Health Science Center South, PO Box 9196,
Morgantown, WV 26506, USA
e-mail: pabostian@hsc.wvu.edu

© Springer International Publishing AG 2017
A.E.M. Eltorai et al. (eds.), *Orthopedic Surgery Clerkship*, DOI 10.1007/978-3-319-52567-9_154

- Metaphyseal enlargement
- Genu varum
- Frontal bossing
- Ulnar deviation of wrists
- Slipped capital femoral epiphysis

Radiologic Findings [5]

Adults

- Nonspecific osteosclerosis
- Chondrocalcinosis – knee, pubic symphysis, or triangular fibrocartilaginous complex of the wrist
- Looser's zones – microfractures or complete fractures similar to that seen in osteoporotic patients
- Bone resorption:
  - Subchondral – distal clavicle, sacroiliac joints, and pubic symphysis
  - Endosteal – long bone diaphysis
  - Subperiosteal – joint margins, especially in the hands and feet

Children

- Rachitic changes
- Widening or elongation of growth plates (due to increased width of zone of provisional calcification)
- Cupping of the metaphyses

Evaluation

Physical Exam

- Common growth disturbances
- Manifestations of hypocalcemia – tetany:
  - Chvostek's sign – facial muscle contractions after tapping facial nerve
  - Trousseau's sign – carpal spasm following compression of the upper arm by blood pressure cuff

Associated Conditions

- Avascular necrosis (commonly of femoral head)
- Tendinitis and tendon rupture

- Carpal tunnel syndrome (due to space-occupying amyloid deposition)
- Brown tumors – due to hyperparathyroidism

Treatment [6]

Medical Management

- Maintenance of calcium and phosphorus homeostasis
- Prevention of soft tissue calcification – dietary restriction of phosphate or ingestion of phosphate binders
- Secondary hyperparathyroidism treated with calcitriol or 1-alpha-hydroxylase – shown to decrease bone pain and increase muscle strength
- Aluminum toxicity – treated with deferoxamine

Surgical Considerations

- Pediatric skeletal deformities:
  - Corrective osteotomies for angular and rotational deformities
  - Prophylactic pinning of contralateral femoral neck following initial slipped capital femoral epiphyses (SCFE) presentation
- Hip arthroplasty:
  - Avascular necrosis secondary to steroid use in renal transplant patients
  - Poor bone stock – more commonly requires cemented prostheses
- Pathologic fractures:
  - Patterns similar to elderly osteoporotic fractures.
  - Poor bone stock may require bone cement, graft, or implant augmentation.
  - Progression to full weight bearing is delayed.

References

1. Martinez I, Saracho R, Montenegro J, Llach F. The importance of dietary calcium and phosphorous in the secondary hyperparathyroidism of patients with early renal failure. Am J Kidney Dis. 1997;29(4):496–502. Epub 1997/04/01. PubMed PMID: 9100037

2. Cannata Andia JB. Adynamic bone and chronic renal failure: an overview. Am J Med Sci. 2000;320(2):81–4. Epub 2000/09/12. PubMed PMID: 10981480

3. Rodino MA, Shane E. Osteoporosis after organ transplantation. Am J Med. 1998;104(5):459–69. Epub 1998/06/17. PubMed PMID: 9626030

4. Mankin HJ. Rickets, osteomalacia, and renal osteodystrophy. An update. Orthop Clin North Am. 1990;21(1):81–96. Epub 1990/01/01. PubMed PMID: 2404238

5. Tigges S, Nance EP, Carpenter WA, Erb R. Renal osteodystrophy: imaging findings that mimic those of other diseases. AJR Am J Roentgenol. 1995;165(1):143–8. doi:10.2214/ajr.165.1.7785573. Epub 1995/07/01. PubMed PMID: 7785573

6. Tejwani NC, Schachter AK, Immerman I, Achan P. Renal osteodystrophy. J Am Acad Orthop Surg. 2006;14(5):303–11. Epub 2006/05/06. PubMed PMID: 16675624

Paget's Disease

155

Kevin Shepet and Colleen Watkins

Epidemiology

- Primarily in adults greater than 40 years old (highest incidence around age 50).
- Men are more affected than women.
- Patients often have one or more family members affected.
- Geographic basis:
  - Higher prevalence in Western Europe and the United States
  - Lower prevalence in Japan and China

Etiology

- Possible link to chronic viral infection (paramyxovirus, RSV) [1]
- Appears to have a possible genetic link although no one single causative genetic mutation has been identified [3]

Pathophysiology

- Characterized by overactivity of osteoclasts (bone resorption).
- Subsequent disorganized bone remodeling.

K. Shepet, MD (✉) • C. Watkins, MD
Department of Orthopaedics, West Virginia University,
Health Science Center – South,
Morgantown, WV, USA
e-mail: khshepet@hsc.wvu.edu

- The bone formed is brittle and prone to fracture.
- Disease phases [4]:
  - Active
    ○ Osteoclasts resorb abnormal amount of bone ("lytic phase").
    ○ Osteoblasts respond by increasing activity level to form new bone ("mixed phase").
    ○ Osteoblasts become dominant over osteoclast-producing bone that is less organized and weaker mechanical properties than normal bone ("sclerotic phase").
  - Inactive
    ○ Osteoclast and osteoblast activity returns to normal levels.
    ○ Areas over sclerotic bone persist.

Clinical Presentation

Location

- Skull
- Spine
- Pelvis
- Femur
- Tibia

Symptoms

- Asymptomatic.
- Bone pain.

A.E.M. Eltorai et al. (eds.), *Orthopedic Surgery Clerkship*, DOI 10.1007/978-3-319-52567-9_155

- Warmth and swelling.
- Acute onset of symptoms – be suspicious of acute pathologic fracture or Paget's sarcoma (see below).

Physical Exam

- Bone tenderness to palpation
- Decreased joint range of motion
- Erythema and warmth
- Gross bony deformity in advanced disease
- Neurologic symptoms (due to spinal stenosis)
- Cranial nerve involvement possible

Imaging

- Radiographs:
  - May see areas of bone resorption ("lytic lesions") and areas of bone formation ("blastic lesions") depending on disease stage (see above) [4]
  - Thickening of bone cortex
  - Bowing of long bones
  - Pathologic fractures
  - Skull lesions – round lytic lesions [3] ("osteoporosis circumscripta")
- Bone scan:
  - Used to survey the entire body for areas of disease involvement.
  - Also can help distinguish active vs. latent stage of disease.
  - Active disease will be "hot" (bright on bone scan).
- MRI (may be useful for evaluation of spinal stenosis)
- CT Scan (better visualization of fracture patterns)

Laboratory Data

- Alkaline phosphatase (ALP – usually elevated, marker for osteoblast activity)
- Calcium (usually normal)
- Urine hydroxyproline [1] (usually elevated – marker for osteoclast activity)

Histology

- Disorganized ("mosaic" pattern) bone
- Large, multinucleated osteoclasts
- Fibrous changes in bone marrow

Treatment

- Observation – appropriate for some asymptomatic patients (see exceptions below)
- Medications:
  - Oral pain medications (responds well to NSAIDs).
  - Bisphosphonates – especially zoledronic acid (inhibit osteoclast activity). Indications for treatment include:
    ○ Active symptomatic disease (elevated ALP)
    ○ Asymptomatic patients with disease located in areas of high risk of deformity or other complications (spine, large joints, weight-bearing joints)
    ○ Prior to planned orthopedic surgery (decreases risk of intraoperative bleeding) [3]
  - Calcitonin (decreases osteoclast activity).
  - Avoid the use of teriparatide (PTH analog) – increases risk of sarcoma.
- Physiotherapy
- Surgery:
  - Open reduction internal fixation (ORIF) of fractures or impending fractures
  - Total joint replacement of arthritic joints (hip/knee)
  - Osteotomy (to correct long bone alignment)
  - Spinal decompression (for symptomatic spinal stenosis)

Paget's Sarcoma

- Secondary sarcoma (most commonly osteosarcoma) may develop from primary Paget's disease.
- Lifetime risk is less than 1% [2].
- Clues include out of control pain, rapidly enlarging mass, and large lytic lesions on radiograph.

- Treatment involves neoadjuvent chemotherapy, surgical resection, and adjuvant chemotherapy.
- Very poor prognosis.

References

1. Allen D. Paget's disease. Orthobullets.com. Accessed 11/2015. http://www.orthobullets.com/pathology/8040/pagets-disease.
2. Miller MD, et al. Review of orthopedics, 6th ed. Phildelphia: Elsevier; 2012.
3. Orthopaedic Knowledge Update: Musculoskeletal Tumors. Rosemont: American Academy of Orthopedic Surgeons. 2014; p 41–42.
4. Singer FR, et al. Paget's disease of bone: pathophysiology, diagnosis, and management. JAAOS. 1995;3(6):336–44.

Osteopetrosis

Michela Rossi, Giulia Battafarano,
Domenico Barbuti, and Andrea Del Fattore

Classification

Autosomal Recessive Osteopetrosis (ARO)

- Infantile form with an average incidence of 1:250.000 [1].
- The most severe osteopetrosis with early fatal outcome.
- Severe increase of bone mass (Fig. 156.2) macrocephaly, hydrocephaly, severe anemia, pancytopenia, and hepatosplenomegaly.
- Blindness and deafness are generally due to cranial nerve compression. Problems with tooth eruption and formation are frequently observed in ARO patients [2, 3].
- Primary degeneration of the brain and retina, due to lysosomal storage disease observed in a subtype of ARO [4–7].
- For this type of osteopetrosis, two different forms of the disease could be distinguished on the histopathological analysis: the osteoclast-rich osteopetrosis is characterized by a high number of osteoclasts, while in the osteoclast-poor forms, no osteoclasts are observed in bone biopsy [8]. Moreover in patients with *loss-of-function* mutations of *TCIRG1* gene, an increase of osteoid surface is observed, resulting in an osteopetro-ricket phenotype [9, 10]. The histopathological analysis of bone biopsy is very important for diagnostic and therapeutic options.
- In Table 156.1, genes involved in the pathogenesis of ARO have been summarized. However, the precise genetic defects remain unknown in about 20% of patients [11].

Intermediate Recessive Osteopetrosis (IRO)

- Milder than ARO.
- Characterized by short stature, bone sclerosis, pathological fractures, dental malformations, and jaw osteomyelitis.
- Brain calcification and renal tubular acidosis in patients with *CAII* mutations display. All patients with this *CAII*-related IRO have a selective defect involving *CAII* expression in erythrocytes [12].
- "Erlenmeyer flask" deformity of the distal femora, bone pain chondrolysis of the left hip in patient with *loss-of-function* mutation of *PLEKHM1* gene [13].

M. Rossi • G. Battafarano • A. Del Fattore (✉)
Bone Physiopathology Group, Multifactorial Disease and Complex Phenotype Research Area, Rome, Italy

D. Barbuti
Imaging Department, Bambino Gesù Children's Hospital, Rome, Italy
e-mail: andrea.delfattore@opbg.net

© Springer International Publishing AG 2017
A.E.M. Eltorai et al. (eds.), *Orthopedic Surgery Clerkship*, DOI 10.1007/978-3-319-52567-9_156

Table 156.1 Genes implicated in osteopetrosis

Gene	Function of the protein	Type of mutations	Osteopetrosis
TCIRG1	Vacuolar V-H+ATPase isoform a3	Loss-of-function	ARO
SNX10	Sortin nexin-10, regulator of endosomal trafficking and V-ATPase recruitment	Loss-of-function	ARO
CLCN7	H+/Cl− exchange transporter 7	Loss-of-function / Dominant negative	ARO / ADO
OSTM1	Osteopetrosis-associated transmembrane protein 1, Beta subunit of ClC7	Loss-of-function	ARO
CAIII	Carbonic anhydrase type II	Loss-of-function	IRO
PLEKHM1	Plekstrin homology domain-containing family M member 1, a protein involved in vesicular trafficking and lysosomal acidification	Loss-of-function	IRO
TNFRSF11A	RANKL receptor	Loss-of-function	ARO
TNFSF11	RANKL	Loss-of-function	ARO
NEMO	Protein involved in the activation of NF-kB	Loss-of-function	X-linked

The Autosomal Dominant Osteopetrosis (ADO)

- Adult form of osteopetrosis with an incidence of 5:100.000.
- Thickness of the skull base, vertebral end plates (sandwich vertebrae or Rugger-Jersey spine) and pelvis, and spontaneous fractures.
- An extremely heterogeneous course ranging from asymptomatic to very severe [1, 14].
- Rare early death, but many patients have a rather poor quality of life [14].
- About 70% of patients harbor heterozygous dominant negative mutation of CLC7 gene, and the remaining 30% still lack genetic diagnosis [15].

X-Linked Form of Osteopetrosis (XLO)

- Ectodermal dysplasia, lymphedema, and immunodeficiency (OL-EDA-ID syndrome). Patients died very young because of complications due to infections [16].

Therapy

ARO

- The only therapeutic approach for this form is the HSCT (hematopoietic stem cell transplantation). Unfortunately, HSCT is not a panacea since the rate of success depends on the degree of HLA match [17]. In oc/oc mice, the feasibility of an osteoclast precursor support therapy was tested, resulting in an improvement of the bone phenotype [18].
- In an experimental study, Frattini et al. tested in utero HSCT using oc/oc mice and showed a clear improvement of bone phenotype in transplanted mice, demonstrating that transient donor engraftment may be sufficient for clinical improvement without any additional therapy [19].
- Patients with loss-of-function mutations of CLC7 and OSTM1 cannot be cured with HSCT. Indeed, it was demonstrated in ostm1−/− and clc7−/− mice and patients, a primary retinal atrophy and degeneration [5, 20, 21].

- Patients with *loss-of-function* mutation of gene encoding RANKL could not benefit of HSCT since the defect is not in hematopoietic lineage. As demonstrated by Sobacchi *et al.* by *in vitro* experiments, this form of osteopetrosis could be cured by RANKL systemic administration, but, unfortunately, there is no financial interest of companies to synthesize a drug for these patients [22].
- High-dose calcitriol has been reported to occasionally ameliorate pathological conditions in osteopetrotic patients [23].
- A long-term treatment with recombinant human interferon gamma increases the bone resorption with a significant decrease in trabecular bone area after 6–18 months of therapy [23].
- High-dose glucocorticoid treatment stabilizes pediatric patients with pancytopenia [24].

ADO

- Unfortunately, there is no therapeutic approach for this form of osteopetrosis.
- The patients are treated to solve the fracture and to reduce the pain [1].
- Experimental therapy tested in an animal model [25].
  - Administration of interferon gamma that significantly reduce the whole body BMD and distal femur bone volume, with increase CTX (collagen type 1 C-telopeptide)/TRAP (tartrate-resistant acid phosphatase) ratio [26].
  - Administration of siRNA (small interfering RNA) specific for *CLC7* mutant transcripts that are able to silence the mutant allele without affecting the wild-type form [27].

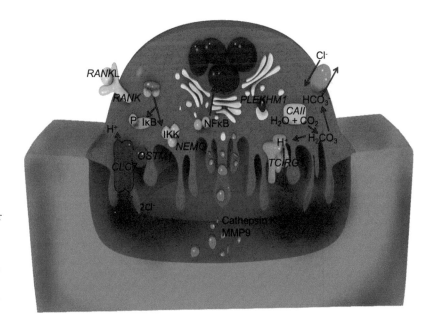

Fig. 156.1 The molecular mechanism of bone resorption and the genes mutated in human osteopetrosis (Thanks to Viola Luciano for her invaluable help to create the figure)

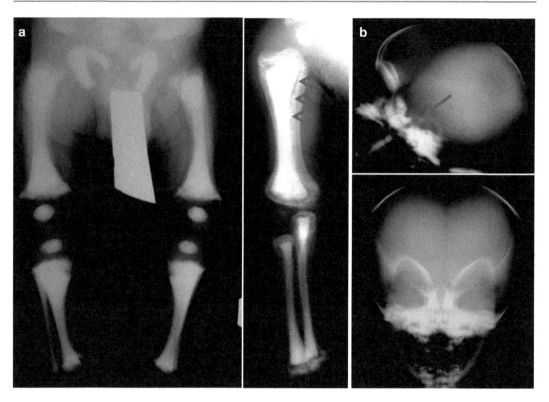

Fig. 156.2 ARO patient. X ray analysis reveals increased bone mass with (**a**) obliterated tibiae and femurs cavities, bone-in-bone appearance (*arrowheads*) and (**b**) sclerosis of the base (*arrow*) and mephistophelic features in anteroposterior view

References

1. Del Fattore A, Cappariello A, Teti A. Genetics, pathogenesis and complications of osteopetrosis. Bone. 2008;42(1):19–29.
2. Frattini A, et al. Defects in TCIRG1 subunit of the vacuolar proton pump are responsible for a subset of human autosomal recessive osteopetrosis. Nat Genet. 2000;25(3):343–6.
3. Kornak U, et al. Mutations in the a3 subunit of the vacuolar H(+)-ATPase cause infantile malignant osteopetrosis. Hum Mol Genet. 2000;9(13):2059–63.
4. Kasper D, et al. Loss of the chloride channel ClC-7 leads to lysosomal storage disease and neurodegeneration. EMBO J. 2005;24(5):1079–91.
5. Kornak U, et al. Loss of the ClC-7 chloride channel leads to osteopetrosis in mice and man. Cell. 2001;104(2):205–15.
6. Lange PF, et al. ClC-7 requires Ostm1 as a beta-subunit to support bone resorption and lysosomal function. Nature. 2006;440(7081):220–3.
7. Chalhoub N, et al. Grey-lethal mutation induces severe malignant autosomal recessive osteopetrosis in mouse and human. Nat Med. 2003;9(4):399–406.
8. Villa A, et al. Infantile malignant, autosomal recessive osteopetrosis: the rich and the poor. Calcif Tissue Int. 2009;84(1):1–12.
9. Barvencik F, et al. CLCN7 and TCIRG1 mutations differentially affect bone matrix mineralization in osteopetrotic individuals. J Bone Miner Res. 2014;29(4):982–91.
10. Schinke T, et al. Impaired gastric acidification negatively affects calcium homeostasis and bone mass. Nat Med. 2009;15(6):674–81.
11. Sobacchi C, et al. Osteopetrosis: genetics, treatment and new insights into osteoclast function. Nat Rev Endocrinol. 2013;9(9):522–36.
12. Jilka RL, et al. Carbonic anhydrase isozymes of osteoclasts and erythrocytes of osteopetrotic microphthalmic mice. Bone. 1985;6(6):445–9.
13. Van Wesenbeeck L, et al. Involvement of PLEKHM1 in osteoclastic vesicular transport and osteopetrosis in incisors absent rats and humans. J Clin Invest. 2007;117(4):919–30.
14. Del Fattore A, et al. Clinical, genetic, and cellular analysis of 49 osteopetrotic patients: implications for diagnosis and treatment. J Med Genet. 2006;43(4):315–25.
15. Del Fattore A, et al. A new heterozygous mutation (R714C) of the osteopetrosis gene, pleckstrin homolog

domain containing family M (with run domain) member 1 (PLEKHM1), impairs vesicular acidification and increases TRACP secretion in osteoclasts. J Bone Miner Res. 2008;23(3):380–91.

16. Smahi A, et al. The NF-kappaB signalling pathway in human diseases: from incontinentia pigmenti to ectodermal dysplasias and immune-deficiency syndromes. Hum Mol Genet. 2002;11(20):2371–5.

17. Driessen GJ, et al. Long-term outcome of haematopoietic stem cell transplantation in autosomal recessive osteopetrosis: an EBMT report. Bone Marrow Transplant. 2003;32(7):657–63.

18. Cappariello A, et al. Committed osteoclast precursors colonize the bone and improve the phenotype of a mouse model of autosomal recessive osteopetrosis. J Bone Miner Res. 2010;25(1):106–13.

19. Frattini A, et al. Rescue of ATPa3-deficient murine malignant osteopetrosis by hematopoietic stem cell transplantation in utero. Proc Natl Acad Sci U S A. 2005;102(41):14629–34.

20. Pangrazio A, et al. Mutations in OSTM1 (grey lethal) define a particularly severe form of autosomal recessive osteopetrosis with neural involvement. J Bone Miner Res. 2006;21(7):1098–105.

21. Ramirez A, et al. Identification of a novel mutation in the coding region of the grey-lethal gene OSTM1 in human malignant infantile osteopetrosis. Hum Mutat. 2004;23(5):471 6.

22. Lo Iacono N, et al. Osteopetrosis rescue upon RANKL administration to Rankl(−/−) mice: a new therapy for human RANKL-dependent ARO. J Bone Miner Res. 2012;27(12):2501–10.

23. Askmyr MK, Fasth A, Richter J. Towards a better understanding and new therapeutics of osteopetrosis. Br J Haematol. 2008;140(6):597–609.

24. Iacobini M, et al. Apparent cure of a newborn with malignant osteopetrosis using prednisone therapy. J Bone Miner Res. 2001;16(12):2356–60.

25. Alam I, et al. Generation of the first autosomal dominant osteopetrosis type II (ADO2) disease models. Bone. 2014;59:66–75.

26. Alam I, et al. Interferon gamma, but not calcitriol improves the osteopetrotic phenotypes in ADO2 mice. J Bone Miner Res. 2015;30(11):2005–13.

27. Capulli M, et al. Effective Small Interfering RNA Therapy to Treat CLCN7-dependent Autosomal Dominant Osteopetrosis Type 2. Mol Ther Nucleic Acids. 2015;4:e248.

Jared L. Harwood and Joel Mayerson

Introduction

Orthopaedic oncologists are tasked with establishing long-term relationships with their patients. Patients will often want you as the medical student to give them the "down low" of imaging studies or labs. Any of these data points given out of context and without an appropriate understanding of each condition and its natural history can be very damaging to the process of establishing a relationship of trust and require a lot of work to undo. Patients have a variety of preferences when it comes to how and how much information they want shared. You should speak with cautious honesty and leave bad news to the attending.

Clinical Workup

The workup of the oncology patient is unique in orthopaedics. Most show up having been told that they have some unwanted lesion in their bone or soft tissues and many have no clinical symptoms.

The only thing they usually have in common is a certainty that they would rather not be seeing an orthopaedic oncologist. When starting each evaluation, you should use what you have available, but "go back to the drawing board," jumping to no conclusions. There is no "one size fits all" in orthopaedic oncology.

Common laboratory examination that will need to be obtained includes complete blood count with manual differential, inflammatory markers (ESR/CRP), alkaline phosphatase, lactic dehydrogenase, and complete metabolic panel. When multiple myeloma is suspected, additional studies include serum protein electrophoresis, urinalysis, urine protein electrophoresis. These additional studies would be expected to demonstrate an M spike, proteinuria, and Bence-Jones proteins respectively.

Clinical Pearls

- Small, superficial, freely mobile, well-circumscribed, long-standing, and fluctuating size are all encouraging physical findings. Conversely, being larger than 5 cm, being deep to fascia, having poorly defined borders, and being rapidly progressing are concerning features.
- Soft tissue sarcomas are often not painful, so the absence of pain should not be overly reassuring. On the other hand, bony lesions usually are painful. Early on dull, achy night pain

The original version of this chapter was revised. An erratum to this chapter can be found at https://doi.org/10.1007/978-3-319-52567-9_159

J.L. Harwood, MD • J. Mayerson, MD (✉)
Department of Orthopaedics, The Ohio State University
Wexner Medical Center, Columbus, OH, USA
e-mail: jared.harwood@osumc.edu;
joel.mayerson@osumc.edu

that wakes patients from sleep can be present. As bony destruction progresses, pain often becomes debilitating, compromising ambulation. In palliative situations, this can be an indication for prophylactic fixation.

Imaging

Imaging is a mainstay of any Oncology patient's workup. X-rays should always be obtained of the area in question and sometimes distantly (i.e. chest X-Ray in the case of surveillance or skeletal survey in the work up of multiple myeloma). MRIs are necessary to adequately evaluate the extent of the primary lesion and the surrounding soft tissues, to include neurovascular structures that will need to be considered with any resection planning. CT scans are helpful in defining bony integrity and are sensitive at picking up metastasis in the lung and abdomen. They also involve a significant amount of radiation (equivalent to 100 to 200 chest X-rays) and are often alternated with X-rays in surveillance situations to minimize lifetime radiation dose and associated risk for secondary malignancies. FDG-PET/CT scans utilize an fluorodeoxyglucose (FDG) tracer measured in standard uptake values (SUVs) that is useful in assessing the tumor's metabolic activity before and after adjuvant therapies, thus gauging response and prognosis.

Imaging Pearls

To help form an appropriate differential diagnosis, you need to ask yourself 6 questions:

1. What type of matrix is being made?
   (a) Calcification
   (b) Bone or osteoid (fluffy, cloud-like densities)
   (c) Cartilage (arcs and rings, popcorn)
   (d) Fibrous (ground-glass)
   (e) Cystic (fallen-leaf)

2. If bone is being made, what type is it?
   (a) Normal
   (b) Reactive
   (c) Tumor

3. What is the bone doing to the lesion and/or what is the lesion doing to the bone (morphology)?
   (a) Border
   (b) Pattern of destruction
   (c) Periosteal reaction
   (d) Matrix
   (e) Soft tissue mass

4. What is the pattern of destruction?
   (a) Geographic
   (b) Moth-eaten
   (c) Permeative

5. What location in the bone is the lesion and which bone (Fig. 157.1)?
   (a) Epiphyseal
   (b) Metaphyseal
   (c) Diaphyseal

6. What is the age of the patient (Table 157.1)?
   (a) <10
   (b) 10–40
   (c) >40

Radiographic Pearls

– Geographic lesions are well-circumscribed. The bone has been able to "contain" the lesion which suggests a more indolent nature
– Sunburst, onion-skinning, or moth-eaten appearances to bone on plain films suggest very aggressive masses that outstrip the bone's ability to contain the lesion despite the periosteum's best efforts.

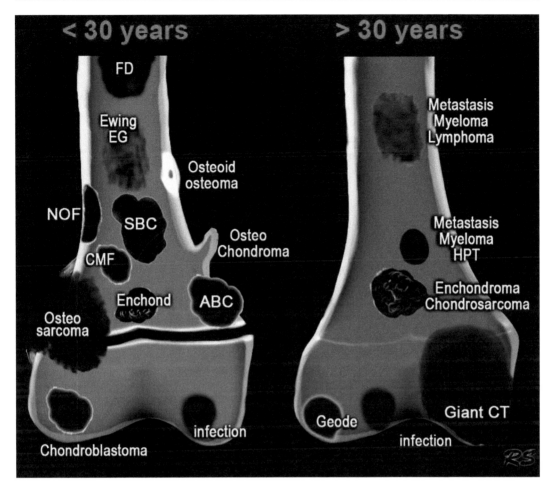

Fig. 157.1 Tumor Type by Location, ABC = Aneurysmal bone cyst, CMF = Chondromyxoid fibroma, EG = Eosinophilic Granuloma, GCT = Giant cell tumor, FD = Fibrous dysplasia, HPT = Hyperparathyroidism with Brown tumor, NOF = Non-Ossifying Fibroma, SBC = Simple Bone Cyst. Reprinted under creative commons license from Radiology Assistant (http://www.radiologyassistant.nl/data/bin/a509797919f47f_TEK-bone-tumor3.jpg)

Table 157.1 Differential by age

Age	Benign	Malignant
0–10 years old	Osteomyelitis Osteofibrous dysplasia	Metastatic rhabdomyosarcoma Metastatic neuroblastoma Leukemia
10–40 years old	NOF Osteoid osteoma Giant cell tumor ABC UBC Osteochondroma MHE Chondroblastoma Fibrous dysplasia Osteomyelitis Eosinophillic granuloma	Osteosarcoma Ewing's sarcoma Desmoplastic fibroma Leukemia Lymphoma
40–80 years old	Enchondroma Bone infarct Bone island Paget's disease Hyperparathyroidism	Metastatic bone disease Myeloma Lymphoma Chondrosarcoma MFH Secondary sarcoma Paget's, irradiation

Staging Systems

Staging is the process of finding out how extensive the cancer is. The most commonly used staging system in Orthopaedic Oncology is the Musculoskeletal Tumor Society or Enneking system [1], which has two different scales depending on whether the lesion is benign or malignant. The Enneking system is a surgical staging system in that it guides surgical management.

Enneking
Roman numerals are used to denote malignant tumors. I – low-grade, II – high-grade, III – metastatic (regional or distant). The letters A and B represent intra and extra-compartmental, respectively. For benign lesions, Arabic numerals are used. 1 - Benign, indolent, or biologically static, 2 - Progressive growth, limited by natural barriers, 3 - Locally aggressive with corresponding soft-tissue mass.

Campanacci staging system [2] is based on radiographic characteristics as follows:
1. Radiographically well-circumscribed lucent lesion with no aggressive features (e.g., periosteal reaction, soft-tissue mass, cortical breach).
2. Relatively well-defined radiographic borders without a radiopaque rim.
3. Indistinct or ill-defined borders with radiographic demonstration of cortical bone destruction, and a soft-tissue mass.

- American Joint Committee on Cancer (AJCC) [3]
- One common staging construct is the AJCC's TNM + G structure where:
  - T1 vs. T2 = tumor size (< or > 5cm)
  - N0 vs. N1 = nodes (no/yes)
  - M0 vs. M1 = metastasis (no/yes)
  - G1 – 3 = grade
  - A tumor's grade is a measure of how likely it is to metastasize and is based on differentiation (1–3), mitotic count (1–3), and tumor necrosis (0–2). Tumors with a score of 2 or 3 are G1, a score of 4 or 5 is G2, while a score of 6 or higher is G3. GX is

used when medical records are incomplete and data insufficient to offer a grade.

Types [3, 4]

Chondrogenic

- *Osteochondroma* – consists of a cartilage capped bony projection on the surface of the bone, containing a marrow cavity that is continuous with that of the underlying bone. The cell of origin is likely a proliferating chondrocyte at the growth plate. Malignant transformation to secondary peripheral chondrosarcoma is estimated at 1% for single lesions and 5% for multiple lesions.
  - Age – most present in the first two decades of life during periods of skeletal growth.
  - Sites – approximately 15% of patients have multiple lesions (multiple hereditary osteochondromatosis). The lesions arise in bones formed by enchondral ossification, most commonly in the metaphysis of the distal femur, upper humerus, and proximal tibia/fibula.
  - Clinical features – often incidentally discovered, symptoms correlate with their size and location. They often present as firm masses. Secondary injuries related to their fracture or impingement on neurovascular structures do occur. Increasing size or pain in a skeletally mature patient may be a sign of malignant degeneration.
  - Imaging features – the cortex is continuous with the bony stalk and shows normal central trabeculation. Large tumors with thick (>1.5 to 2 cm in an adult), unmineralized, cartilaginous caps should raise concern for malignant transformation. This does not occur in patients with open growth plates. The size of the cartilage cap is best seen on T2-weighted MRI.
  - Histology – the lesion has three layers: the perichondrium, cartilage, and bone. The outer layer is nonneoplastic. Below

this is the hyaline cartilage cap that mimics disorganized growth plate-like cartilage.

- Genetics – biallelic inactivation of the EXT1 or EXT2 gene within the cartilage cap. This is thought to destabilize the bony collar and provide a proliferative advantage. As a result EXT-mutated cells may grow out of the bone and recruit normal cells to form osteochondromas.
- Prognosis – excision is usually curative.

• *Chondroma*: *enchondroma* (inside the bone – common) and *periosteal chondroma* (on surface of the bone – uncommon) – tumors of hyaline cartilage. Both lesions are usually solitary and sporadic. Most are <5 cm in size.

- Age – most present in the second to fifth decades of life.
- Sites – the short tubular bones of the hand are most often affected (40%). Next most common are the tubular long bones.
- Clinical features – hand lesions can present as a swelling, with or without pain, and pathologic fractures. Long bone lesions are more often asymptomatic. Most are discovered incidentally.
- Imaging features – enchondromas are usually "hot" on bone scan. When present, the mineralization pattern is highly characteristic, consisting of punctate, flocculent, or ring and arc patterns. Lesions can completely replace the medullary cavity. In large, long bones endosteal erosion or scalloping may be present; however, cortical thickening and/or bone expansion should raise the suspicion of chondrosarcoma.
- Histology – enchondromas are hypocellular, avascular tumors with abundant hyaline cartilage matrix. The chondrocytes are situated within sharp-edged lacunar spaces. Lesions in the hands and feet can be more cellular and cytologically atypical than long bone tumors.
- Genetics – IDH1/IDH2 mutations.
- Prognosis – most often treated with observation. Treat with local curettage when symptomatic. Recurrence is uncommon. Occasionally there can be delayed recur-

rences and they can rarely recur as a low-grade chondrosarcoma.

• *Synovial chondromatosis* – presents as multiple hyaline nodules, typically present in the subsynovial tissue.

- Age – third to fifth decade.
- Sites – two-thirds of cases involve the knee joint although any joint can be involved.
- Clinical features – pain, swelling, palpable nodules, joint clicking, locking or movement restriction, as well as secondary osteoarthritis.
- Imaging features – on X-ray and CT demonstrate small masses, round and calcified at the periphery that are visible inside the joint.
- Histology – nodules consist of hyaline cartilage in which the chondrocytes are clustered. Nodules are often surrounded by synovial tissue.
- Genetics – expression levels of the hedgehog target genes PTCH1 and GLI1 are substantially higher than in normal synovial tissue. IDH1 and IDH2 mutations are absent.
- Prognosis – recurrence is found in 15–20% of cases. Malignant transformation is extremely rare, and metastases are only seen in 29% of cases.

• *Chondroblastoma* – composed of chondroblasts. It usually arises in the epiphyses or apophysis of skeletally immature patients.

- Age – most patients are between 10–25 years at diagnosis.
- Sites – 75% of cases involve the long bones including the epiphyseal regions of the distal and proximal femur, proximal tibia, and proximal humerus. Chondroblastomas almost invariably involve a single bone.
- Clinical features – localized pain, often mild, and sometimes for several years prior to presentation.
- Imaging features – lytic, centrally or eccentrically placed, sharply demarcated, small (3–6 cm), occupying less than half of the epiphysis. There is generally no expansion of the bone. On MRI, extensive edema can be seen.

- Histology – the characteristic cells are uniform, round to polygonal with well-demarcated cytoplasmic borders. Mature hyaline cartilage is relatively uncommon. Chicken wire calcifications are characteristic.
- Genetics – generally express S100 and SOX9. Positivity for keratins and p63 is frequently observed. IDH1 and IDH2 mutations are absent.
- Prognosis – between 80 and 90% are successfully treated by simple curettage with bone grafting. Local recurrence rates are between 14 and 18%. Rarely pulmonary metastases may develop, although they tend to be clinically nonprogressive.

Osteogenic

- *Osteoid osteoma*
  - Age – generally children and adolescents.
  - Sites – most common in long bones, especially the proximal femur, and cortically based lesion.
  - Clinical features – disproportionate pain that is usually (80%) completely responsive to NSAIDs. Osteoid osteomas are usually exquisitely tender to palpation. When close to a joint, effusions can be associated. In the spine the lesions usually affect the neural arch and can lead to painful scoliosis secondary to spasm.
  - Imaging features – usually small in size (<2 cm). Characterized by a dense cortical sclerosis surrounded by radiolucent nidus, best imaged with CT scan.
  - Histology – nidus demonstrates differentiated osteoblastic activity surrounded by hypervascular sclerotic bone.
  - Genetics – strong nuclear staining for Runx2 and Osterix, common pathways in normal skeletal development.
  - Prognosis – recurrences are uncommon. Surgical techniques are being supplanted by less invasive treatments that include CT-guided core drill excision, percutaneous radiofrequency ablation, cryoablation, and laser photocoagulation.

- *Osteoblastoma* – benign bone-forming tumor that is >2 cm and produces woven bone spicules that are bordered by prominent osteoblasts.
  - Age – 10–30 years predominantly with a 2.5:1 male to female ratio.
  - Sites – posterior elements of the spine and pelvis in 40–55% of cases. Most appendicular sites are in the lower extremities and most occur intramedullary.
  - Clinical features – similar to osteoid osteoma, back pain, scoliosis, and nerve compression. Does not respond to NSAIDs.
  - Imaging features – large (most often 3–10 cm), lytic, well circumscribed, and oval or round almost always confined by a periosteal shell of reactive bone.
  - Histology – identical to osteoid osteoma, composed of woven bone spicules and trabeculae that are haphazardly arranged. There is no infiltration of surrounding the bone like you would see in osteosarcoma.
  - Prognosis – excellent, often treated with curettage. Recurrences are unusual.

Fibrohistiocytic

- *Non-ossifying fibroma* (*NOF*) – fibroblastic proliferation admixed with osteoclast-type giant cells.
  - Age – children.
  - Sites – vast majority arise from the metaphysis of lower extremity long bones.
  - Clinical features – most lesions are asymptomatic and undergo spontaneous resolution at skeletal maturity. These lesions are usually discovered incidentally after a musculoskeletal injury prompts radiographic evaluation. Estimates are that 30–40% of children have one or more occult lesions.
  - Imaging features – radiolucent lesions centered on the cortex and usually in the distal metaphysis of the involved long bone. They can be loculated. The lesions can expand or destroy the cortex, which can be thinned or expanded. Periosteal reaction is absent unless pathologic fracture has occurred.

- Histology – consists of bland, spindle-shaped fibroblasts that are arranged in a storiform growth pattern. The stromal cells can demonstrate hemosiderin deposition and foamy histiocytes. Multinucleated giant cells can often be found.
- Prognosis – excellent. Treatment is usually observation. Larger lesions, when painful, should be treated with curettage. Recurrences are rare.

Giant Cell

- *Giant cell tumor of bone (GCT)* – a locally aggressive tumor composed of a proliferation of mononuclear cells among which are scattered macrophages and osteoclast-like giant cells
  - Age – peak incidence is between 20 and 45 years of age.
  - Sites – typically involves the epiphysis/metaphysis of long bones. Most common sites are the distal femur, proximal tibia, distal radius, and proximal humerus. It can also occur in the vertebral bodies of the spine, most often in the sacrum.
  - Clinical features – typically present with pain and swelling. Five to 10% can presents with pathologic fracture, <1% with benign pulmonary implants in lungs.
  - Imaging features – expansile, eccentric, and often lobulated area of osteolysis with a narrow zone of transition. The tumor often extends up to the subchondral bone.
  - Histology – characterized by very large numbers of giant cells (oftentimes with 20–50 nuclei) that appear uniformly scattered among numerous round or spindled-shaped mononuclear cells. While mitotic figures can be present they should be typical. Any atypical mitotic figures should raise one's suspicion for a diagnosis of sarcoma.
  - Genetics – generally positive for normal osteoclast markers like CD51 and a host of macrophage markers like CD45, CD33, and CD68. They are negative for CD14, CD163, and HLA-DR.

- Prognosis – malignant transformation can occur in less than 1% of cases. GCT behaves as a benign, but locally aggressive tumor. Pulmonary metastases (called benign pulmonary implants) are present in 1–2% of patients, typically 3–4 years after primary diagnosis. Local recurrence occurs in 15–50% of cases after curettage with adjuvant treatment.

Undefined

- *Aneurysmal bone cyst* – destructive, expansile neoplasms composed of multiloculated blood-filled cystic spaces.
  - Age – most common during the first two decades of life (80%).
  - Sites – metaphysis of long bones, especially the femur, tibia, and humerus and posterior elements of vertebral bodies.
  - Clinical features – pain and swelling.
  - Imaging features – lytic, eccentric, expansile masses with well-defined margins. Most tumors contain thin shell of subperiosteal, reactive bone. CT shows a cystic, expansile, and radiolucent tumor. MRI studies show internal septa and the characteristic fluid-fluid levels, created by the different densities of the cyst fluid, caused by settling of erythrocytes.
  - Histology – the fibrous septa are composed of bland fibroblasts with scattered, multinucleated, giant cells and reactive woven bone rimmed by osteoblasts.
  - Genetics – contains cytogenetic rearrangements of the USP6 gene at chromosome band 17p13. The most common translocation t (16; 17) leads to fusion of the cadherin 11 gene with USP6.
  - Prognosis – recurrence rate following curettage is variable (20–70%). Spontaneous regression following incomplete removal is very unusual.
- *Simple bone cyst* – intramedullary, usually unilocular cystic bone cavity lined by a fibrous membrane and filled with serous or serosanguinous fluid. Males predominate 3:1.
  - Age – about 80% of the patients are in the first two decades of life.

- Sites – the proximal humerus (50%), proximal femur (25%), and proximal tibia.
- Clinical features – most are asymptomatic but can also be discovered after pathologic fracture or incidentally.
- Imaging features – well-outlined, centrally located, metaphyseal-diaphyseal lucency, expanding and thinning the cortices, not wider than the epiphyseal plate. It usually abuts but rarely violates the growth plate. Cysts located near the plate are called "active," while those separated by normal cancellous bone are termed "inactive" or "latent."
- Histology – inner lining and septae of the cyst consist of connective tissue, containing foci of reactive new bone, hemosiderin pigment, and scattered giant cells.
- Genetics – case reports have been published demonstrating a complex karyotype.
- Prognosis – recurrence is reported in 10–20% of cases, especially in younger patients and in large cysts. Large cysts are also related to limb shortening.
- *Fibrous dysplasia* – medullary, fibro-osseous lesion.
  - Age – usually present in childhood or adolescence. The polyostotic form often presents earlier in life.
  - Sites – the monostotic form is six to ten times more common than the polyostotic form. Craniofacial bones and the femur are the two most common sites. In the monostotic from, a substantial number of cases involve the femur, skull, and tibia and an additional 20% in the ribs. In the polyostotic form, the femur, pelvis, and tibia are involved in the majority of cases.
  - Clinical features – lesions are often asymptomatic, although pain and fractures are common presentations.
  - Imaging features – nonaggressive geographical lesion with a ground-glass matrix. The "shepherd crook" deformity of the proximal femur is highly diagnostic when present. Generally there is neither soft tissue extension nor periosteal reaction. Bone scintigraphy, CT, and MRI best delineate the features and extent of the disease.
  - Histology – fibrous and osseous tissue are present in varying proportions. The fibrous

tissue is composed principally of bland fibroblastic cells. The osseous component is comprised of irregular, curvilinear, and trabeculae of woven bone.
  - Genetics – caused by post-zygotic, activating missense mutations in the GNAS gene. These activating mutations have been detected in up to 93% of cases.
  - Prognosis – excellent. Monostotic fibrous dysplasia can cause skeletal deformities, leg-length discrepancies, or impinge on cranial nerves, while extensive polyostotic disease may be crippling. Malignant transformation very rarely occurs.
- *Osteofibrous dysplasia* (OFD) – usually self-limiting but reported to progress to adamantinoma in some cases. It characteristically involves the cortical bone of the anterior midshaft of the tibia during infancy and childhood. Most cases of OFD arise de novo.
  - Age – most commonly detected during the first two decades of life. Extremely rare after skeletal maturity.
  - Sites – the proximal or middle third of the tibial cortex is the most frequent site. Ipsilateral involvement of the fibula is seen in about 20% of cases.
  - Clinical features – swelling or painless deforming anterior bowing of the tibia.
  - Imaging features – may involve the entire bone with significant bowing deformity. The lesion is well-demarcated and associated with thinning, expanding or even missing cortex. The expanding cortex is often sclerotically rimmed. Separate or confluent oval, scalloped, saw-toothed or bubbly multiloculated, lytic lesions are often noted. Perilesional sclerosis may be considerable. Periosteal reactions and soft tissue extensions are unusual. Bone scans are typically hot.
  - Histology – irregular fragments of woven bone often rimmed by lamellar layers of bone laid down by well-defined osteoblasts. The fibrous component consists of bland spindle cells with callogen production. Zonal architecture has been described with fibrous tissue near the center and anastomosing and lamellar bone peripherally.
  - Genetics – positive for vimentin and occasionally S100 and Leu7. Trisomies of chro-

mosomes 7, 8, and 12. Proto-oncogenes FOS and JUN are expressed. GNAS mutations are absent.

– Prognosis – gradual growth during the first decade of life with stabilization at about 15 years of age, followed by healing or spontaneous resolution. Risk of significant deformity or pseudoarthrosis, impending or existing pathologic fracture, the desire for definitive diagnosis and possibly the severity of symptoms warrant surgical intervention.

• *Langerhans cell histiocytosis* – a clonal and likely neoplastic proliferation of pathologic Langerhans cells.

– Age – birth to eighth decade of life, although 80% of cases are seen in patients under the age of 30. There is a 2:1 male to female ratio.

– Sites – most commonly involves the bones of the skull, notably the calvarium. Other frequently involved sites are the femur, pelvis, and mandible. In adults the rib is the most frequently involved site. Monostotic disease is three to four times more common than polyostotic disease.

– Clinical features – pain and swelling.

– Imaging features – purely lytic, well-demarcated lesion, usually associated with thick periosteal new bone formation.

– Histology – the diagnosis depends on the recognition of lesional Langerhans cells which are of intermediate size. Chromatin is either diffusely dispersed or condensed along the nuclear membrane. Inflammatory cells are usually present, and necrosis is common. "Tennis racket"-shaped inclusions are known as Birbeck granules.

– Genetics – CD1a and CD207/Langerin membrane positivity as well as nuclear and cytoplasmic expression of S100 and CD45 negative immunostaining

– Prognosis – good. Spontaneous healing is not uncommon; however reactivations may occur in approximately 10% of monostotic cases and 25% of polyostotic cases. Mortality is associated with disseminated disease involving viscera and usually occurs in individuals aged <2 years at diagnosis.

Treatment Principles

• Interventions span from observation to amputation depending on the behavior of the tumor. While some tumors can be diagnosed by history, exam, and imaging alone, most surgical interventions should be preceded with biopsy for tissue diagnosis. Biopsy principles are a crucial take away from an orthopaedic oncology clerkship. A well-planned biopsy, especially in malignant tumors can make the difference between someone keeping their extremity or not. In malignant bone tumors, a negative margin is directly correlated to the patient's risk for local recurrence and metastasis. The following are some principles that will serve you well:

– Biopsies should be performed at the same facility where they will be treated if they are malignant.

– All malignant tumor patients should be transferred as expeditiously as possible to their tertiary care facility for further evaluation and treatment, as to not delay the appropriate treatment.

– Biopsy tracts should be longitudinal in the extremity and always in line with the definitive procedure incision, and should a more extensive surgery be required.

– Unlike many approaches, tissue planes should not be dissected as this will allow for broader contamination necessitating a more extensive re-excision if needed.

– Exact hemostasis should be maintained throughout the procedure. Any area of hematoma is presumed contaminated for resection purposes.

– Complication rates are at least four times higher when malignant tumors are treated outside a tertiary referral center. Unnecessary amputation of extremities affected by malignant bone tumors is the ultimate complication that occurs in 4% cases treated outside tertiary referral centers.

• Limb salvage options do exist and allow for keeping the limb in many cases. Examples include megaprostheses, internal hemipelvectomy, and rotationplasty in the lower extremity. See Table 157.2.

Table 157.2 Nonoperative and operative differential by treatment

Nonoperative	
Observation	Fibrous dysplasia
	Osteofibrous dysplasia
	Enchondroma
	Ollier's
	Marfucci's
	Osteochondroma
	MHE
	NOF
	Jaffe-Campanacci
	Paget's
	Eosiniphillic granuloma
	Lipoma
Bisphosphonate therapy	Metastatic bone disease (with wide resection and radiation)
	Myeloma (with chemotherapy)
	Paget's disease (with observation)
	Fibrous dysplasia (with observation)
Radiation alone	Solitary myeloma
Chemotherapy alone	Lymphoma
	Multiple myeloma
Operative	
Radiofrequency ablation	Osteoid osteoma
Aspiration and injection	UBC
Curettage and bone grafting	GCT
	ABC
	Chondroblastoma
	Chondromyxoid fibroma
	Osteoblastoma
	NOF (if symptomatic)
Marginal resection	Periosteal chondroma
	Neurilemoma (soft tissue)
	Nodular fasciitis (soft tissue)
	Epidermal inclusion cyst
	Glomus tumor
Wide resection alone	Chondrosarcoma
	Parosteal osteosarcoma
	Chordoma
	Adamantinoma
	Squamous cell (if no metastases)
Wide resection + irradiation	Metastatic bone disease
	High-grade soft tissue sarcoma (angiosarcoma, synovial sarcoma, liposarcoma, desmoid tumor, MFH/fibrosarcoma)
Wide resection + chemotherapy	Osteosarcoma
	Periosteal osteosarcoma
	Ewing's sarcoma
	MFH
	Fibrosarcoma
	Secondary sarcoma
	Dedifferentiated chondrosarcoma
	Rhabdomyosarcoma (exception to soft tissue sarcoma)

Resection types are classified as:

- Intralesional or debulking – plane of dissection is within the tumor. Leaves gross tumor. Appropriate for symptomatic benign lesions where a more aggressive dissection might sacrifice neurovascular structures.
- Marginal – plane of dissection is in the pseudo-capsule that surrounds satellite lesions. Acceptable for most benign lesions and low-grade malignancies.
- Wide – plane of dissection is through normal tissue, leaving a cuff of tissue around the tumor. Preferred for most high-grade malignancies. Combined with adjuvant and/or neoadjuvant treatments in cases where wide margins (2 cm) cannot be achieved. These additive treatments include radiation, chemotherapy, and increasingly immunotherapy.
- Radical – the entire involved compartment is excised. Mostly replaced by wide resection as there has been no proven survival benefit to justify the added morbidity.
- Amputation – the entire limb is removed. Its corollary in the pelvis is the external hemipelvectomy.

References

1. Enneking WF. A system of staging musculoskeletal neoplasms. Clin Orthop Relat Res. 1986;204:9–24.
2. Campanacci M. Giant cell tumor of bone. In: Campanacci M. Bone and soft tissue tumors. 2nd ed. Berlin: Springer; 1999. p. 99–132.
3. American Cancer Society. How are soft tissue sarcomas staged? Available at: https://www.cancer.org/cancer/soft-tissue-sarcoma/detection-diagnosis-staging/staging.html. Accessed on Mar 2017.
4. Tumours of bone. WHO classification of tumours of soft tissue and bone. 4th ed. Fletcher CDM, Unni KK, Mertens F., editors. Lyon: International Agency for Research on Cancer, 2013. p. 239–394.

Malignant Bone Tumors

Jared L. Harwood and Joel Mayerson

Introduction

Orthopaedic oncologists are tasked with establishing long-term relationships with their patients. Patients will often want you as the medical student to give them the "down low" of imaging studies or labs. Any of these data points given out of context and without an appropriate understanding of each condition and its natural history can be very damaging to the process of establishing a relationship of trust and require a lot of work to undo. Patients have a variety of preferences when it comes to how and how much information they want shared. You should speak with cautious honesty and leave bad news to the attending.

Clinical Workup

The workup of the oncology patient is unique in orthopaedics. Most show up having been told that they have some unwanted lesion in their bone or soft tissues and many have no clinical symptoms.

The original version of this chapter was revised. An erratum to this chapter can be found at https://doi.org/10.1007/978-3-319-52567-9_159

J.L. Harwood, MD • J. Mayerson, MD (✉)
Department of Orthopaedics, The Ohio State University Wexner Medical Center,
Columbus, OH, USA
e-mail: jared.harwood@osumc.edu;
joel.mayerson@osumc.edu

The only thing they usually have in common is a certainty that they would rather not be seeing an orthopaedic oncologist. When starting each evaluation, you should use what you have available, but "go back to the drawing board," jumping to no conclusions. There is no "one size fits all" in orthopaedic oncology.

Common laboratory examination that will need to be obtained includes complete blood count with manual differential, inflammatory markers (ESR/CRP), alkaline phosphatase, lactic dehydrogenase, and complete metabolic panel. When multiple myeloma is suspected, additional studies include serum protein electrophoresis, urinalysis, urine protein electrophoresis. These additional studies would be expected to demonstrate an M spike, proteinuria, and Bence-Jones proteins respectively.

Clinical Pearls

– Small, superficial, freely mobile, well-circumscribed, long-standing, and fluctuating size are all encouraging physical findings. Conversely, being larger than 5 cm, being deep to fascia, having poorly defined borders, and being rapidly progressing are concerning features.
– Soft tissue sarcomas are often not painful, so the absence of pain should not be overly reassuring. On the other hand, bony lesions usually are painful. Early on dull, achy night pain

that wakes patients from sleep can be present. As bony destruction progresses, pain often becomes debilitating, compromising ambulation. In palliative situations, this can be an indication for prophylactic fixation.

Imaging

Imaging is a mainstay of any Oncology patient's workup. X-rays should always be obtained of the area in question and sometimes distantly (i.e. chest X-Ray in the case of surveillance or skeletal survey in the work up of multiple myeloma). MRIs are necessary to adequately evaluate the extent of the primary lesion and the surrounding soft tissues, to include neurovascular structures that will need to be considered with any resection planning. CT scans are helpful in defining bony integrity and are sensitive at picking up metastasis in the lung and abdomen. They also involve a significant amount of radiation (equivalent to 100 to 200 chest x-rays) and are often alternated with X-rays in surveillance situations to minimize lifetime radiation dose and associated risk for secondary malignancies. FDG-PET/CT scans utilize an fluorodeoxyglucose (FDG) tracer measured in standard uptake values (SUVs) that is useful in assessing the tumor's metabolic activity before and after adjuvant therapies, thus gauging response and prognosis.

Imaging Pearls

To help form an appropriate differential diagnosis, you need to ask yourself 6 questions:

1. What type of matrix is being made?
   (a) Calcification
   (b) Bone or osteoid (fluffy, cloud-like densities)
   (c) Cartilage (arcs and rings, popcorn)

   (d) Fibrous (ground-glass)
   (e) Cystic (fallen-leaf)
2. If bone is being made, what type is it?
   (a) Normal
   (b) Reactive
   (c) Tumor
3. What is the bone doing to the lesion and/or what is the lesion doing to the bone (morphology)?
   (a) Border
   (b) Pattern of destruction
   (c) Periosteal reaction
   (d) Matrix
   (e) Soft tissue mass
4. What is the pattern of destruction?
   (a) Geographic
   (b) Moth-eaten
   (c) Permeative
5. What location in the bone is the lesion and which bone (Fig. 158.1)?
   (a) Epiphyseal
   (b) Metaphyseal
   (c) Diaphyseal
6. What is the age of the patient (Table 158.1)?
   (a) <10
   (b) 10–40
   (c) >40

Radiographic Pearls

– Geographic lesions are well-circumscribed. The bone has been able to "contain" the lesion which suggests a more indolent nature
– Sunburst, onion-skinning, or moth-eaten appearances to bone on plain films suggest very aggressive masses that outstrip the bone's ability to contain the lesion despite the periosteum's best efforts.

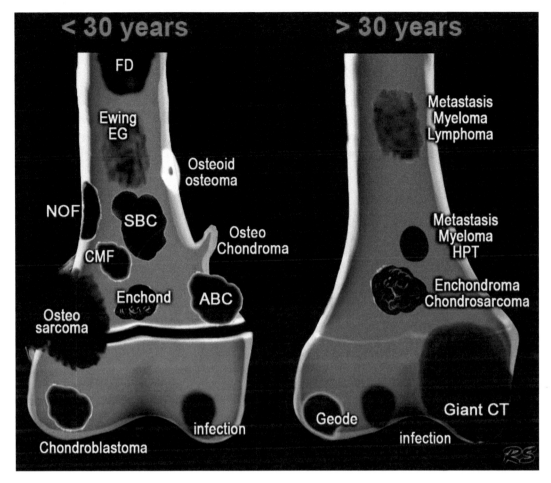

Fig. 158.1 Tumor Type by Location, ABC = Aneurysmal bone cyst, CMF = Chondromyxoid fibroma, EG = Eosinophilic Granuloma, GCT = Giant cell tumor, FD = Fibrous dysplasia, HPT = Hyperparathyroidism with Brown tumor, NOF = Non-Ossifying Fibroma, SBC = Simple Bone Cyst. Reprinted under creative commons license from Radiology Assistant (http://www.radiologyassistant.nl/data/bin/a509797919f47f_TEK-bone-tumor3.jpg)

Table 158.1 Differential by age

Age	Benign	Malignant
0–10 years old	Osteomyelitis Osteofibrous dysplasia	Metastatic rhabdomyosarcoma Metastatic neuroblastoma Leukemia
10–40 years old	NOF Osteoid osteoma Giant cell tumor ABC UBC Osteochondroma MHE Chondroblastoma Fibrous dysplasia Osteomyelitis Eosinophillic granuloma	Osteosarcoma Ewing's sarcoma Desmoplastic fibroma Leukemia Lymphoma
40–80 years old	Enchondroma Bone infarct Bone island Paget's disease Hyperparathyroidism	Metastatic bone disease Myeloma Lymphoma Chondrosarcoma MFH Secondary sarcoma Paget's, irradiation

Staging Systems

Staging is the process of finding out how extensive the cancer is. The most commonly used staging system in Orthopaedic Oncology is the Musculoskeletal Tumor Society or Enneking system [1], which has two different scales depending on whether the lesion is benign or malignant. The Enneking system is a surgical staging system in that it guides surgical management.

Enneking
Roman numerals are used to denote malignant tumors. I – low-grade, II – high-grade, III – metastatic (regional or distant). The letters A and B represent intra and extra-compartmental, respectively. For benign lesions, Arabic numerals are used. 1 - Benign, indolent, or biologically static, 2 - Progressive growth, limited by natural barriers, 3 - Locally aggressive with corresponding soft-tissue mass.

Campanacci staging system [2, 3] is based on radiographic characteristics as follows:
1. Radiographically well-circumscribed lucent lesion with no aggressive features (e.g., periosteal reaction, soft-tissue mass, cortical breach).
2. Relatively well-defined radiographic borders without a radiopaque rim.
3. Indistinct or ill-defined borders with radiographic demonstration of cortical bone destruction, and a soft-tissue mass.

- American Joint Committee on Cancer (AJCC) [3]
- One common staging construct is the AJCC's TNM + G structure where:
  - T1 vs. T2 = tumor size (< or > 5 cm)
  - N0 vs. N1 = nodes (no/yes)
  - M0 vs. M1 = metastasis (no/yes)
  - G1 – 3 = grade
  - A tumor's grade is a measure of how likely it is to metastasize and is based on differentiation (1–3), mitotic count (1–3), and tumor necrosis (0–2). Tumors with a score of 2 or 3 are G1, a score of 4 or 5 is G2, while a score of 6 or higher is G3. GX is used when medical records are incomplete and data insufficient to offer a grade.

Types [1–3]

Chondrogenic

- *Chondrosarcoma*
  - Age – 50–70 years old.
  - Sites – the pelvis (most frequently the ilium), femur, proximal humerus, and ribs. Can occur in any bone derived from enchondral ossification.
  - Clinical features – local swelling and pain of months to years of duration.
  - Imaging features – most frequently in the metaphysis and diaphysis of long bones. Variable presence of "arcs/rings," "popcorn-like" calcifications.
  - Histology – abundant blue-gray cartilage matrix with atypical chondrocytes. Increased grades have increasing cellularity and atypia.
  - Genetics – IDH1 and IDH2 mutations. The myxoid variant has the translocation t(9:22) and fusion protein EWS-CHN.
  - Prognosis – histologic grade is the single most important predictor of local recurrence and metastases (grade 1–83% 5-year survival, grade 2/3–53%). Pelvis tumors carry a poor prognosis as well.
  - Associated conditions – Ollier disease and Maffucci syndrome patients have a markedly increased risk of developing secondary chondrosarcomas, around 40% and 53%, respectively.
  - Subtypes – rare.
  - Dedifferentiated, mesenchymal, and clear cell – 5-year survival rates ~10%, 40–50%, and 80–90%, respectively.

Osteogenic

- *Conventional osteosarcoma* – most common high-grade primary malignant bone tumor that involves a high-grade intraosseous neoplasm in which the cells produce osteoid. It is termed primary when the underlying bone is normal and secondary when the underlying bone has been altered such as with previous radiation or Paget's disease.

- Age – most cases develop between 10 and 14 years with a second peak (30%) > 40 years old.
- Sites – vast majority occur in the metaphyseal region (90%) of the extremity long bones, especially the distal femur (30%), proximal tibia (15%), and proximal humerus (15%).
- Clinical features – presents as a painful, enlarging mass. Pain is deep, progressive, and usually present for weeks to months by diagnosis. Night pain is common.
- Imaging features – typically presents as a large, destructive, poorly-defined, mixed lytic and blastic mass that violates the cortex and forms a large soft tissue component. Periosteal reaction forms Codman's triangle.
- Histology – the presence of malignant osteoid in the setting of a pleiomorphic spindle cell matrix is essential to the diagnosis. Mitotic figures are common.
- Genetics – immunoprofile lacks diagnostic specificity and is positive for osteocalcin, osteonectin, S100, actin, SMA, NSE, and CD 99. It is negative for factor VIII, CD 31, and CD 45. There are no characteristic translocations.
- Prognosis – survival improved with the advent of multi-agent chemotherapy. Most patients who present for cure are treated with surgery (usually wide margin, limb-salvage procedures) with overall ~65% 5-year survival rate. Those that are present with metastatic disease have an overall survival of <20%. Localized distal disease, >90% tumor necrosis, and complete resection are associated with a 5-year survival of >80%. Paget osteosarcoma has a 5-year survival of 10%. Radiation-induced osteosarcoma has a similar survival to conventional osteosarcoma.
- Associated conditions – Paget's disease (transformation occurs in approximately 1% of patients and accounts for roughly 50% of osteosarcoma in patients >60 years old), Li-Fraumeni syndrome, hereditary retinoblastoma, Rothmund-Thomson syndrome. Most post-radiation patients have received >20 Gy.

- Subtypes:
  ○ Low-grade central (1–2% of osteosarcomas) – low-grade neoplasm that arises in the medullary canal.
  ○ Telangiectatic (4%) – characterized by large septated spaces filled with blood, high fracture risk.
  ○ Small cell (1.5%) – characterized by the presence of small round blue cells.
  ○ Parosteal (4%) – low-grade that arises from the surface of bone. Seventy percent involve the distal posterior femur. The prognosis is excellent with a 91% 5-year overall survival. The treatment is surgery only, no chemotherapy.
  ○ Periosteal (<2%) – intermediate-grade that arises from the surface of bone. Tend to occur in a more diaphyseal location of the distal femur and proximal tibia in nearly 80% of cases. Chemotherapy controversial.
  ○ High-grade surface (<1%) – histology same as conventional but on surface of bone only.
- Ewing's sarcoma – a small, round blue cell neoplasm. It is the second most common sarcoma of bone in children and young adults.
  - Age – nearly 80% occur in patients younger than 20 years old.
  - Sites – most commonly occur in the diaphysis or metaphyseal-diaphyseal portion of long bones.
  - Clinical features – pain severe enough to wake patients up with or without a mass are the most common symptoms. Intermittent fever can also be seen.
  - Imaging features – ill-defined, osteolytic appearance that can often be described as "moth eaten" or permeative. Onion skin-type periosteal reaction is common.
  - Histology – in classic Ewing's there are uniform sheets of small round blue cells with round nuclei containing fine chromatin, scanty clear or eosinophilic, and PAS-positive cytoplasm.
  - Genetics – EWSR1-ETS gene on chromosome 22 (11; 22) translocation leads to the fusion protein EWS-FLI1 and formation of

oncogenes. The cell of origin appears to be mesenchymal and neural crest-derived stem cells. There is a diffuse CD99 positivity, which is similar to lymphoma.

- Prognosis – Approximately 2/3 of patients are cured from their disease with the presence of metastases being the major prognostic factor. Treatment includes systemic chemotherapy. Local control is obtained with surgery and/or radiation therapy. Survival rates are affected by percent necrosis similar, to osteosarcoma.

Hematopoietic

- *Primary non-Hodgkin lymphoma of the bone* – lymphoid cell (typically B-cell lymphomas) neoplasm that produces one or more bony masses without any supraregional lymph node involvement or other extranodal lesions.
  - Age – adult.
  - Sites – the femur is the most commonly involved single site.
  - Clinical features – bone pain with or without a mass.
  - Imaging features – favors the diaphysis of long bones and is usually poorly demarcated with a wide transition to normal bone. The cortex is usually destroyed with a large soft tissue mass. If the cortex is less involved, the radiographs can be completely normal. Bone scans are almost always hot.
  - Histology – Small round blue cell tumor. Nuclei tend to be large and irregular with cleaved and/or multilobulated appearance. Histology can be mistaken for sarcoma or primary lymphoma. Primary Hodgkin lymphoma of the bone requires the presence of Reed-Sternberg cells.
  - Genetics – strong staining for CD20.
  - Prognosis – excellent. Overall survival with the use of chemotherapy is approaching 90%

Notochordal

- *Chordoma* – demonstrates notochordal differentiation. There is a 1.8:1 male to female ratio. These tumors are rare in the African American population. Vast majority are sporadic in nature.
  - Age – typically the fifth to seventh decades of life.
  - Sites – chiefly located in the base of the skull, vertebral bodies, and sacrococcygeal bones in fairly equal proportions.
  - Clinical features – often painful but differs based on its site (i.e., headache, neck pain, diplopia, and facial nerve palsy when skull based) and can have bowel/bladder dysfunction with sacral lesions.
  - Imaging features – midline sacral structure often difficult to see on plain films secondary to bowel gas. CT demonstrates midline bone destruction and soft tissue mass with calcifications. Lesion is bright on MRI T2.
  - Histology – typically composed of large cells with clear to eosinophilic cytoplasm separated into lobules by fibrous septa. The tumor cells have copious "bubbly" cytoplasm referred to as "physaliferous cells." Atypia is variable.
  - Genetics – express keratin and are usually immunoreactive for EMA, and S100. Brachyury (a protein that in humans is encoded by the T gene) is a highly specific marker for chordoma.
  - Prognosis – the overall median survival is 7 years. Up to 40% of non-cranial tumors metastasize to the lung, bone, lymph nodes, and subcutaneous tissue.

Vascular

- *Angiosarcoma* – high-grade neoplasm made of cells that demonstrate endothelial differentiation.
  - Age – almost even distribution between the second and eighth decades.

- Sites – demonstrate a preference for short and long tubular bones (74%), especially the femur.
- Clinical features – pain with or without a mass.
- Imaging features – manifests as a single or regionally multifocal, osteolytic tumor. Cortical destruction and extension into soft tissues is common. Periosteal reaction is usually absent. An MRI usually demonstrates a heterogenous lesion with extensive reactive changes.
- Histology – most often epithelioid in appearance and less frequently spindled. The cytoplasm is deeply eosinophilic with vacuoles that may be empty or hold intact erythrocytes. Mitotic figures are numerous.
- Genetics – expresses a number of endothelial markers including CD31, vWF, ERG, FLI1, SMA, keratin, and EMA.
- Prognosis – 5-year survival is approximately 33%. Surgery with negative margins is needed for cure.

Myogenic, Lipogenic, and Epithelial

- *Leiomyosarcoma* – cell shows smooth muscle differentiation. A small subset of patients have a prior exposure to radiation or EBV infection.
  - Age – peak incidence in fifth decade.
  - Sites – most lesions occur in the lower extremity about the knee.
  - Clinical features – pain with occasional pathologic fracture, often with soft tissue mass.
  - Imaging features – lytic, aggressive lesions with a permeative growth pattern and cortical destruction on x-ray.
  - Histology – cells are arranged in long, intersecting fascicles, growing in an infiltrative pattern. The tumor cells have a distinctive fibrillary, eosinophilic cytoplasm and elongated, cigar-shaped nuclei with blunted ends.

- Genetics – diffuse staining for desmin, h-Caldesmon, and SMA.
- Prognosis – grade correlates well with clinical outcome with high-grade lesions tending to spread distantly with 50% of patients finally succumbing to disease.
- Treatment – see osteosarcoma.

- *Adamantinoma* – a biphasic tumor characterized by a variety of morphological patterns, most commonly clusters of epithelial cells, surrounded by a relatively bland spindle-cell osteofibrous component.
  - Age – median age is 25–35 years old.
  - Sites – the anterior tibial metaphysis or diaphysis is involved in 85–90% of cases.
  - Clinical features – main complaint is usually swelling with or without pain.
  - Imaging features – the tumor is typically well circumscribed, cortical, lobulated, and osteolytic. Multifocality within the same bone or in the fibula can be seen. It commonly remains within the cortex and spreads longitudinally but may destroy the cortex or extend into the medullary canal.
  - Histology – intermingled epithelial and osteofibrous components. Four main differentiation patterns are basaloid, tubular, spindle cell, and squamous. A "zonal" architecture has been described with the center and periphery of the lesion having different characteristics.
  - Genetics – the fibrous tissue is positive for vimentin, while the epithelial cells showing coexpression of keratin, EMA, vimentin, p63, and podoplanin.
  - Prognosis – risk factors for recurrence include intralesional and marginal surgery and extracompartmental extension which can rise to up to 90%. These tumors metastasize in 12–29% of patients to regional lymph nodes and the lungs. Overall survival is 75–80%.
- *Undifferentiated high-grade pleomorphic sarcoma* – name given when specific differenti-

ated tissue type cannot be determined. Usually in middle aged or older adults. Survival similar to osteosarcoma as well.

- Age – diagnosis usually from second to eighth decade with higher incidence in adults > 40 years old.
- Sites – long bones of the lower extremities, particularly the femur (30–45%), followed by the tibia and humerus. The knee is a common location. Almost all are solitary lesions.
- Clinical features – pain and less frequently swelling, varying from 1 week to 3 years.
- Imaging features – lytic, aggressive, and poorly limited with cortical destruction and soft-tissue involvement.
- Histology – appearance is quite heterogeneous with mainly spindle-shaped cells and varying numbers of multinucleated giant cells, often frankly atypical.
- Genetics – complex karyotypes with TP53 mutations, MDM2 amplifications, and CDKN1A expression in the minority of cases.
- Prognosis – highly malignant with metastases, particularly to the lungs. Treated as osteosarcoma in most cases with tumor necrosis after chemotherapy being an important prognostic factor. In patients with localized disease, 5-year survival is >50%.

Treatment Principles

- Interventions span from observation to amputation depending on the behavior of the tumor (Table 158.2). While some tumors can be diagnosed by history, exam, and imaging alone most surgical interventions should be preceded with a biopsy for tissue diagnosis. Biopsy principles are a crucial take away from an orthopaedic oncology clerkship. A well-planned biopsy, especially in malignant tumors can make the difference between someone keeping their extremity or not. In malignant tumors, a negative margin is directly correlated to the patient's risk for local recurrence and metastasis. The following are some principles that will serve you well:
  - Biopsies should be performed at the same facility where they will be treated if they are malignant.

Table 158.2 Nonoperative and operative differential by treatment

Nonoperative	
Observation	Fibrous dysplasia Osteofibrous dysplasia Enchondroma Ollier's Marfucci's Osteochondroma MHE NOF Jaffe-Campanacci Paget's Eosiniphillic granuloma Lipoma
Bisphosphonate therapy	Metastatic bone disease (with wide resection and radiation) Myeloma (with chemotherapy) Paget's disease (with observation) Fibrous dysplasia (with observation)
Radiation alone	Solitary myeloma
Chemotherapy alone	Lymphoma Multiple myeloma
Operative	
Radiofrequency ablation	Osteoid osteoma
Aspiration and injection	UBC
Curettage and bone grafting	GCT ABC Chondroblastoma Chondromyxoid fibroma Osteoblastoma NOF (if symptomatic)
Marginal resection	Periosteal chondroma Neurilemoma (soft tissue) Nodular fasciitis (soft tissue) Epidermal inclusion cyst Glomus tumor
Wide resection alone	Chondrosarcoma Parosteal osteosarcoma Chordoma Adamantinoma Squamous cell (if no metastases)
Wide resection + irradiation	Metastatic bone disease High-grade soft tissue sarcoma (angiosarcoma, synovial sarcoma, liposarcoma, desmoid tumor, MFH/fibrosarcoma)
Wide resection + chemotherapy	Osteosarcoma Periosteal osteosarcoma Ewing's sarcoma MFH Fibrosarcoma Secondary sarcoma Dedifferentiated chondrosarcoma Rhabdomyosarcoma (exception to soft tissue sarcoma)

- All malignant tumor patients should be transferred as expeditiously as possible to their tertiary care facility for further evaluation and treatment, as to not delay the appropriate treatment.
- Biopsy tracts should be longitudinal in the extremity and always in line with the definitive procedure, should a more extensive surgery be required.
- Unlike many approaches, tissue planes should not be dissected as this will allow for broader contamination, necessitating a more extensive re-excision if needed.
- Exact hemostasis should be maintained throughout the procedure. Any area of hematoma is presumed contaminated for resection purposes.

Limb salvage options do exist and allow for keeping the limb in many cases. Examples include megaprostheses, internal hemipelvectomy, and rotationplasty in the lower extremity.

Resection types are classified as:

- Intralesional or debulking – plane of dissection is within the tumor. Leaves gross tumor. Appropriate for symptomatic benign lesions where a more aggressive dissection might sacrifice neurovascular structures.
- Marginal – plane of dissection is in the pseudo-capsule that surrounds satellite lesions. Acceptable for most benign lesions and lowgrade malignancies
- Wide – plane of dissection is through normal tissue, leaving a cuff of tissue around the tumor. Preferred for most high-grade malignancies. Combined with adjuvant and/or neoadjuvant treatments in cases where wide margins (2 cm) cannot be achieved. These additive treatments include radiation, chemotherapy, and increasingly immunotherapy.
- Radical – the entire involved compartment is excised. Mostly replaced by wide resection as there has been no proven survival benefit to justify the added morbidity.
- Amputation – the entire limb is removed. Its corollary in the pelvis is the external hemipelvectomy.

References

1. Enneking WF. A system of staging musculoskeletal neoplasms. Clin Orthop Relat Res. 1986;(204):9–24.
2. Tumours of bone. WHO classification of tumours of soft tissue and bone. 4th ed. Fletcher CDM, Unni KK, Mertens F, editors. Lyon: International Agency for Research on Cancer; 2013. p. 239–394.
3. Campanacci M. Giant cell tumor of bone. In: Bone and soft tissue tumors. 2nd ed. Berlin: Springer; 1999. p. 99–132.

Erratum to: Orthopedic Surgery Clerkship

Erratum to A.E.M. Eltorai et al. (eds.), *Orthopedic Surgery Clerkship*,
https://doi.org/10.1007/978-3-319-52567-9

This book was inadvertently published missing the authors and corrections listed below.

The original chapters have been updated accordingly.

Authors:

(Chapter 10) Christopher E. Urband

The correct order of authors and affiliation are given below:

Christopher E. Urband, William M. Wind and Leslie J. Bisson

C. E. Urband, MD
Department of Orthopaedics, Jacobs School of
Medicine and Biomedical Sciences, Buffalo, NY, USA

W.M. Wind, MD • L.J. Bisson (✉)
Jacobs School of Medicine and Biomedical Sciences,
University at Buffalo, 4949 Harlem Road, Amherst,
NY 14226, USA
e-mail: ljbisson@buffalo.edu

The updated online versions of these chapters can be found at
https://doi.org/10.1007/978-3-319-52567-9_10
https://doi.org/10.1007/978-3-319-52567-9_121
https://doi.org/10.1007/978-3-319-52567-9_133
https://doi.org/10.1007/978-3-319-52567-9_157
https://doi.org/10.1007/978-3-319-52567-9_158

(Chapter 121) Ettore Vulcano, Alexander J. Kish, Tonya W. An, Amiethab A. Aiyer

The correct order of authors and affiliation are given below:

Matthew A.Varacallo, Ettore Vulcano, Alexander J. Kish, Tonya W. An, Amiethab A. Aiyer

M.A. Varacallo, MD (✉)
Department of Orthopaedic Surgery,
Hahnemann University Hospital,
245 N. 15th Street, M.S. 420, Philadelphia, PA, USA
e-mail: matt.varacallo@tenethealth.com

E. Vulcano, MD
Orthopedics, Mount Sinai Health System,
New York, NY, USA

A.J. Kish, MD
Department of Orthopaedic Surgery,
University of Maryland Medical Center, Baltimore, MD, USA

T.W. An
Orthopedics Cedars-Sinai Medical Center,
Los Angeles, CA, USA

A.A. Aiyer
Department of Orthopaedic Surgery,
University of Miami, Miami, FL, USA

(Chapter 133) Ettore Vulcano, Matthew A.Varacallo, Tonya W. An, Amiethab A. Aiyer

The correct order of authors and affiliation are given below:

Alexander J. Kish, Ettore Vulcano, Matthew A.Varacallo, Tonya W. An, Amiethab A. Aiyer

A.J. Kish, MD (✉)
Department of Orthopaedic Surgery,
University of Maryland Medical Center, Baltimore, MD, USA
e-mail: alexanderjkish@gmail.com

E. Vulcano, MD
Orthopedics, Mount Sinai Health System,
New York, NY, USA

M.A. Varacallo, MD
Department of Orthopaedic Surgery,
Hahnemann University Hospital,
245 N. 15th Street, M.S. 420, Philadelphia,
PA, USA

T.W. An
Orthopedics Cedars-Sinai Medical Center,
Los Angeles, CA, USA

A.A. Aiyer
Department of Orthopaedic Surgery,
University of Miami, Miami, FL, USA

Corrections:

Page 766, Line starting with "Radiographically" should be started as new paragraph.
Page 766, Start "American Joint Committee on Cancer (AJCC) [3]" in a new line without indentation.
Page 766, Omit "Rare" that appears above point 2.
Page 771, Omit "by and large should be done" under the first point of heading "**Treatment Principles**"
Page 776, Line starting with "Radiographically" should be started as new paragraph.
Page 776, Start "American Joint Committee on Cancer (AJCC) [3]" in a new line without indentation.
Page 776, Omit "Rare" that appears above point 1.

Index

© Springer International Publishing AG 2017
A.E.M. Eltorai et al. (eds.), *Orthopedic Surgery Clerkship*, DOI 10.1007/978-3-319-52567-9